Illustrated textbook of
Paediatrics

THIRD EDITION

Commissioning Editor: *Ellen Green/Pauline Graham*
Development Editor: *Clive Hewat*
Project Manager: *Morven Dean*
Design Direction: *Stewart Larking*
Illustrations Manager: *Bruce Hogarth*
Illustrator: *Cactus*

Illustrated Textbook of
Paediatrics

THIRD EDITION

Dr Tom Lissauer MB BChir FRCPCH

Consultant Paediatrician
St. Mary's Hospital
London
UK

Dr Graham Clayden MD FRCPCH

Reader in Paediatrics
Kings College London
School of Medicine at Guy's, Kings and St Thomas' Hospitals
Evelina Children's Hospital
London
UK

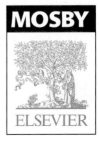

MOSBY

ELSEVIER

Edinburgh   London   New York   Oxford   Philadelphia   St Louis   Sydney   Toronto 2007

MOSBY
ELSEVIER

An imprint of Elsevier Limited

First edition 1997
Second edition 2001
Third edition 2007

ISBN-13: 978 0 7234 3397 2
ISBN-10: 0 7234 3397 6

International Student Edition
ISBN: 978 0 7234 3398 9

British Library Cataloguing in Publication Data
A catalogue record for this book is available from the British Library

Library of Congress Cataloging in Publication Data
A catalog record for this book is available from the Library of Congress

Note
Knowledge and best practice in this field are constantly changing. As new research and experience broaden our knowledge, changes in practice, treatment and drug therapy may become necessary or appropriate. Readers are advised to check the most current information provided (i) on procedures featured or (ii) by the manufacturer of each product to be administered, to verify the recommended dose or formula, the method and duration of administration, and contraindications. It is the responsibility of the practitioner, relying on their own experience and knowledge of the patient, to make diagnoses, to determine dosages and the best treatment for each individual patient, and to take all appropriate safety precautions. To the fullest extent of the law, neither the Publisher nor the Editors assumes any liability for any injury and/or damage to persons or property arising out or related to any use of the material contained in this book.

The Publisher

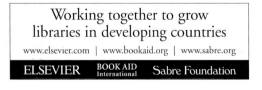

ELSEVIER — your source for books, journals and multimedia in the health sciences

www.elsevierhealth.com

Working together to grow libraries in developing countries

www.elsevier.com | www.bookaid.org | www.sabre.org

ELSEVIER   BOOK AID International   Sabre Foundation

Printed in Spain

Contents

Foreword
to the third edition

The publication of this book has proved to be an important milestone in paediatric undergraduate education. It has become enormously popular with medical students, its distinctive cover the hallmark of students on their paediatric clinical attachment. The authors, both well known for their contribution to undergraduate and postgraduate medical education and examinations, have produced an outstanding book, covering core information for paediatrics and child health in a concise but informative manner, without overburdening the reader with more obscure conditions. The large number of colour photographs and drawings which enliven most pages of the book both hold the reader's attention and help to guide one to the most fundamental points described in the text. Furthermore, the book successfully captures the fundamental elements of humanity, sensitivity and emotional understanding required by all professionals who care for children and their families. It was not surprising that the book received awards for innovation and excellence in the British Medical Association and Royal Society of Medicine Book Competitions and has been translated into several languages.

Medical students beginning clinical paediatrics face a daunting task. Children are affected by the full range of medical and surgical conditions which affect adults but in addition suffer from a large number of inherited or acquired disorders which occur uniquely in the early years of life. In the few weeks allocated to paediatrics in the crowded medical school curriculum, the student must acquire knowledge not only of the diagnosis and management of common paediatric disorders but also of the complex social, developmental, educational and emotional problems faced by them. Meticulous care has been taken in this book to distil to essentials the information required for paediatric undergraduate training, highlighting the important differences between paediatrics and adult medicine.

This third edition has enabled the authors to keep the information up to date and to incorporate some extra material on paediatric allergy and adolescent medicine to reflect the current ethos of paediatric medicine.

Professor Michael Levin
Professor of International Child Health,
Imperial College School of Medicine, London

Foreword
to the first edition

You are about to read a textbook unlike any you have ever read before. It is unique in its presentation, organization, graphics and design. I predict that the *Illustrated Textbook of Paediatrics* will become a standard by which all other medical textbooks will be judged. The plethora of information which every medical student is expected to absorb and integrate is unending. Therefore, it is incumbent on teachers and texts to be innovative and creatively selective in their presentation of information and wisdom. The editors, Tom Lissauer and Graham Clayden, have been successful in achieving this.

The information is presented in a clear, concise fashion and has been supplemented by original illustrations and colourful, easy-to-read charts and graphs.

Each section of the book deserves praise. The chapter on genetics is noteworthy because it does not present overwhelming details of biochemical/molecular biology but presents a comprehensive compendium of the subject, the importance of which is undisputed in the 20th century. Perinatology and nutrition offer the student important information that has occasionally been slighted in older texts.

The reader will find both enjoyment and instruction in this new introduction to clinical paediatrics. The text is practical and the information is easily accessible.

In conclusion, I salute the authors and editors. I wish I had written this book.

The late Frank A Oski, MD
Distinguished Service Professor,
The Johns Hopkins University School of Medicine,
Baltimore, Maryland

Acknowledgements

We would like to acknowledge the major contribution made to previous editions by the following contributors:

First edition:
Lynn Ball (Haematological disorders), Nigel Curtis (Paediatric Emergencies, Infection and Immunity), Gill Du Mont (Skin), Tony Hulse (Growth and puberty; and Endocrine and metabolic disorders), Nigel Klein (Paediatric emergencies), Nicholas Madden (Genitalia), Angus Nicoll (Development, language, hearing and vision), Karen Simmer (Perinatal medicine; and neonatal medicine), Elizabeth Thompson (Genetics).

Second edition:
Paula Bolton-Maggs (Haematological disorders), Jon Couriel (Respiratory disorders), Ruth Gilbert (Evidence-based medicine), Dennis Gill (History and examination), Raanan Gillon (Ethics), Peter Hill (Emotions and behaviour), Nigel Klein (Infection and immunity), Simon Nadel (Paediatric emergencies), Barbara Phillips (Environment), Andrew Redington (Cardiac disorders), John Sills (Bones and joints), Rashmin Tamhne (The child in society), Michael Weindling (Perinatal medicine, Neonatal medicine).

The contributors to this edition have extensively drawn on the material prepared for previous editions.

Preface

This textbook has been written for undergraduates. Our aim has been to provide the core information required by medical students for the 6–10 weeks assigned to paediatrics in the curriculum of most undergraduate medical schools. We are delighted that it has become so widely used not only in the UK but also in northern Europe, India, Pakistan, Australia, South Africa and other countries. We are also pleased that nurses, therapists and other health professionals who care for children have found the book helpful. It will also be of assistance to doctors preparing for postgraduate examinations such as the Diploma of Child Health (DCH) and Membership of the Royal College of Paediatrics and Child Health (MRCPCH).

The huge amount of positive feedback we have received on the first two editions from medical students in the UK and abroad has spurred us on to produce this new edition. We have updated the text and added two new chapters, one on allergy and another on adolescent medicine.

In order to make learning from this book easier we have followed a lecture-note style using short sentences and lists of important features. Illustrations have been used to help the student recognise important signs or clinical features and to make the book more attractive and interesting to use. Key Learning points have been identified with a ✤. Case histories have been chosen to highlight points within their clinical context. Summary boxes of important facts, highlighted with a 🔘, have been added in this edition to help with revision. To further facilitate learning and revision, self-assessment questions and answers have been produced and are available on the internet (www.studentconsult.com) to purchasers of this book. They include case scenarios, clinical photographs and images, and a number of different methods of assessment, to make them more instructive and enjoyable.

The male gender for children has been used throughout the book for stylistic simplicity.

We would like to thank all our contributors and Ellen Green at Elsevier for their assistance in producing this new edition. Thanks also to Ann, Rachel and David Lissauer for their ideas and assistance, and for their understanding of the time taken away from the family in the preparation of this new edition.

We welcome any comments about the book.

Tom Lissauer and Graham Clayden

Contributors

Dr Ulrich Baumann
Consultant Paediatric Hepatologist
Birmingham Children's Hospital, Birmingham
Ch. 20: Liver disorders

Dr Mitch Blair
Reader in Paediatrics and Child Public Health
Imperial College, Northwick Park & St Marks'
NHS Trust Campus, Harrow, Middlesex
Ch. 1: The child in society

Dr Tom Blyth
Consultant Paediatrician
Pembury Hospital, Tunbridge Wells
Honorary Consultant in Paediatric Allergy
Guy's and St. Thomas's Hospital, London
Ch. 15: Allergy and immunity

Professor Ian Booth
Leonard Parsons Professor of Paediatrics & Child
Health and Director, Institute of Child Health,
Birmingham Children's Hospital, Birmingham
Ch. 12: Nutrition
Ch. 13: Gastroenterology

Dr Graham Clayden
Reader in Paediatrics
Kings College London School of Medicine at
Guy's, Kings and St. Thomas's Hospitals,
Evelina Children's Hospital, London

Dr Michelle Cummins
Consultant Paediatric Haematologist
Bristol Royal Hospital for Children, Bristol
Ch. 22: Haematological disorders

Dr Iolo Doull
Consultant Respiratory Paediatrician
Children's Hospital of Wales, Cardiff
Ch. 16: Respiratory disorders

Dr Saul Faust
Senior Lecturer in Paediatric Infectious Diseases
University of Southampton, Southampton
Ch. 14: Infection

Professor Elena Garralda
Professor in Child and Adolescent Psychiatry
Imperial College, St Mary's Hospital, London
Ch. 23: Emotions and behaviour

Professor George Haycock
Emeritus Professor of Paediatrics
The Kings College London School of Medicine at
Guy's, Kings & St Thomas' Hospitals, Evelina
Children's Hospital, London
Ch. 18: Kidney and urinary tract

Dr Helen Jenkinson
Consultant Paediatric Oncologist
Birmingham Children's Hospital, Birmingham
Ch. 21: Malignant disease

Professor Deirdre Kelly
Professor of Paediatric Hepatology
Birmingham Children's Hospital, Birmingham
Ch. 20: Liver disorders

Dr Helen Kingston
Consultant Clinical Geneticist
St Mary's Hospital, Manchester
Ch. 8: Genetics

Professor Gideon Lack
Professor in Paediatric Allergy and Immunology
The Kings College London School of Medicine at
Guy's, Kings & St Thomas' Hospitals,
Evelina Children's Hospital, London
Ch. 15: Allergy and immunity

Mr Anthony Lander
Consultant Paediatric Surgeon
Birmingham Children's Hospital, Birmingham
Ch. 13: Gastroenterology

Dr Vic Larcher
Consultant Paediatrician
Great Ormond Street Hospital for Children,
London
Ch. 5: Care of the sick child (ethics)

Dr Tom Lissauer
Consultant Paediatrician
St Mary's Hospital, London
Ch. 1: The child in society
Ch. 2: History and examination
Ch. 5: Care of the sick child
Ch. 9: Perinatal medicine
Ch. 10: Neonatal medicine

Dr Hermione Lyall
Consultant in Paediatric Infectious Diseases
St. Mary's Hospital, London
Ch. 14: Infection

Dr Ian Maconochie
Consultant in Paediatric Accident & Emergency
Medicine
St Mary's Hospital, London
Ch. 7: Environment

Dr Maud Meates-Dennis
Senior Lecturer in Paediatrics
Christchurch School of Medicine and Health
Sciences, Christchurch, New Zealand
Ch. 5: Care of the sick child (evidence-based medicine)

Dr Richard Newton
Consultant Paediatric Neurologist
Royal Manchester Children's Hospital,
Pendlebury, Manchester
Ch. 27: Neurological disorders

Dr Lesley Rees
Consultant Paediatric Nephrologist
Great Ormond Street Hospital for Children,
London
Ch. 18: Kidney and urinary tract

Professor Irene Roberts
Professor in Paediatric Haematology
Imperial College, St Mary's and Hammersmith
Hospitals, London
Ch. 22: Haematological disorders

Dr Terry Segal
Consultant Paediatrician
University College Hospital, London
Ch. 28: Adolescent medicine

Professor Jo Sibert
Emeritus Professor of Child Health
Cardiff University, Cardiff
Ch. 7: Environment

Dr Diane P. L. Smyth
Consultant Paediatrician in Neurology and
Neurodisability
St Mary's Hospital, London
Ch. 3: Normal child development, hearing and vision
*Ch. 4: Developmental problems and the child with
special needs*

Professor Tauny Southwood
Professor of Paediatric Rheumatology
Institute of Child Health, Birmingham Children's
Hospital, Birmingham
Ch. 2: History and examination
Ch. 26: Bones, joints and rheumatic disorders

Professor Mike Stevens
CLIC Professor of Paediatric Oncology
Bristol Royal Hospital for Children, Bristol
Ch. 21: Malignant disease

Mr Mark Stringer
Clinical Anatomist
University of Otago, Dunedin, New Zealand
Formerly Professor of Paediatric Surgery,
St James' University Hospital, Leeds
Ch. 19: Genitalia

Dr Rob Tasker
Consultant Paediatrician Intensivist
Addenbrooke's Hospital, Cambridge
Ch. 6: Paediatric emergencies

Dr Sharon Taylor
Consultant in Child and Adolescent Psychiatry
Imperial College, St Mary's Hospital, London
Ch. 23: Emotions and behaviour

Professor David Thomas
Consultant Paediatric Urologist
St James' University Hospital, Leeds
Ch. 19: Genitalia

Dr Robert M. R. Tulloh
Consultant Paediatric Cardiologist
Department of Congenital Heart Disease,
Bristol Royal Hospital for Children, Bristol
Ch. 16: Respiratory disorders
Ch. 17: Cardiac disorders

Professor Julian Verbov
Professor of Dermatology
Alder Hey Children's Hospital, Liverpool
Ch. 24: Skin

Dr Russell Viner
Consultant in Adolescent Medicine and
Endocrinology
University College London Hospital and Great
Ormond Street Hospital, London
Ch. 28: Adolescent medicine

Dr Jerry Wales
Senior Lecturer in Paediatric Endocrinology
Sheffield Children's Hospital, Sheffield
Ch. 11: Growth and puberty
Ch. 25: Endocrine and metabolic disorders (endocrine)

Professor Andrew Whitelaw
Professor of Neonatal Medicine
University of Bristol
Southmead Hospital, Bristol
Ch. 9: Perinatal medicine
Ch. 10: Neonatal medicine

Dr Ed Wraith
Consultant Paediatrician and Director of Willink
Biochemical Genetics Unit
Royal Manchester Children's Hospital,
Pendlebury, Manchester
*Ch. 25: Endocrine and metabolic disorders (metabolic
disorders)*

The child in society

Most medical encounters with children involve an individual child presenting to a doctor with a symptom, such as diarrhoea. After taking a history, examining the child and performing any necessary investigations, the doctor arrives at a diagnosis or differential diagnosis and makes a management plan. This disease-oriented approach plays an important part in ensuring the immediate and long-term well-being of an individual. However, the nature of the child's illness needs to be seen within the wider context of the society in which he or she lives. This will affect the likely cause (if the diarrhoea is likely to be from a viral illness or contaminated water supply), the severity of the child's illness (the organism likely to be responsible and the child's nutritional status) and management options (who will take care of the child when ill, is preprepared oral rehydration therapy available, is hospital treatment possible and what facilities can it offer?). In order to be a truly effective clinician, the doctor must be able to place the child's clinical problems within the context of the family and of the society in which they live.

The way in which the environment impacts on a child is exemplified by the contrast between the major child health problems in developed and developing countries. In developed countries they are a range of complex, often previously fatal, chronic disorders and behavioural, emotional or developmental problems. By contrast, in developing countries the predominant problems are infection and malnutrition (Fig. 1.1, Box 1.1).

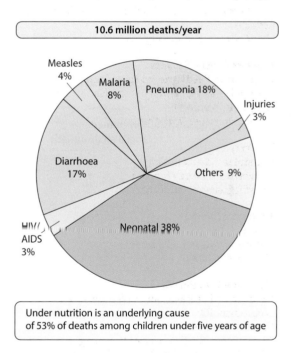

10.6 million deaths/year

Measles 4%
Malaria 8%
Pneumonia 18%
Injuries 3%
Diarrhoea 17%
Others 9%
HIV/AIDS 3%
Neonatal 38%

Under nutrition is an underlying cause of 53% of deaths among children under five years of age

Figure 1.1 Causes of death of the 10.6 million children less than 5-years-old dying annually throughout the world. Infection, often combined with undernutrition, is the main cause of death. (Source: Bryce J et al. WHO estimates of the cause of death in children. *Lancet* 2005; 365:1147–1152.)

Box 1.1 Contrast between main child health problems in developed and developing countries

Developed countries

- Severe, often previously fatal chronic disorders – malignant disease, cystic fibrosis
- Provision of paediatric and neonatal intensive care, organ transplantation and other specialist services
- Behavioural and emotional disorders – attention deficit disorder, anorexia nervosa
- Neurodevelopmental disorders – language delay, reading difficulties, clumsiness, cerebral palsy
- Road traffic and other accidents
- Lack of family cohesion
- Socioeconomic disadvantage among the 'have-nots' – lack of money, unemployment, inadequate housing and education
- Inequality of access to health services
- Excessive consumption – obesity
- Drug and alcohol abuse, smoking, teenage pregnancies

Developing countries

- Infection – respiratory tract, diarrhoea, malaria, tuberculosis, HIV
- Malnutrition – marasmus, kwashiorkor, severe iron deficiency anaemia
- Developmental and learning problems of organic pathology – Down's syndrome, congenital anomalies
- Sanitation, water supply, food hygiene, housing and education
- Poverty and unemployment
- Health care – not available or poor quality
- High birth rate – children constitute high proportion of population

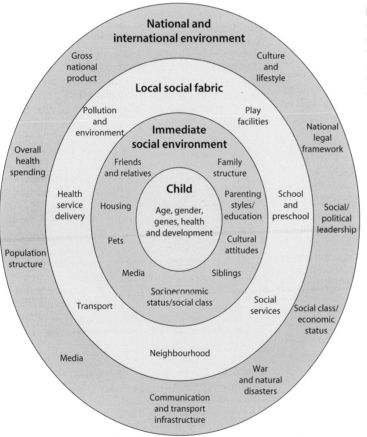

Figure 1.2 A child's world consists of overlapping, interconnected and expanding socio-environmental layers, which influence children's health and development. (After Bronfenbrenner U, Contexts of child rearing – problems and prospects. *American Psychologist* 1979; 34: 844–850.)

The child's world

It is clear from the difference in the major child health problems in developed and developing countries that children's health is profoundly influenced by their social, cultural and physical environment. This can be considered in terms of the child himself, the family and immediate social environment, the local social fabric and the national and international environment (Fig. 1.2). Our ability to intervene as clinicians needs to be seen within this context of complex interrelating influences on health.

The child

The child's world will be affected by gender, genes, physical health, temperament and development. It will also vary markedly with age; the life of an infant or toddler is mainly determined by the home environment, and that of the young child by school and friends, whereas the teenager will be aware of and influenced by events not only nationally but also internationally, e.g. in music, sport, fashion or politics.

Immediate social environment

Family structure

Although the 'two biological parent family' remains the norm, there are many variations in family structure. In the UK this has changed markedly over the last 30 years (Fig. 1.3). One in four children now live in a single-parent household. There are 1.4 million single parents in England and Wales. Disadvantages of single parenthood include a higher level of unemployment, poor housing and financial hardship (Table 1.1). These social adversities may affect parenting resources, e.g. vigilance about safety, adequacy of nutrition, take-up of preventive services such as immunisation and regular screening, and ability to cope with an acutely sick child at home. The increase in the number of parents who change partners and the accompanying rise in reconstituted families (1 in 10 children live in a stepfamily) mean that children are having to cope with a range of new and complex parental and sibling relationships. This may result in emotional, behavioural and social difficulties.

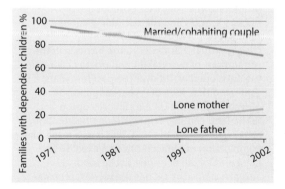

Figure 1.3 Changing structure of the family 1971–2002 (ONS, General Household Survey 2002).

Table 1.1 Percentage of families on low gross weekly household income in UK (ONS, General Household Survey 2002)

	<£100	£100–£500	<£500
Married couple	3	26	71
Single parent	10	74	16

The trend towards smaller families provides an increased standard of living. With many parents now leaving home in order to work, there is a greater demand for professional child care. This may be in the form of child-minding or preschool nurseries. Increasing attention is being paid to the quality of day-care facilities in terms of supervision of the children and improving the opportunities they provide for social interaction and learning.

Approximately 3% of children under 16 years old in the UK live away from their original family home; 50 000 of these are 'looked after' by social services, and the remainder live in temporary housing.

Refugees are often placed in temporary housing and may be moved repeatedly into areas unfamiliar to them. They often encounter additional problems as a result of communication difficulties, poverty, fragmentation of families, loss of family members causing post-traumatic stress syndrome, racism and uncertainty regarding the safety of friends and family. Raising children under these circumstances is fraught with difficulties.

Parenting styles

Parenting that is warm and receptive to the child, whilst imposing reasonable and consistent boundaries, will promote the development of an autonomous and self-reliant adult. Some parents are either excessively authoritarian or permissive. Children's emotional development may be damaged by parents who neglect or abuse their children.

The child's temperament is also important, especially when there is a mismatch with the parenting style of the parents; for example, a child with a very determined temperament may be in constant conflict with an authoritarian parent and this may result in tantrums and other behavioural problems.

Siblings have a marked influence on the family dynamics. The arrival of a new baby may engender a feeling of insecurity in older brothers and sisters and result in attention-seeking behaviour. How siblings affect each other appears to be determined by the emotional quality of their relationships with each other and also with other members of the family, including their parents. The role of grandparents and other family members varies widely and is influenced by the family's culture; in some, they are the main caregivers, while in others they play only a peripheral role, exacerbated by geographical separation.

Cultural attitudes to child-rearing

The way in which children are brought up evolves within a community over generations. An example is the use of physical punishment by parents to discipline their children. This is seen as acceptable or even desirable by a high proportion of parents in the UK and the USA, where there is strong public opinion against making 'reasonable chastisement' by parents illegal. However, such legislative measures have been adopted in countries such as

3

Sweden, where they have been largely successful in changing cultural practice.

Peers

Peers exert a major influence on children. Peer relationships and activities provide a 'sense of group belonging' and have potentially long-term benefits for the child. Relationships can also go wrong, e.g. persistent bullying, which may result in or contribute to psychosomatic symptoms, misery and even, in extreme cases, suicide.

Socioeconomic status/social class

Poverty is a key determinant of health and well-being of children. Healthcare problems in which the UK prevalence rates are increased by poverty and deprivation include:

- low-birthweight infants
- injuries
- hospital admissions
- asthma
- behavioural problems
- special educational needs
- child abuse.

Socioeconomic status is usually described by a comparison between the family income and the national median income. For example, taking poverty as below 50% of the national median income after adjustment for household size and composition, 20% of children in the UK in 2003/4 were poor (2.5 million children) (Fig. 1.4). Low socioeconomic status is often associated with multiple disadvantages, e.g. food of inadequate quantity and nutritional value, substandard housing or homelessness, lack of 'good enough' parenting and poor access to health care and educational facilities. Poor housing may restrict opportunities for play and this may adversely affect the child's development. In general, higher levels of maternal education benefit children's development;

maternal low intelligence and mental illness have an adverse effect. There are marked differences in living experiences between ethnic groups: 42% of Muslim children experience overcrowding compared to the 12% average, whereas 50% of Afro-Caribbean children live in single-parent households compared to 15% of white children and less than 10% of those from the Indian subcontinent. In 1992, in England and Wales, 12% of births were to mothers born outside the UK; in 2002 it was nearly 18%.

Local social fabric

Neighbourhood

Cohesive communities and amicable neighbourhoods are positive influences on children. Racial tension and other social adversities, such as gang violence and drugs, will adversely affect the emotional and social development of children, as well as their physical health. Parental concern about safety may create tensions in balancing their children's freedom with overprotection and restriction of their lifestyles.

Lifestyle issues concerning children include:

- *Poor nutrition* – the National Diet and Nutrition Survey in 2000 in the UK found that 4 out of 5 teenagers ate a diet predominantly consisting of chips, white bread, crisps, biscuits, ketchup and fizzy drinks; 16% of 15–18-year-old females were on a diet and 1 in 5 ate no fruit at all, with some living in inner city estates saying that they had easier access to illegal drugs than to fresh fruit and vegetables! In order to improve children's nutrition in the UK, healthy eating is being vigorously promoted, free daily fruit portions are provided in primary schools and the nutritional content of school meals is being improved.
- *Obesity* – there has been a large increase in the proportions of overweight and obese children in the developed world over the past few years; it is estimated that 6.5% of 9 year olds and 15% of 15-year-olds in the UK are clinically obese (BMI >90th centile). The figures are nearer 25% for 15-year-olds in the USA. This is as a result of a combination of reduced physical exercise and increased intake of calorie dense foods.
- *Sexual health* – the UK has the highest teenage pregnancy rate in western Europe: twice that of Germany, three times that of France and six times that of the Netherlands. There has been a marked increase in sexually transmitted diseases amongst 16–19-year-olds.
- *Smoking and alcohol* – in the UK 12% of girls aged 11–15 years smoke regularly compared to 9% of boys, rising to 30% in 16–19-year-olds. One in four children of the same age regularly drink alcohol, with binge-drinking becoming increasingly problematic.
- *Drug abuse* – nearly 30% of 15-year-olds have had personal experience of using drugs in England and Wales.

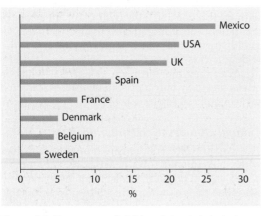

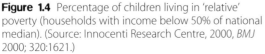

Figure 1.4 Percentage of children living in 'relative' poverty (households with income below 50% of national median). (Source: Innocenti Research Centre, 2000, *BMJ* 2000; 320:1621.)

These lifestyle issues follow a complex interaction between attitudes and practices in the home and in the community. Their prevalence tends to be greater in deprived communities.

Health service delivery

The variation in the quality of health care is an important component in preventing morbidity and mortality in children. In all countries, health services for children are increasingly provided within primary care. Some aspects of specialist paediatric care are also increasingly provided within the child's home, local community or local hospital through shared care arrangements and specialist community nursing and medical teams. However, access to and the range of these services varies widely.

Schools

Schools provide a powerful influence on children's emotional and intellectual development and their subsequent lives. Differences in the quality of schools in different areas can accentuate inequalities already present in society. Good education also provides the opportunity for children brought up in poverty to improve their social circumstances.

> To educate a girl is to educate a whole family. And what is true of families is also true of communities and, ultimately, whole countries. Study after study has taught us that there is no tool for development more effective than the education of girls. No other policy is as likely to raise economic productivity, lower infant and maternal mortality, improve nutrition and promote health – including helping to prevent the spread of HIV/AIDS. No other policy is as powerful in increasing the chances of education for the next generation.
> (Kofi Annan, Secretary General UN, 2004)

Travel

The increasing ease of travel can broaden children's horizons and opportunities. Especially in rural areas, the ease and availability of transport allow greater access to medical care and influence the pattern of provision of both primary and specialist medical services. However, a consequence of the increasing use of motor vehicles is the large number of injuries sustained by children from road traffic accidents, mainly as pedestrians. Attention to accident prevention, such as calming traffic in residential areas and separating cars from pedestrians and cyclists, is helping to reduce the number of children injured. The widespread use of cars also contributes to a reduction in children's levels of exercise. Whereas 80% of children in the UK went to school by foot or bicycle in 1971, this has dropped to less than 10%.

National and international environment

Economic wealth

There is a relationship between a country's gross national product and child health; some examples of this are shown in Table 1.2. It shows that the lower the gross national product:

- the greater the proportion of the population who are children
- the higher the childhood mortality
- the higher the proportion of newborn infants with low birthweight
- the lower the immunisation rate.

However, even in countries with a high gross national product, many children live in financially deprived circumstances.

Worldwide, there has been an enormous improvement in children's health over the last 50 years. It is estimated that the proportion of children who die before reaching 5 years of age is now less than half the level of 1960. The dramatic reduction in childhood mortality in England over the last century is shown in Figure 1.5.

The largest reductions in under-fives mortality are primarily related to improvements in living conditions such as improved sanitation and

Table 1.2 National socioeconomic conditions and child health (based on UNICEF, *State of the World's Children*, 2006)

Category of countries	Health and socioeconomic indicators					
	Gross national income (in US$, per person)	% of world population (6.8×10⁹)	Under 5 years (% of population)	Mortality rate <5 years old (per 1000 live births)	Nutrition – low birth-weight (% of births <2.5 kg)	Immunisation – diphtheria, pertussis, tetanus (DPT) at 1 year (%)
Industrialised	32 232	14	5.5	9	7	95
Developing	1 524	75	10.5	72	17	73
Least developed	345	11	15	115	19	63

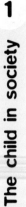
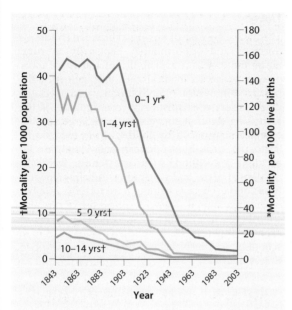

Figure 1.5 Marked reduction in mortality of children aged 0–14 years between 1843 and 2003. In 1900, 15% of babies born in England died by 1 year of age and 23% by 14 years of age; in 2003 the figures were 0.6% and 0.64%, respectively.

housing, and access to food and water. These have dramatically reduced fatalities from infectious disease. More recent contributions to this reduction, but of less relative impact over a long timescale, have included increased availability and uptake of immunisation and major medical improvements in perinatal and infant care. In all countries difficult choices need to be made about the allocation of scarce resources. Should a developing country provide expensive drugs and care for the small number of children with malignant disease or allocate its resources to preventive programmes for many children? In developed countries, difficult decisions also have to be faced in deciding the affordability of very expensive procedures, such as heart or liver transplantation, and certain drugs, such as the genetically engineered enzyme replacement therapy for Gaucher's disease. The public are becoming more engaged in these debates.

Media

The media has a powerful influence on children. It can be positive and educational. However, the impact of television, video and film can be negative owing to reduced opportunities for social interaction and active learning, lack of physical exercise as well as exposure to undesirable influences, such as violence, sex and cultural stereotypes, e.g. an expectation that teenage girls should be slim. The extent to which the aggressive tendencies of children may be exacerbated or encouraged by exposure to violence in films and television is an unresolved issue of widely held concern.

Box 1.2 Children and war: worldwide, devastating effect of war on children in the last decade

- Mortality – >2 million children died
- Morbidity – >6 million children disabled, mainly paraplegia and sensory deficits
- Loss of home and refugee status – 20 million children homeless and living as refugees
- Orphans – 1 million children orphaned
- Psychological trauma – 10 million children estimated to have post-traumatic stress syndrome; rape and sexual humiliation of females widely used as a strategy of conflict
- Children as soldiers – estimated 300 000 child soldiers in more than 30 conflicts worldwide
- Disruption of healthcare system – immunisation and child health surveillance programmes interrupted or disbanded
- Anti-personnel mines – 8000–10 000 killed or maimed each year

Source: State of World's Children, UNICEF, 2005.

The internet is enabling parents and children to become better informed about their children's medical problems. This is especially beneficial for the many rare conditions encountered in paediatrics. Parents and children can now access the latest information from around the world and can also communicate directly with other affected children or families. A disadvantage is that it may result in the dissemination of information which is incorrect or presented from a biased viewpoint, and may result in requests for inappropriate investigations or treatment and demands for 'new interventions', even before their safety and efficacy have been established.

War and natural disasters

Children are especially vulnerable when there is war, civil unrest or natural disasters (Box 1.2). Not only are they at greater risk from infectious diseases and malnutrition but they may lose their caregivers and other members of their families and are likely to have been exposed to highly traumatic events. Their lives will have been uprooted, socially and culturally, especially if they are forced to flee from their homes and become refugees.

Children's rights

Children are now recognised as having their own human rights. These are laid down in the United Nations Convention on the Rights of the Child, which has been ratified by all members of the United Nations, including the UK, but excluding the USA and Somalia (Fig. 1.6, Box 1.3). Implications of the convention include the involvement of children in clinical decision-making and in issues of consent.

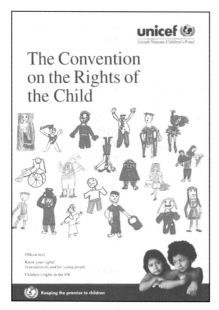

Figure 1.6 United Nations Convention on the Rights of the Child (1989).

<table>
<tr><td></td></tr>
</table>

Box 1.3 Summary of the United Nations Convention on the Rights of the Child (1989)

1. Survival rights
The child's right to life and to the most basic needs – food, shelter and access to health care

2. Developmental rights
To achieve their full potential – education, play, freedom of thought, conscience and religion. Those with disabilities to receive special services

3. Protection rights
Against all forms of abuse, neglect, exploitation and discrimination

4. Participation rights
To take an active role in their communities and nations

The new paediatrics and child health

In developed countries, there has been a marked shift in emphasis of paediatric practice from children with acute infections, which are now mostly prevented by immunisation or easily treated, to complex, multi-system physical disorders and disabilities and emotional and behavioural problems. This necessitates a more holistic approach to their care (Fig. 1.7). Instead of care being decided solely by doctors, the child and family are increasingly involved in a partnership determining the pattern of this care, based on the information provided to them. Other services are often involved, including the primary healthcare team, paediatric community nurses, the playschool/nursery or school, social services, religious community, the voluntary services and complementary health practitioners. Specialist services may be from secondary or tertiary care paediatric centres, which are forming collaborative networks with district general hospitals or community services over a wide geographical area. Good communication and close cooperation is required between all the parties involved. A designated key worker is often chosen to help families with this. Information may also be obtained from professional or voluntary organisations or parent support groups, which may be national or, increasingly, international.

Doctors can also play an important role in the population-based approach to improving child health. This also requires consideration not only of healthcare issues but also of social welfare,

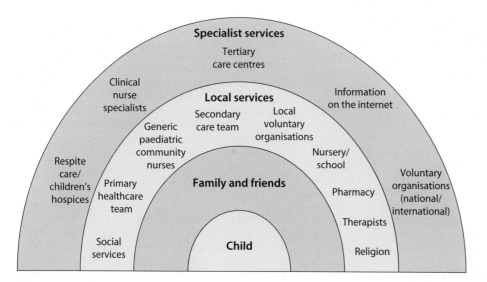

Figure 1.7 Health care is now centred around the child and family. It is adapted according to the child's condition. Good communication and cooperation between professionals is crucial. A key worker is often appointed to assist the family with this. (Courtesy of Dr Ann Goldman.)

Summary

Child health:

- For the individual child – depends on the child himself, the immediate social environment (family, parenting, peers, socioeconomic status), the local social fabric and the national and international environment.
- The main problems in developed countries are: chronic medical disorders, behavioural and emotional disorders, neurodevelopmental disorders, accidents, socioeconomic disadvantage, excessive consumption of food, drug and alcohol abuse, smoking, teenage pregnancies.
- The main problems in developing countries are: infection, malnutrition, poverty, sanitation, water supply, food hygiene, housing and education, availability and quality of health care, high birth rate, war.
- The United Nations Convention on the Rights of the Child provides children with rights to be provided with their basic needs, to be able to achieve their full potential, not to be subjected to abuse, neglect, exploitation or discrimination and to be able to take an active role in their community.

education and the local community, the voluntary sector and the general public as well as parents and children. Doctors can also help children through advocacy, when public awareness is raised about children's issues and information is provided to inform public debate. Examples of this are child labour, gun control and tobacco advertising.

Further reading

Blair M, Stewart-Brown S, Waterston T, Crowther R 2003 Child public health. Oxford University Press, Oxford

United Nation Children's Fund 1989 The convention on the rights of the child. UNICEF

Internet

www.doh.gov.uk (National Service Framework for Children)
www.statistics.gov.uk/children/
www.unicef.org
www.who.int

History and examination

The cornerstone of clinical practice continues to be history-taking and clinical examination. Good doctors will continue to be admired for their ability to distil the important information from the history, for their clinical skills, for their attitude towards patients, and for their knowledge of diseases, disorders and behaviour problems.

Parents are acutely interested in and anxious about their children. They will quickly recognise doctors who demonstrate interest, empathy and concern. They will seek out doctors who possess the appropriate skills and attitudes towards their children.

In approaching clinical history and examination of children, it is helpful to visualise some common clinical scenarios in which children are seen by doctors:

- an acute illness, e.g. respiratory tract infection, meningitis, appendicitis
- a chronic problem, e.g. failure to thrive, chronic cough
- a newborn infant with a congenital malformation or abnormality, e.g. developmental dysplasia of the hip, Down's syndrome
- suspected delay in development, e.g. slow to walk, talk or acquire skills
- behaviour problems, e.g. temper tantrums, hyperactivity, eating disorders.

The aims and objectives are:

- to establish the relevant facts of the history; this is always the most fruitful source of diagnostic information
- to elicit all relevant clinical findings
- to collate the findings from the history and examination

- to formulate a working diagnosis or differential diagnosis on the basis of logical deduction
- to assemble a problem list and management plan.

The above can be summarised by the acronym HELP:

H = history
E = examination
L = logical deduction
P = plan of management.

Key points in paediatric history and examination are:

- the child's age is always a key feature in the history and examination (Fig. 2.1) as it determines:
  - the nature and presentation of illnesses, developmental or behaviour problems
  - the way in which the history-taking (Fig. 2.2) and examination are conducted
  - the way in which any subsequent management is organised.
- parents are astute observers of their children. Never ignore or dismiss what they say.

Taking a history

Introduction

- Make sure you have read any referral letter and scanned the notes *before* the start of the interview.
- Observe the child at play in the waiting area and observe their appearance, behaviour and gait as they come into the clinic room. The continued observation of the child during the whole

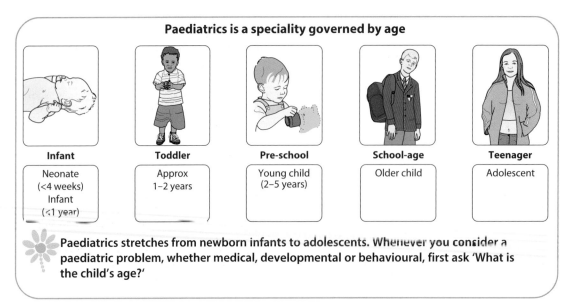

Paediatrics is a speciality governed by age

Infant	Toddler	Pre-school	School-age	Teenager
Neonate (<4 weeks) Infant (<1 year)	Approx 1–2 years	Young child (2–5 years)	Older child	Adolescent

🌼 Paediatrics stretches from newborn infants to adolescents. Whenever you consider a paediatric problem, whether medical, developmental or behavioural, first ask 'What is the child's age?'

Figure 2.1 The illnesses and problems children encounter are highly age-dependent. The child's age will determine the questions you ask on history-taking, how you conduct the examination, the diagnosis or differential diagnosis and your management plan.

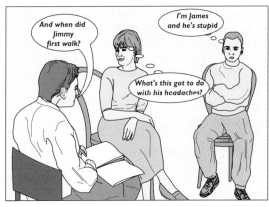

Figure 2.2 The history must be adapted to the child's age. The age when a child first walks is highly relevant when taking the history of a toddler but irrelevant for a teenager with headaches.

interview may provide important clues to the diagnosis and management.

- When you welcome the child, parents and siblings, check that you know the child's first name and gender. Ask how the child prefers to be addressed.
- Introduce yourself.
- Determine the relationship of the adults to the child.
- Establish eye contact and rapport with the family. Infants and some toddlers are most secure in parents' arms or laps. Young children may need some time to get to know you.
- Ensure that the interview environment is as welcoming and unthreatening as possible. Avoid having desks or beds between you and the family, but keep a comfortable distance.
- Have toys available. Observe how the child separates, plays and interacts with any siblings present.
- Don't forget to address questions to the child, when appropriate.

- There will be occasions when the parents will not want the child present or when the child should be seen alone. This is usually to avoid embarrassing older children or teenagers or to impart sensitive information. It must be handled tactfully, often by negotiating to talk separately to each in turn.

Presenting symptoms

Full details are required of the presenting symptoms. Let the parents and child recount the presenting complaints in their own words and at their own pace. Note the parent's words about the presenting complaint: onset, duration, previous episodes, what relieves/aggravates them, time course of the problem, if getting worse and any associated symptoms. Has the child's or the family's lifestyle been affected? What has the family done about it?

Make sure you know:

- what prompted referral to a doctor
- what the parents think or fear is the matter.

The scope and detail of further history-taking are determined by the nature and severity of the presenting complaint and the child's age. Whilst the comprehensive assessment listed here is sometimes required, usually a selective approach is more appropriate (Fig. 2.3). This is not an excuse for a short, slipshod history, but instead allows one to focus on the areas where a thorough, detailed history is required.

General enquiry

Check:

- general health – how active and lively?
- normal growth
- pubertal development (if appropriate)
- feeding/drinking/appetite
- any recent change in behaviour or personality.

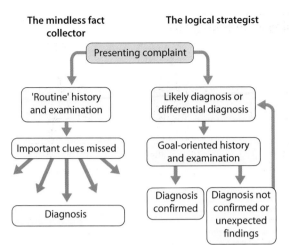

Figure 2.3 The history and examination should be goal-oriented, based on the presenting complaint. Comprehensive history-taking is best reserved for training or for complex, multi-system disorders. (Adapted from Hutson J M, Beasley S W, *The Surgical Examination of Children*, Heinemann Medical Books, London, 1988.)

Systems review

Selected, as appropriate:

- general rashes, fever (if measured)
- respiratory – cough, wheeze, breathing problems
- ENT – throat infections, snoring, noisy breathing (stridor)
- cardiovascular – heart murmur, cyanosis, exercise tolerance
- gastrointestinal – vomiting, diarrhoea/constipation, abdominal pain
- genitourinary – dysuria, frequency, wetting, toilet-trained
- neurological – seizures, headaches, abnormal movements
- musculoskeletal – disturbance of gait, limb pain or swelling, other functional abnormalities.

Make sure that you and the parent or child mean the same thing when describing a problem.

Past medical history

Check:

- maternal obstetric problems, delivery
- birthweight and gestation
- perinatal problems, whether admitted to special care baby unit
- immunisations (ideally from the personal child health record)
- past illnesses, hospital admissions and operations, accidents and injuries.

Medication

Check:
- past and present medications
- known allergies.

Family history

Families share houses, genes and diseases!

- Have any members of the family or friends had similar problems or any serious disorder?
- Draw a family tree. If there is a positive family history, extend family pedigree over several generations.
- Is there consanguinity?

Social history

Check:

- Relevant information about the family and its community – parental occupation, economic status, housing, relationships, parental smoking, marital stresses.
- Is the child happy at home? What are the child's preferred play or leisure activities?
- Is the child happy at nursery/school?

This 'social snapshot' is crucial since many childhood illnesses or conditions are permeated by adult problems, e.g.:

- alcohol and drug abuse
- long-term unemployment/poverty
- poor, damp, cramped housing
- parental psychiatric disorders
- unstable partnership.

Development

Check:

- parental worries about vision, hearing, development
- key developmental milestones (Fig. 2.4)
- previous child health surveillance developmental checks
- bladder and bowel control
- child's temperament, behaviour
- sleeping problems
- concerns and progress at nursery/school.

Look through the personal child health record.

An approach to examining children

Obtaining the child's cooperation

- Make friends with the child.
- Be confident but gentle.
- Avoid dominating the child.
- Short mock examinations, e.g. auscultating a teddy or the mother's hand, may allay a young child's fears.
- When first examining a young child, start at a non-threatening area, such as a hand or knee.
- Explain what you are about to do and what you want the child to do, in language he can understand. As the examination is essential, not optional, it is best not to ask his permission, as it may well be refused!

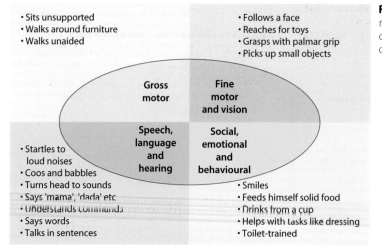

- Sits unsupported
- Walks around furniture
- Walks unaided

- Follows a face
- Reaches for toys
- Grasps with palmar grip
- Picks up small objects

Gross motor

Fine motor and vision

Speech, language and hearing

Social, emotional and behavioural

- Startles to loud noises
- Coos and babbles
- Turns head to sounds
- Says 'mama', 'dada' etc
- Understands commands
- Says words
- Talks in sentences

- Smiles
- Feeds himself solid food
- Drinks from a cup
- Helps with tasks like dressing
- Toilet-trained

Figure 2.4 Some key developmental milestones in infants and young children. These are considered in detail in Chapter 3.

- A smiling, talking doctor appears less threatening, but this should not be overdone as it can interfere with one's relationship with the parents.
- Leave unpleasant procedures until last.

Adapting to the child's age

Adapt the examination to suit the child's age. Whilst it may be difficult to examine some toddlers and young children fully, it is usually possible with resourcefulness and imagination on the doctor's part.

- Babies in the first few months are best examined on an examination couch with a parent next to them.
- A toddler is best initially examined on his mother's lap or occasionally over a parent's shoulder. Parents are reassuring for the child and helpful in facilitating the examination if guided as to what to do (Fig. 2.5).
- Preschool children may initially be examined whilst they are playing.
- Older children and teenagers are often concerned about privacy. Teenage girls should normally be examined in the presence of their mother, or a nurse or suitable chaperone. Be aware of cultural sensitivities in different ethnic groups.

Undressing children

Be sensitive to children's modesty. The area to be examined must be inspected fully, but this is best done in stages, re-dressing the child when each stage has been completed. It is easiest and kindest to ask the child or parent to do the undressing.

Warm, clean hands

Hands must be washed before (and after) examining a child. Warm smile, warm hands and a warm stethoscope all help!

Developmental skills

A good overview of developmental skills can be obtained by watching the child play. A few simple

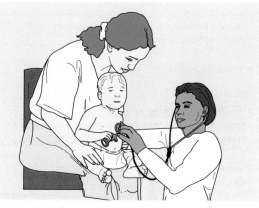

Figure 2.5 Distracting a toddler with a toy allows auscultation of the heart.

toys, such as some bricks, a car, doll, ball, pencil and paper, pegboard, miniature toys and a picture book, are all that is required, as they can be adapted for any age. If developmental assessment (see Ch. 3) is the focus of the examination, it is advisable to assess this before the physical examination, as cooperation may then be lost.

Examination

Initial observations

Careful observation is usually the key to success in examining children. Look before touching the child. Inspection will provide information on:

- severity of illness
- growth and nutrition
- behaviour and social responsiveness
- level of hygiene and care.

Severity of illness

Is the child sick or well? If sick, how sick? For the acutely ill infant or child, perform the '60-second rapid assessment':

- Airway and Breathing – respiration rate and effort, presence of stridor or wheeze, cyanosis
- Circulation – heart rate, pulse volume, peripheral temperature, capillary refill time
- Disability – level of consciousness.

The care of the seriously ill child is described in Chapter 6.

Measurements

As abnormal growth may be the first manifestation of illness in children, always measure and plot growth on centile charts for:

- weight, noting previous measurements from personal child health record
- length (in infants, if indicated) or height in older children
- head circumference in infants.

As appropriate:

- temperature
- blood pressure
- peak expiratory flow rate.

General appearance

The face, head and neck, and hands are examined. The general morphological appearance may suggest a chromosomal or dysmorphic syndrome. In infants, palpate the fontanelle and sutures.

Respiratory system

Cyanosis

Central cyanosis is best observed on the tongue.

Clubbing of the fingers and/or toes

Clubbing (Fig. 2.6a) is usually associated with chronic suppurative lung disease, e.g. cystic fibrosis, or cyanotic congenital heart disease. It is occasionally seen in inflammatory bowel disease or cirrhosis.

Tachypnoea

Rate of respiration is age-dependent (Table 2.1).

Respiratory system

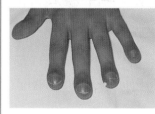

Figure 2.6a Clubbing of the fingers. There is increased curvature, loss of nail angle and fluctuation. This child had cystic fibrosis.

Table 2.1 Respiratory rate in children (breaths/min)

Age	Normal	Tachypnoea
Neonate	30–50	>60
Infants	20–30	>50
Young children	20–30	>40
Older children	15–20	>30

Table 2.2 Chest signs of some common chest disorders of children

	Chest movement	Percussion	Auscultation
Bronchiolitis	Laboured breathing Hyperinflated chest Chest recession	Hyper-resonant	Fine crackles in all zones Wheezes may/may not be present
Pneumonia	Reduced on affected side Rapid, shallow breaths	Dull	Bronchial breathing Crackles
Asthma	Reduced but hyperinflated Use of accessory muscles Chest wall retraction	Hyper-resonant	Wheeze

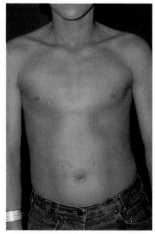

Figure 2.6b Hyperexpanded chest from chronic obstructive airways disease. This boy had severe asthma.

Infants with pneumonia may not have any abnormal signs on auscultation.

Sputum is rarely produced by children, as they swallow it. The main exception is suppurative lung disease from cystic fibrosis.

Dyspnoea

Laboured breathing. Increased work of breathing is judged by:

- nasal flaring
- expiratory grunting – to increase positive end-expiratory pressure
- use of accessory muscles, especially sternomastoids
- retraction (recession) of the chest wall, from use of suprasternal, intercostal and subcostal muscles
- difficulty speaking (or feeding).

Chest shape

- hyperexpansion or barrel shape (Fig. 2.6b), e.g. asthma
- *pectus excavatum* (hollow chest) or *pectus carinatum* (pigeon chest)
- Harrison's sulcus (indrawing of the chest wall from diaphragmatic tug), e.g. from poorly controlled asthma
- asymmetry of chest movements.

Palpation

- Chest expansion – this is 3–5 cm in school-aged children. Measure maximal chest expansion with tape measure. Check for symmetry.
- Trachea – checking that it is central is seldom helpful and is disliked by children. To be done selectively.
- Location of apex beat to detect mediastinal shift.

Percussion

- Needs to be done gently, comparing like with like, using middle fingers.
- Seldom informative in infants.
- Localised dullness – collapse, consolidation, fluid.

Auscultation, i.e. ears and stethoscope

- Note quality and symmetry of breath sounds and any added sounds.
- Harsh breath sounds from the upper airways are readily transmitted to the upper chest in infants.
- Hoarse voice – abnormality of the vocal cords.
- Stridor – harsh, low-pitched, mainly inspiratory sound from upper airways obstruction.
- Breath sounds – normal are vesicular; bronchial breathing is higher-pitched and the lengths of inspiration and expiration are equal.
- Wheeze – high-pitched, expiratory sound from distal airway obstruction (Table 2.2).
- Crackles – discontinuous 'moist' sounds from the opening of bronchioles (Table 2.2).

Cardiovascular system

Cyanosis

Observe the tongue for central cyanosis.

Clubbing of fingers or toes

Check if present.

Pulse

Check:

- rate (Table 2.3)
- rhythm – sinus arrhythmia (variation of pulse rate with respiration) is normal
- volume – small in circulatory insufficiency or aortic stenosis; increased in high-output states (stress, anaemia); collapsing in patent ductus arteriosus, aortic regurgitation.

Inspection

Look for:

- respiratory distress
- precordial bulge – caused by cardiac enlargement
- ventricular impulse – visible if thin, hyperdynamic circulation or left ventricular hypertrophy
- operative scars – mostly sternotomy or left lateral thoracotomy.

Palpation

Thrill = palpable murmur.
Apex (4th–5th intercostal space, mid-clavicular line):

- not palpable in some normal infants, plump children or dextrocardia
- heave from left ventricular hypertrophy.

Right ventricular heave at lower left sternal edge – right ventricular hypertrophy.

Percussion

Cardiac border percussion is rarely helpful in children.

Auscultation

Listen for heart sounds and murmurs.

Heart sounds

- Splitting of second sound is usually easily heard and is normal (Fig. 2.7).
- Fixed splitting of second heart sound in atrial septal defects.
- Third heart sound in mitral area is normal in young children.

Murmurs

- Timing – systolic/diastolic/continuous
- Duration – mid-systolic (ejection)/pansystolic
- Loudness – systolic murmurs graded:
  1–2: soft, difficult to hear
  3: easily audible, no thrill
  4–6: loud with thrill
- Site of maximal intensity – mitral/pulmonary/aortic/tricuspid areas
- Radiation:
  – to neck in aortic stenosis
  – to back in coarctation of the aorta or pulmonary stenosis.

Cardiovascular system

Table 2.3 Normal resting pulse rate in children

Age	Beats/min
<1 year	110–160
2–5 years	95–140
5–12 years	80–120
>12 years	60–100

Increased with stress, exercise, fever, arrhythmia.

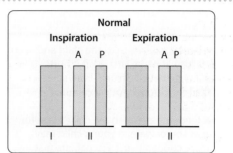

Figure 2.7 The splitting of the second heart sound is easily heard in children.

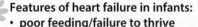 **Features of heart failure in infants:**
- poor feeding/failure to thrive
- sweating
- tachypnoea
- tachycardia
- gallop rhythm
- cardiomegaly
- hepatomegaly.

Features suggesting a murmur is significant:
- conducted all over the precordium
- loud
- thrill (equals grade 4–6 murmur)
- any diastolic murmur
- accompanied by other abnormal cardiac signs.

Draw your findings (see Ch. 17 on cardiac disorders).

Hepatomegaly

Important sign of heart failure in infants. An infant's liver is normally palpable 1–2 cm below the costal margin.

Femoral pulses

In coarctation of the aorta:

- decreased volume or may be impalpable in infants
- brachiofemoral delay in older children.

Blood pressure (see p. 15)

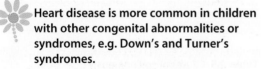 **Heart disease is more common in children with other congenital abnormalities or syndromes, e.g. Down's and Turner's syndromes.**

Abdomen

Abdominal examination is performed in three major clinical settings:

- the routine part of the examination
- an 'acute abdomen' – ?cause (see p. 211)
- recurrent abdominal pain/distension/constipation mass.

Associated signs

Examine:

- the eyes for signs of jaundice and anaemia
- the tongue for coating and colour
- the fingers for clubbing.

Inspection

The abdomen is protuberant in normal toddlers and young children. The abdominal wall muscles must be relaxed for palpation.

Generalised abdominal distension is most often explained by the five 'F's:

- fat
- fluid (ascites – uncommon in children, most often from nephrotic syndrome)
- faeces (constipation)
- flatus (malabsorption, intestinal obstruction)
- fetus (not to be forgotten after puberty).

Occasionally, it is caused by a grossly enlarged liver and/or spleen or muscle hypotonia.

Causes of localised abdominal distension are:

- upper abdomen – gastric dilatation from pyloric stenosis, hepato/splenomegaly
- lower abdomen – distended bladder, masses.

Other signs:

- dilated veins in liver disease, abdominal striae
- operative scars (draw a diagram)
- peristalsis – from pyloric stenosis, intestinal obstruction.

Are the buttocks normally rounded, or wasted as in malabsorption, e.g. coeliac disease or malnutrition?

Palpation

- Use warm hands, explain, relax the child and keep the parent close at hand. First ask if it hurts.
- Palpate in a systematic fashion – liver, spleen, kidneys, bladder, through four abdominal quadrants.
- Ask about tenderness. Watch the child's face for grimacing as you palpate. A young child may become more cooperative if you palpate first with their hand or by putting your hand on top of theirs.

Tenderness

- *Location* – localised in appendicitis, hepatitis, pyelonephritis; generalised in mesenteric adenitis, peritonitis
- *Guarding* – often unimpressive on direct palpation in children. Pain on coughing, on moving about/ walking/bumps during car journey suggests peritoneal irritation. Back bent on walking may be from psoas inflammation in appendicitis.

Hepatomegaly (Table 2.4, Fig. 2.8)

- Palpate from right iliac fossa.
- Locate edge with tips or side of finger.
- Edge may be soft or firm.
- Unable to get above it.
- Moves with respiration.
- Measure (in cm) extension below costal margin in mid-clavicular line.

Liver tenderness is likely to be due to inflammation from hepatitis.

Splenomegaly (Table 2.5)

- Palpate from right iliac fossa.
- Edge is usually soft.
- Unable to get above it.
- Notch occasionally palpable if markedly enlarged.
- Moves on respiration (ask the child to take a deep breath).

Abdomen

Table 2.4   Causes of hepatomegaly

Infection	Congenital, infectious mononucleosis, hepatitis, malaria, parasitic infection
Haematological	Sickle cell anaemia, thalassaemia
Liver disease	Chronic active hepatitis, portal hypertension, polycystic disease
Malignancy	Leukaemia, lymphoma, neuroblastoma, Wilms' tumour, hepatoblastoma
Metabolic	Glycogen and lipid storage disorders, mucopolysaccharidoses
Cardiovascular	Heart failure
Apparent	Chest hyperexpansion from bronchiolitis or asthma

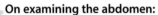

On examining the abdomen:
- **inspect first, palpate later**
- **superficial palpation first, deep palpation later**
- **guarding is unimpressive in children**
- **silent abdomen – serious!**
- **immobile abdomen – serious!**

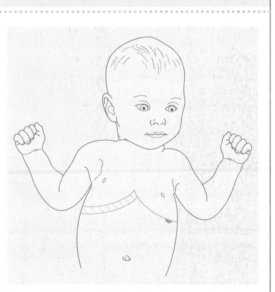

Figure 2.8 Normal findings. The liver edge is 1–2 cm below the costal margin in infants and young children. The spleen may be 1–2 cm below the costal margin in infants.

Table 2.5 Causes of splenomegaly

Infection	Viral, bacterial, protozoal (malaria, leishmaniasis), parasites, infective endocarditis
Haematological	Haemolytic anaemia
Malignancy	Leukaemia, lymphoma
Other	Portal hypertension, systemic juvenile idiopathic arthritis (Still's disease)

- Measure size below costal margin (in cm) in mid-clavicular line.

If uncertain whether it is palpable:

- use bimanual approach to spleen
- turn child onto right side.

A palpable spleen is at least twice its normal size!

Kidneys

These are not usually palpable beyond the neonatal period unless enlarged or the abdominal muscles are hypotonic.

On examination:

- palpate by balloting bimanually
- they move on respiration
- one can get above them.

Tenderness implies inflammation.

Abnormal masses

- *Wilms' tumour* – renal mass, sometimes visible, does not cross midline.
- *Neuroblastoma* – irregular firm mass, may cross midline; the child is usually very unwell.
- *Faecal masses* – mobile, non-tender, indentable.
- *Intussusception* – acutely unwell, mass may be palpable, most often in right upper quadrant.

Percussion

- *Liver* – dullness delineates upper and lower border. Record span.
- *Spleen* – dullness delineates lower border.
- *Ascites* – shifting dullness. Percuss from most resonant spot to most dull spot.

Auscultation

Not very useful in 'routine' examination, but important in 'acute abdomen':

- increased bowel sounds – intestinal obstruction, acute diarrhoea
- reduced or absent bowel sounds – paralytic ileus, peritonitis.

Genital area

The genital area is examined routinely in young children, but in older children and teenagers this is done only if relevant, e.g. vaginal discharge. Is there an inguinal hernia or a perineal rash?

In *males*:

- Is the penis of normal size?
- Is the scrotum well developed?
- Are the testes palpable? With one hand over the inguinal region, palpate with the other hand. Record if the testis is descended, retractile or impalpable.
- Is there any scrotal swelling (hydrocele or hernia)?

In *females*:

- Do the external genitalia look normal?

Does the anus look normal? Any evidence of a fissure?

Rectal examination

- Not part of routine examination.
- Unpleasant and disliked by children.
- Its usefulness in the 'acute abdomen' (e.g. appendicitis) is debatable in children, as they have a thin abdominal wall and so tenderness and masses can be identified on palpation of the abdomen. Some surgeons advocate it to identify a retrocaecal appendix, but interpretation is problematic as most children will complain of pain from the procedure.
- If intussusception is suspected, the mass may be palpable and stools looking like redcurrant jelly may be revealed on rectal examination.

Urinalysis

- Checked if appropriate.
- Clean catch urine specimen preferred.
- Dipstick testing for proteinuria, haematuria, glycosuria, leukocyturia.
- Examination of the microscopic appearance of urine is helpful for determining the origin of haematuria (crenated red cells, red cell casts).

A hyperexpanded chest in bronchiolitis or asthma may displace the liver and spleen downwards, mimicking hepato/splenomegaly.

Neurology/neurodevelopment

Brief neurological screen

A quick neurological and developmental overview should be performed in all children. When doing this:

- use common sense to avoid unnecessary examination
- adapt it to the child's age
- take into consideration the parent's account of developmental milestones.

Watch the child play, draw or write. Are the manipulative skills normal? Can he walk, run, climb, hop, skip, dance? Are the child's language skills and speech satisfactory? Are the social interactions appropriate? Does vision and hearing appear to be normal?

In infants, assess primarily by observation:

- Observe posture and movements of the limbs.
- When picking the infant up, note their tone. The limbs and body may feel normal, floppy or stiff. Head control may be poor, with abnormal head lag on pulling to sitting.

Most children are neurologically intact and do not require formal neurological examination of reflexes, tone, etc. More detailed neurological assessment is performed only if indicated. Specific neurological

17

concerns or problems in development or behaviour require detailed assessment.

More detailed neurological examination

If the child has a neurological problem, a detailed and systematic neurological examination is required.

Patterns of movement

Observe walking and running: normal walking is with a heel–toe gait. A toe–heel pattern of walking (toe-walkers) although often idiopathic, may suggest pyramidal tract (corticospinal) dysfunction causing spasticity and tight Achilles tendon, spinal pathology (diastematomyelia) or neuropathy. Children with myopathy may also develop tight Achilles tendon due to weakness. If you are unsure whether a gait is heel–toe or toe–heel, look at the pattern of shoe wear.

A broad-based gait may be due to an immature gait (normal in a toddler) or secondary to a cerebellar disorder. Proximal muscle weakness around the hip girdle can cause a waddling gait. Unilateral weakness or hemiparesis of the leg will manifest as circumduction of the affected leg. Look for asymmetry, style of gait and arm swing (see Fig. 4.4).

Observe standing from lying down supine. Children up to 3 years of age will turn prone in order to stand because of poor pelvic muscle fixation; beyond this age, it suggests neuromuscular weakness (e.g. Duchenne's muscular dystrophy) or low tone which could be due to a central (brain) cause. The need to turn prone to rise or, later, as weakness progresses, to push off the ground with straightened arms and then climb up the legs is known as Gower's sign (see Fig. 27.12).

Coordination

Assess this by:

- asking the child to build one brick upon another or using a peg-board, and do up and undo buttons, draw, copy patterns, write
- asking the child to hold his arms out straight and close his eyes, and then observing for drift or tremor (this is really looking for asymmetry, position sense, and neglect of one side with visual cues removed)
- finger–nose testing (use teddy's nose to reach out and touch if necessary)
- rapid alternating movements of hands and fingers
- touching tip of each finger in turn with thumb
- asking the child to walk heel–toe, jump and hop.

Subtle asymmetries in gait may be revealed by Fogge's test – children are asked to walk on their heels, the outside and then the inside of their feet. Watch for the pattern of abnormal movement in the upper limbs. Observe them running.

Inspection of limbs

Muscle bulk

- Wasting may be secondary to cerebral palsy, meningomyelocele, muscle disorder or from previous poliomyelitis.

- Increased bulk of calf muscles may indicate Duchenne's muscular dystrophy, or myotonic conditions.

Muscle tone

Tone, in limbs

- Best assessed by taking the weight of the whole limb and then bending and extending it around a single joint. Testing is easiest at the knee and ankle joints. Assess the resistance to passive movement as well as the range of movement.
- Increased tone (spasticity) in adductors and internal rotators of the hips, clonus at the ankles or increased tone on pronation of the forearms at rest is usually the result of pyramidal dysfunction. This can be differentiated from the cog-wheel rigidity seen in extrapyramidal conditions.
- The posture of the limbs may give a clue as to the underlying tone, e.g. scissoring of the legs (see Figs 4.3 and 4.4), pronated forearms, fisting, extended legs suggests increased tone. Sitting in a frog-like posture of the legs suggests hypotonia (see Fig. 8.2a), whilst abnormal posturing and extension suggests fluctuating tone (dyskinesia).

Truncal tone

- In pyramidal tract disorders, the trunk and head tend to arch backwards (extensor posturing).
- In muscle disease and some central brain disorders, the trunk may be hypotonic (see Fig. 27.13). The child feels floppy to handle and cannot support the trunk in sitting.

Head lag

- This is best tested by pulling the child up by the arms from the supine position.

Power

Difficult to test in babies. Watch for antigravity movements and note motor function. Both will tell you a lot about power. From 6 months onwards, watch the pattern of mobility and gait. Watch the child standing up from lying and climbing stairs. From the age of 4 years, power can be tested formally against gravity and resistance, first testing proximal muscle and then distal muscle power and comparing sides.

Reflexes

Test with the child in a relaxed position and explain what you are about to do before approaching with a tendon hammer, or demonstrate on parent or toy first. Brisk reflexes may reflect anxiety in the child or a pyramidal disorder. Absent reflexes may be due to a neuromuscular problem or a lesion within the spinal cord, but may also be due to inexpert examination technique. Children will reinforce reflexes if asked.

Plantar responses

In children the responses are often equivocal and unpopular as it is unpleasant. They are unreliable under 1 year of age. Upgoing plantar responses provide additional evidence of pyramidal dysfunction.

Sensation

Testing the ability to withdraw to tickle is usually adequate as a screening test. If loss of sensation is likely, e.g. meningomyelocele or spinal lesion (transverse myelitis etc.), more detailed sensory testing is performed as in adults. In spinal and cauda equina lesions there may be a palpable bladder or absent perineal sensation.

Cranial nerves

Before about 4 years old you need some ingenuity to test for abnormal or asymmetric signs – make it a game; ask them to mimic you:

- **I** Need not be tested in routine practice. Can be done by recognising the smell of a hidden mint sweet.
- **II** Visual acuity – determined according to age. Direct and consensual pupillary response tested to light and accommodation. Visual fields can be tested if the child is old enough to cooperate.
- **III,IV,VI** Full eye movement through horizontal and vertical planes. Is there a squint? Nystagmus – avoid extreme lateral gaze, as it can induce nystagmus in normal children.
- **V** Clench teeth and waggle jaw from side to side against resistance.
- **VII** Close eyes tight, smile and show teeth.
- **VIII** Hearing – ask parents, although unilateral deafness could be missed this way. If in doubt, needs formal assessment in a suitable environment.
- **IX** Levator palati – saying 'aagh'. Look for deviation of uvula.
- **X** Recurrent laryngeal nerve – listen for hoarseness or stridor.
- **XI** Trapezius and sternomastoid power – shrug shoulders and turn head against resistance.
- **XII** Put out tongue and look for any atrophy or deviation.

Bones and joints

Presentation of bone and joint disorders varies:

- Inspect for – swelling from a joint effusion (loss of joint outline) or synovial thickening, redness, pain on movement, loss of function, muscle wasting above and below any swollen joints.
- Palpate for – heat (comparing joints), tenderness, fluctuation of effusion.
- Movements – active before passive in order not to hurt the child. Explain movements in child-friendly words. If necessary, show on your own joints the movements you wish to test. Record joint movement in degrees.
- Limp – may be due to hip, knee or ankle pain. Hip pain may be referred from the knee or vice versa.
- Scoliosis – inspect the spine, especially in older children/adolescents. Ask to stand straight (as a soldier!) and then to touch toes (see Fig. 26.11).

Neck

Thyroid

- Inspect – swelling uncommon in childhood; occasionally at puberty.
- Palpate from behind and front for swelling, nodule, thrill.
- Auscultate if enlarged.
- Look for signs of hypo/hyperthyroidism.

Lymph nodes

Examine systematically – occipital, cervical, axillary, inguinal. Note size, number, consistency of any glands felt:

- Small, discrete, pea-sized, mobile nodes in the neck, groin and axilla – common in normal children, especially if thin.
- Small, multiple nodes in the neck – common after upper respiratory tract infections (viral/bacterial).
- Multiple lymph nodes of variable size in children with extensive atopic eczema – frequent finding, no action required.
- Large, hot, tender, sometimes fluctuant node, usually in neck – infected/abscess.
- Variable size and shape:
  - infections: viral, e.g. infectious mononucleosis, or TB
  - rare causes: malignant disease (usually non-tender), Kawasaki's disease, cat-scratch.

Blood pressure

Indications

Must be closely monitored (Box 2.1) if critically ill, if there is renal or cardiac disease or diabetes mellitus, or if receiving drug therapy which may cause hypertension, e.g. corticosteroids. Not measured often enough in children.

Technique

When measured with a sphygmomanometer:

- Show the child that there is a balloon in the cuff and demonstrate how it is blown up.
- Use largest cuff which fits comfortably, covering at least two-thirds of the upper arm. (Too small a cuff often causes an abnormally high reading.)
- The child must be relaxed and not crying.
- Systolic pressure is the easiest to determine in young children and clinically the most useful.

Box 2.1 Measuring blood pressure in children

- Sphygmomanometer
  - stethoscope in older children
  - Doppler ultrasound in infants
- Oscillometric (e.g. Dynamapp) – helpful in infants and young children
- Invasive – direct measurement from an arterial catheter is preferable if critically ill

- Diastolic pressure is when the sounds disappear. May not be possible to discern in young children.

Measurement

Must be interpreted according to a centile chart (see Fig. A.3, in the Appendix). Blood pressure is increased by tall stature and obesity. Charts relating blood pressure to height are available and preferable; however, for convenience, charts relating blood pressure to age are often used. An abnormally high reading must be repeated, with the child relaxed, on at least three separate occasions.

Eyes

Examination

Inspect eyes, pupils, iris and sclerae. Are eye movements full and symmetrical? Is nystagmus detectable? If so, may have ocular or cerebellar cause, or testing may be too lateral to the child. Are the pupils round (absence of posterior synechiae), equal, central and reactive to light? Is there a squint?

Epicanthic folds are common in Asian ethnic groups.

Ophthalmoscopy

- In infants, the red reflex is seen from a distance of 20–30 cm. Absence of red reflex occurs in corneal clouding, cataract, retinoblastoma.
- Fundoscopy – difficult. Requires experience and cooperation. In infants, mydriatics are needed and an ophthalmological opinion may be required. Retinopathy of prematurity and retinopathy of congenital infections and choroido-retinal degeneration show characteristic findings. Retinal

haemorrhages may be seen in head trauma or in 'shaken baby syndrome' (non-accidental injury).
- In older children with headaches, diabetes mellitus or hypertension, optic fundi should be examined. Mydriatics are not usually needed.

Ears and throat

Examination is usually left until last, as it can be unpleasant. Explain what you are going to do. Show the parent how to hold and gently restrain a younger child to ensure success and avoid possible injury (Figs 2.9, 2.10).

Throat

Try quickly to get a look at the tonsils, uvula, pharynx and posterior palate. Older children (5 years +) will open their mouths as wide as possible without a spatula. A spatula is required for young children. Look for redness, swelling, pus or palatal petechiae. Also check the teeth for dental caries and other gross abnormalities.

Ears

Examine ear canals and drums gently, trying not to hurt the child. Look for anatomical landmarks on the ear drum and for swelling, redness, perforation, dullness, fluid.

Communicating with children

Throughout the consultation, make sure that your communication with the child is appropriate for the child's age and stage of development (Table 2.6).

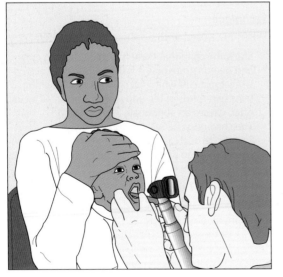

Figure 2.9 Holding a young child to examine the throat. The mother has one hand on the head and the other across the child's arms.

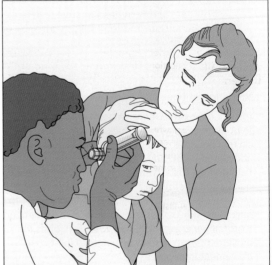

Figure 2.10 Holding a young child correctly is essential for successful examination of the ear with an auroscope. The mother has one hand on the child's head and the other hand holding the upper arm.

The reasons for talking with children

Why talk to children when you can get the information from the parent? The reasons are:

- To establish rapport
- To obtain the child's own views about their problems
- To know how the child feels about their health and life
- To reduce anxiety and fear and to improve compliance with assessment and treatment
- To determine the presence of associated emotional or psychiatric problems

	Preschool child (2–5 years)	School-age child (6–11 years)	Adolescent (12–18 years)
Thought processes	When I close my eyes, Mum goes away (world viewed differently, from own perspective) I am asleep, so everyone is asleep (centre of their world) When I fell, the floor hurt me (objects are alive) My toy elephant is crying because the other elephants won't play with him (involvement in pretend play)	I have been invited to Katie and Jane's parties - maybe I could go for some time to each (able to start solving concrete problems Am I going to be chosen for the school choir? (develops worries about the future) Mum gets really upset when Dad gets drunk, but Dad does not care (able to see another person's point of view and take on more than one perspective)	I can handle things without Mum's help (seeking autonomy and separation) Should our country be at war? (develops concern about social issues)
Effect on the way we talk to them	Use short, concrete questions within their immediate experience. To avoid yes/no answers use a choice of options, e.g. when you go to nursery, what do you like to do – draw or dress up or something else? Use toys or puppets whilst interviewing, e.g. to represent different people in the child's life	Use familiar examples of experience of others to explore the child's feelings and behaviour, e.g. when a boy was bullying another boy at school, he came to see me so we could talk about how he controls his temper. Do you ever get angry and bully others? You can get at their hopes and dreams by asking them, ' if I was a magician and could give you three wishes, what would they be?'	Should be given an opportunity to be seen alone as they may have problems and difficulties not known to the parents and that the adolescent does not want to share with them Upsetting thoughts can be explored in some adolescents using metaphors

⊚ Summary

In taking a history and performing a clinical examination:

- the child's age is a key feature – it will determine the nature of the problem, how the consultation is conducted, the likely diagnosis and its management
- the interview environment should be welcoming – with suitable toys for young children
- most information is usually obtained from a focused history and observation rather than detailed examination although examination is also important
- check growth, including charts in personal child health record, and development
- with young children – be confident but gentle, don't ask their permission to examine them or they may say 'no' and leave unpleasant procedures (ears and throat) until last
- involve children with the consultation, as appropriate to their age.

Summary and management plan

At the end of the history and examination:

- Summarise the key problems (in physical, emotional, social and family terms, if relevant).
- List the diagnoses or differential diagnoses.
- Draw up a management plan to address the problems, both short- and long-term. This could be reassurance, a period of observation, performing investigations or therapeutic intervention.
- Provide explanation to the parents and to the child, if old enough. Consider providing further information, either written or on the internet.
- If relevant, discuss what to tell other members of the family.
- Consider which other professionals should be informed.
- Write a brief summary in the child's personal child health record.
- Ensure your notes are dated and signed.

Further reading

Gill D, O'Brien N 2003 Paediatric clinical examination made easy. 4th edn. Churchill Livingstone, Edinburgh

Normal child development, hearing and vision

Children acquire functional skills throughout childhood. The term 'child development' is used to describe the skills acquired by children between birth and about 5 years of age, when there is a rapid progress in mobility, speech and language, communication and independence skills. During school age, evidence of developmental progression is predominantly through cognitive development, abstract thinking and skills of conceptualisation, although there is also some further maturation of early developmental skills.

Normal development in the first few years of life is monitored:

- by parents, who are provided with guidance about normal development in their child's personal child health record
- at regular child health surveillance checks
- whenever a young child is seen by a health care professional, when a brief opportunistic overview is made.

The main objective of assessing a young child's development is the early detection of delayed or abnormal development in order to:

- help children achieve their maximum potential
- provide treatment or therapy promptly (particularly important for impairment of hearing and vision)

- act as an entry point for the care and management of the child with special needs.

This chapter covers normal development, whilst delayed or abnormal development and the child with special needs are considered in Chapter 4.

Influence of heredity and environment

A child's development represents the interaction of heredity and the environment on the developing brain. Heredity determines the potential of the child, while the environment influences the extent to which that potential is achieved. For optimal development, the environment has to meet the child's physical and psychological needs (Fig. 3.1). These vary with age and stage of development:

- infants are totally physically dependent on their parents and require a limited number of carers to meet their psychological needs
- primary school age children can meet some of their physical needs and cope with many social relationships
- adolescents are able to meet most of their physical needs while experiencing increasingly complex emotional needs.

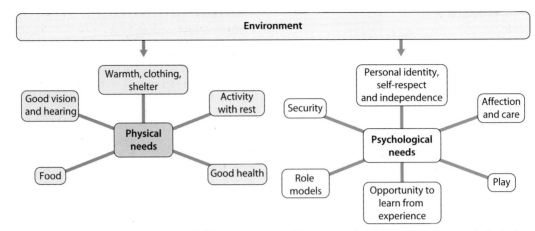

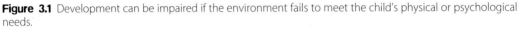

Figure 3.1 Development can be impaired if the environment fails to meet the child's physical or psychological needs.

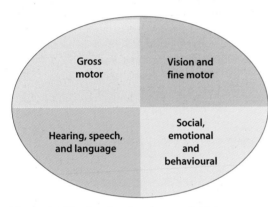

Figure 3.2 The four functional areas of child development and their core features.

Fields of development

There are four fields of developmental skills to consider whenever a young child is seen (Fig. 3.2). These are:

- gross motor
- vision and fine motor
- hearing, speech and language
- social, emotional and behavioural.

Gross motor skills are the most obvious initial area of developmental progress. As fine motor skills require good vision, these are grouped together; similarly, normal speech and language development depends on reasonable hearing and so these are also considered together. Social, emotional and behavioural skills are a spectrum of psychological development.

The acquisition of developmental abilities for each skill field follows a remarkably constant pattern between children, but may vary in rate. It is like a sequential story. Thus the pattern of acquisition of skills:

- is sequentially constant
- should always be considered longitudinally,

relating each stage to what has gone before and what lies ahead
- varies in rate between children.

A deficiency in any one skill area can have an impact on other areas. For instance, a hearing impairment may affect a child's language, social and communication skills and behaviour. As a child grows, additional skills become important, such as attention and concentration and how an individual child manages to integrate his skills.

Developmental milestones

Chronological age, physical growth and developmental skills usually evolve hand in hand. Just as there are normal ranges for changes in body size with age, so there are ranges over which new skills are acquired. Important developmental skills are called developmental milestones.

When considering developmental milestones:

- The *median age* is the age when half of a standard population of children achieve that level; it serves as a guide to when stages of development are likely to be reached but does not tell us if the child's skills are outside the normal range.
- *Limit ages* are the age by which they should have been achieved. Limit ages are usually 2 standard deviations from the mean. They are more useful as a guide to whether a child's development is normal than the median ages. Failure to meet them gives guidance for action regarding more detailed assessment, investigation or intervention.

Median and limit ages

The difference between median and limit ages can be demonstrated by considering the age range for the important developmental milestone of walking unsupported. The percentage of children who take their first steps unsupported is:

- 25% by 11 months
- 50% by 12 months

- 75% by 13 months
- 90% by 15 months
- 97.5% by 18 months.

The median age is 12 months and is a guide to the common pattern to expect, although the age range is wide. The limit age is 18 months (two standard deviations from the mean). Of those not achieving the limit age, many will be normal late walkers, but a proportion will have an underlying medical problem, such as cerebral palsy, a primary muscle disorder or global developmental delay. A few may be understimulated from social deprivation. Hence, any child who is not walking by 18 months should be assessed and examined. Thus 18 months can be set as a 'limit age' for children not walking. Setting the limit age earlier may allow earlier identification of problems, but will also increase the number of children labelled as 'delayed' who are in fact normal.

Variation in the pattern of motor development

There is variation in the pattern of motor development between children. For example, normal motor development is the progression from immobility to walking, but not all children do so in the same way. Whilst most achieve mobility by crawling (83%), some bottom-shuffle and others crawl with their abdomen on the floor, so-called commando crawling (creeping) (Fig. 3.3). A very few just stand up and walk. The locomotor pattern (crawling, creeping, shuffling, just standing up) determines the age of sitting, standing or walking.

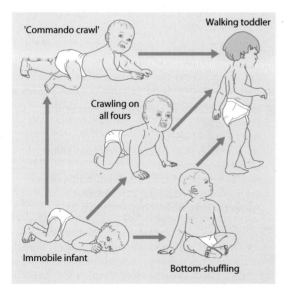

Figure 3.3 Early locomotor patterns. Most children crawl on all fours en route to walking, but some 'bottom-shuffle' and others 'commando crawl' (creep). Bottom-shuffling often runs in families, but the late walking that often goes with the locomotor variant needs to be differentiated from an abnormality such as cerebral palsy.

The limit age of 18 months for walking applies predominantly to children who have had crawling as their early mobility pattern. Children who bottom-shuffle or commando crawl tend to walk later than crawlers, so that within those not walking at 18 months there will be some children who demonstrate a locomotor variant pattern, with their developmental progress still being normal. For example, of children who become mobile by bottom-shuffling, 50% will walk independently by 18 months and 97.5% by 27 months of age, with even later ages for those who initially commando crawl.

Adjusting for prematurity

If a child has been born preterm, this should be allowed for when assessing developmental age by calculating it from the expected date of delivery. Thus the anticipated developmental skills of a 9-month baby (chronological age) born 3 months early at 28 weeks' gestation are more like those of a 6-month baby (corrected age). Correction is not required after about 2 years of age when the number of weeks early the child was born no longer represents a significant proportion of the child's life.

Is development normal?

When evaluating a child's developmental progress and whether it is normal or not:

- Concentrate on each field of development (gross motor; vision and fine motor; hearing and speech/language; social, emotional and behavioural) separately.
- Consider the pattern of development reached by thinking longitudinally about each developmental field. Ask about the sequence of development already achieved as well as those skills to be anticipated shortly.
- Determine the stage the child has reached for each skill field.
- Relate the progress of each developmental field to the others. Is the child progressing similarly through each skill field, or does one or more field of development lag behind the others?
- Then relate the child's developmental achievements to his age (chronological or corrected).

This will enable you to decide if the child's developmental progress is normal or delayed. Normal development implies steady progress in all four developmental fields with acquisition of skills occurring before recognised limit ages are reached. If there is developmental delay, does it affect all four developmental fields (global delay), or one or more developmental field only (specific developmental delay)? As children grow older and acquire further skills, it becomes easier to make a more accurate assessment of their abilities and developmental status.

◎ Summary

Assessing child development

When assessing a young child's development:

- consider the four fields of developmental skills – gross motor; vision and fine motor; hearing and speech/language; social, emotional, behavioural
- the acquisition of developmental abilities follows a similar pattern between children, but may vary in rate, and still be normal.

Terms used are:

- developmental milestones: the acquisition of important developmental skills
- median age: when half the population acquire a skill; serves as a guide to normal pattern of development
- limit age: when a skill should have been acquired; further assessment is indicated if not achieved.

When evaluating a child's development, consider:

- the stage the child has reached for each skill field
- the sequence of developmental progress
- if progress is similar in each skill field
- how the child's developmental achievements relate to age.

Table 3.1 Some primitive reflexes present at birth. (These should disappear by 4–6 months)

Reflex – mode of eliciting it	Description
Moro – sudden head extension	Symmetrical extension, then flexion of all limbs
Grasp – an object is placed in the palm at the base of the fingers	Flexion of the fingers of the hand
Rooting – stimulus near the mouth	Turning of the head towards the stimulus
Placing – infant held vertically and the dorsum of the feet brought into contact with a surface	Lifts first one foot, placing it on the surface, followed by the other
Positive supporting reflex – infant held vertically, feet on a surface	Legs take body weight, may push up against gravity
Atonic neck reflex (ATNR) – lying supine, the head is turned by the examiner to one side	Infant adopts a 'fencing' posture, with the arm outstretched on the side to which the head is turned

Pattern of child development

This is described in detail for each field of development, including key developmental milestones and limit ages:

- gross motor development (Fig. 3.4 and Table 3.1)
- vision and fine motor (Fig. 3.5)
- hearing, speech and language (Fig. 3.6)
- social, emotional and behavioural (Fig. 3.7).

In order to screen a young child's development, it is necessary to know only a limited number of key developmental milestones and their limit ages.

Cognitive development

Cognition refers to higher mental function. This progresses with age. In infancy, thought processes are centred around immediate experiences. The thought processes of preschool children (which have been called preoperational thought by Piaget), tend to be:

- that they are the centre of the world
- that inanimate objects are alive and have feelings and motives
- that events have a magical element
- that everything has a purpose. Toys and other objects are used in imaginative play as aids to thought to help make sense of experience and social relationships.

In middle school children, the dominant mode of thought is practical and orderly, tied to immediate circumstances and specific experiences. (This has been called operational thought.)

It is only in the mid-teens that an adult style of abstract thought (formal operational thought) begins to develop, with the ability for abstract reasoning, testing hypotheses and manipulating abstract concepts.

Intelligence testing (IQ)

Cognitive function can be assessed objectively by formal IQ tests but disadvantages are that the tests:

- may be affected by cultural background and linguistic skills
- do not test all skill areas
- do not necessarily reflect an individual child's ultimate potential
- may be compromised by individual disabilities, such as a motor disorder as in cerebral palsy, necessitating care in interpreting results.

'Performance' or 'non-verbal' intelligence tests assess abilities independent of language. 'Verbal' intelligence tests, especially those for younger children, reflect general intellectual skills, particularly relating to language. Performance and verbal intelligence testing allows formulation of a performance IQ (PIQ) and verbal IQ (VIQ) which together give an overall IQ figure. Children with disabilities may have problems such as with speech or hand skills that may compromise testing so that results in these situations have to be interpreted with care.

Gross motor development (median ages)

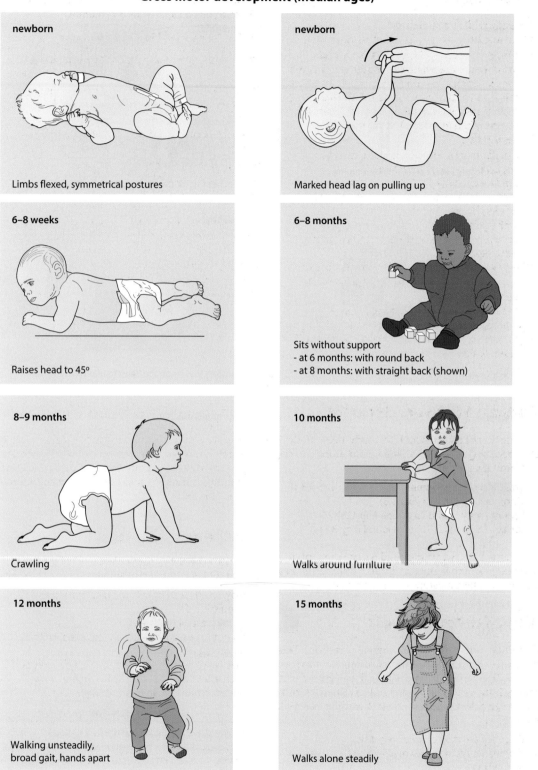

newborn

Limbs flexed, symmetrical postures

newborn

Marked head lag on pulling up

6–8 weeks

Raises head to 45°

6–8 months

Sits without support
- at 6 months: with round back
- at 8 months: with straight back (shown)

8–9 months

Crawling

10 months

Walks around furniture

12 months

Walking unsteadily, broad gait, hands apart

15 months

Walks alone steadily

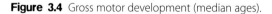

Figure 3.4 Gross motor development (median ages).

Vision and fine motor (median ages)

6 weeks

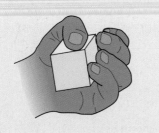

Newborn – follows face in midline.
Follows moving object or face by turning the head (illustrated).

4 months

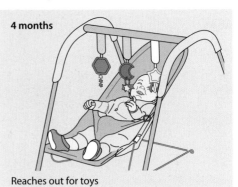

Reaches out for toys

6 months

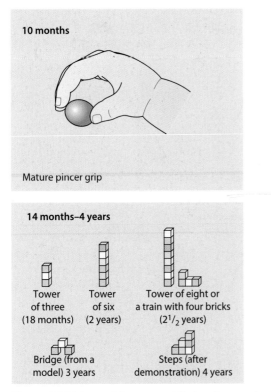

Palmar grasp

7 months

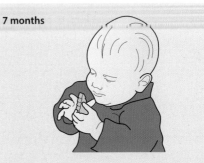

Transfers toys from one hand to another

10 months

Mature pincer grip

16–18 months

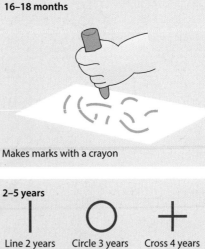

Makes marks with a crayon

14 months–4 years

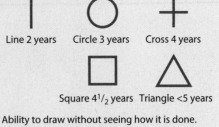

Tower of three (18 months)

Tower of six (2 years)

Tower of eight or a train with four bricks (2¹/₂ years)

Bridge (from a model) 3 years

Steps (after demonstration) 4 years

2–5 years

Line 2 years	Circle 3 years	Cross 4 years

Square 4¹/₂ years   Triangle <5 years

Ability to draw without seeing how it is done. Can copy (draw after seeing it done) 6 months earlier.

Figure 3.5 Vision and fine motor skills (median ages).

Hearing, speech and language (median ages)

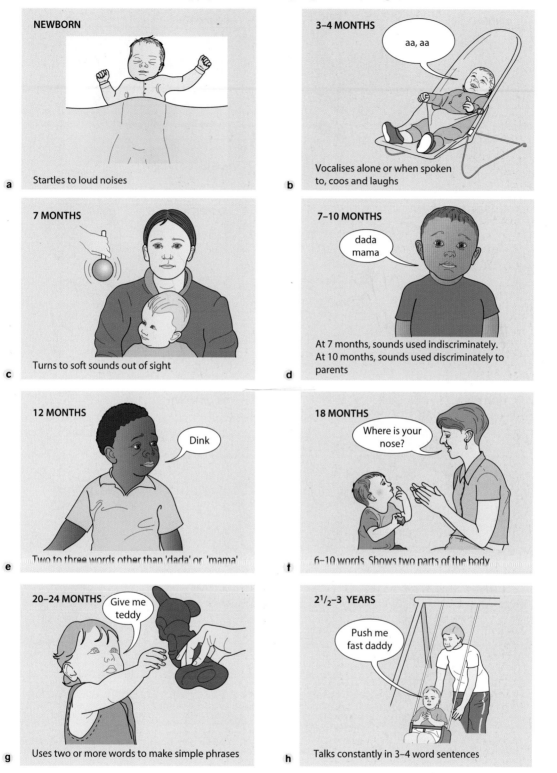

Figure 3.6 Hearing, speech and language (median ages).

Social, emotional and behavioural development (median ages)

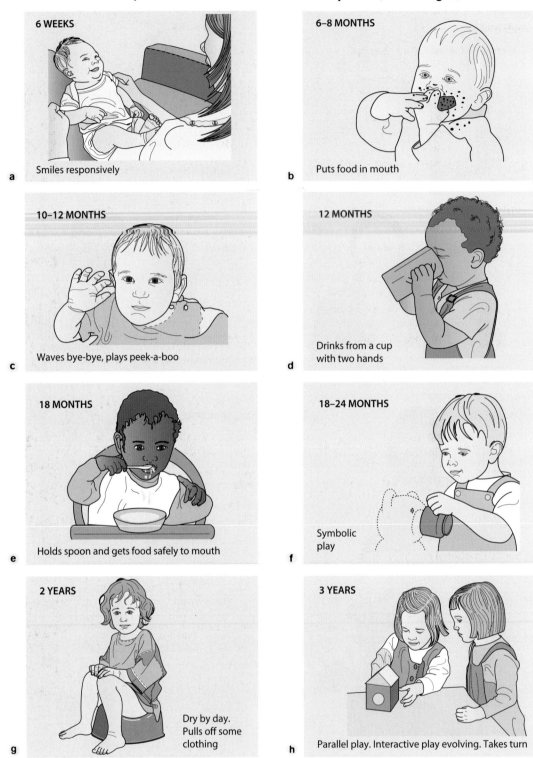

Figure 3.7 Social, emotional and behavioural development (median ages).

Fields of development

Overview of developmental stages

- Acquisition of tone and head control
- Primitive reflexes disappear
- Sitting
- Standing, walking, running
- Hopping, jumping, pedaling

Vision and fine motor

- Visual alertness, fixing and following
- Grasp reflex, hand regard
- Voluntary grasping, pincer, points
- Handles objects with both hands, transfers from hand to hand
- Writing, cutting, dressing

Hearing, speech and language

- Sound recognition, vocalisation
- Babbling
- Single words, understands simple requests
- Joining words, phrases
- Simple and complex conversation

Social, emotional and behavioural

- Smiling, socially responsive
- Separation anxiety
- Self help skills, feeding, dressing, toileting
- Peer group relationships
- Symbolic play
- Social/communication behaviour

Limit ages

Gross motor	Limit ages
Head control	4 months
Sits unsupported	9 months
Stands independently	12 months
Walks independently	18 months

Vision and fine motor	Limit ages
Fixes and follows visually	3 months
Reaches for objects	6 months
Transfers	8 months
Pincer grip	12 months

Hearing, speech and language	Limit ages
Polysyllabic babble	7 months
Consonant babble	10 months
Saying 6 words with meaning	18 months
Joins words	2 years
3-word sentences	2.5 years

Social behaviour	Limit ages
Smiles	8 weeks
Fear of strangers	10 months
Feeds self/spoon	18 months
Symbolic play	2–2.5 years
Interactive play	3–3.5 years

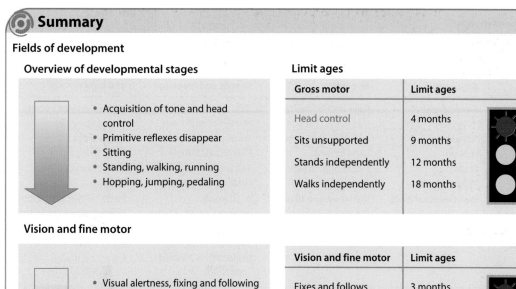

Pattern of child development

31

Summary

Developmental milestones by age median

Age	Gross motor	Vision and fine motor	Hearing and speech and language	Social, emotional and behavioural
Newborn	Flexed posture	Fixes and follows face	Stills to voice Startles to loud noise	Smiles – only at 6 weeks
7 months	Sits without support	Transfers objects from hand to hand	Turns to voice Polysyllabic babble	Finger feeds Fears strangers
1 year	Stands independently	Pincer grip 10 months Points	1–2 words Understands name	Drinks from cup Waves
18 months	Walks independently	Immature grip of pencil Random scribble	6–10 words Points to 4 body parts	Feeds himself with spoon Beginning to help with dressing
2½ years	Runs and jumps	Draws	3–4 word sentences Understands 2 joined commands	Parallel play Clean and dry

Analysing developmental progress

Detailed assessment

So far, emphasis has been mainly on thinking about developmental progress in a longitudinal way, taking each skill field and its progression individually, and then relating the progress in each to the others and to chronological age. This is the fundamental concept of learning how to think about developmental assessment of children. Detailed questioning and observation is required to assess children with developmental problems but is unnecessary when checking developmental progress in normal clinical practice, when a short cut approach can be adopted.

The short cut approach

This concentrates on the most actively changing skills for the child's age. The age at which developmental progress accelerates differs in each of the developmental fields. In Figure 3.8, this is represented diagrammatically for each developmental field by representing the rate of developmental change according the intensity of the colour; the more intense the colour, the more rapid the developmental change. This means there is for:

- gross motor development: an explosion of skills during the first year of life
- vision and fine motor development: more evident acquisition of skills from 1 year onwards
- hearing, speech and language: a big expansion of skills from 18 months
- social, emotional and behavioural development: expansion in skills is most obvious from 2.5 years.

Understanding the time when acceleration in each skill field becomes more obvious and knowing the child's age helps guide the direction of initial developmental questioning. Thus for a child aged:

- <18 months – it is likely to be most useful to begin questions around gross motor abilities, acquisition of vision and hearing skills, followed by questions about hand skills.
- 18 months to 2.5 years – initial developmental questioning is likely to be most usefully directed at acquisition of speech and language and fine motor (hand) skills with only later and brief questioning about gross motor skills (as it is likely the child would have presented earlier if these were of concern).
- 2.5 to 3.5 years – initial questions are best focused around speech and language and social/emotional/behavioural skills.

Developmental questioning needs to cover the whole area of developmental progression but this more focused way of taking a developmental history allows a quicker and more appropriate assessment. It directs the assessment to current abilities instead of concentrating on parents trying to remember the age when their child acquired developmental milestones some time in the past.

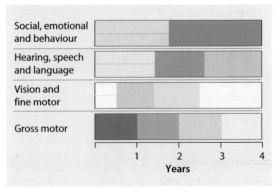
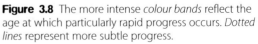

Figure 3.8 The more intense *colour bands* reflect the age at which particularly rapid progress occurs. *Dotted lines* represent more subtle progress.

Observation during questioning

Of equal importance to taking the developmental history is the examiner's ability to observe the child throughout any visit. Not only will this provide an almost immediate guide to where to begin questioning, it will offer the opportunity for a rapid overview of the child's abilities, behaviour, peer group and parent–child relationships, all of which will go towards determining the overall picture about the child and his developmental abilities.

Equipment for developmental testing

Simple basic equipment is all that is needed for most developmental assessment. Equipment is aimed at bringing out the child's skills using play. Cubes, a ball, picture book, doll and miniature toys such as a tea-set, crayons and paper will allow a quick, but useful screen of mobility, hand skills, play, speech and language. These items allow the child to relax by having fun at the same time as facilitating observer assessment of his skills.

Developmental screening and assessment

Developmental screening (checks of whole populations of children at set ages by trained professionals) is a formal process within the child health surveillance and promotion programme. It is also an essential role of all health professionals to screen a young child's developmental progress opportunistically at every health contact, e.g. by the general practitioner for a sore throat, in the accident and emergency department for a fall or on admission to a paediatric ward. In this way, every child contact is optimised to check that development is progressing normally.

There are a number of problems inherent in developmental screening:

- It is based on clinical opinion, which is subjective and therefore has its limitations.
- A single observation of development may be limited by the child being tired, hungry, shy or simply not wishing to take part.
- Whilst much of the focus of early development and progress in infants is centred on motor development, this is a poor predictor of problems in cognitive function and later school performance. Development of speech and language is a better predictor of cognitive function but is less easy to assess rapidly.

The reliability of screening tests can be improved by adding a questionnaire completed by parents beforehand. Increasingly, screening is being targeted towards children at high risk or when there are parental concerns. If an abnormal pattern of development has been identified, the child should be referred to a therapist for an early intervention programme.

Summary

Pattern of child development
When analysing a young child's developmental progress:
- consider the child's age and then concentrate your questions on the areas of likely maximum developmental progress
- offer the child suitable toys to find out about his skills
- observe how the child uses the toys and interacts with people.

Developmental assessment is the detailed analysis of a particular area of development and follows concern after screening that a child's developmental progress is abnormal in some way. It is part of the diagnostic process and relates to investigation, therapy and counselling. Developmental assessment is by referral to a specialist service and this may be the developmental paediatrician, therapy disciplines, or the local multidisciplinary child development service, which will include a paediatrician.

A range of tests have been developed to screen development in a formal reproducible manner (e.g. the Schedule of Growing Skills and the Denver Developmental Screening Test). There are also standardised tests to assess the development of infants and young children, such as the Griffiths and the Bailey Infant Development Scales. They are used, for example, in follow-up studies of preterm infants. There are also standardised tests concentrating on specific aspects of development (e.g. the Reynell language scale, the Gross Motor Function Measure (GMFM) and the Autism Diagnostic Interview). All but the screening tests are time-consuming and require training for reliable results.

Cognitive (higher mental function) assessment of school-age children using IQ and other tests is carried out by clinical or educational psychologists.

Summary

Developmental screening and assessment
- *Developmental screening* – checks of whole populations or groups of children at set ages by trained professionals.
- *Developmental assessment* – detailed analysis of overall development or specific areas of development.

Child health surveillance and promotion programme

The programme of child health surveillance and promotion provides an overview of all aspects of health and development for all young children. The programme has three main elements:

- immunisation
- health promotion – to minimise hazards and promote optimum physical and mental health
- screening for the early detection and intervention of physical and developmental problems.

The programme is a compromise between the desire to detect problems and potentially intervene early whilst avoiding an excessive number of visits. The way it is organised in the UK is shown in Table 3.2. At each review, a check is made for specific physical abnormalities and on the child's overall development, health and growth. Selected health promotion topics are considered (Table 3.2). There is an emphasis on parental opinion for vision, hearing, speech and language, as parents are usually excellent at the early detection of any problems. Details of each review are entered in the child's personal child health record. These books are kept by the parents and they are asked to bring them whenever the child is seen by a health professional.

The child health promotion programme is carried out in primary care by general practitioners or health visitors. If problems are identified, an action plan is made for the child, which could involve giving advice and monitoring progress or referral to a specialist.

> ⊙ **SUMMARY**
>
> **The child health surveillance and promotion programme:**
> - is provided in primary care
> - includes immunisation, health promotion and developmental screening
> - emphasises the role of parents in the early detection of developmental problems.

Hearing

During the later stages of pregnancy, the fetus responds to sound. At birth, a baby startles to sound, but there is a marked preference for voices. The ability to locate and turn towards sounds comes later in the first year. A checklist for parents of normal hearing responses during infancy is shown in Box 3.1.

Box 3.1 Hearing checklist for parents (used with permission from Dr Barry McCormick, Children's Hearing Assessment Centre, Nottingham)

Shortly after birth	Startles and blinks at a sudden noise, e.g. slamming of door
By 1 month	Notices sudden prolonged sounds, e.g. a vacuum cleaner, and pauses and listens when they begin
By 4 months	Quietens or smiles to the sound of your voice even when he cannot see you. He may also turn his head or eyes towards you if you come up from behind and speak to him from the side
By 7 months	Turns immediately to your voice across the room or to very quiet noises made on each side, so long as he is not too occupied with other things
By 9 months	Listens attentively to familiar everyday sounds and searches for very quiet sounds made out of sight. Should also show pleasure in babbling loudly and tunefully
By 12 months	Shows some response to his own name and to other familiar words. May respond when you say 'no' and 'bye-bye' even when he cannot see any accompanying gesture

If you suspect that your baby is not hearing normally, seek advice from your health visitor or doctor.

Hearing tests

Newborn

Early detection and treatment of hearing impairment improves the outcome for speech and language and behaviour. In order to detect hearing impairment in the newborn period, hearing can be tested by:

- evoked otoacoustic emission (EOAE) (Fig. 3.9a) – an earpiece is inserted into the ear canal and produces a sound which evokes an echo or emission from the ear if cochlear function is normal.
- auditory brainstem response (ABR) audiometry (Fig. 3.9b) – computer analysis of EEG waveforms evoked in response to a series of clicks.

Universal neonatal hearing screening has been introduced in the UK and other countries. In the UK, initial screening is performed using different

Table 3.2 The child health surveillance and promotion programme in the UK

Age (by whom)	Screening	General examination and immunisation	Health promotion
Newborn Usually hospital doctor; may be trained midwife, neonatal nurse practitioner or GP	Developmental dysplasia of the hips (DDH) Testicular descent in boys Red reflex of fundus Hearing screening	Full physical examination Weight, head circumference and plot centiles BCG offered if at risk Hepatitis B vaccine, if indicated, (and repeat at 1, 2, 12 months)	Feeding and nutrition Back to sleep, avoid overheating and parental smoking to reduce risk of sudden infant death syndrome Sibling management Car seats
5–6 days Midwife	Blood test for biochemical screening (Guthrie test)		
New birth visit Home visit by midwife or health visitor usually around 12 days	Assess child and family health needs, including parental mental health needs		Distributes 'Birth to Five' guide and personal child health record, if not already provided
8 weeks General practitioner	Heart murmurs and femoral pulses Development dysplasia of the hips (DDH) Testicular descent in boys Red reflex of fundus	Full physical examination Weight, head circumference and plot centiles Vision/hearing – parental concern? First immunisation – diphtheria, tetanus, pertussis, polio (DTaP/IPV), Hib, pneumococcal (PCV)	Nutrition Immunisation Recognition of illness Avoid passive smoking Crying and sleep problems
3 months Child health clinic	General review of progress	Second immunisation – DTaP/IPV/Hib, MenC	Weaning
4 months Child health clinic	General review of progress	Third immunisation – DTaP/IPV/Hib, PCV MenC	
8 months Health visiting team	Systematic assessment of the child's physical, emotional and social development and family needs	If parental concern – hearing, vision, development	Accident prevention – choking, scalds and burns, safety gates, car seats Nutrition and dental care Avoid sunburn
12 months		Immunisation – Hib, MenC	Weaning
13 months Child health clinic	General review of progress	Immunisation – MMR (measles, mumps and rubella), PCV	
2–3 years Health visiting team, if indicated	General review of progress	Parental concerns – behaviour, hearing, vision and general development	Accident prevention Behaviour problems Toilet training
4–5 years (preschool) Orthoptist		Assessment of vision	
4–5 years Child health clinic	General review of progress	Immunisation – MMR, diphtheria, tetanus, pertussis, polio (DTaP/IPV)	
5 years – school entry School nurse	Vision (phased out if already tested) Hearing (audiometry)	Measure height and weight, plot centiles Examination – only if problem identified or parental concern	Check immunisations up-to-date
Primary and secondary schools School nurse	Access at open sessions or clinics by a child, parents or teachers	Nursing care provided according to needs	
Secondary school School nurse		Immunisation (13–16 years) – diphtheria, tetanus, polio (Td/IPV)	

Adapted from Hall D B M and Elliman D, *Health for All Children*, Oxford University Press, Oxford, 2003, and Key Issues for Primary Care, National Service Framework for Children, Young People and Maternity Services, Department Of Health, 2004.

Hearing

Hearing screening of newborn infants

a Evoked otoacoustic emissions (EOAE)

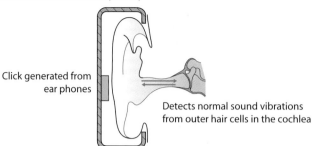

Click generated from ear phones

Detects normal sound vibrations from outer hair cells in the cochlea

Advantages:
- Simple and quick to perform, though is affected by ambient noise

Disadvantages:
- Misses auditory neuropathy as function of auditory nerve or brain not tested
- Relatively high false positive rate in first 24 hours after birth as vernix or amniotic fluid are still in ear canal
- Not a test of hearing but a test of cochlear function

b Automated auditory brainstem response (AABR)

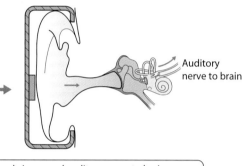

Auditory nerve to brain

Auditory stimulus – short duration clicks at different intensities via earphones

Signal via ear and auditory nerve to brain

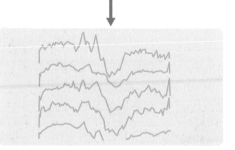

EEG waveforms – computerised analysis determines if normal or abnormal

Advantages:
- Screens entire hearing pathway from ear to brainstem
- Low false positive rate

Disadvantages:
- Affected by movement, so infants need to be asleep or very quiet, so time consuming
- Complex computerised equipment, but is mobile
- Requires electrodes applied to infant's head, which parents may dislike

Figure 3.9 Universal neonatal hearing screening is usually performed using **(a)** otoacoustic emission testing or **(b)** auditory brainstem response audiometry.

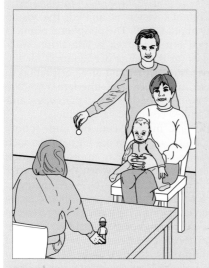

Figure 3.10 Distraction hearing test. The test is hard to perform reliably as babies with hearing difficulties learn to compensate by using shadows, smells and guesswork to locate the presenter. The test must be done by well-trained professionals.

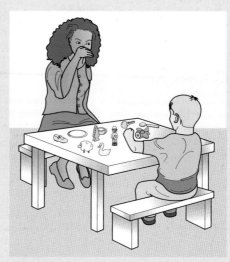

Figure 3.12 Speech discrimination testing using miniature toys to detect hearing loss in children between 18 months and 4 years of age.

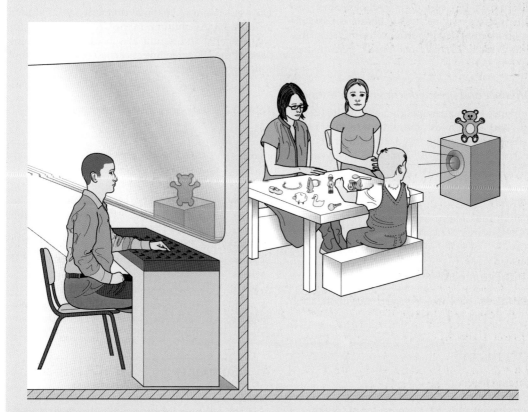

Figure 3.11 Visual reinforcement audiometry. While an assistant plays with the child, sounds of a specific frequency are emitted from a speaker. When the child turns to it, the tester lights up a toy by the speaker to reinforce the sound with a visual reward. This test is particularly useful at 10–18 months.

combinations of evoked otoacoustic emission (EOAE) testing or auditory brainstem response (ABR) audiometry. If a normal response cannot be obtained, the child is referred to an audiologist.

Distraction testing

This has been the mainstay of hearing screening but has been replaced by universal neonatal screening. It is now only used as a screening test for infants who have not had newborn screening, or as a diagnostic test. It is performed at 7–9 months of age (Fig. 3.10). The test relies on the baby locating and turning appropriately towards sounds. High and low frequency sounds are presented out of the infant's field of vision. Testing is unreliable if not carried out by properly trained staff since it can be difficult to identify hearing-impaired infants as they are particularly adept at using non-auditory cues.

Visual reinforcement audiometry

This is particularly useful to assess impairment in infants between 10 and 18 months, although it can be used between the age of 6 months and 3 years. Hearing thresholds are established using visual rewards (illumination of toys) to reinforce the child's head turn to stimuli of different frequencies. Localisation of the stimuli is not necessary and insert earphones may be used to obtain ear specific information, thus making it more useful than free field tests such as distraction and performance testing (Fig. 3.11).

Performance and speech discrimination testing

Performance testing using high- and low-frequency stimuli and speech discrimination testing using miniature toys can be used for children with suspected hearing loss at 18 months to 4 years of age (Fig. 3.12).

Audiometry

Threshold audiometry can be used to detect and assess the severity of hearing loss in children from 4 years old.

Parental concern

At all ages, parental concern about hearing warrants further assessment.

⊚ Summary

Regarding hearing:
- Early detection and treatment of hearing impairment improves the outcome of speech and language and behaviour.
- Newborn hearing screening is performed for the early identification of hearing impairment.
- If there is parental concern about hearing, further assessment is warranted.

Vision

A newborn infant's vision is limited; the visual acuity is only about 6/200. The peripheral retina is well developed but the fovea is immature. Well-focused images on the retina are required for the acquisition of visual acuity and any obstruction to this, e.g. from a cataract, will interfere with the normal development of the optic pathways and visual cortex unless corrected early in life.

Most newborn infants can fix and follow horizontally. There is a preference for patterns such as faces. Initially the eyes may appear to squint; this is particularly noticeable when the baby tries to look at near objects and the eyes over-converge.

By about 6 weeks of age, both eyes should move together when following a light source. By 12 weeks no squint should be present. Babies slowly develop the ability to focus at different distances. Visual acuity also improves: from 6/60 at 3 months to being able to poke at 1 cm objects at 8 months and at 1 mm objects (e.g. hundreds and thousands) at 15 months. Adult levels are reached by 3–4 years of age, when they can match letters at 6/6 using both eyes together.

Vision testing

The assessment of vision at different ages is shown in Table 3.3. All children in the UK are screened for visual acuity and squint at school entry. In some parts of the UK screening is carried out in preschool children at 4–5 years.

Table 3.3 Testing vision at different ages

Age	Test
Birth	Face fixation and following Preferential looking – preference for patterned objects to plain ones
6 weeks	Optokinetic nystagmus (normal) demonstrated on looking at a moving, striped target
6 months	Reaches well for toys
2 years	Can identify pictures of reducing size
3 years onwards	Letter matching using single letter charts (log MAR)
5 years onwards	Can identify a line of letters on a log MAR or Snellen chart by name or matching

⊚ Summary

Vision
- Term newborn infants can fix and follow horizontally and prefer to watch faces.
- Visual acuity is poor in the newborn but increases to adult levels by 3 years of age.
- Vision screening is performed in preschool children or at school entry.

4

Developmental problems and the child with special needs

Any child whose development is delayed or disordered needs assessment to determine the cause and management. Neurodevelopmental problems present at all ages, with an increasing number now recognised antenatally (Table 4.1). Many are identified in the neonatal period because of abnormal neurology or dysmorphic features. During infancy and early childhood, problems often present at an age when a specific area of development is most rapid and prominent, i.e. motor problems during the first 18 months of age, speech and language problems between 18 months and 3 years and social and communication disorders between 2 and 4 years. Abnormal development may be caused not only by neurodevelopmental problems but also by ill health or if the child's physical or psychological needs are not met.

When performing a clinical examination on a young child with a developmental problem:

- Ask the parent what their child can and cannot do.

- *Observe* the child from the first moment seen.
- Make it fun. Your examination should be perceived as a game by the child although he may not always follow your rules.
- Toys to use are cubes, a ball, car, doll, pencil, paper, pegboard, miniature toys, picture book, adapting their use to the child.
- Formulate a developmental picture in terms of gross motor; vision and fine motor; hearing, speech and language; and social, emotional and behaviour. You will be screening all of these skills simultaneously.
- At the end of developmental screening you should be able to describe what a child is able to do and what the child cannot do, if his abilities are within normal limits for their age and, if not, which developmental fields are outside the normal range.
- Clinical signs to look for that may aid diagnosis or guide investigation are:
  - patterns of growth – height, weight, head circumference with centile plotting

Table 4.1 Presentation of neurodevelopmental concerns by age

Prenatal	Positive family history, e.g. affected siblings or family members; ethnicity, e.g. Tay–Sachs disease in Jewish parents Antenatal screening tests, e.g. ultrasound for spina bifida or hydrocephalus, amniocentesis for Down's syndrome
Perinatal	Following birth asphyxia/neonatal encephalopathy Preterm infants with intraventricular haemorrhage/periventricular leucomalacia, post haemorrhagic hydrocephalus Dysmorphic features Abnormal neurological behaviour – tone, feeding, movement, seizures, visual inattention
Infancy	Global developmental delay Delayed or asymmetric motor development Visual or auditory concerns by parent or after screening Neurocutaneous/dysmorphic features
Preschool	Speech and language delay Abnormal gait Loss of skills
School age	Problems with balance and coordination Learning difficulties Attention control Hyperactivity Specific learning difficulties, e.g. dyslexia, dyspraxia
Any age	Acquired brain injury, e.g. after meningitis, head injury

- dysmorphic features – face, limbs, body proportions, cardiac, genitalia
- skin – neurocutaneous stigmata, injuries, cleanliness nutrition
- central nervous system examination – wasting, abnormal posture/symmetry, power tone, deep tendon reflexes, clonus, plantar responses, sensory examination, cranial nerves
- cardiovascular examination – abnormalities are associated with many dysmorphic syndromes
- visual function and ocular abnormalities
- hearing – by questioning parents about hearing and language development and checking if neonatal hearing screening was done
- patterns of mobility, dexterity, communication and social skills, general behaviour
- cognition.

Many examination findings can be predicted from *observation* of functional skills.

The choice of investigations is influenced by the child's age, the history and clinical findings (Table 4.2). In some children no cause can be identified even after extensive investigation.

Many parental concerns about their child's development are found to be variations of normal, in which case the parents should be reassured. If in doubt, observe the child's progress over a period of time.

Abnormal development – key concepts

The terminology can be can be confusing, but:

- *Delay* – implies slow acquisition of all skills (global delay) or of one particular field or area of skill (specific delay), particularly in relation to developmental problems in the 0–5 years age group.
- *Learning difficulty* – used in relation to children of school age and may be cognitive, physical or both (complex).
- *Disorder* – maldevelopment of a skill.

The following are agreed definitions:

- *Impairment* – loss or abnormality of physiological function or anatomical structure.
- *Disability* – any restriction or lack of ability due to the impairment.
- *Handicap* – a disadvantage from a disability which limits or prevents fulfilment of a normal role.

The term handicap is now discouraged as it can imply a person deserves pity. Difficulty and disability are often used interchangeably, but difficulty is used particularly in an educational context.

The *pattern* of abnormal development (global or specific) can be categorised as (Fig. 4.1):

- slow but steady
- plateau effect
- showing regression.

The *severity* can be categorised as:

- mild
- moderate
- severe
- profound.

Other features of developmental delay are:

- the gap between normal and abnormal development becomes greater with increasing age

Table 4.2 Investigations or assessment to consider for abnormal development

Cytogenetic	*Chromosome karyotype *Fragile X analysis DNA FISH analysis, e.g. for chromosome 7, 15, 22 deletions
Metabolic	*Thyroid function tests, liver function tests, bone chemistry, urea and electrolytes, plasma amino acids Creatine kinase, blood lactate, VLCFA (very long chain fatty acids), ammonia, blood gases, white cell (lysosomal) enzymes, urine amino and organic acids, urine mucopolysaccharides (GAG) and oligosaccharide screen, urine reducing substances Maternal amino acids for raised phenylalanine
Infection	Congenital infection screen
Imaging	Cranial ultrasound in newborn CT and MRI brain scans Skeletal survey
Neurophysiology	EEG (may be specific for seizures, some progressive neurological disorders) Nerve conduction studies, EMG, VEP (visual evoked potentials), ERG (electroretinogram)
Histopathology/histochemistry	Nerve and muscle biopsy
Other	*Hearing *Vision Clinical genetics Cognitive assessment Therapy assessment Child psychiatry Nursery/school reports

Basic screening tests are marked with an asterisk*.

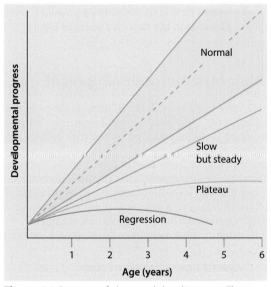

Figure 4.1 Patterns of abnormal development. These may be slow but steady, plateau or regression.

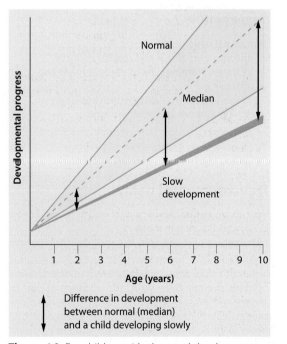

Difference in development between normal (median) and a child developing slowly

Figure 4.2 For children with abnormal development, the gap between their abilities and what is normal widens with age.

and therefore becomes more apparent over time (Fig. 4.2)

- it may be the presentation of a wide variety of underlying conditions (Table 4.3).
- the site and severity of brain damage influences the clinical outcome, i.e. whether there is specific or global developmental delay, learning and/or physical disability

- it may be genetic, with important implications for the family
- there is a wide age band across which it can be normal to achieve a developmental skill. Limit ages denote beyond normal range.

Table 4.3 Conditions which cause developmental delay and learning difficulty. The site and severity of brain damage influences the clinical outcome, i.e. whether specific or global developmental delay, learning and/or physical disability

Prenatal

Genetic	Chromosome/DNA disorders, e.g. Down's syndrome, fragile X syndrome
	Cerebral dysgenesis, e.g. microcephaly, absent corpus callosum, hydrocephalus, neuronal migration disorder, vascular occlusion
Metabolic	Hypothyroidism, phenylketonuria
Teratogenic	Alcohol and drug abuse
Congenital infection	Rubella, cytomegalovirus, toxoplasmosis
Neurocutaneous syndromes	Tuberous sclerosis, neurofibromatosis

Perinatal

Extreme prematurity	Intraventricular haemorrhage/periventricular leucomalacia
Birth asphyxia	Hypoxic-ischaemic encephalopathy
Metabolic	Symptomatic hypoglycaemia, hyperbilirubinaemia

Postnatal

Infection	Meningitis, encephalitis
Anoxia	Suffocation, near drowning, seizures
Trauma	Head injury – accidental or non-accidental
Metabolic	Hypoglycaemia, inborn errors of metabolism

Other

Unknown (about 25%)

Summary

Abnormal development:

- incorporates global and specific delay or disorder, learning difficulty, impairment and disability.
- varies in pattern of progression and severity
- becomes more apparent with age.

Developmental delay

Global developmental delay implies delay in acquisition of all skill fields (gross motor, vision and fine motor, hearing and speech/language, social/emotional and behaviour). It usually becomes apparent in the first 2 years of life. However, some children present later with, for instance, delay in speech and language but review of their developmental history may reveal delayed gross and fine motor skills (but insufficient at the time to generate referral), and a diagnostic label of global developmental delay may then be more appropriate than specific language delay. Global developmental delay is likely to be associated with cognitive difficulties although these may only become apparent several years later. Causes of global developmental delay are listed in Table 4.3.

Specific developmental delay is when one field of development or skill area is more delayed than others or is developing in a disordered way.

Global developmental delay usually presents in the first two years of life.

Abnormal motor development

This may present as delay in acquisition of motor milestones, e.g. head control, rolling, sitting, standing, walking or as problems with balance, an abnormal gait, asymmetry of hand use, involuntary movements or rarely loss of motor skills. Concern about motor development usually presents between 6 months and 2 years of age when acquisition of motor skills is occurring most rapidly. Examination may reveal underlying abnormal motor signs.

Causes of abnormal motor development include:

- cerebral palsy
- congenital myopathy/primary muscle disease
- spinal cord lesions, e.g. spina bifida
- global developmental delay as in many syndromes or of unidentified cause.

As hand dominance is not acquired until 1–2 years or later, asymmetry of motor skills during the first year of life is always abnormal and may suggest an underlying hemiplegia.

Late walking (>18 months old) may be caused by any of the above but also needs to be differentiated from children who display the locomotor variants of bottom-shuffling or commando crawling (see Ch. 3) and needs to be differentiated from organic causes such as cerebral palsy.

Concern about abnormal motor development needs assessment by a neurodevelopmental paediatrician and physiotherapist. Ongoing physiotherapy input and subsequent involvement of an occupational therapist is likely to be needed.

Cerebral palsy

Cerebral palsy is a disorder of movement and posture due to a non-progressive lesion of motor pathways in the developing brain. Although the lesion is non-progressive, the clinical manifestations emerge over time, reflecting the balance between normal and abnormal cerebral maturation. Cerebral palsy is the most common cause of motor impairment in children, affecting about 2 per 1000 live births. In addition to disorders of movement and posture, children with cerebral palsy often have other problems reflecting more widespread brain dysfunction. These include:

- learning difficulties (about 60%)
- epilepsy (40%)
- squints (30%)
- visual impairment from errors of refraction and cortical damage (20%)
- hearing impairment (20%)
- speech and language disorders (due to hearing loss, oro-motor incoordination and learning difficulties)
- behaviour disorders
- feeding problems
- joint contractures, hip subluxation, scoliosis.

Causes

About 80% of cerebral palsy is antenatal in origin due to vascular occlusion, cortical migration disorders or structural maldevelopment of the brain during gestation. Some of these problems are linked to gene deletions. Other antenatal causes are genetic syndromes and congenital infection.

Only about 10% of cases are thought to be due to hypoxic-ischaemic injury at birth and this proportion has remained relatively constant over the last decade.

About 10% are postnatal in origin. Preterm infants are especially vulnerable to brain damage from periventricular leucomalacia (PVL) secondary to ischaemia and/or severe intraventricular haemorrhage. The rise in survival of extremely preterm infants has been accompanied by an increase in survivors with cerebral palsy, although the number of such children is relatively small. Other postnatal causes are meningitis/encephalitis/encephalopathy, head trauma from accidental or non-accidental injury, symptomatic hypoglycaemia, hydrocephalus and hyperbilirubinaemia.

MRI brain scans may assist in identifying the cause of the cerebral palsy. Haematological problems due to thrombophilia or clotting disorders should be excluded in neonatal stroke.

Clinical presentation

Many children who develop cerebral palsy will have been identified as being at risk in the neonatal period. Early features of cerebral palsy are:

- abnormal limb tone and limb and/or trunk posture in infancy with delayed motor milestones (Fig. 4.3); may be accompanied by slowing of head growth
- feeding difficulties, with oromotor incoordination, slow feeding, gagging and vomiting
- abnormal gait once walking is achieved
- asymmetric hand function before 12 months of age.

In cerebral palsy, primitive reflexes, which facilitate the emergence of normal patterns of movement and which need to disappear for motor development to progress, may persist and become obligatory (see Ch. 3).

The diagnosis is made by clinical examination, with particular attention to assessment of the pattern of tone in the limbs and trunk, posture, hand function and gait. There are three main clinical types of cerebral palsy, each reflecting dysfunction of a specific motor pathway, namely spastic (70%), ataxic hypotonic (10%), dyskinetic (10%). There may also be a mixed pattern (10%).

Spastic cerebral palsy

In this type, there is damage to the upper motor neuron (pyramidal or corticospinal tract) pathway. Limb tone is increased (spasticity) with associated brisk deep tendon reflexes and extensor plantar responses. The increased limb tone may suddenly yield under pressure in a 'clasp knife' fashion. Spasticity tends to present early and may even be seen in the neonatal period. Sometimes there is initial hypotonia, particularly of the head and trunk. There are three main types of spastic cerebral palsy:

- *Hemiplegia* – unilateral involvement of the arm and leg (Fig. 4.4). The arm is usually affected more than the leg, with the face spared. Affected children often present at 4–12 months of age with fisting of the affected hand, a flexed arm, a pronated forearm, asymmetric reaching or hand function. Subsequently a tiptoe walk (toe–heel gait) on the affected side may become evident. Affected limbs may initially be flaccid and hypotonic, but increased tone soon emerges as the predominant sign. The past medical history is usually normal, with an unremarkable birth history with no evidence of hypoxic-ischaemic encephalopathy. However, in some the condition is caused by a neonatal stroke.
- *Quadriplegia* – all four limbs are affected, often severely. The arms may be affected more than the legs. The trunk is involved with extensor posturing and poor head control and low central tone (Fig. 4.5). This form of cerebral palsy is often associated with seizures, microcephaly and moderate or severe intellectual impairment. There may have been a history of hypoxic-ischaemic encephalopathy after birth.
- *Diplegia* – all four limbs, but the legs are affected to a much greater degree than the arms, so that hand function may appear to be relatively normal. It is with functional use of the hands that motor difficulties in the arms are most apparent. Walking is abnormal.

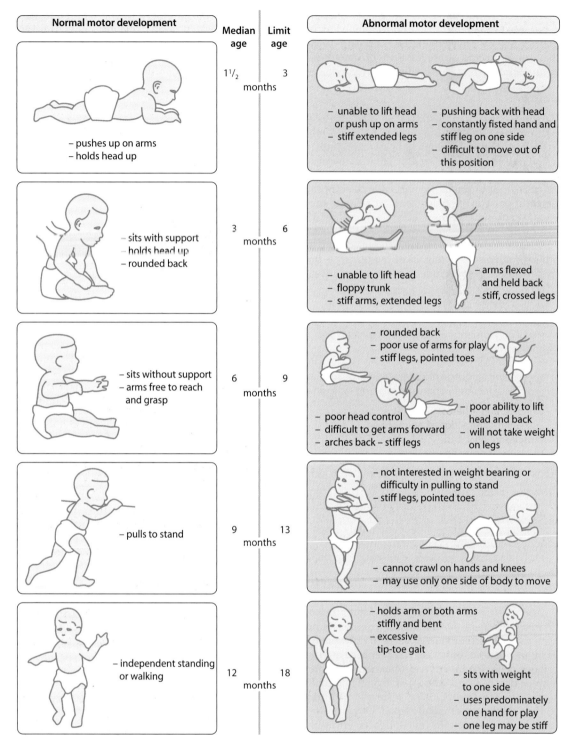

Normal motor development	Median age	Limit age	Abnormal motor development
– pushes up on arms – holds head up	1½ months	3	– unable to lift head or push up on arms – stiff extended legs	– pushing back with head – constantly fisted hand and stiff leg on one side – difficult to move out of this position
– sits with support – holds head up – rounded back	3 months	6	– unable to lift head – floppy trunk – stiff arms, extended legs	– arms flexed and held back – stiff, crossed legs
– sits without support – arms free to reach and grasp	6 months	9	– rounded back – poor use of arms for play – stiff legs, pointed toes – poor head control – difficult to get arms forward – arches back – stiff legs	– poor ability to lift head and back – will not take weight on legs
– pulls to stand	9 months	13	– not interested in weight bearing or difficulty in pulling to stand – stiff legs, pointed toes – cannot crawl on hands and knees – may use only one side of body to move	
– independent standing or walking	12 months	18	– holds arm or both arms stiffly and bent – excessive tip-toe gait – sits with weight to one side – uses predominately one hand for play – one leg may be stiff	

Figure 4.3 Normal motor milestones and patterns of abnormal motor development. Cerebral palsy (hemiplegia or quadriplegia) is the commonest cause of the developmental problems shown. (Adapted from Pathways Awareness Foundation, 123 North Wacker Drive, Chicago, IL. Tel. (+1) 800-326-8154, Internet: www.pathwaysawareness.org.)

Ataxic hypotonic cerebral palsy

Signs are relatively symmetrical. There is early trunk and limb hypotonia, poor balance and delayed motor development. Incoordinate movements, intention tremor and an ataxic gait may be evident later, reflecting dysfunction in the cerebellum or its connections.

Dyskinetic cerebral palsy

There is dyskinesia (fluctuating tone) leading to frequent involuntary movements (generally of all four limbs) especially evident with movement or stress. These involuntary movements may be:

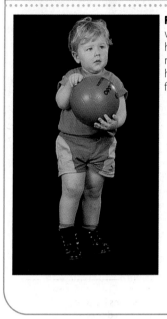

Figure 4.4 A child with a right spastic hemiplegia. His right arm is hyperpronated, flexed, hand fisted.

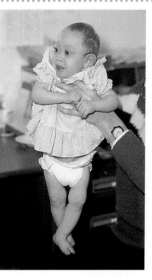

Figure 4.5 A child with spastic quadriplegia showing scissoring of the legs from excessive adduction of the hips, pronated forearms and 'fisted' hands.

- chorea – irregular, sudden and brief non-repetitive movements
- dystonia and athetosis – simultaneous and sustained contraction of agonist and antagonist muscles involving the trunk or proximal limbs (dystonia) or distal parts of the limb (athetosis).

Intellect may be relatively unimpaired. Affected children often present with floppiness, poor trunk control and delayed motor development in infancy, with abnormal movements sometimes not appearing before 1 year of age. The signs are due to damage to the basal ganglia or their associated pathways (extrapyramidal). In the past, hyperbilirubinaemia due to rhesus disease of the newborn was a common cause.

Management

Parents should be given details of the diagnosis as early as possible, but prognosis is difficult during infancy until the severity and pattern of evolving signs and the child's developmental progress have become clearer over several months or years of life. Children with cerebral palsy are likely to have a wide range of associated medical, psychological and social problems, making it essential to adopt a multidisciplinary approach to assessment and management, as described later in this chapter.

Abnormal speech and language development

A child may have a deficit in either receptive or expressive speech and language, or both. The deficit may be a delay or a disorder.

Speech and language *delay* may be due to

- hearing loss
- global developmental delay
- difficulty in speech production from an anatomical deficit, e.g. cleft palate, or oromotor incoordination, e.g. cerebral palsy
- environmental deprivation/lack of opportunity for social interaction
- normal variant/familial pattern.

Speech and language *disorders* include disorders of:

- language comprehension (receptive dysphasia) – inability or difficulty in comprehending speech and language
- language expression (expressive dysphasia) – inability or difficulty in producing speech whilst knowing what is needing to be said
- phonation and speech production such as stammering (dysfluency), dysarthria or verbal dyspraxia
- pragmatics, (difference between sentence meaning and speaker's meaning) construction of sentences, semantics, grammar
- social/communication skills (autistic spectrum disorder).

Summary

Cerebral palsy:
- has many causes. Only about 10% follow hypoxic-ischaemic encephalopathy
- usually presents in infancy with abnormal tone and posture, delayed motor milestones and feeding difficulties
- may be spastic, ataxic hypotonic, dyskinetic or mixed pattern.

Speech and language problems are usually first suspected by parents or primary healthcare professionals. A hearing test and assessment by a speech and language therapist are the initial steps. In early years there is considerable overlap between language and cognitive (intellectual) development. Involvement of a neurodevelopmental paediatrician and paediatric audiological physician is indicated. Speech and language therapy may be provided on a continuous, burst or review basis. Special schooling (usually language units attached to a mainstream primary school) are available but only appropriate for a very few. Many children with early speech and language problems will need learning support at school entry.

There are many tests of language development including:

- the Symbolic Toy test – assesses very early language development
- the Reynell test for receptive and expressive language – used for preschool children.

Abnormal development of social/communication skills (autistic spectrum disorder)

Children who fail to acquire normal social and communication skills may have an autistic spectrum disorder. The prevalence of autistic spectrum disorder is 3–6/1000 live births. It is more common in boys. Presentation is usually between 2 and 4 years of age when language and social skills normally rapidly expand. The children present with a triad of difficulties and associated co-morbidities (Box 4.1).

Where only some of the behaviours are present, the child is described as having autistic features but not the full spectrum.

Asperger's syndrome refers to a child with the social impairments of an autistic spectrum disorder but at the milder end, and near-normal speech development. Such children still have major difficulties with the give-and-take of ordinary social encounters, a stilted way of speaking and narrow, strange interests which they do not share with others, and are often clumsy. In reality autistic spectrum disorders are a continuum of behavioural states ranging from the severe form of autism with or without severe learning difficulties to the milder Asperger's syndrome to autistic features occurring secondary to other clinical problems. No cause has been identified; there is probably multiple aetiology with a genetic component in at least some. The condition is not the result of emotional trauma or deviant parenting. There is no evidence for a suggested link with the MMR vaccine.

Management

The condition has lifelong consequences of varying degree for the child's social/communication skills. Parents need a great deal of support. They often feel initial guilt that they did not recognise the problem earlier. A wide range of interventions have been

Box 4.1 Features of autistic spectrum disorders

Impaired social interaction:
- does not seek comfort, share pleasure, form close friendships
- prefers own company, no interest or ability in interacting with peers (play or emotions)
- gaze avoidance
- socially and emotionally inappropriate behaviour
- does not appreciate that others have thoughts and feelings
- lack of appreciation of social cues

Speech and language disorder:
- delayed development, may be severe
- limited use of gestures and facial expression
- formal pedantic language
- impaired comprehension with over-literal interpretation of speech
- echoes questions, repeats instructions, refers to self as 'you'
- superficially perfect expressive speech

Imposition of routines with ritualistic and repetitive behaviour:
- on self and others, with violent temper tantrums if disrupted
- unusual stereotypical movements such as hand flapping and tip toe gait
- poverty of imagination in play and general activities
- peculiar interests and repetitive adherence
- restriction in behaviour repertoire

Co-morbidities:
- general learning and attention difficulties (about two thirds)
- seizures (about one quarter, often not until adolescence)

promoted over the last ten years but with little evidence base except for applied behavioural analysis (ABA), a behaviour modification approach that helps to reduce ritualistic behaviour, develop language, social skills and play and to generalise use of all these skills. It is currently the most widely accepted treatment approach but requires 25–30 hours of individual therapy each week, so is costly and time-consuming. An appropriate educational placement needs to be sought; some schools incorporate an ABA approach. Less than 10% of children with autism are able to function independently as adults.

- **Autistic spectrum disorder:**
- **presents at 2–4 years with impaired social interaction, speech and language disorder and imposition of routines with ritualistic and repetitive behaviour**
- **is usually managed by behaviour modification using applied behavioural analysis (ABA).**

Table 4.4 Causes and management of hearing loss

	Sensorineural	Conductive
Causes	Genetic (the majority) Antenatal and perinatal: • Congenital infection • Preterm • Hypoxic-ischaemic encephalopathy • Hyperbilirubinaemia Postnatal: • Meningitis/encephalitis • Head injury • Drugs, e.g. aminoglycosides, furosemide (frusemide) • Neurodegenerative disorders	Otitis media with effusion (glue ear) Eustachian tube dysfunction: • Down's syndrome • Cleft palate • Pierre Robin sequence • Mid-facial hypoplasia Wax (only rarely a cause of hearing loss)
Hearing loss	May be profound (>95 dB hearing loss)	Maximum of 60 dB hearing loss
Natural history	Does not improve and may progress	Intermittent or resolves
Management	Amplification or cochlear implant if necessary	Conservative, amplification or surgery

Hearing impairment

Any concern about hearing impairment should be taken seriously. Any child with delayed language or speech, learning difficulties or behavioural problems should have their hearing tested, as a mild hearing loss may be the underlying cause without parents or other carers realising it. Hearing loss may be:

• sensorineural – caused by a lesion in the cochlea or auditory nerve and its central connections and usually present at birth
• conductive – from abnormalities of the ear canal or the middle ear, most often from otitis media with effusion.

The causes, natural history and management of hearing loss are listed in Table 4.4. Hearing tests are described in Chapter 3. The typical audiogram in sensorineural and conductive hearing loss is shown in Figure 4.6.

Sensorineural hearing loss

This type of hearing loss is uncommon (1 in 1000 of all live births; 1 in 100 in extremely low birthweight infants). It is usually present at birth or develops in the first few months of life. It is irreversible and can be of any severity, including profound.

The child with severe bilateral sensorineural hearing impairment will need early amplification with hearing aids for optimal speech and language development. Hearing aid use requires close supervision, beginning in the home together with the parents and continuing into school. Children often resist wearing hearing aids because background noise can be amplified unpleasantly. Cochlear implants may be required where hearing aids give insufficient amplification.

Many children with moderate hearing impairment can be educated within the mainstream school system or in partial hearing units attached to mainstream schools. Children with hearing impairment should be placed in the front of the classroom so that they can readily see the teacher. Gesture, visual context and lip movement will also allow children to develop language concepts. Speech may be delayed, but with appropriate therapy can be of good quality. Modified and simplified signing such as Makaton can be helpful for children who are both hearing-impaired and learning-disabled. Specialist teaching and support in preschool and school years is provided by peripatetic teachers for children with hearing impairment. Those with profound hearing impairment may need to attend a school for children who are deaf.

Conductive hearing loss

Conductive hearing loss from middle ear disease is usually mild or moderate but may be severe. It is much more common than sensorineural hearing loss. In association with upper respiratory tract infections, many children have episodes of hearing loss which are usually self-limiting. In some cases of chronic otitis media with effusion, the hearing loss may last many months or years. In most affected children there are no identifiable risk factors present but children with Down's syndrome, cleft palate and atopy are particularly prone to hearing loss from middle ear disease.

Impedance audiometry tests, which measure the air pressure within the middle ear and the compliance of the tympanic membrane, determine if the middle ear is functioning normally. If the condition does not improve spontaneously, medical treatment (decongestant or a long course of antibiotics or treatment of nasal allergy) can be given. If that fails, surgery is considered, with insertion of tympanostomy tubes (grommets) with or without the removal of adenoids. Hearing aids are used in cases where problems recur after surgery.

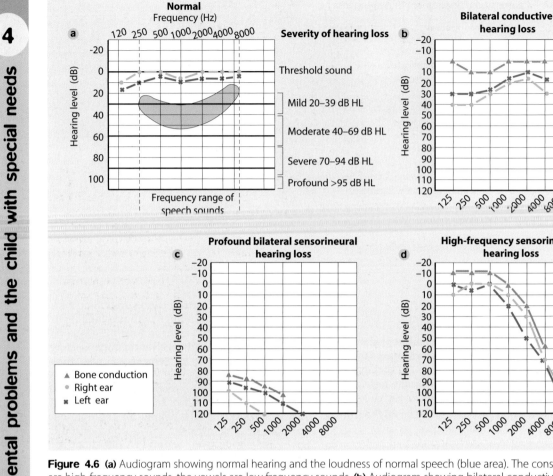

Figure 4.6 **(a)** Audiogram showing normal hearing and the loudness of normal speech (blue area). The consonants are high-frequency sounds, the vowels are low frequency sounds. **(b)** Audiogram showing bilateral conductive hearing loss. There is a 30–40 dB hearing loss in both the right and left ears. **(c)** Audiogram showing bilateral profound sensorineural hearing loss. **(d)** Audiogram showing bilateral high-frequency sensorineural hearing loss.

The decision whether to intervene surgically should be based on the degree of functional disability rather than on absolute hearing loss.

> Any child with poor or delayed speech or language must have their hearing assessed.

Summary

Hearing loss
Sensorineural hearing loss:
- is usually present at birth and is irreversible
- for severe hearing impairment, early amplification with hearing aids or cochlear implants is needed for optimal speech and language development
- assistance from peripatetic teachers for children with hearing impairment may be required.

Conductive hearing loss:
- is usually due to middle ear disease, often otitis media with effusion
- is usually mild or moderate and transient
- if it does not resolve, insertion of tympanostomy tubes (grommets) with or without the removal of adenoids will need to be considered.

Abnormalities of vision

Normal visual development and tests of vision are described in Chapter 3.

Visual impairment may present in infancy with:

- loss of red reflex from a cataract
- a white reflex in the pupil, which may be due to retinoblastoma, cataract or retinopathy of prematurity (ROP).
- not smiling responsively by 6 weeks post-term
- lack of eye contact with parents
- visual inattention
- random eye movements
- nystagmus
- squint
- photophobia

Box 4.2 Causes of visual impairment

Genetic	**Antenatal and perinatal**	**Postnatal**
Cataract	Congenital infection	Trauma
Albinism	Retinopathy of prematurity	Infection
Retinal dystrophy	Hypoxic-ischaemic encephalopathy	Juvenile idiopathic arthritis
Retinoblastoma	Cerebral abnormality/damage	
	Optic nerve hypoplasia	

Severe visual impairment

This affects 1 in 1000 live births in the UK but is higher in developing countries. A family history of severe visual impairment, developmental delay or extreme prematurity places the infant at an increased risk. The causes are listed in Box 4.2. In developed countries, about 50% of severe visual impairment is genetic; in developing countries acquired causes such as infection are more prevalent. When visual impairment is of cortical origin, resulting from cerebral damage, examination of the eye, including the pupillary responses, may be normal.

Although few causes of severe visual impairment can be cured, early detection is important as certain elements may require treatment and much can be done to help the child and parents. Parents of a partially sighted or severely visually impaired child need appropriate advice on how to provide non-visual stimulation using speech and touch, on providing a safe home environment and on how to build the child's confidence. In the UK this is usually provided by peripatetic teachers for children with visual impairment. The teachers provide input at both preschool and school ages. Partially sighted children may be able to attend a mainstream school but require special assistance with low vision aids, which include filtered lenses, high powered magnifiers and small telescopic devices and computers. Severely visually impaired children may need special schooling. Some will need to be taught Braille to enable them to read. While many severely visually impaired children have a visual disability alone, at least half have additional neurodevelopmental problems.

Squint (strabismus)

In this common condition there is misalignment of the visual axes. The history may be helpful as squints are often intermittent. The parents are usually correct if they report deviation of the eyes. There may be a history of squint in the family. Newborn babies often give the appearance of having a squint. In older infants and young children, marked epicanthic folds may cause confusion (pseudosquint). Any infant with a squint persisting beyond 2 months of age should be referred for a specialist ophthalmological opinion. A squint is usually caused by failure to develop binocular vision due to refractive errors, but cataracts, retinoblastoma and other intraocular causes must be excluded.

Squints are commonly divided into:

- *Concomitant* (non-paralytic, common) – usually due to a refractive error in one or both eyes which is often treated by correction with glasses but may require surgery. These squints are particularly common in children with neurodevelopmental delay. The squinting eye most often turns inwards (convergent), but there can be outward (divergent) or, rarely, vertical deviation.
- *Paralytic* (rare) – due to paralysis of the motor nerves. When rapid in onset, this can be sinister because of the possibility of an underlying space-occupying lesion such as a brain tumour.

Corneal light reflex test

For the non-specialist, the light reflex test is used to detect squints (Fig. 4.7). It is easiest to use a pen torch held at a distance to produce reflections on both corneas simultaneously. The light reflection should appear in the same position in the two eyes. If it does not, a squint is present. However, a minor squint may be difficult to detect.

Cover test

When a squint is present and the fixing eye is covered, the squinting eye moves to take up fixation (Fig. 4.8). The child's interest can be attracted with a toy or light. The test should be performed with the object near (33 cm) and distant (at least 6 m), as certain squints are present only at one distance. Occlusion should be with a card or plastic occluder. These tests are difficult to perform and reliable results are best obtained by an orthoptist or ophthalmologist.

Refractive errors

Hypermetropia

This is the most common refractive error in young children and should be corrected early to avoid irreversible damage to vision (amblyopia). This is more likely if accompanied by a squint but may occur without.

Myopia

This is relatively uncommon in young children and is less likely to cause amblyopia unless it is severe or only one eye is affected.

Amblyopia

This is a potentially permanent loss of visual acuity in an eye that has not received a clear image. It

Squints

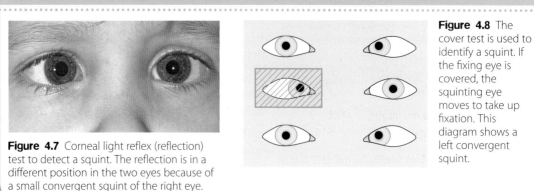

Figure 4.7 Corneal light reflex (reflection) test to detect a squint. The reflection is in a different position in the two eyes because of a small convergent squint of the right eye.

Figure 4.8 The cover test is used to identify a squint. If the fixing eye is covered, the squinting eye moves to take up fixation. This diagram shows a left convergent squint.

affects 2–3% of children. In most cases, it affects one eye; rarely, both are involved. Any interference with visual development may cause amblyopia, such as unilateral or bilateral refractive errors, squint or visual deprivation, e.g. ptosis or cataract. Treatment is by correction of any refractive error with glasses, together with patching of the 'good' eye for specific periods of the day to force the 'lazy' eye to work and therefore develop better vision. It is continued until the vision in the 'lazy' eye no longer improves. The longer treatment is delayed, the less likely it is that normal vision will be obtained. Early treatment is essential, as after 7 years of age improvement is unlikely. Considerable encouragement and support often need to be given to both the child and parents, as young children usually dislike having their eye patched, particularly if vision in the unpatched eye is poor.

⊚ Summary

Regarding vision:

- Abnormal eye movements in a newborn infant or not smiling responsively by 6 weeks post-term – can the infant see?
- Any infant with a squint (fixed or otherwise) after 2 months of age – refer for an ophthalmological opinion.
- Concomitant squint – common, usually due to a refractive error in one or both eyes.
- Paralytic squint – rare, due to paralysis of the motor nerves; if rapid onset, consider space-occupying lesion.
- Testing for squints – corneal light reflex (reflection) test for the non-specialist, cover test for the specialist.

Slow acquisition of cognitive skills/ general learning difficulty

The term 'learning difficulty' (reflecting cognitive learning difficulties) is now preferred to 'mental retardation' or 'mental handicap'. In the UK learning difficulties are classified as:

- mild (IQ 70–90)
- moderate (IQ 50–70)
- severe (IQ 20–50)
- profound (IQ less than 20).

Children with mild learning difficulties are usually supported by additional helpers (learning support assistants, LSA) in mainstream schools, whereas children with moderate, severe and profound learning difficulties are likely to need the resources of special schools.

Severe or profound learning difficulties are usually apparent from infancy as marked global developmental delay whereas moderate learning difficulties emerge only as delay in speech and language becomes apparent. Mild learning difficulties may only become apparent when the child starts school.

A child with profound learning difficulties will have no significant language and be completely dependent for all of his needs. A child with severe learning difficulties is likely to be able to learn minimal self care skills and acquire simple speech and language. Both will need high or total supervision and support throughout life.

The prevalence of severe learning difficulty is about 3–4 per 1000 children. Most have an organic cause irrespective of social class, in contrast to moderate learning difficulty (30 per 1000 children) in which children of parents from lower socio-economic classes are over-represented.

Common causes of developmental delay and learning difficulty are listed in Table 4.3.

Specific learning disorders

Developmental coordination disorder (DCD) or dyspraxia

Developmental coordination disorder (dyspraxia) is a disorder of motor planning and/or execution with no significant findings on standard neurological examination. It is a disorder of the higher cortical processes and there may be associated problems of perception (how the child interprets what he sees and hears), use of language and putting thoughts together.

Children may have:

- planning dyspraxia, where there are difficulties with:
  - planning a sequence or order of coordinated movements
  - actions that involve manipulation of objects
- executive dyspraxia, where there are difficulties with:
  - knowing what to do but being unable to do it
  - moving from one activity to another
  - copying actions.

The difficulties may impact on educational progress and self-esteem and suggest the child has greater academic difficulties than may be the case. Features include problems with:

- handwriting, which is typically awkward, messy, irregular and poorly spaced
- dressing (buttons, laces, clothes)
- cutting up food
- poorly established laterality
- copying and drawing
- messy eating from difficulty in coordinating biting, chewing and swallowing (oromotor dyspraxia). Dribbling of saliva is common.

Assessment and advice is primarily from an occupational therapist. A visual assessment may also be helpful. Dyspraxia in its milder form often goes undetected during the first few years of life as the child achieves gross motor milestones at the normal times. With therapy (emphasis on sensory integration, sequencing and executive planning) and maturity, the condition should improve.

Dyslexia

Dyslexia is a disorder of reading skills disproportionate to the child's IQ. The term is often used when the child's reading age is more than 2 years behind his chronological age. Assessment needs to include vision and hearing and involves an educational psychologist.

Dyscalculia, dysgraphia

These are disorders in the development of calculation or writing skills.

Associated co-morbidities of specific learning disorders

These are:

- attention deficit disorder
- hyperactivity
- poor sensory integration skills (touch, balance)
- depression, conduct disorders.

Management of specific learning disorders

Assessment may include vision and hearing and assessment by an occupational therapist, physiotherapist and educational psychologist. Co-morbidities need to be identified. Treatment is aimed at improving skill acquisition, with educational and information technology support as appropriate.

Problems with concentration and attention

Attention deficit disorder (ADD) and attention deficit hyperactivity disorder (ADHD) are considered in Chapter 23.

Multidisciplinary child development services

Although children with a wide range of conditions have additional needs, the term 'special needs' is usually used for children with developmental problems and disabilities. In order to optimise their assessment and care on an ongoing basis, child development services have been developed nationally on a geographic area as a secondary care service.

A child developmental service (CDS):

- is multidisciplinary with predominantly health professionals (paediatrician, physiotherapist, occupational therapist, speech and language therapist, clinical psychologist, specialist health visitor, dietician) in the team but often also includes a social worker (Fig. 4.9)
- is multi-agency (Fig. 4.10) and may include health, social services, education, volunteers, voluntary agencies, parent support groups
- aims to provide a coordinated service with good interagency liaison to meet the functional needs of the child
- predominantly sees preschool children with moderate or severe difficulties but may have resources to support children with milder problems
- may provide multidisciplinary support and monitor children up to school-leaving age (16–19 years)
- maintains a register of children with disabilities and special needs (this may be held by Social Services, but there is an increasing trend to single multi-agency Special Needs registers)
- is community or hospital based but has emphasis on children's needs within the community (home, nursery, school), regardless of its location
- often has a nominated key worker for a child, to facilitate parents getting access to information and services their child may need.

Emphasis is on:

- diagnosis
- assessment of functional skills

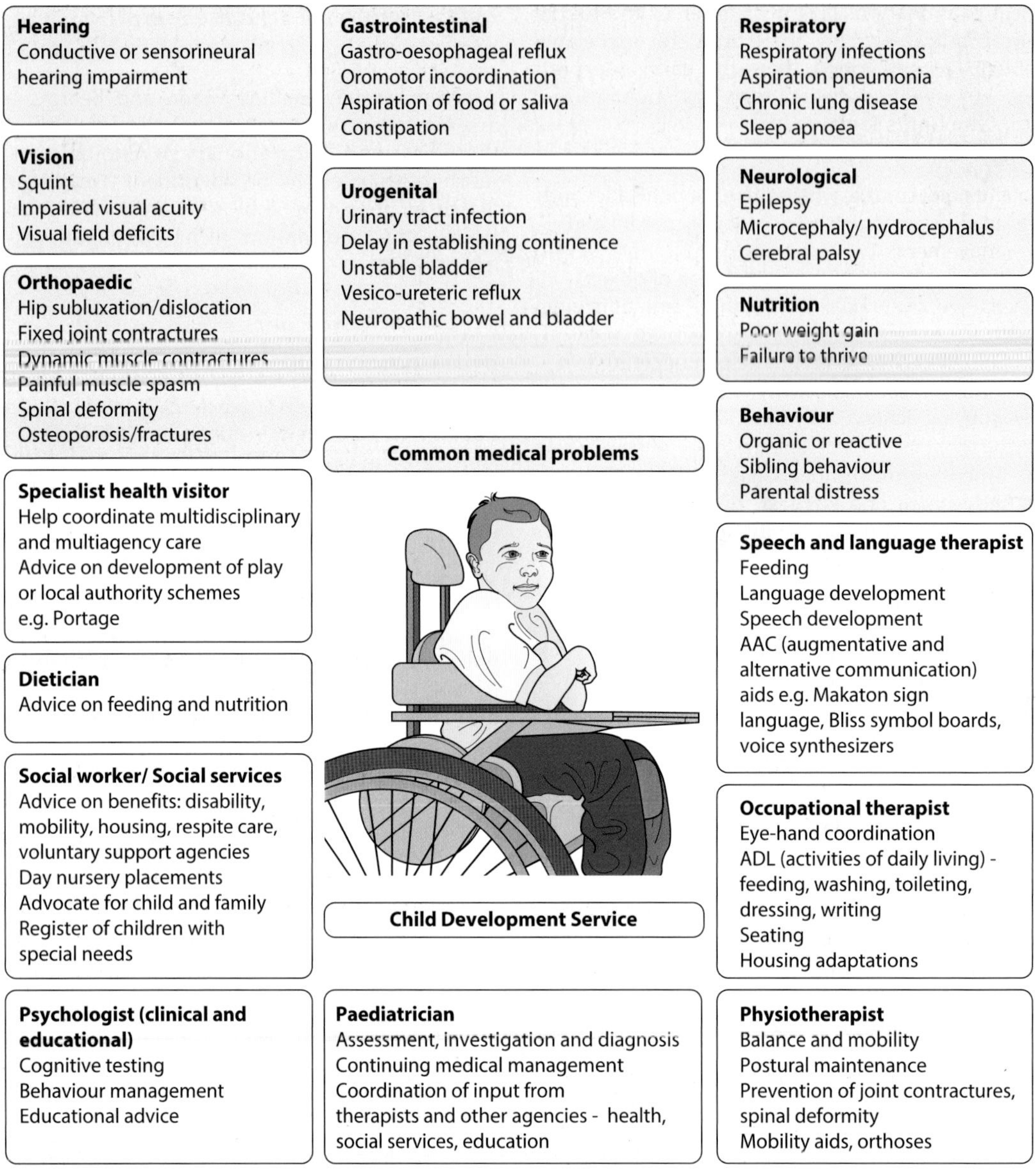

Hearing
Conductive or sensorineural hearing impairment

Vision
Squint
Impaired visual acuity
Visual field deficits

Orthopaedic
Hip subluxation/dislocation
Fixed joint contractures
Dynamic muscle contractures
Painful muscle spasm
Spinal deformity
Osteoporosis/fractures

Specialist health visitor
Help coordinate multidisciplinary and multiagency care
Advice on development of play or local authority schemes
e.g. Portage

Dietician
Advice on feeding and nutrition

Social worker/ Social services
Advice on benefits: disability, mobility, housing, respite care, voluntary support agencies
Day nursery placements
Advocate for child and family
Register of children with special needs

Psychologist (clinical and educational)
Cognitive testing
Behaviour management
Educational advice

Gastrointestinal
Gastro-oesophageal reflux
Oromotor incoordination
Aspiration of food or saliva
Constipation

Urogenital
Urinary tract infection
Delay in establishing continence
Unstable bladder
Vesico-ureteric reflux
Neuropathic bowel and bladder

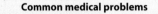

Common medical problems

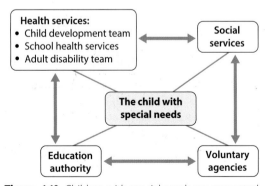

Child Development Service

Paediatrician
Assessment, investigation and diagnosis
Continuing medical management
Coordination of input from therapists and other agencies - health, social services, education

Respiratory
Respiratory infections
Aspiration pneumonia
Chronic lung disease
Sleep apnoea

Neurological
Epilepsy
Microcephaly/ hydrocephalus
Cerebral palsy

Nutrition
Poor weight gain
Failure to thrive

Behaviour
Organic or reactive
Sibling behaviour
Parental distress

Speech and language therapist
Feeding
Language development
Speech development
AAC (augmentative and alternative communication) aids e.g. Makaton sign language, Bliss symbol boards, voice synthesizers

Occupational therapist
Eye-hand coordination
ADL (activities of daily living) - feeding, washing, toileting, dressing, writing
Seating
Housing adaptations

Physiotherapist
Balance and mobility
Postural maintenance
Prevention of joint contractures, spinal deformity
Mobility aids, orthoses

Figure 4.9 Summary of the common medical conditions and the many health professionals in the child development service involved in the care of children with developmental problems.

Health services:
- Child development team
- School health services
- Adult disability team

Social services

The child with special needs

Education authority

Voluntary agencies

Figure 4.10 Children with special needs are supported by the integrated input of health and social services, local education authorities and voluntary agencies.

- provision of therapy
- regular review
- a coordinated approach to care (multidisciplinary, multi-agency).

Functional skills kept under review include:

- mobility
- hand function
- vision
- hearing
- speech, language and communication including social/communication skills
- behaviour, social and emotional skills
- self help skills including continence
- learning.

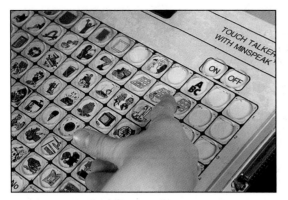

Figure 4.11 A touch pad communication system using symbols. This child with dystonic posturing can still press the desired key.

Many children with special needs have medical problems (Fig. 4.9) which require investigation, treatment and review. Good inter-professional communication is vital for well-coordinated care. This will be assisted by all professionals keeping entries in the child's Personal Child Health Record up-to-date.

In addition to locally organised child development services, specialist neurodisability services are required for:

- rehabilitation following acquired brain injury
- surgery for cerebral palsy, scoliosis
- gait analysis
- spasticity management including botulinum toxin
- epilepsy unresponsive to two or more anticonvulsants or where there is severe cognitive and behavioural regression related to epilepsy
- complex communication disorders, diagnosis and therapeutic intervention
- mixed complex learning problems, often with neuropsychiatric co-morbid symptoms
- provision of communication aids (Fig. 4.11)
- sensory impairments, e.g. cochlear implants
- services for severe visual and hearing impairment
- specialised seating/wheelchairs and orthoses (Fig. 4.12)
- management of movement disorders, e.g. intrathecal baclofen.

Needs are likely to change over time with key stages being at transition to school and adult services. A care plan should be developed at each stage and needs to be shared with the child and family and then regularly reviewed. Involvement with specialist services may be of variable frequency throughout childhood. Collaboration across services is vital in promoting a service tailored around the child and family.

Summary

Children with developmental problems and disabilities

- are looked after by local multidisciplinary Child Development Services
- often have complex medical needs
- need regular review, as needs change with time
- require coordination of care between the family and the many professionals involved, as well as close liaison with education and social services.

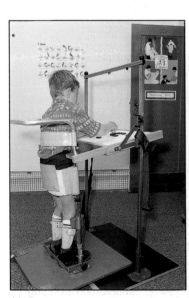
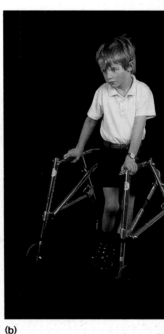
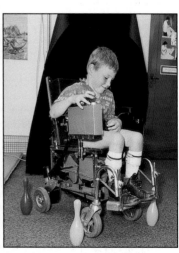

(a)　　　　　　(b)　　　　　　(c)

Figure 4.12 (a) A standing frame assisting a boy with cerebral palsy to be upright. **(b)** A boy with athetoid cerebral palsy is able to walk with the help of a frame. **(c)** A 6-year-old boy with four-limb spasticity is able to steer this electric wheelchair. (Reproduced from Newton R, *Color Atlas of Pediatric Neurology*, Mosby–Wolfe, London, 1995.)

Education

In England and Wales, several Education Acts and the 2000 Code of Practice have made provision for children with special educational needs to receive educational input appropriate to their requirements. This includes their right to integration into mainstream education whenever possible. Education authorities have a duty to identify children whose special educational needs will require additional resources.

Initial recognition that a child may have special educational needs (SEN) may occur at the preschool stage in children with specific or global developmental delay or with specific disabilities, or may only become evident when the child is of school age. Early identification maximises the child's opportunity to progress. The Local Education Authority (LEA) is informed of these children by a process called 'notification', usually by the paediatrician if preschool or by an education professional if at school.

The 2000 Code of Practice suggests that pupils' needs may fall within four broad areas:

- cognition and learning
- communication and interaction
- behaviour, emotional and social development
- sensory and/or physical needs.

Where a child is identified as having special educational needs, a special educational needs coordinator (SENCO) within the teaching staff is responsible for formulating an individual education plan (IEP) for the child within the school or nursery or for seeking help from external services, e.g. educational psychology.

If a child's needs are so severe that they cannot be met effectively within the resources normally available to the school or nursery school, the Local Education Authority (LEA) is asked to conduct a statutory assessment of a child's educational needs. This may lead to production of a Statement of Special Educational Needs for the child which identifies the extra help the child should have and which has to be reviewed annually. Parents can also request such an assessment.

Although children are integrated into mainstream school where practicable, special schools or units are usually more suitable for children with severe learning difficulties and sometimes for those with severe physical, sensory, communication or behaviour problems. Many special educational placements will have a need for therapy input (physiotherapy, occupational and speech/language therapy) as well as specialised teaching resources. Support for the behavioural needs of a child may come from a clinical or educational psychologist.

Transition of care to adult services

In the UK, adult disability services are in general poorly developed by comparison to those provided for children. Young adults with severe learning and physical disabilities are supported by Adult Learning Disability Teams, but there is only limited national provision for those with mild or moderate learning disabilities or with a predominantly physical disability. Major issues for young adults with disabilities include social challenges; namely care, housing, mobility, finance, leisure, employment, genetic and sexual counselling. Health information must be properly transferred from child to adult health services if reinvestigation of already well-clarified conditions is to be avoided.

The rights of disabled children

Irrespective of their disability, the aspirations and rights of children as affirmed by the United Nations Convention on the Rights of the Child need to be respected (see Ch. 1). Technological advances to improve mobility, communication and emotional expression are helping enable disabled people to better achieve their full potential, rather than being held back by their disability. However, this requires skilled assistance and adequate resources. Prominent public figures who function effectively despite disabilities help to make the pubic appreciate what can be achieved and serve as an inspiration to those with disabilities.

Further reading

Department for Education and Science 2002 Together from the start: practical guidance for professionals working with disabled children and their families. DfES

Department of Health 2003 National Service Framework for Children, Young People and Maternity Services: Disabled Children and Young People and those with Complex Health Needs. DoH

Hall D, Elliman D 2003 Health for all children, 4th edn. Oxford University Press, Oxford

Hall D, Hill P, Elliman D 1999 The child surveillance handbook. Radcliffe Medical Press, Oxford. *A practical handbook*

Meggitt C 2006 Child development. An illustrated guide 2nd edn. Heinemann Educational, Oxford

Polnay L 2002 Community paediatrics. Churchill Livingstone, Edinburgh

Internet

National Autistic Society (national recommendations for management of autistic spectrum disorder 2003 and national plan for autism): www.nas.org.uk

Care of the sick child

Most sick children are cared for by their parents at home. Medical management is initially given by general practitioners or, in some countries, primary care paediatricians. Most hospital admissions are at secondary care level. A smaller number of children will require tertiary care in a specialist centre, e.g. paediatric intensive care unit, cardiac or oncology unit. There are a few national centres for very rare and complex treatments, e.g. organ transplantation, craniofacial surgery (Fig. 5.1).

Primary care

The majority of acute illness in children is mild and transient (e.g. upper respiratory tract infection, gastroenteritis) or readily treatable (e.g. urinary tract infection). Although serious conditions are uncommon (Fig. 5.2), they must be identified promptly. The condition of sick children, especially infants, may deteriorate rapidly, and parents require rapid access to a general practitioner or other healthcare professionals working in primary care, who in turn require ready access to secondary care. Acutely ill children may also attend walk-in centres, be seen at home by emergency care practitioners (trained nurses or paramedics working in the pre-hospital setting). Advice may also be obtained from a health professional by telephone via NHS Direct, via the internet with NHS Direct Online or by NHS Direct cable TV services. Although an individual general practitioner will care for relatively few children with serious chronic illnesses (e.g. cystic fibrosis, diabetes mellitus) or disability (e.g. cerebral palsy), each affected child and family are likely to require considerable input from the whole of the primary care team.

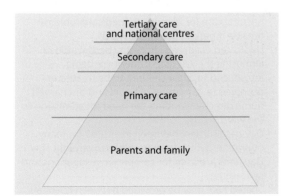

Figure 5.1 Schematic representation of the 'clinical iceberg' of the provision of care for sick children. (Adapted from Audit Commission, *Children First*, 1993.)

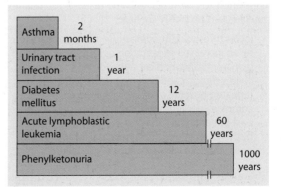

Figure 5.2 Number of years a general practitioner needs to work before encountering a child newly presenting with these conditions.

Box 5.1 Services which should be available for children attending an Accident and Emergency department

Environment	**Staff**	**Medical care**
Separate waiting area, play facilities, child friendly treatment and recovery areas	Medical and nursing staff trained and experienced in the care and treatment of children	Resuscitation and other equipment for children
Access for parents to examination, X-ray and anaesthetic rooms	Non-paediatric staff trained in communicating with children and families	Priority for prompt treatment
		Rapid transfer if inpatient admission is needed
	Effective communication with other health professionals	Child protection policies
		Procedures and counselling are in place following the sudden death of a child

Adapted from *Welfare of Children in Hospital*, HMSO, London, 1991.

Hospital care

Accident and Emergency

Approximately 3.5 million children attend an Accident and Emergency (A&E) department each year in England and Wales, 1 in 4 children. The services which should be provided for children are shown in Box 5.1. The number of departments able to meet these expectations is increasing, often by creating a dedicated children's A&E department.

Hospital admission

In England and Wales, 1 in 11 children is admitted to hospital each year, representing 16% of all hospital admissions. About 42% of acute admissions are under the care of paediatricians, and the remainder are surgical patients (although a paediatrician is also involved in their care whilst they are in hospital, to oversee any medical requirements). Most paediatric admissions are of infants and young children under 5 years of age and are emergencies, whereas surgical admissions peak at 5 years of age, one-third of which are elective (Fig. 5.3). The reasons for medical admission are shown in Table 5.1.

Although primary and community health services for children have improved markedly over the last decade, the hospital admission rate has continued to rise (Fig. 5.4). The reasons for this are unclear, but probably include:

- lower threshold for admission – there appears to be an increased expectation of hospital admission by parents and medical staff worried that the child's clinical condition may deteriorate
- repeated hospital admission of children with complex conditions who would have died in the past but are now surviving, e.g. very low birthweight infants from neonatal intensive care units, children with cancer or organ failure.

Strenuous efforts are being made to reduce the rate and length of hospitalisation:

- The new speciality of ambulatory paediatrics encompasses specialist paediatricians providing

Table 5.1 Reason for paediatric medical admissions to a district general hospital

Respiratory 31%	Asthma 11%
	URTI 6%
	Croup 4%
	Bronchiolitis 4%
	Pneumonia 3%
	Tonsillitis 2.5%
Environment 22%	Head injury 12%
	Poisoning 8%
	Child protection 1.5%
Gastroenterology 15%	Gastroenteritis 7%
	Constipation/soiling 2%
	Abdominal pain/vomiting 2%
	Failure to thrive 1%
Infection 10%	Viral infection 6%
	Septicaemia/meningitis 1.5%
Neurology 8%	Febrile convulsions 3%
	Epilepsy 3%
	Apnoea/cyanotic attacks 2%
Kidney and urinary tract 3%	Urinary tract infection 2.5%
Other 11%	

Data based on 2160 consecutive admissions to Pinderfields Hospital, Wakefield. Courtesy of Dr Roddy MacFaul.

hospital care for immediate medical problems outside inpatient paediatric wards.

- Dedicated children's short stay beds within or alongside the A&E department are being introduced to allow children to be treated or observed for a number of hours and discharged home directly, avoiding the need for admission to the ward.
- Day-case surgery has been instituted for many operations which used to require overnight stay. Day units are used for complex investigations and procedures.
- Shared care may be provided between hospitals and primary care, with paediatricians and other healthcare professionals seeing children at home or in primary care settings.

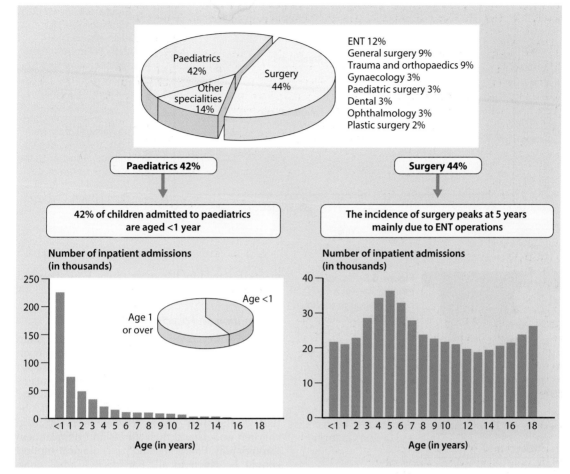

Figure 5.3 Hospital admissions as inpatients of children aged 0–18 years in England and Wales in 1990–91. (Adapted from Audit Commission, *Children First*, 1993.)

- Home care teams aim to provide care in the child's home and thereby reduce hospital attendance, admission and length of stay. Most teams comprise community paediatric nurses, but some include doctors, and they either cover all aspects of paediatric care within a geographical area or are for a specific condition, e.g. cystic fibrosis or malignancy, usually centred around a tertiary referral centre. The problems managed at home by such teams include:
  – changing postoperative wound dressings or managing burns
  – day-to-day management and support for the family for chronic illnesses, e.g. diabetes mellitus, asthma and eczema
  – specialist care, e.g. home oxygen therapy, intravenous infusions via a central venous catheter (e.g. antibiotics or chemotherapy) or peritoneal dialysis
  – symptom and pain control and emotional support of terminally ill children (Fig. 5.5).

Some teams provide a 'hospital at home' service for children who are acutely ill, in order to avoid hospitalisation.

Hospital admission of children:
- **should be avoided whenever possible**
- **most medical admissions are infants and young children, surgical admissions occur throughout childhood.**

Children in hospital

Children should only be admitted to hospital if their care cannot be provided safely at home. Removing young children from their familiar environment to a strange ward is stressful and frightening for the child, parents and family. Ill or injured children may regress in their behaviour, acting younger than their actual age. It also disrupts family routines, not only of the child in hospital but also of siblings who still need to be looked after at home and transported to and from nursery or school.

Family-centred care

Care in hospital should be child- and family-centred. Parents and siblings should be involved in the child's care, which should be appropriate for the child's physical and emotional maturity and needs.

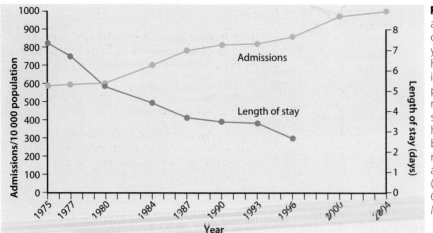

Figure 5.4 Inpatient admission rates for children aged 0–14 years in England. There has been a marked increase in the paediatric admission rate, whereas the surgical admission rate has fallen slightly. In both, there has been a marked reduction in the average length of stay. (Adapted from Audit Commission, *Children First*, 1993.)

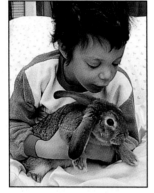

Figure 5.5 Providing terminal care in a child's home. Although this child required a subcutaneous morphine infusion to control her pain from malignant disease, she was able to remain at home and enjoyed playing with her pet rabbit. (By kind permission of her parents and Dr Ann Goldman.)

A holistic approach should be adopted towards the child and his family rather than simply focusing on the medical condition. Young children may interpret the pain experienced in hospital and separation from their home or parents as punishment. In general, the distress arising from separating children from their mothers is greatest in young children, and increases the longer the length of stay and the more frequently the child is admitted. Parents of infants and young children should be encouraged to stay with their child overnight and continue to provide the care and support they would give at home. Parents know best about their child's usual behaviour and habits and due attention must be paid to their worries or comments. Many parents rapidly learn some of the nursing skills, e.g. tube feeding, required by their child. Good communication is needed between staff and parents to arrive at a mutually agreed plan of responsibilities for looking after the child. This will avoid parents either feeling pressurised to accept responsibilities they are not confident about or feeling brushed aside and undervalued by staff. Parents should be able to stay overnight with their child.

Child-orientated environment

Children should be cared for within a children's ward. Adolescents should be with others of their own age and not forced to accept ward arrangements designed for babies or adults. Education and facilities for play should be provided.

Information and psychosocial support

Detailed information should be provided, given personally and preferably also written and available in appropriate ethnic languages. Staff should be sensitive to the family's individual needs according to their social, educational, cultural and religious background. Play specialists should be part of the ward team because they can help children understand their illness and its treatment through play. Emotional and psychological support should be given to all. For elective admissions, children and their families should be offered an advance visit and have details of proposed treatment and management explained at an appropriate level.

Skilled staff

Children in hospital should be cared for by specially trained medical, nursing and support staff. Every child admitted to hospital should be supervised by a children's physician or surgeon. Children constitute only a relatively small proportion of the workload in acute surgical specialities, so surgeons and anaesthetists should treat a sufficient number of children to maintain their skills. There should be a 'named nurse' responsible for planning and coordinating care by other nurses to ensure that families receive all the information they need and provide a link with staff involved in discharge planning and post-discharge arrangements.

Multidisciplinary care

Successful management of paediatric conditions often relies on a network of multidisciplinary care, with all the professionals working well together as a coordinated team. If this breaks down, particularly when dealing with complex issues such as child protection, the consequences may be disastrous for the child, family and professionals involved. Child psychiatrists, the community paediatric team and social services are important members of the team.

Tertiary care

As the number of children requiring tertiary care is relatively small, it is concentrated in specialist centres. Increasingly, the centre is linked to several district general hospitals to form a clinical network. These centres have the advantage of having a wide range of specialists, not only medical staff but also nursing and other healthcare profes-sionals, and diagnostic and other services. A disadvantage is that they are often some distance from the child's home and hospital stay may be prolonged, e.g. following a bone marrow transplant. Accommoda-tion for parents should be provided. Shared care arrangements between tertiary centres and local hospitals are designed to minimise the need for the child to travel to the specialist centre. For example, a child with malignant disease would attend a tertiary centre for the initial diagnostic assessment and treatment, and subsequently for specialised treatment and periodic review, but much of the maintenance therapy would be provided by the local hospital together with monitoring of their health and regular blood and other tests performed by a specialist nurse at home.

⊙ Summary

Children in hospital should be provided with:
- family centred care – holistic approach to family, parent able to stay and provide parental care
- child oriented environment – geared for child's age, together with education and play facilities
- information and psychosocial support – verbal and written information for both parents and child
- the opportunity to have their views and fears listened to, if old enough
- skilled staff – specially trained to care for children
- multidisciplinary care
- access to tertiary care – with shared care arrangements with local hospital and primary care.

Pain

It is easy to ignore or underestimate pain in children. Pain should ideally be anticipated and prevented.

Acute pain

This may be caused by:

- tissue damage, e.g. burns or trauma
- specific disease process, e.g. sickle cell crisis
- medical intervention – investigations or procedures
- surgery.

Chronic pain

In children, chronic severe pain sometimes occurs as a result of disease such as malignant disease or juvenile idiopathic arthritis (juvenile chronic arthritis). Intermittent pain of mild or moderate severity, e.g. headache or recurrent abdominal pain, is more common.

Older children can describe the nature and severity of the pain they are experiencing. In younger children, assessing pain is more difficult. Observation and parental impression are commonly used and a number of self-assessment tools have been designed for children over 3 years old (Fig. 5.6).

Management

The approaches to pain management are listed in Box 5.2. This should allow pain to be prevented or kept to a minimum. Age-appropriate explanation should be given when possible and the approach be reassuring; however, it is imperative not to lie to children, otherwise they will not believe what they are told in the future. Distraction techniques such as blowing bubbles, telling stories, holding family toys or playing computer games, as well as the involvement of trained play specialists, can be highly successful in ameliorating pain in children. Some children develop particular preferences for a particular venepuncture site or distraction technique, and this should be accommodated as far as possible.

For minor medical procedures, e.g. vene-puncture or inserting an intravenous cannula, pain can be alleviated by explanation and the use of a topical anaesthetic. Additional and appropriate use of inhalation agents such as nitrous oxide (laughing

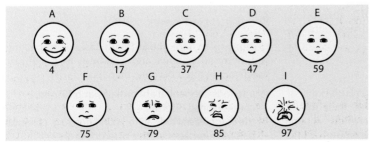

Figure 5.6 An example of a scoring system for pain assessment in children where '0' represents extremely happy and '100' extremely sad. (From McGrath P A, DeVeber L L, Hearn M T, Multidimensional pain assessment in children. In: Fields H, Dubner R, Cervero F (eds) *Advances in Pain Research and Therapy*, Raven Press, New York, 1985; p 387–393.)

• •
Box 5.2 Approaches to pain management

Explanation and information

Psychological, by the parent, doctor, nurse or play specialist
Behavioural
Distraction
Hypnosis

Medical
Local: anaesthetic cream, local anaesthetic infiltration, nerve blocks, warmth or cold, physiotherapy, transcutaneous electrical nerve stimulation (TENS)
Analgesics:
    Mild – paracetamol, NSAIDs
    Moderate – codeine, NSAIDs
    Strong – morphine
Sedatives and anaesthetic agents:
    Intranasal midazolam, nitrous oxide, general anaesthetic
Anti-epileptic and antidepressant drugs for neuropathic pain

Consider the route for analgesics – oral if possible, otherwise intravenous, subcutaneous or rectal.
NSAIDs, non-steroidal anti-inflammatory drugs.

gas) or the adjunctive use of mild sedation alongside pain relief, e.g. intranasal midazolam, can be helpful for more painful procedures such as suturing a wound. For more invasive procedures, e.g. bronchoscopy, a general anaesthetic should be given.

Postoperative pain can be markedly reduced by local infiltration of the wound, nerve blocks and postoperative analgesics. For severe pain, there was reluctance in the past to use morphine in children for fear of depressing breathing. This should not occur when morphine is given in appropriate dosage under nursing supervision to children with a normal respiratory drive. Intravenous morphine can be given using a patient-controlled delivery system in older children or a nurse-controlled system in young children.

 Pain should be anticipated and prevented rather than treated.

Prescribing medicines for children

There are marked differences in the absorption, distribution and elimination of drugs between children and adults.

Absorption

In the neonate and infant, oral formulations of drugs are given as liquids. However, their intake cannot be guaranteed and absorption is unpredictable as it is affected by gastric emptying and acidity, gut motility and the effects of milk in the stomach. In acutely ill neonates and infants, drugs are given intravenously to ensure reliable and adequate blood and tissue concentrations. Intramuscular injections should be avoided if possible as there is little muscle bulk available for injection, absorption is variable and they are painful. Rectal administration can be used for some drugs; absorption is more reliable, but this route is not popular in the UK. Significant systemic absorption can occur across the skin, particularly in preterm infants. Occasionally this can be used therapeutically, but is a potential cause of toxicity, e.g. alcohol and iodine absorption from cleansing solutions applied to the skin for procedures.

Young children find it difficult to take tablets and a liquid formulation is required. Most are glucose-free. Persuading children to take medicines is often a problem, especially if the preparation has an unpleasant taste. Adherence (compliance) is improved when medicines are only required once or twice a day and if regimens are kept simple.

Distribution

Water comprises a larger percentage of the body in the neonate (80%) than in older children and adults (55%). Drugs which distribute within the extracellular fluid will require a larger dose relative to body weight in infants than in adults. As extracellular fluid correlates with body surface area, this is used when accurate drug dosage is required, e.g. cytotoxic agents. For drugs with a high margin of safety, drug dosages are expressed per kilogram body weight or based on age, with the assumption that the child is of average size. Weight-based dosages should not simply be extrapolated to older children, as the dosage will be excessively large.

In the first few months of life, the plasma protein is low. More of the drug may be unbound and pharmacologically active. In jaundiced babies, bilirubin may compete with some drugs, e.g. sulphonamides, for albumin binding sites, making such drugs unsuitable for use in this situation.

Elimination

In neonates, drug biotransformation is reduced, as microsomal enzymes in the liver are immature. This leads to a prolonged half-life of drugs metabolised in the liver, e.g. theophylline. Renal excretion is reduced by the low glomerular filtration rate which increases the half-life of some drugs, e.g. vancomycin. Measuring the plasma drug concentration is necessary under these circumstances.

Breaking bad news

Doctors often face the difficult task of imparting bad news to parents and children. In paediatric practice it is often because there is:

- a serious congenital abnormality at birth, e.g. chromosomal disorder
- the diagnosis of a disabling condition, e.g. cerebral palsy, neurodegenerative disorder, gross

Summary

Regarding medicines for children:

- oral formulations need to be given as liquids in infants and young children
- are usually prescribed per kilogram of body weight, but check the maximum dose
- intramuscular drugs should be avoided if at all possible
- intravenous drug dosages can easily be miscalculated as they vary widely in children because of their different size and drugs often need to be diluted; all dosages and dilutions must be checked independently by two trained members of staff
- to improve compliance use formulations requiring the least number of times to be taken per day
- always check drug dosage in the BNF (British National Formulary) for Children.

intracranial abnormality seen at ultrasound in preterm infants
- a serious illness, e.g. meningitis or malignant disease, or an accident, e.g. head injury
- the sudden death of a child, e.g. sudden infant death syndrome (SIDS).

Initial interview

The manner in which the initial interview is conducted is very important. It may have a profound influence on the parents' ability to cope with the problem and their subsequent relationship with health professionals. Parents often continue to recall and recount, for many years, details of the initial interview when they were informed that their child had a serious problem. Parents of children with life-threatening illnesses have said that what they valued most was open, sympathetic, direct and uninterrupted discussion in private that allowed sufficient time for doctors to repeat and clarify information and for them to ask questions (Box 5.3).

Box 5.3 How parents wish to be told the diagnosis of a life-threatening illness

Setting
In private
Uninterrupted
Unhurried
Both parents (or friend/relative) present if possible
Senior doctor
Nurse or social worker present

Establish contact
Find out what the family knows or suspects
Respect family's vulnerability
Use the child's name
Do not avoid looking at them
Be direct, open, sympathetic

Provide information
Flexibility is essential
Pace rather than protect from bad news
Name the illness
Describe symptoms relevant to child's condition
Discuss aetiology – parents will usually want to know
Anticipate and answer questions. Don't avoid difficult issues because parents have not thought to ask

Explain long-term prognosis
If child is likely to die, listen to concerns about time, place and nature of death
Outline the support/treatment available

Address feelings
Be prepared to tolerate reactions of shock, especially anger or weeping
Acknowledge uncertainty
How is it likely to affect the family?
What and how to tell other children, relatives and friends?

Concluding the interview
Elicit what parents have understood
Clarify and repeat
Acknowledge that it may be difficult for parents to absorb all the information
Mention sources of support
If possible, give parents contact telephone number
Give address of self-help group

Follow-up
Offer early follow-up
Suggest to families that they write down questions in preparation for next appointment
Ensure adequate communication of content of interview to:
- other members of staff
- general practitioner and health visitor
- other professionals, e.g. a referring paediatrician

Adapted from Woolley H, Stein A, Forrest G C, Baum J D, 1989 Imparting the diagnosis of life-threatening illness in children. *British Medical Journal* 298: 1623–1626.

Discharge from hospital

Children should be discharged from hospital as soon as clinically and socially appropriate. Although there is increasing pressure to reduce the length of hospital stay to a minimum, this must not allow discharge planning to be neglected. Before discharge from hospital, parents and children should be informed of:

- the reason for admission and any implications for the future
- details of medication and other treatment
- any clinical features which should prompt them to seek medical advice, and how this should be obtained
- the existence of any voluntary self-help groups if appropriate
- problems or questions likely to be asked by other family members or in the community. These should be anticipated by the doctor and discussed. What do the nursery or school, baby-sitters or friends need to know? What about sports, etc.?

In addition:

- Suitability of home circumstances needs to be assessed, particularly when the home requires adaptation for special needs.
- Social support may need to be arranged, especially in relation to child protection.
- Medical information should be added to the child's personal child health record.
- Consider who else should be informed about the admission and what information it is relevant for them to receive. This must be done before or at the time of discharge. The aim is to provide a seamless service of care, treatment and support, with the family and all the professionals fully informed (Fig. 5.7). This can be facilitated for children with a chronic illness or disability by having a key worker to coordinate their care.

Ethics

Situations arise in paediatric practice in which the course of action that should be followed is unclear. Knowledge of the ethical theories and principles which underpin medical practice is helpful in understanding the issues involved. It is important to justify decisions to investigate or treat in accordance with these principles, and in language that is clear to all concerned.

Definitions of the principles of medical ethics

These are:

- *non-maleficence* – do no harm (psychological and/or physical)
- *beneficence* –positive obligation to do good (these two principles have been part of medical ethics since the Hippocratic Oath)
- *justice* – fairness for all, equity and equality of care
- *respect for autonomy* – respect for individuals' rights to make informed and thought-out decisions for themselves in accordance with their capabilities
- *truth-telling and confidentiality* – important aspects of autonomy that support trust, essential in the doctor–patient relationship
- *duty* – the moral obligation to act irrespective of the consequences in accordance with moral laws which are universal, apply equally to all and which respect persons as autonomous beings
- *utility* – the obligation to do the greatest good for the greatest number
- *rights* – justifiable moral claims, e.g. the right to life, respect, education, which impose moral obligations upon others.

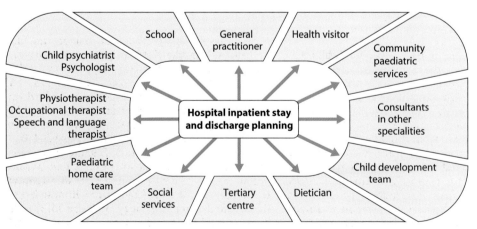

Figure 5.7 Some of the professionals who may need to be informed on admission or discharge about a child admitted to hospital.

Application of ethical principles to paediatrics

Non-maleficence

Children are more vulnerable to harm. This includes their suffering from fear of procedures, which they may be too young to express verbally. Doctors may do harm from lack of skill or knowledge, especially if they do not treat children frequently.

Beneficence

The child's interest is paramount. In the UK, this is enshrined in the Children Act 1989 and the UN Convention on the Rights of the Child. This may sometimes conflict with parental autonomy, such as the emergency treatment of a child where the parent is not immediately available or when details are given to social workers in suspected child abuse.

Justice

This involves ensuring a comprehensive child health service, including the prevention of illness and equal access to health care even when poverty, language barriers and parental disability are present.

Autonomy

Children have restricted but developing rights in law. Parents are trusted to make decisions on their child's behalf because they will usually act in the child's best interests, but there may be circumstances, e.g. child abuse, in which this is not the case.

Truth-telling

It is more difficult with children than adults to be sure that they understand what is happening to them. For example, it is easy to reassure children falsely that procedures will not hurt; when they find this is untrue, trust will be lost for future occasions.

Consent

Valid consent is required for all medical interventions other than emergencies or when urgent intervention is necessary to prevent serious risk of present or future harm. It provides the ethical and legal authority for action which would otherwise be a common assault or interfere with the right of individuals to decide what should be done to them (autonomous choice). To be valid, consent must be sufficiently informed, and freely given by a person who is competent to do so. Clinicians have a duty to provide sufficient information to enable a reasonable person to make the decision and must answer all questions honestly. Information has to be given in language that is clear and understandable. In UK law, the legal age of consent to medical treatment is 16 years. The right of children below this age to give consent depends on their competence rather than their age. They may consent to medical examination and treatment provided they can demonstrate that they have the maturity and judgement to understand and appraise the nature and implications of the proposed treatment, including the risks and alternative courses of action. This is known as Gillick competence.

When a child lacks the maturity and judgement to give consent, this capacity is given to a person having parental responsibility – usually a natural parent, or to a court. In practice, problems occur only when there is disagreement between the child and the parents and clinicians over treatment, e.g. contraception for under 16-year-olds.

When a girl less than 16 years of age requests contraception without parental knowledge, a professional can provide it if satisfied that she cannot be persuaded to inform her parents, that she is likely to have sex with or without contraception and that receiving contraception is in her best interests. These are known as the Fraser guidelines.

Despite these provisos, legal judgments have not supported children who refuse treatment that parents and clinicians feel to be in their best interests, especially if its purpose is to save life or prevent serious harm, e.g. heart transplantation for acute cardiomyopathy in an intelligent 15-year-old. Where disputes cannot be resolved by negotiation or mediation, or there is doubt over the legality of what is proposed, legal advice should be sought. Whatever the outcome children should have their views heard and be given reasons as to why they are being over-ridden.

Confidentiality

Children are owed the same duty of confidentiality as adults irrespective of their legal capacity. In general, personal information about them should not be shared without their consent or agreement unless it is necessary for their health or to protect them from serious harm, e.g. in actual or suspected child abuse.

Best interests

It is a general ethical and legal maxim that the best interests of the child are paramount. Doctors therefore have a duty to save life, restore health and prevent disease by treatments that confer maximum benefit and minimal harm and which respect the autonomy of the child as far as possible. Parents have the ethical and legal duty to make decisions on behalf of their child, provided that they act in their best interests. Disputes may arise over what constitutes best interest and who should decide them; these may require legal intervention especially when the withholding or withdrawing of life-sustaining treatment may be involved. Courts have generally been supportive of the position that in some circumstances the burdens of providing life-sustaining treatment outweigh its benefits.

Ethics

Case History
5.1 Meningococcal septicaemia

Jack, aged 5 years, has a fever and purpuric rash and you suspect he may have potentially fatal meningococcal septicaemia. Jack hates needles and makes it clear that he rejects any sort of injection. 'No I don't want an injection, go away' is the message, loud and clear, when you try to take blood, do a lumbar puncture, and insert an indwelling intravenous cannula for his antibiotics. Yet with the full and anxious approval of his parents, you go ahead and do these things anyway. But if Jack was 25 years old and made it clear that he refused your interventions, while you'd strongly urge him to give permission and explain that he was in real danger of dying as a result of such refusal, you would not (presumably) treat him against his will, even if his mother and father still urged you to do so.

In contrast to normal adult medical ethics, in paediatrics the autonomy of the patient either is not present at all (as in babies and young infants) or is often not sufficiently developed to be respected if the child's decision conflicts with what appropriate other people consider to be in that child's best interests. The decisions about the child's medical care are generally entrusted to his parents. Why the parents? They are given the privilege and responsibility of making decisions on behalf of their children largely because they are most likely to protect and promote the interests of their children. The normal assumption in paediatric practice is that doctors should work closely with parents and give advice that parents may or may not accept. Wherever possible, a mutually trusting and respectful working relationship should be developed and maintained, both because it will be in the best interests of the child and because it will tend to lead to far better experiences of medical care for all involved.

Also, consider whether your decision would have been the same about performing an extra venepuncture for a special blood test for an ethically approved research project.

Case histories 5.1 and 5.2 demonstrate some of the ethical problems encountered in paediatrics.

The ethics of research in paediatrics

Research involving children is important in promoting children's health and well-being and may provide an evidence base for practice. Children differ from adults in their anatomy, physiology, disease patterns and responses to therapy, but many drugs in current use have not been tested on them. However, children are perhaps more vulnerable to the harm which may be produced by research and should be protected against it.

Distinction is often made between therapeutic research, where there is an intention to benefit the individual subject, and non-therapeutic research, which carries a wider societal benefit but without intent to benefit individuals. However, research that fails to benefit individuals may be ethical provided that it involves an acceptable level of risk.

Where a child suffers from a particular disease, e.g. acute lymphoblastic leukaemia, randomised clinical trials may be used to compare treatment regimens. The ethical justification for such trials is that there is no good reason to believe that one of the treatments would be better than the other – 'therapeutic equipoise' – and that the standard treatment used for comparative purposes is the best currently available.

The situation is different when an investigation, e.g. blood test, X-ray or intervention, is proposed for normal children as part of a control group in a trial or for the purpose of establishing a normal range. Both can be ethically justified provided that the procedure in question carries no more risk than generally encountered and accepted in everyday life.

Whatever the nature of the research a number of criteria must be met:

- Appropriate research should be first carried out in adults or older children.
- The project should have a sound scientific basis and be well designed.
- The researchers should be competent to carry it out in the time specified.
- Sufficient information should be given in a form comprehensible to the child and family to enable them to give valid consent to participation, e.g. by

Summary

Ethics in paediatrics:
- both clinicians and parents aim to do what is in their child's best interests
- conflicting views can usually be resolved by good communication
- if not resolved – help may be sought from further, wider communication, or a second, truly independent opinion, or sometimes from hospital ethical committees, or may go to court.
- older children who understand the issues and have strong views as to what should or should not be done to them – there is increasing ethical and legal support for them to exercise as much autonomy as they are capable of.

5.2 Acute lymphatic leukaemia, truth-telling and stopping treatment

Jane, aged 10 years, has acute lymphoblastic leukaemia which was diagnosed 4 years ago. She has relapsed, with early involvement of the central nervous system. She is well known to the staff of her local children's ward as she has had four relapses of her leukaemia and a previous bone marrow transplant. It is the opinion of her paediatric consultant that no further medical treatment is likely to be curative. Jane asks one of the junior paediatric doctors why her parents had been so upset following a recent discussion with the consultant, at which she had not been present. The parents had made it very clear to all the staff that they did not want their child to be informed of the poor prognosis, nor would they tell her why she was not having further chemotherapy.

The parents have heard of a new drug which is claimed, in some reports on the internet, to help such children. However, it is very expensive, there is evidence that it does not cross the blood–brain barrier and the doctors consider it highly unlikely to be of benefit. The parents insist on a trial of the drug.

Ethical issues to consider are:
Autonomy – the parents claim the right to control the information reaching their child on the grounds that it is in her best interests as judged by them.

Truth-telling – the staff feel that it would be wrong to reassure her falsely.

Non-maleficence – the parents wish to avoid the shock of the news and the loss of hope in their daughter.

Beneficence – the staff wish to support the child effectively, which would be difficult if she were to be isolated by ignorance of what is upsetting her family and carers.

Justice – should scarce resources be used on this new drug? Because her parents are desperate, should Jane be given a drug which, in the specialist's opinion, will not benefit her?

Best interests – what are Jane's best interests and who should decide them? What weight should be given to Jane's own views based on her experience of her illness?

In such situations, further discussion between the parents and staff whom they trust is usually the key to resolving the situation. The parents will need to understand the mutual benefits of adopting as open a pattern of communication as possible. They may be helped by a member of staff being present or helping them talk or listen to the child, who will usually understand more than the parents suspect.

Parents almost always wish to do the best for their child. Detailed explanation is likely to help them see that the child's best interests may not be to seek further cure but to accept a change of focus towards palliative care. A second opinion from an independent specialist may be helpful, as may a specific ethical review. If, despite all efforts to reach agreement, the parents reject the doctor's advice, it is fairest to let a court of law decide whether or not to accept the parents' demands.

provision of information sheets in an appropriate form and language or by the use of independent translators.
- Parents must have the option to withdraw their child from the research at any stage without prejudice.
- The project must be reviewed and approved by an independent scientific and ethical process (Research Ethics Committee).

Evidence-based paediatrics

Clinicians have always sought to base their decisions on the best available evidence. However, such decisions have often been made intuitively, given as clinical opinion, which is difficult to generalise, scrutinise or challenge. Evidence-based practice provides a systematic approach to enable clinicians to efficiently use the best available evidence, usually from research, to help them solve their clinical problems. The difference between this approach and old-style clinical practice is that clinicians need to know how to turn their clinical problems into questions that can be answered by the research literature, to search the literature efficiently, and to analyse the evidence, using epidemiological and biostatistical rules (Figs 5.8 and 5.9). Sometimes, the best available evidence will be a high-quality, systematic review of randomised controlled trials, which are directly applicable to a particular patient. For other questions, lack of more valid studies may mean that one has to base one's decision on previous experience with a small number of similar patients. The important factor is that, for any decision, clinicians know the strength of the evidence, and therefore the degree of uncertainty. As this approach requires clinicians to be explicit about the evidence they use, others involved in the decisions (patients, parents, managers and other clinicians) can debate and judge the evidence for themselves.

Application of evidence-based medicine to clinical problems

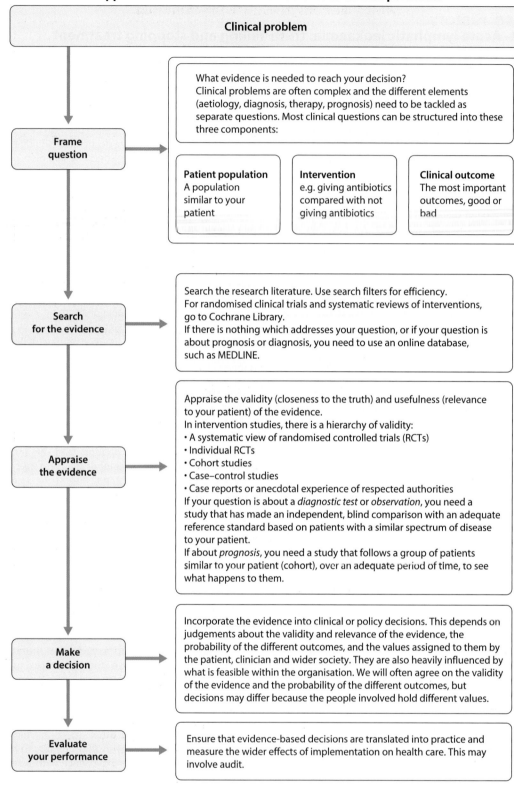

Clinical problem

Frame question

What evidence is needed to reach your decision?
Clinical problems are often complex and the different elements (aetiology, diagnosis, therapy, prognosis) need to be tackled as separate questions. Most clinical questions can be structured into these three components:

Patient population
A population similar to your patient

Intervention
e.g. giving antibiotics compared with not giving antibiotics

Clinical outcome
The most important outcomes, good or bad

Search for the evidence

Search the research literature. Use search filters for efficiency.
For randomised clinical trials and systematic reviews of interventions, go to Cochrane Library.
If there is nothing which addresses your question, or if your question is about prognosis or diagnosis, you need to use an online database, such as MEDLINE.

Appraise the evidence

Appraise the validity (closeness to the truth) and usefulness (relevance to your patient) of the evidence.
In intervention studies, there is a hierarchy of validity:
• A systematic view of randomised controlled trials (RCTs)
• Individual RCTs
• Cohort studies
• Case–control studies
• Case reports or anecdotal experience of respected authorities
If your question is about a *diagnostic test* or *observation*, you need a study that has made an independent, blind comparison with an adequate reference standard based on patients with a similar spectrum of disease to your patient.
If about *prognosis*, you need a study that follows a group of patients similar to your patient (cohort), over an adequate period of time, to see what happens to them.

Make a decision

Incorporate the evidence into clinical or policy decisions. This depends on judgements about the validity and relevance of the evidence, the probability of the different outcomes, and the values assigned to them by the patient, clinician and wider society. They are also heavily influenced by what is feasible within the organisation. We will often agree on the validity of the evidence and the probability of the different outcomes, but decisions may differ because the people involved hold different values.

Evaluate your performance

Ensure that evidence-based decisions are translated into practice and measure the wider effects of implementation on health care. This may involve audit.

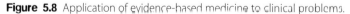

Figure 5.8 Application of evidence-based medicine to clinical problems.

Example of evidence-based practice in solving a clinical problem – the management of acute otitis media

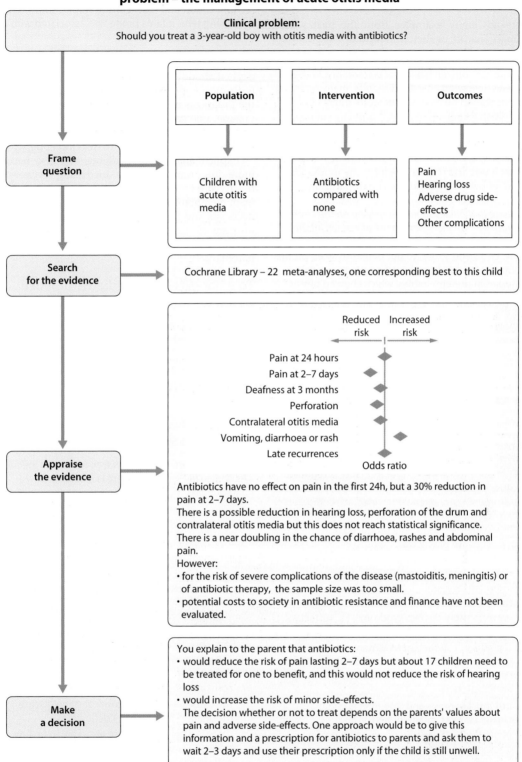

Figure 5.9 An example of an evidence-based medicine approach to a clinical problem – the treatment of acute otitis media with antibiotics.

Why practise evidence-based paediatrics?

There are many examples from the past where, through lack of evidence, clinicians have harmed children, e.g.:

- *Blindness from retinopathy of prematurity*. In the 1950s, following anecdotal reports, many neonatal units started nursing all premature infants in additional ambient oxygen, irrespective of need. This reduced mortality, but as no properly conducted trials were performed of this new therapy, it took several years for it to be realised that it was also responsible for many thousands of babies becoming blind from retinopathy of prematurity.
- *Advice that babies should sleep lying on their front (prone), which increases the risk of sudden infant death syndrome (SIDS)*. Medical advice given during the 1970s and 1980s, to put babies to sleep prone, appears to have been based on physiological studies in preterm babies, which showed better oxygenation when nursed prone. Furthermore, autopsies on some infants who died of SIDS showed milk in the trachea, which was assumed to have been aspirated and this was thought to be more likely if they were lying on their back. However, an accumulation of more valid evidence from cohort and case–control studies showed that nursing term infants prone was associated with an increased risk of SIDS.

Evidence-based medicine allows clinicians to be explicit about the probability (or risk) of important outcomes. For example, in discussing with parents the prognosis of a child who has had a febrile convulsion, one can state that 'the risk of developing epilepsy is 1 in 100' instead of using vague terms, such as 'he/she is unlikely to develop epilepsy'.

Explicit analysis of evidence has also become more important with the increasing delivery of health care by teams rather than individuals. Each team member needs to understand the rationale for decisions and the probability of different outcomes in order to make their own clinical decisions and to provide consistent information to patients and parents.

To what extent is paediatric practice based on sound evidence?

There are two paediatric specialities in which there is a considerable body of reliable, high-quality

---

Box 5.4 Examples of the range of evidence available in paediatrics

1. Clear evidence of benefit

Surfactant therapy in preterm infants
The meta-analysis (see Fig. 10.12) from a Cochrane systematic review shows that mortality is reduced by 40% in preterm infants with respiratory distress syndrome (RDS) treated with surfactant compared with placebo.

This evidence was rapidly produced and introduced into practice as:

- respiratory distress syndrome is a common cause of death and morbidity in a neonatal intensive care unit
- there is a clearly understood disease mechanism for respiratory distress syndrome, i.e. surfactant deficiency
- the effect of surfactant treatment was immediately obvious at the cot-side – ventilator settings usually have to be reduced shortly after administration
- potential benefits and side-effects could be clearly defined and identified
- neonatologists are a relatively small group of doctors who meet regularly – national and international studies could be organised and their results quickly disseminated
- there was widespread financial support and involvement from the pharmaceutical industry.

2. Clear evidence, but need to balance benefits and harms

Antibiotic treatment for children with otitis media
As shown in Figure 5.9, there is a balance of risk and benefits.

3. No clear evidence

Bulk forming laxatives for constipation
Bulk forming laxatives, such as methylcellulose or ispaghula husk, are used in children with constipation. However, this is not based on clear evidence. There are no systematic reviews and no randomised controlled studies of these agents in children.

Some possible reasons for the lack of evidence on the use of these laxatives in this common condition are:

- constipation is not a life-threatening disorder
- the causes are multifactorial and the disease mechanism is not clearly defined
- there is a belief that there are likely to be few side-effects to the use of bulk forming laxatives and clinicians are prepared to prescribe them without clear evidence
- there is limited support for studies from the pharmaceutical industry
- the research agenda is not driven by such clinical problems.

evidence underpinning clinical practice, namely paediatric oncology and, to a lesser extent, neonatology. Management protocols of virtually all children with cancer are part of multicentre trials designed to identify which treatment gives the best possible results. The trials are national or, increasingly, international, and include short- and long-term follow-up. Examples of the range of evidence available in paediatrics are given in Box 5.4. In general, the evidence base for paediatrics is poorer than in adult medicine. Reasons for this include:

- The relatively small number of children with significant illness requiring investigation and treatment. To overcome this, multicentre trials are required, which are more difficult to organise and expensive.
- Additional ethical limitations
    - subjecting children to additional investigations or giving a new treatment is severely limited by the inability of the child to give consent. Some parents are concerned that participating in a trial could mean that their child could receive treatment that turns out to be inferior to the standard treatment and could have unknown side-effects.
    - there is concern over the ability of parents to give truly informed consent immediately after the acute onset of serious illness, e.g. the birth of a preterm infant, meningococcal septicaemia or meningitis.
- Limited investment by the pharmaceutical industry in drug trials, as drug use in children is insufficient to justify the cost and ethical difficulties of conducting trials. As a result, approximately 50% of drug treatments in children are unlicensed ('off label').

The consequence is that there is less of a culture of randomised controlled trials in paediatrics compared with adult medicine.

For evidence-based practice to become more widespread, clinicians must recognise the need to ask questions, particularly about procedures or interventions which are common practice. However, evidence-based medicine is not cookbook medicine. Incontrovertible evidence is rare, and clinical decisions complex, which is why clinical care is provided by clinicians and not technicians. Evidence-based health care cannot change this, but is an essential tool to help clinicians make rational, informed decisions together with their patients. In addition, evidence-based paediatrics provides a way for clinicians to articulate their priorities for research and thereby set a research agenda which is relevant to service needs.

Summary

Evidence-based paediatrics:
- requires clinical problems to be framed into questions, to search the literature and then appraise the evidence in order to make a decision
- is less well developed than in adult medicine
- should be adopted whenever possible; however, clinical decisions are complex and the evidence base usually informs rather than determines clinical decision-making.

Further reading

Department of Health 2004 National Service Framework for Children, Young People and Maternity Services – Core Standards, Children and Young People who are Ill, Standards for Hospital Services, Disabled Children and Young People and those with Complex Health Needs, The Mental Health and Psychological Well-being of Children and Young People, Maternity Services. Department of Health

Glasziou P P, Del Mar C B, Sanders S L, Hayem M 2007 Antibiotics for acute otitis media in children. The Cochrane Database of Systematic Reviews

Moyer V A, Elliot E J, Davis R L et al 2000 Evidence based paediatrics and child health. BMJ Books, London

Nelson K B, Ellenberg J H 1978 Prognosis in children with febrile seizures. Pediatrics 61:720–727

Internet

Search filters:
http://www.ihs.ox.ac.uk/library/filters.html
www.nelh.nhs.uk/
www.cebm.net/
Evidence based medicine:
www.tripdatabase.com
www.clinicalevidence.com
www.cochrane.org
Consent:
www.dh.gov.uk/PolicyAndGuidance/HealthAndSocial CareTopics/Consent

Paediatric emergencies

There are few situations that provoke greater anxiety than being called to see a child who is seriously ill. This chapter outlines a basic approach to the emergency management of seriously ill children.

 Doctors should be able to provide life support for children of all ages, from newborn to adolescents.

The seriously ill child

The rapid clinical assessment of the seriously ill child will identify if there is potential respiratory, circulatory or neurological failure. This should take less than 1 minute. Normal vital signs are shown in Figure 6.1 and how a rapid assessment is performed in Figure 6.2. Resuscitation is given immediately if necessary, followed by secondary assessment and other emergency treatment.

The seriously ill child may present with shock, respiratory distress, as a drowsy/unconscious or fitting child or with a surgical emergency. Their causes are listed in Figure 6.4. In children, the key to successful outcome is the early recognition and active management of conditions that are life-threatening and potentially reversible.

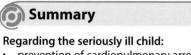 **Summary**

Regarding the seriously ill child:
- prevention of cardiopulmonary arrest is by early recognition and treatment of respiratory distress, respiratory or circulatory failure.

Vital signs

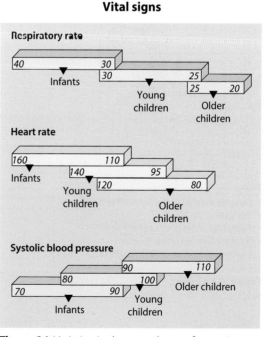

Figure 6.1 Variation in the normal range for respiratory rate, heart rate and systolic blood pressure with age.

Assessment of the seriously ill child

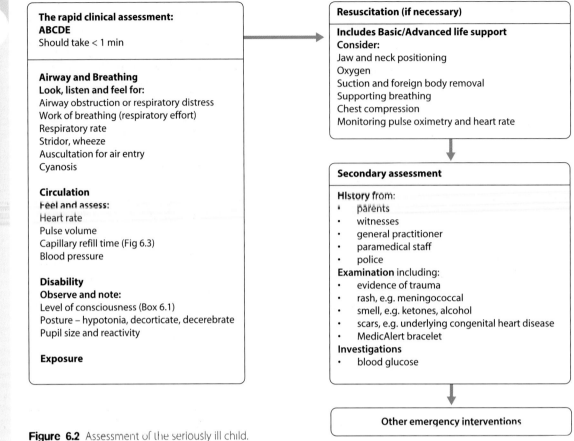

The rapid clinical assessment:
ABCDE
Should take < 1 min

Airway and Breathing
Look, listen and feel for:
Airway obstruction or respiratory distress
Work of breathing (respiratory effort)
Respiratory rate
Stridor, wheeze
Auscultation for air entry
Cyanosis

Circulation
Feel and assess:
Heart rate
Pulse volume
Capillary refill time (Fig 6.3)
Blood pressure

Disability
Observe and note:
Level of consciousness (Box 6.1)
Posture – hypotonia, decorticate, decerebrate
Pupil size and reactivity

Exposure

Resuscitation (if necessary)

Includes Basic/Advanced life support
Consider:
Jaw and neck positioning
Oxygen
Suction and foreign body removal
Supporting breathing
Chest compression
Monitoring pulse oximetry and heart rate

Secondary assessment

History from:
• parents
• witnesses
• general practitioner
• paramedical staff
• police
Examination including:
• evidence of trauma
• rash, e.g. meningococcal
• smell, e.g. ketones, alcohol
• scars, e.g. underlying congenital heart disease
• MedicAlert bracelet
Investigations
• blood glucose

Other emergency interventions

Figure 6.2 Assessment of the seriously ill child.

Capillary refill time

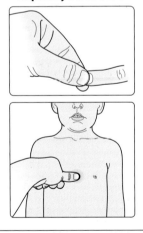

Press on the skin of the sternum or a digit at the level of the heart
Apply blanching pressure for 5 seconds
Measure time for blush to return
Prolonged capillary refill if >2 seconds

Figure 6.3 Capillary refill time. Digital pressure for 5 seconds. Normal <2 seconds.

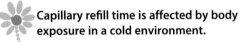 **Capillary refill time is affected by body exposure in a cold environment.**

Box 6.1 AVPU rapid assessment of level of consciousness – more detailed evaluation is with the Glasgow Coma Scale (see Table 6.2)

A	ALERT
V	Responds to VOICE
P	Responds to PAIN
U	UNRESPONSIVE

A score of P means that the child's airway is at risk and will need to be maintained by a manoeuvre or adjunct.

Cardiopulmonary resuscitation

In adults, cardiopulmonary arrest is often cardiac in origin, secondary to ischaemic heart disease. In contrast, children usually have healthy hearts but experience hypoxia from respiratory or neurological failure or shock. If this occurs, irrespective of the cause, basic life support must be started immediately.

Basic life support (Fig. 6.5)

Advanced life support (Fig. 6.6)

Children who have been resuscitated successfully should be transferred to a paediatric high-dependency or intensive care unit.

Presentation and causes of serious illness in children

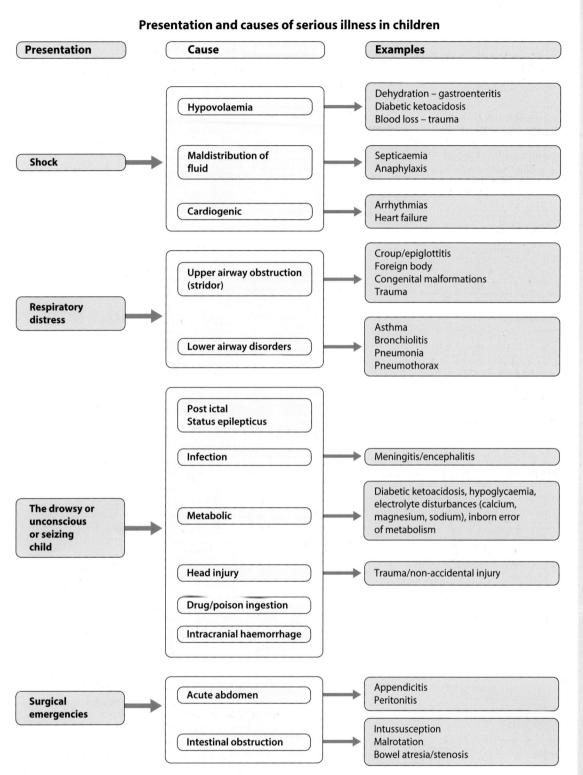

Figure 6.4 The main modes of presentation of serious illness in children and their causes.

Basic life support

SAFE approach → Shout for help
Approach with care
Free from danger
Evaluate **ABC**

Check responsiveness:
Ask 'Are you all right?'
Stimulate
Do not shake children with
suspected cervical spine injury

No response

Open airway:
• Head tilt, chin lift
• Jaw thrust (if unsuccessful)

No breathing

Check breathing for max 10 secs:
• Look, listen, feel

Breathe
Remove any obvious obstruction
Give 5 initial rescue breaths

Check pulse for max 10 secs:
>1 year old – carotid
<1 year old – brachial

No pulse or <60/min

Compress chest
Rate: 100 compressions/min
Compression: Ventilation ratio for
all children:
Two rescuers – 15:2
Lone rescuer – 30:2

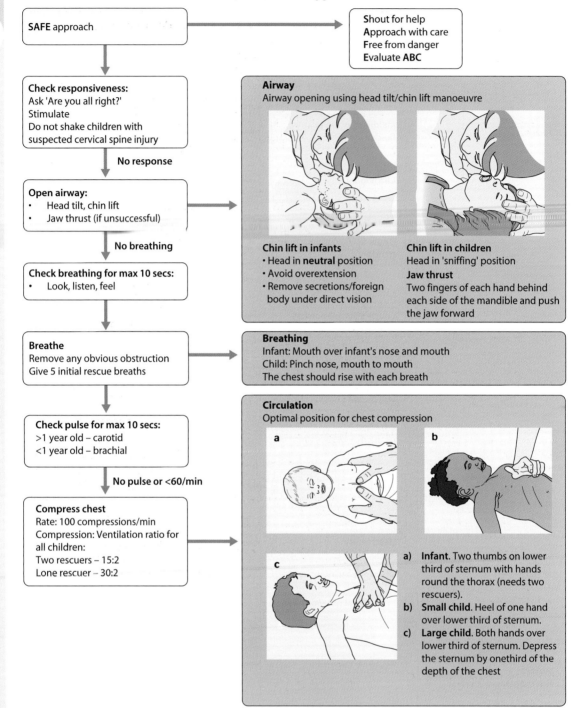

Airway
Airway opening using head tilt/chin lift manoeuvre

Chin lift in infants
• Head in **neutral** position
• Avoid overextension
• Remove secretions/foreign
  body under direct vision

Chin lift in children
Head in 'sniffing' position
Jaw thrust
Two fingers of each hand behind
each side of the mandible and push
the jaw forward

Breathing
Infant: Mouth over infant's nose and mouth
Child: Pinch nose, mouth to mouth
The chest should rise with each breath

Circulation
Optimal position for chest compression

a) **Infant.** Two thumbs on lower
    third of sternum with hands
    round the thorax (needs two
    rescuers).
b) **Small child.** Heel of one hand
    over lower third of sternum.
c) **Large child.** Both hands over
    lower third of sternum. Depress
    the sternum by onethird of the
    depth of the chest

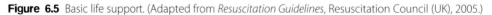

Figure 6.5 Basic life support. (Adapted from *Resuscitation Guidelines*, Resuscitation Council (UK), 2005.)

Advanced life support

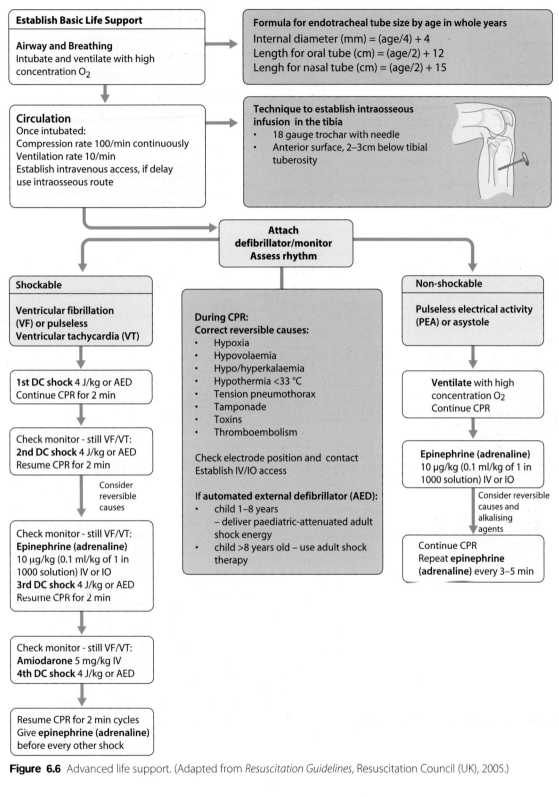

Establish Basic Life Support

Airway and Breathing
Intubate and ventilate with high concentration O₂

Formula for endotracheal tube size by age in whole years
Internal diameter (mm) = (age/4) + 4
Length for oral tube (cm) = (age/2) + 12
Lengh for nasal tube (cm) = (age/2) + 15

Circulation
Once intubated:
Compression rate 100/min continuously
Ventilation rate 10/min
Establish intravenous access, if delay use intraosseous route

Technique to establish intraosseous infusion in the tibia
- 18 gauge trochar with needle
- Anterior surface, 2–3cm below tibial tuberosity

Attach defibrillator/monitor Assess rhythm

Shockable

Ventricular fibrillation (VF) or pulseless Ventricular tachycardia (VT)

1st DC shock 4 J/kg or AED
Continue CPR for 2 min

Check monitor - still VF/VT:
2nd DC shock 4 J/kg or AED
Resume CPR for 2 min

Consider reversible causes

Check monitor - still VF/VT:
Epinephrine (adrenaline)
10 µg/kg (0.1 ml/kg of 1 in 1000 solution) IV or IO
3rd DC shock 4 J/kg or AED
Resume CPR for 2 min

Check monitor - still VF/VT:
Amiodarone 5 mg/kg IV
4th DC shock 4 J/kg or AED

Resume CPR for 2 min cycles
Give **epinephrine (adrenaline)** before every other shock

During CPR:
Correct reversible causes:
- Hypoxia
- Hypovolaemia
- Hypo/hyperkalaemia
- Hypothermia <33 °C
- Tension pneumothorax
- Tamponade
- Toxins
- Thromboembolism

Check electrode position and contact
Establish IV/IO access

If **automated external defibrillator (AED):**
- child 1–8 years
  – deliver paediatric-attenuated adult shock energy
- child >8 years old – use adult shock therapy

Non-shockable

Pulseless electrical activity (PEA) or asystole

Ventilate with high concentration O₂
Continue CPR

Epinephrine (adrenaline)
10 µg/kg (0.1 ml/kg of 1 in 1000 solution) IV or IO

Consider reversible causes and alkalising agents

Continue CPR
Repeat **epinephrine (adrenaline)** every 3–5 min

Figure 6.6 Advanced life support. (Adapted from *Resuscitation Guidelines*, Resuscitation Council (UK), 2005.)

Management of the seriously injured child

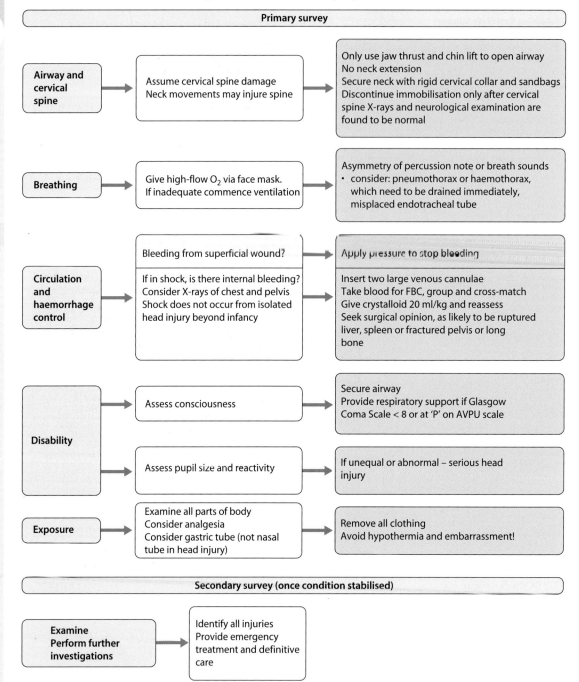

Figure 6.7 Management of the seriously injured child.

The seriously injured child

Management of the seriously injured child must take account of potential injury to the cervical spine and other bones and internal injuries (Fig. 6.7).

Shock

Shock is present when the circulation is inadequate to meet the demands of the tissues. Critically ill children are often in shock, usually because of hypovolaemia due to fluid loss or maldistribution of fluid, as occurs in sepsis or intestinal obstruction.

Why are children so susceptible to fluid loss?

Children normally require a much higher fluid intake per kilogram of body weight than adults (Table 6.1). This is because they have a higher surface area to volume ratio and a higher basal metabolic rate. Children may therefore become dehydrated if:

- they are unable to take oral fluids
- there are additional fluid losses due to fever, diarrhoea or increased insensible losses (e.g. due to increased sweating or tachypnoea)
- there is loss of the normal fluid-retaining mechanisms, e.g. burns, the permeable skin of premature infants, increased urinary losses or capillary leak.

Clinical features

The clinical features of shock are due to compensatory physiological mechanisms to maintain the circulation and the direct effects of poor perfusion of tissues and organs (Box 6.2). In early, compensated shock, the blood pressure is maintained by increased heart and respiratory rates, redistribution of blood from venous reserve volume and diversion of blood flow from non-essential tissues such as the skin in the peripheries, which become cold. In shock due to dehydration, there is usually >10% loss of body weight (see Ch. 13) and a profound metabolic acidosis and it is compounded by failure to feed and drink whilst severely ill. After acute blood loss or redistribution of blood volume because of infection, low blood pressure is a late feature. It signifies that compensatory responses are failing. In late or uncompensated shock, compensatory mechanisms fail and blood pressure falls and lactic acidosis increases. It is important to recognise early, compensated shock, as this is reversible, in contrast to uncompensated shock, which may be irreversible.

Management priorities

Fluid resuscitation

Rapid restoration of the intravascular circulating volume is the priority (Fig. 6.8). This will usually be with 0.9% saline, or blood if following trauma.

Subsequent management

If there is no improvement following fluid resuscitation or there is progression of shock and respiratory failure, a paediatric intensive care unit should be involved and transfer arranged as the child may need:

Box 6.2 Clinical signs of shock

Early (compensated)	Late (decompensated)
Tachypnoea	Acidotic (Kussmaul)
Tachycardia	breathing
Decreased skin turgor	Bradycardia
Sunken eyes and	Confusion/depressed
fontanelle	cerebral state
Delayed capillary refill	Blue peripheries
(>2 s)	Absent urine output
Mottled, pale, cold skin	Hypotension
Core–peripheral	
temperature gap (>4°C)	
Decreased urinary output	

Summary

Shock in children:
- is often from hypovolaemia
- the early signs of compensated shock are from increased sympathetic tone – tachycardia, pallor and peripheral vasoconstriction (prolonged capillary refill time); its recognition is important as at this stage it is reversible
- fluid therapy is the key to its successful treatment.

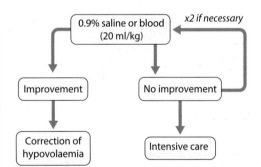

Figure 6.8 Initial fluid resuscitation in shock.

Table 6.1 Fluid intake at different ages

Body weight	Fluid requirement/24 h	Volume/kg per hour (approximate)
First 10 kg	100 ml/kg	4 ml/kg
Second 10 kg	50 ml/kg	2 ml/kg
Subsequent kg	20 ml/kg	1 ml/kg

Examples of calculations		
Weight of child	**Fluid requirement/24 h**	**Volume per hour (approximate)**
Infant 7 kg	700 ml	28 ml/h
Child 18 kg	1000 + 400 = 1400 ml	40 + 16 = 56 ml/h
Adolescent 62 kg	1000 + 500 + 840 = 2340 ml	40 + 20 + 42 = 102 ml/h

- tracheal intubation and mechanical ventilation
- invasive monitoring of blood pressure
- inotropic support
- correction of haematological, biochemical and metabolic derangements
- support for renal or liver failure.

The febrile child

Most febrile children have a brief, self-limiting viral infection. Mild localised infections, e.g. otitis media or tonsillitis, may be diagnosed clinically. The clinical problem lies in identifying the relatively few children with a serious invasive bacterial infection which needs prompt treatment.

Factors which need to be considered are:

- past medical history
- illness of other family members
- if a specific illness is prevalent in the community

- immunisation status
- recent travel abroad, e.g. malaria, typhoid
- contact with animals, e.g. brucellosis
- predisposition to infection, e.g. nephrotic syndrome, sickle cell disease, HIV infection, chemotherapy for malignant disease or, rarely, a primary immunodeficiency.

Initial assessment, investigations and management

Some diagnostic clues to evaluating the febrile child are shown in Figures 6.9 and 6.10. Infants and toddlers often present with non-specific signs. If they are suspected of having a severe bacterial infection, urgent investigations called a septic screen (Box 6.3) are performed and intravenous antibiotic therapy given immediately to avoid the illness becoming more severe and to prevent rapid spread to other sites of the body. In febrile infants less

The febrile child

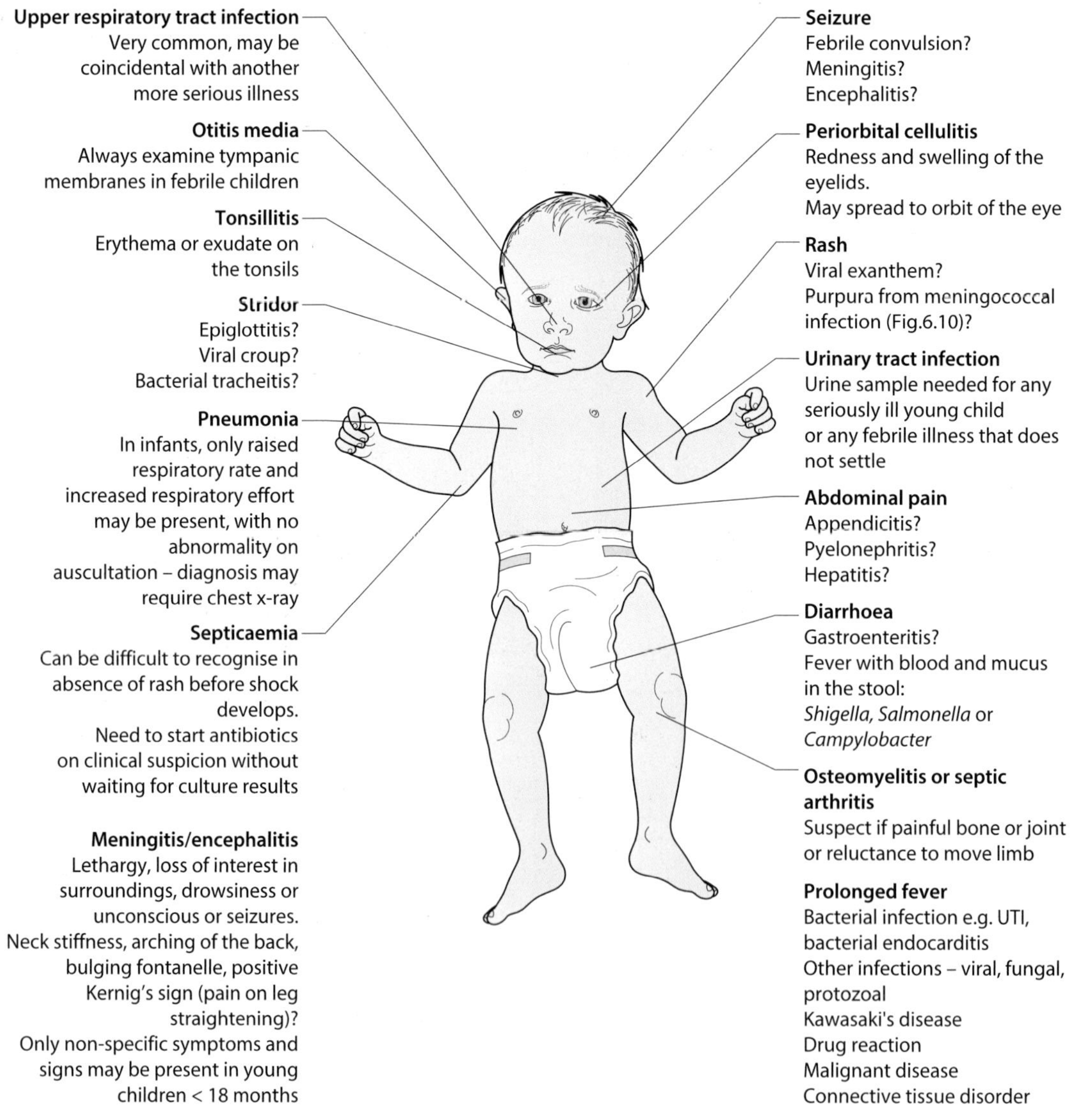

Upper respiratory tract infection
Very common, may be coincidental with another more serious illness

Otitis media
Always examine tympanic membranes in febrile children

Tonsillitis
Erythema or exudate on the tonsils

Stridor
Epiglottitis?
Viral croup?
Bacterial tracheitis?

Pneumonia
In infants, only raised respiratory rate and increased respiratory effort may be present, with no abnormality on auscultation – diagnosis may require chest x-ray

Septicaemia
Can be difficult to recognise in absence of rash before shock develops.
Need to start antibiotics on clinical suspicion without waiting for culture results

Meningitis/encephalitis
Lethargy, loss of interest in surroundings, drowsiness or unconscious or seizures.
Neck stiffness, arching of the back, bulging fontanelle, positive Kernig's sign (pain on leg straightening)?
Only non-specific symptoms and signs may be present in young children < 18 months

Seizure
Febrile convulsion?
Meningitis?
Encephalitis?

Periorbital cellulitis
Redness and swelling of the eyelids.
May spread to orbit of the eye

Rash
Viral exanthem?
Purpura from meningococcal infection (Fig.6.10)?

Urinary tract infection
Urine sample needed for any seriously ill young child or any febrile illness that does not settle

Abdominal pain
Appendicitis?
Pyelonephritis?
Hepatitis?

Diarrhoea
Gastroenteritis?
Fever with blood and mucus in the stool:
Shigella, Salmonella or *Campylobacter*

Osteomyelitis or septic arthritis
Suspect if painful bone or joint or reluctance to move limb

Prolonged fever
Bacterial infection e.g. UTI, bacterial endocarditis
Other infections – viral, fungal, protozoal
Kawasaki's disease
Drug reaction
Malignant disease
Connective tissue disorder

Figure 6.9 Some diagnostic clues to evaluating the febrile child.

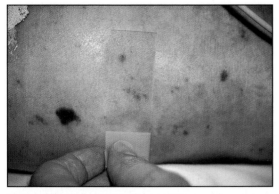

Figure 6.10 The glass test for meningococcal purpura. Parents are advised to suspect meningococcal disease if their child is febrile and has a rash that does not blanche when pressed under a glass. (Courtesy of Dr Parviz Habibi.)

Box 6.3 Septic screen

Full blood count including differential white cell count
Blood culture
Acute-phase reactant, e.g. C-reactive protein
Urine for microscopy, culture and sensitivity
CSF (unless contraindicated) for microscopy, culture and sensitivity
Chest X-ray

Summary

The febrile child:
- upper respiratory tract infection (URTI) is an extremely common cause
- check for otitis media
- serious bacterial infection must be considered
- if fever in an infant is unexplained, exclude a urinary tract infection
- the younger the child the lower the threshold for performing a septic screen and starting antibiotics.

than 2 months old, identifying serious bacterial infection is unreliable from clinical examination alone, and a septic screen and antibiotic therapy are indicated. Other factors which influence the selection of which children to investigate and treat are shown in Figure 6.11. Children who are not seriously ill can be managed at home with regular review by the parents as long as they are given clear instructions (e.g. what clinical features should prompt reassessment by a doctor).

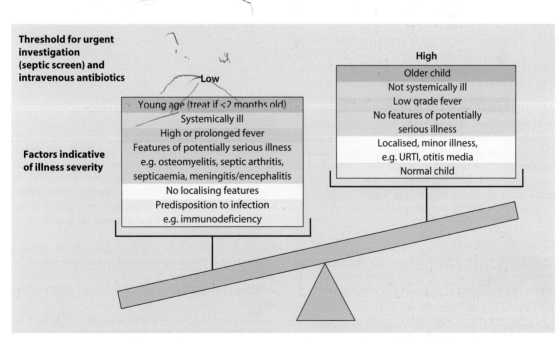

Figure 6.11 Evaluation of the need for urgent investigation and treatment in the febrile child.

Septicaemia

Bacteria may cause a focal infection or proliferate in the bloodstream, leading to septicaemia. In septicaemia, the host response includes the release of inflammatory cytokines and activation of endothelial cells which may lead to septic shock. The commonest cause of septic shock in childhood is meningococcal infection, which may or may not be accompanied by meningitis. Fortunately, its incidence in the UK has fallen markedly since immunisation was introduced. *Pneumococcus* is the commonest organism causing bacteraemia, but it is unusual for it to cause septic shock. In neonates, the commonest causes of septicaemia are group B streptococcus or Gram-negative organisms acquired from the birth canal.

Clinical features

See Box 6.4.

Management priorities

Children with septic shock will need to be rapidly stabilised and may require transfer to a paediatric intensive care unit.

Antibiotics

Choice depends on the child's age and any predisposition to infection.

Fluids

Significant hypovolaemia is often present, owing to fluid maldistribution, which occurs due to the release of vasoactive mediators by host inflammatory and endothelial cells. There is loss of intravascular proteins and fluid which may occur due to the development of a 'capillary leak' caused by endothelial cell dysfunction. Circulating plasma volume is lost into the interstitial fluid. Central venous pressure monitoring and urinary catheterisation may be required to guide the assessment of fluid balance. Capillary leak into the lungs causes pulmonary oedema, which may lead to respiratory failure, necessitating mechanical ventilation.

Circulatory support

Myocardial dysfunction occurs as inflammatory cytokines and circulating toxins depress myocardial contractility. Inotropic support may be required.

Disseminated intravascular coagulation (DIC)

Abnormal blood clotting causes widespread microvascular thrombosis and consumption of clotting factors. If bleeding occurs, clotting derangement should be corrected with fresh frozen plasma and platelet transfusions.

Steroids

There is no evidence that steroids are of benefit in septic shock.

Box 6.4 Clinical features of septicaemia

History	Examination
Fever	Fever
Poor feeding	Purpuric rash
Miserable	(meningococcal
Lethargy	septicaemia)
History of focal infection, e.g.	Irritability
meningitis, osteomyelitis,	Shock
gastroenteritis, cellulitis	Multi-organ failure
Predisposing conditions,	
e.g. sickle cell disease,	
immunodeficiency	

Summary

Septicaemia:
- the most common cause of septic shock in children is meningococcal disease
- may occur without meningitis
- early antibiotic therapy and fluid resuscitation are life-saving
- may need admission to paediatric intensive care for multi-organ failure.

Coma

In coma, there is disturbance of the functioning of the cerebral hemispheres and/or the reticular activating system of the brainstem. The level of awareness may range from excessive drowsiness to unconsciousness. It is assessed by rapidly using AVPU or the Glasgow Coma Scale (Table 6.2).

The immediate assessment of a child in coma is shown in Figures 6.12 and 6.13. The causes, clinical features and investigations of coma are listed in Table 6.3. In contrast to adults, most children have a diffuse metabolic insult rather than a structural lesion.

The history, examination and investigation of coma are directed towards the cause. Treatment should be directed to treatable causes, especially infection.

Table 6.2 Glasgow Coma Scale, incorporating Children's Coma Scale

| | Glasgow Coma Scale (4-15 years) | Children's Coma Scale (<4 years) | |
	Response	Response	Score
Eyes	Open spontaneously	Open spontaneously	4
	Verbal command	React to speech	3
	Pain	React to pain	2
	No response	No response	1
Best motor response			
Verbal command	Obeys	Spontaneous or obeys verbal command	6
Painful stimulus	Localises pain	Localises pain	5
	Withdraws	Withdraws	4
	Abnormal flexion	Abnormal flexion (decorticate posture)	3
	Extension	Abnormal extension (decerebrate posture)	2
	No response	No response	1
Best verbal response	Oriented and converses	Smiles, orientated to sounds, follows objects, interacts	5
	Disoriented and converses	Fewer than usual words, spontaneous irritable cry	4
	Inappropriate words	Cries only to pain	3
	Incomprehensible sounds	Moans to pain	2
	No response	No response to pain	1

A score of <8 out of 15 means that the child's airway is at risk and will need to be maintained by a manoeuvre or adjunct.

Initial assessment and management of coma

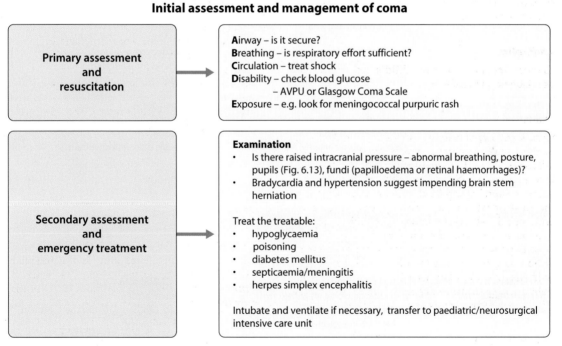

Primary assessment and resuscitation

Airway – is it secure?
Breathing – is respiratory effort sufficient?
Circulation – treat shock
Disability – check blood glucose
　　　　　– AVPU or Glasgow Coma Scale
Exposure – e.g. look for meningococcal purpuric rash

Secondary assessment and emergency treatment

Examination
- Is there raised intracranial pressure – abnormal breathing, posture, pupils (Fig. 6.13), fundi (papilloedema or retinal haemorrhages)?
- Bradycardia and hypertension suggest impending brain stem herniation

Treat the treatable:
- hypoglycaemia
- poisoning
- diabetes mellitus
- septicaemia/meningitis
- herpes simplex encephalitis

Intubate and ventilate if necessary, transfer to paediatric/neurosurgical intensive care unit

Figure 6.12 Initial assessment and management of coma.

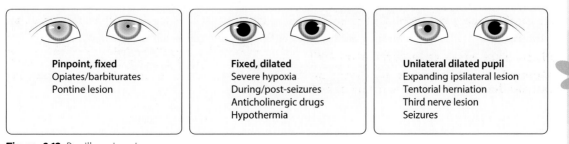

Pinpoint, fixed
Opiates/barbiturates
Pontine lesion

Fixed, dilated
Severe hypoxia
During/post-seizures
Anticholinergic drugs
Hypothermia

Unilateral dilated pupil
Expanding ipsilateral lesion
Tentorial herniation
Third nerve lesion
Seizures

Figure 6.13 Pupillary signs in coma.

Table 6.3 Causes, history and examination, and investigation of coma

Cause	History and examination	Diagnostic investigations
Infection Meningitis or meningoencephalitis	Fever Irritability, lethargy, drowsiness Poor feeding Rash, e.g. meningococcal purpura Seizures Overseas travel	Full blood count Culture of blood, urine, infected sites, CSF (unless contraindicated) for bacteria and viruses Acute-phase reactant Rapid bacterial antigen/PCR tests for organisms
Metabolic Diabetes mellitus	Previously diagnosed diabetes mellitus Diabetic ketoacidosis	Blood glucose, plasma electrolytes Urine for glucose and ketones Blood gas analysis
Inborn errors of metabolism	Previous history of loss of consciousness Sudden collapse Consanguinity Developmental delay Death or illness of siblings Hepatomegaly	Blood glucose Blood gas analysis Blood ammonia, lactate Urine amino and organic acids Plasma amino acids
Hepatic failure	Jaundice Abnormal bleeding	Abnormal liver function tests Prolonged prothrombin time
Acute renal failure	Oliguria Hypertension	Abnormal creatinine
Hypoglycaemia	Any acutely ill child Known diabetes mellitus Sudden onset of coma	Low blood glucose
Poisoning	Accidental – poison usually identified Deliberate – tablets may be found, also illicit drugs and alcohol	Toxicology screen Plasma level for paracetamol and salicylates
Status epilepticus or post-ictal	Past history of seizures Neurocutaneous lesions on the skin Developmental delay Ongoing seizure activity, e.g. abnormal eye movements Focal neurological signs	Blood glucose Electrolytes – sodium, potassium, calcium, magnesium Drug levels if on anticonvulsants EEG CT scan
Trauma – accidental/ non-accidental	History of road traffic accident, fall, etc. Bruising, haemorrhage Fractures – cervical spine, etc. Focal neurology Retinal haemorrhages	Radiological – plain X-rays or CT/MRI scans
Intracranial tumour or haemorrhage/infarct/ abscess	Raised intracranial pressure: • headache worse on lying down • early morning vomiting • focal neurological signs, e.g. squint, ataxia • personality change • papilloedema/retinal haemorrhage • hypertension	Cranial CT/MRI scan Coagulation screen Screen for procoagulant disorders (protein C and S deficiency) Echocardiogram to exclude infective endocarditis
Hypertension	Symptoms and signs of raised intracranial pressure Fundoscopy – hypertensive changes High blood pressure	Left ventricular hypertrophy on ECG or echocardiography Creatinine and electrolytes

Status epilepticus

This is a seizure lasting 30 minutes or longer, or when successive seizures occur so frequently that the patient does not recover consciousness between them. After immediate primary assessment and resuscitation, the priority is to stop the seizure as quickly as possible (Fig. 6.14).

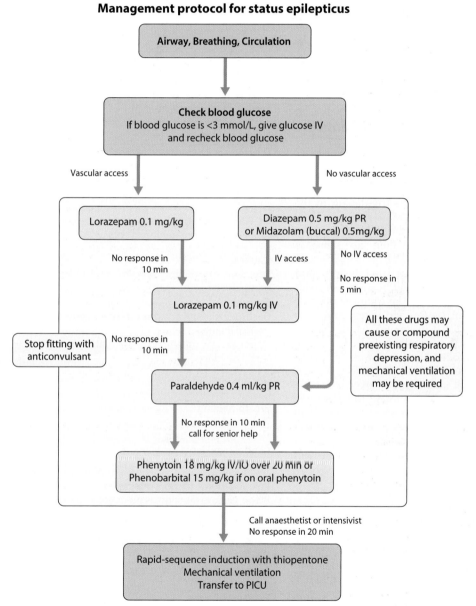

Figure 6.14 Management protocol for status epilepticus. (Adapted from *Advanced Paediatric Life Support*, BMJ Publishing Group, London, 2005.)

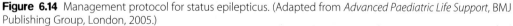

Anaphylaxis

In children, the most common causes are ingestion or contact with nuts, egg, milk or drugs. Urticaria and angioedema causing facial swelling are treated with an oral antihistamine (e.g. chlorphenamine) and observed over 2 hours for possible complications. Anaphylaxis is life-threatening, from laryngeal oedema, brochoconstriction and shock. Its management is outlined in Figure 6.15. Children who have had a serious allergic reaction should carry an epinephrine (adrenaline) auto-injector (e.g. Epipen) with them so that treatment can be initiated immediately.

Apparent life-threatening events (ALTE)

These occur in infants and are a combination of apnoea, colour change, alteration in muscle tone, choking or gagging, which are frightening to the observer. They may occur on more than one occasion. ALTEs may be the presentation of a potentially serious disorder, although often no cause is identified.

Management requires a detailed history and thorough examination to identify problems with the baby or in care-giving. The infant should be admitted to hospital. Causes and investigations to be considered are listed in Box 6.5. Multi-channel overnight monitoring is usually indicated.

In most, the episode is brief, with rapid recovery, and the baby is well clinically. Baseline investigations and overnight monitoring of oxygen saturation, respiration and ECG are found to be normal. The parents should be taught resuscitation and will find it helpful to receive follow-up from a specialist paediatric nurse and paediatrician.

Detailed specialist investigation and assessment will be required if clinical, biochemical or physiological abnormalities are identified.

The death of a child

The risk of death is four times greater during infancy than at any other age in childhood. In many, a serious condition will have been diagnosed before or after birth, such as a congenital abnormality or complications of prematurity. Deaths which occur suddenly and unexpectedly in infancy are known as sudden unexpected death in infancy (SUDI). In some, a previously undiagnosed congenital abnormality, e.g. congenital heart disease, will be found at autopsy. Rarely, an inherited metabolic

Immediate management of anaphylaxis

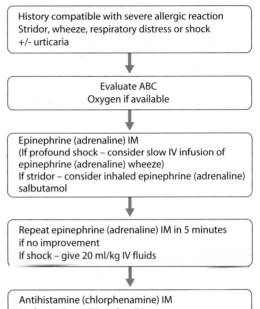

Figure 6.15 Management of anaphylaxis.

Box 6.5 Causes and investigations to be considered in apparent life-threatening events

Causes
Infections – respiratory syncytial virus (RSV), pertussis
Seizures
Gastro-oesophageal reflux (present in one-third of normal infants)
Upper airways obstruction – natural or imposed
No cause identified

Uncommon
Cardiac arrhythmia
Breath-holding
Anaemia
Heavy wrapping/heat stress
Central hypoventilation syndrome
Cyanotic spells from intrapulmonary shunting

Investigations to be considered
Blood glucose (as soon as possible)
Blood gas (as soon as possible)
Oxygen saturation monitoring
Cardiorespiratory monitoring
EEG
Oesophageal pH monitoring
Barium swallow
Full blood count
Urea and electrolytes, liver function tests
Lactate
Urine (collect and freeze first sample)
– metabolic studies
– microscopy and culture
– toxicology
ECG – for QT_c conduction pathway abnormality
Chest X-ray
Lumbar puncture

disorder is identified, in particular the fatty acid oxidation defect medium-chain acyl-CoA dehydrogenase deficiency (MCAD), which can very rarely result in sudden death in infants, but is increasingly identified in the UK from routine biochemical screening (Guthrie test) as the test for this disorder is being introduced more widely. After 1 month of age, in most instances of sudden and unexplained death, no cause is identified and the death is classified as sudden infant death syndrome (SIDS). The vast majority of such deaths, even when occurring several times in the same family, are due to natural causes. Rarely, the death may be due to suffocation or other forms of non-accidental injury. In 2003, in the UK, three mothers imprisoned after the loss of more than one infant had their convictions overturned. This followed concern about the standard of proof required from medical expert witnesses in the absence of eye witness evidence of harmful conduct and about the quality of the procedures adopted during the investigation of the deaths. Since then, new procedures have been recommended in order to prevent unwarranted incrimination of parents whilst also protecting other infants and children in the family from risk of injury.

Sudden infant death syndrome

This is defined as the sudden and unexpected death of an infant or young child for which no adequate cause is found after a thorough postmortem examination. There is marked variation in the incidence of SIDS in different countries, suggesting that environmental factors are important (Box 6.6). SIDS occurs most commonly at 2–4 months of age (Fig. 6.16). The risk for subsequent children is slightly increased.

In the UK, the incidence of SIDS has fallen dramatically during the last few years (Fig. 6.17), coinciding with a national 'Back to Sleep' campaign (Fig. 6.18). This advocates that:

- infants should be put to sleep on their back (not their front or side)
- overheating by heavy wrapping and high room temperature should be avoided
- infants should be placed in the 'feet to foot' position
- parents should not smoke near their infants

● ●

Box 6.6 Factors associated with SIDS (based on data from Fleming P et al, *Sudden unexpected deaths in infancy*, The Stationery Office, London, 2000, with permission)

The infant
Age 1–6 months, peak at 12 weeks
Low birthweight and preterm (but 60% are normal birthweight term infants)
Sex (boys 60%)
Multiple births

The parents
Low income*
Poor or overcrowded housing
Maternal age (mother aged <20 years has three times the risk of a mother aged 25–29 years, but 80% of affected mothers are >20 years old)*
Single unsupported mother (twice the rate of supported mothers)
High maternal parity*
Maternal smoking during pregnancy (1–9 cigarettes/day doubles the risk: >20/day increases the risk fivefold)*
Parental smoking after baby's birth

The environment
The infant sleeps lying prone
The infant is overheated from high room temperature and too may clothes and covers, particularly when ill

*Three of these four factors are present in over 40% of SIDS but only 8% of control families.

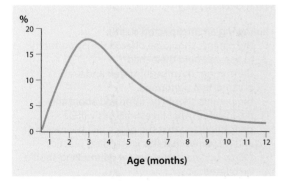

Figure 6.16 Age distribution of SIDS. (Based on data from Fleming P et al, *Sudden unexpected deaths in infancy*, The Stationery Office, London, 2000, with permission.)

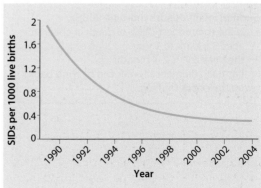

Figure 6.17 Decline in the number of deaths from SIDS in the UK from 1.9/1000 live births in 1989 to 0.41 in 2004.

Prevention of sudden infant death syndrome

Figure 6.18 Key features of the 'Back to Sleep' campaign.

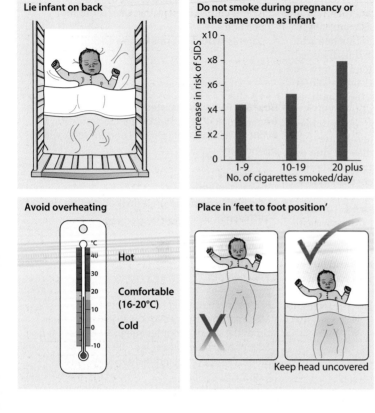

- parents should seek medical advice promptly if their infant becomes unwell
- parents should have the baby in their bedroom for the first 6 months of life
- parents should avoid bringing the baby into their bed when they are tired or have taken alcohol, sedative medicines or drugs
- parents should avoid sleeping with their infant on a sofa, settee or armchair.

Summary

Sudden infant death syndrome (SIDS):
- is the commonest cause of death in children aged 1 month to 1 year
- the peak age is 2–4 months
- has been dramatically reduced by lying babies on their back to sleep.

Following the sudden death of a child

The sudden death of a child is one of the most distressing events that can happen to a family. If close family members are absent, arrangements should be made for them to come, if this is possible. The family should be spoken to sympathetically and in private (see Ch. 5). An outline of the recommended management after an infant has died suddenly and unexpectedly is shown in Figure 6.19.

Summary

Following an unexpected death:
- the parents should be offered the opportunity to see and hold their child
- the coroner must be informed and a postmortem performed
- the parents should be informed about the postmortem, that investigations will be performed and that the police will be involved and reassured that this is standard practice
- follow-up and bereavement counselling should be offered.

Management of the sudden unexpected death of an infant

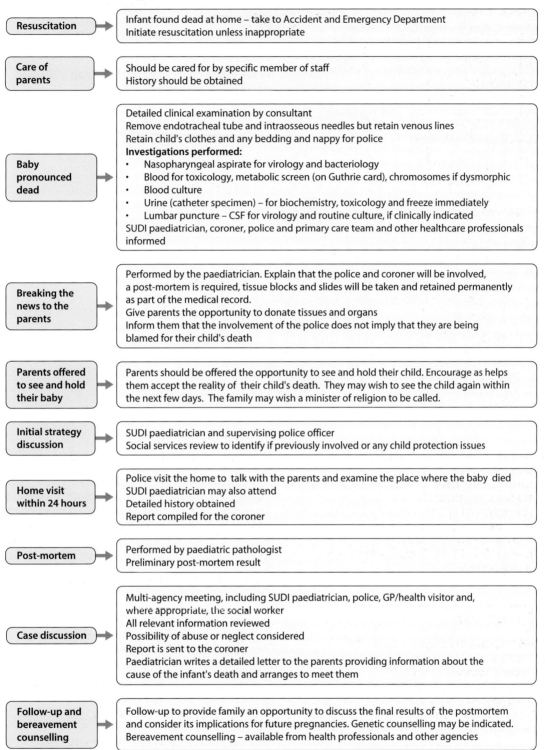

Resuscitation	Infant found dead at home – take to Accident and Emergency Department Initiate resuscitation unless inappropriate
Care of parents	Should be cared for by specific member of staff History should be obtained
Baby pronounced dead	Detailed clinical examination by consultant Remove endotracheal tube and intraosseous needles but retain venous lines Retain child's clothes and any bedding and nappy for police **Investigations performed:** • Nasopharyngeal aspirate for virology and bacteriology • Blood for toxicology, metabolic screen (on Guthrie card), chromosomes if dysmorphic • Blood culture • Urine (catheter specimen) – for biochemistry, toxicology and freeze immediately • Lumbar puncture – CSF for virology and routine culture, if clinically indicated SUDI paediatrician, coroner, police and primary care team and other healthcare professionals informed
Breaking the news to the parents	Performed by the paediatrician. Explain that the police and coroner will be involved, a post-mortem is required, tissue blocks and slides will be taken and retained permanently as part of the medical record. Give parents the opportunity to donate tissues and organs Inform them that the involvement of the police does not imply that they are being blamed for their child's death
Parents offered to see and hold their baby	Parents should be offered the opportunity to see and hold their child. Encourage as helps them accept the reality of their child's death. They may wish to see the child again within the next few days. The family may wish a minister of religion to be called.
Initial strategy discussion	SUDI paediatrician and supervising police officer Social services review to identify if previously involved or any child protection issues
Home visit within 24 hours	Police visit the home to talk with the parents and examine the place where the baby died SUDI paediatrician may also attend Detailed history obtained Report compiled for the coroner
Post-mortem	Performed by paediatric pathologist Preliminary post-mortem result
Case discussion	Multi-agency meeting, including SUDI paediatrician, police, GP/health visitor and, where appropriate, the social worker All relevant information reviewed Possibility of abuse or neglect considered Report is sent to the coroner Paediatrician writes a detailed letter to the parents providing information about the cause of the infant's death and arranges to meet them
Follow-up and bereavement counselling	Follow-up to provide family an opportunity to discuss the final results of the postmortem and consider its implications for future pregnancies. Genetic counselling may be indicated. Bereavement counselling – available from health professionals and other agencies

Figure 6.19 A recommended approach to the management of the sudden unexpected death of an infant. There are local variations in its implementation. (Adapted from *Sudden Unexpected Death in Infancy*. RCPCH, London, 2004.)

The death of a child

Further reading

Goldman A, Hain R, Lieben S 2005 The Oxford textbook of palliative care in children. Oxford University Press, Oxford. *Medical, psychological and practical issues of caring for terminally ill children and their families*

Advanced Life Support Group 2005 Advanced Paediatric Life Support. The Practical Approach, 4th Edn. Blackwell BMJ Books

RCPCH 2004 Sudden unexpected death in infancy. The report of a working group convened by the Royal College of Pathologists and The Royal College of Paediatrics and Child Health. RCPCH, London (www.rcpath.org and www.rcpch.ac.uk).

Resuscitation Council (UK) 2005 Updated guidelines on paediatric life support

Environment

Children need a safe, healthy and nurturing environment to achieve their full potential. Environmental hazards include accidents, poisons and abuse. As far as possible, children should be protected from harm. This is mainly the responsibility of parents, families and carers, but doctors, other professionals and society also play a role in advocating for safe environments for children. The risk of environmental hazards is increased by:

- poverty
- poor quality, overcrowded homes
- lack of a safe environment for play
- poor parenting skills, which may be due to parental psychiatric illness, drug and alcohol abuse, violent temperament, poor education or lack of social support.

Accidents

Accidents (now often called 'unintentional injuries') are extremely common. In the UK, 1 in 4 children attend an A&E department each year; about half because of an accident. Most accidents cause only minor injury but they can be fatal. Accidents are a major cause of death in children over a year of age (Figs 7.1 and 7.2) and also cause significant disability and suffering, including post-traumatic stress disorder. Head injury with brain damage is the major cause of disability from accidents. Cosmetic damage following burns, scalds and other accidents may cause the child profound psychological harm. Trauma to children of nursery age is more common in summer, and in boys.

> **Accidents are the second most common cause of death in children over a year of age.**

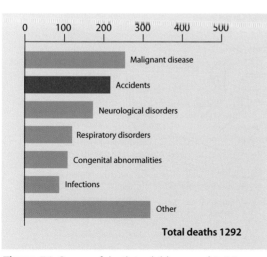

Figure 7.1 Causes of death in children aged 1–14 years in England and Wales (2004).

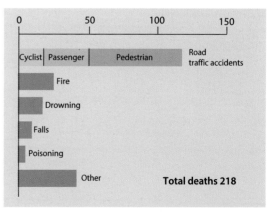

Figure 7.2 Causes of fatal accidents in children in England and Wales (2004). The most common cause is road traffic accidents.

Types of accident affecting children

The type of accident affecting a child depends on the child's age and stage of development. Babies can drown if left unsupervised in the bath because they cannot get back to a sitting position if they fall. Toddlers constantly explore their immediate environment, usually the home, and are unaware of the consequences of their actions. They are prone to falls, scalds, ingestion of potentially harmful substances and may wander off and drown in ponds, pools or other open water. Most serious accidents in babies and toddlers can be anticipated by an observant adult and prevented by vigilant supervision. Older children experience a different range of accidents, mainly as pedestrians or cyclists, while playing sport or from falls while climbing.

Accident prevention

The prevention of childhood accidents is clearly important. Doctors who treat children and see the effects of accidents are particularly well placed to provide the community with advice on appropriate preventive measures (Fig. 7.3). In order to prevent accidents:

- the relationship between an individual type of accident and the child's developmental level must be considered
- specific solutions should be based on detailed epidemiology, e.g. child-resistant containers are

the best method to limit children's access to medicines
- changes backed by legislation are the most successful.

Organisations such as the Royal Society for the Prevention of Accidents and the Children Accident Prevention Trust are important resources in helping reduce accidents by providing education and lobbying for legislative changes, e.g. bicycle helmet wearing.

> **The number of children killed in accidents has declined markedly over the past 20 years.**

Road traffic accidents

Road traffic accidents (RTAs) are the most common cause of accidental death in childhood and can be divided into several types.

Pedestrian road traffic accidents

Children's involvement in road traffic accidents is mostly as pedestrians. Boys between the ages of 5 and 9 years are at maximum risk, particularly after school. Children are unable to estimate the speed or dangers of traffic and to foresee dangerous situations. Although it is important to make

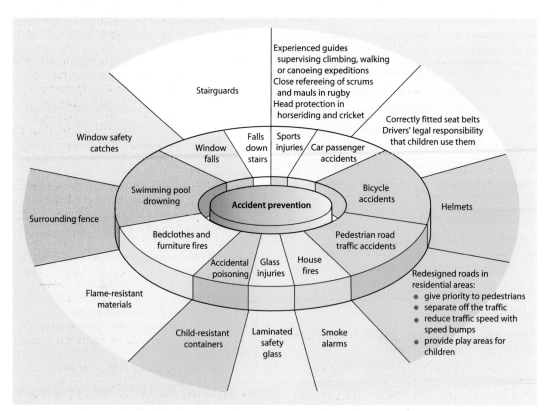

Figure 7.3 Examples of accident prevention.

children aware of the dangers, education about road safety has proved to be of limited value in reducing the number of accidents. Primary prevention is required; i.e. modifying the environment.

Child passengers in cars

Unrestrained children become missiles inside cars during crashes, even at low speeds. There is good evidence that child restraint systems prevent injury and death.

Bicycle accidents

Bicycle accidents are common during childhood. A boy has a 1 in 80 chance of having a cycling-related head injury severe enough to warrant admission to hospital during childhood. Studies have shown that the wearing of bicycle helmets reduces the severity of head injury.

Head injuries

Minor head injuries in childhood are common, and the vast majority of children recover without suffering any ill effect. However, about 1 in 800 of these children develop serious problems. The aim of the management of head injuries is to identify those children requiring treatment and to avoid secondary damage to the brain from hypoxia or poor cerebral perfusion (Fig. 7.4). In infants, as their skull sutures have not fused, cranial volume may increase from an extradural or subdural bleed before neurological signs or symptoms develop. The haemoglobin concentration may fall and they may become shocked. In infants and young children, unexplained head injuries may be the result of child abuse. The combination of retinal haemorrhages and widespread bruising is highly suggestive of a shaking injury, most likely from non-accidental injury or severe trauma.

> **Summary**
>
> **Head injury management:**
> - mild – discharge home with written advice
> - potentially severe – monitor to avoid secondary damage
> - severe – resuscitate, CT scan and neurosurgical referral.

Internal injuries

Children may suffer internal injuries associated with severe trauma. These include:

- Abdominal injuries, including a ruptured spleen, ruptured liver, kidney and bowel. There should be a high index of suspicion for these internal injuries if there has been abdominal trauma. The child needs close observation. Abdominal ultrasound and X-rays, including CT scan, may be helpful. If there is any doubt, a laparotomy is undertaken. Children may also sustain abdominal injuries from child abuse.
- Chest injuries, including pneumothorax and haemopericardium, which may require emergency treatment.

These children should be managed in a paediatric intensive care unit. Intra-abdominal injuries such as a contained splenic bleed are increasingly managed conservatively with close monitoring, but paediatric surgical support must be available immediately in case surgery is required.

Burns and scalds

Burns and scalds are a significant accidental cause of death, although most of the deaths occurring in house fires are caused by gas and smoke inhalation rather than thermal injury. Scalds in toddlers are common, from knocking over cups of hot liquid or grabbing the handle of a saucepan of boiling water on a cooker, or from bath water which is too hot.

Management

The severity of the injury is assessed:

- Is the *airway, breathing and circulation* satisfactory?
- *Was there any smoke inhalation?* If this has occurred, there is a danger of subsequent respiratory complications and carbon monoxide poisoning. All affected children should be observed and managed in hospital, with a low threshold to protect the airway before secondary problems develop.
- *Depth of the burn.* In superficial burns, the skin will be epithelialised from surviving cells. In partial thickness burns, there is some damage to the dermis with blistering, and the skin is pink or mottled; regeneration for superficial and partial thickness burns is from the margins of the wound and from the residual epithelial layer surrounding the hair follicles deep within the dermis. In deep (full thickness) burns, the skin is destroyed down to and including the dermis and looks white or charred, is painless and involves hair follicles, hence skin grafting is often required. Deep burns need assessment and treatment in hospital.
- *Surface area of the burn.* This should be calculated from a surface area chart (Fig. 7.5). The palm and adducted fingers cover about 1% of the body surface. Burns covering more than 5% full thickness, and 10% partial thickness need assessment by burns specialists. Involvement of more than 70% of the body surface carries a poor chance of survival.
- *Involvement of special sites.* Burns to the face may be disfiguring, those to the mouth may compromise the airway from oedema, and those to the hand may cause functional loss from scarring.

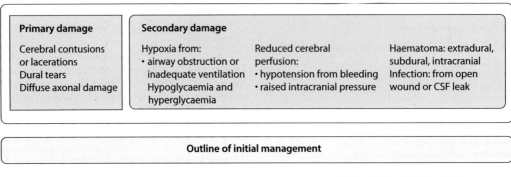

Head injuries in children

Damage caused by head injuries

Primary damage

Cerebral contusions
or lacerations
Dural tears
Diffuse axonal damage

Secondary damage

Hypoxia from:
• airway obstruction or
  inadequate ventilation
Hypoglycaemia and
hyperglycaemia

Reduced cerebral
perfusion:
• hypotension from bleeding
• raised intracranial pressure

Haematoma: extradural,
subdural, intracranial
Infection: from open
wound or CSF leak

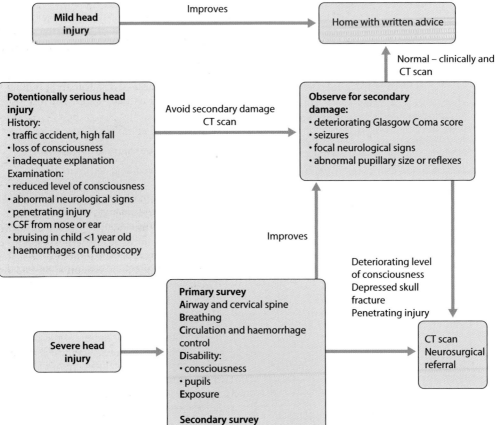

Outline of initial management

Mild head injury → Improves → Home with written advice

Normal – clinically and CT scan

Potentially serious head injury
History:
• traffic accident, high fall
• loss of consciousness
• inadequate explanation
Examination:
• reduced level of consciousness
• abnormal neurological signs
• penetrating injury
• CSF from nose or ear
• bruising in child <1 year old
• haemorrhages on fundoscopy

Avoid secondary damage
CT scan →

Observe for secondary damage:
• deteriorating Glasgow Coma score
• seizures
• focal neurological signs
• abnormal pupillary size or reflexes

Improves

Deteriorating level
of consciousness
Depressed skull
fracture
Penetrating injury

Severe head injury →

Primary survey
Airway and cervical spine
Breathing
Circulation and haemorrhage
control
Disability:
• consciousness
• pupils
Exposure

Secondary survey

**CT scan
Neurosurgical
referral**

Figure 7.4 Head injuries in children.

Treatment

This should be directed at:

* Relieving pain, assessed with a pain score, may require the use of strong analgesics such as intravenous morphine.
* Treating shock with intravenous fluids, preferably plasma expanders, and close monitoring of haematocrit and urinary output. Children with more than 10% burns will require intravenous fluids.
* Providing wound care. Burns should be covered with cling film (plastic wrapping), which reduces

pain from contact with cold air and reduces the risk of infection. Blisters should be left alone. Irrigation with cold water should only be used briefly to superficial or partial thickness burns covering less than 10% of the body as it may rapidly cause excessive cooling. Tetanus immunisation status must be ascertained and a booster given if required.

Severe burns or significant burns to special sites are best dealt with in specialist units. Plastic surgeons will often need to embark on a programme of skin grafts and treatment of contractures. The

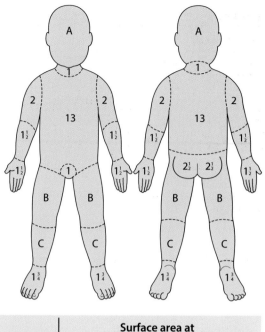

Area indicated	Surface area at			
	1 year	5 years	10 years	15 years
A	8.5	6.5	5.5	4.5
B	3.25	4.0	4.5	4.5
C	2.5	2.75	3.0	3.25

Figure 7.5 Method of calculating the surface area of a burn (Lund and Browder chart).

psychological sequelae of severe burns are often marked and long-lasting, and appropriate psychological support is required.

> ## Summary
>
> **Burns and scalds:**
> * assess – need for resuscitation, if any smoke inhalation, depth and surface area of burns and if special sites involved
> * management – pain control, treat shock, provide wound care (cling film), refer to specialist centre if more than 5% full thickness, 10% partial thickness or significant burns to special sites.

Drowning and near-drowning

Drowning is a significant cause of accidental death in children in the UK. Most victims are young children. Drowning is three times more common in boys than in girls. Warmer affluent countries tend to have a higher incidence of drowning than in the UK, particularly because of drowning in domestic swimming pools. Babies may drown in the bath, toddlers may wander into domestic ponds or swimming pools, and older children may get into difficulty in swimming pools, rivers, canals, lakes and in the sea. Children should always be supervised when swimming.

Near-drowning

Up to 30% of fatalities can be prevented by skilled on-site resuscitation. Even children who are unconscious with fixed dilated pupils can survive near-drowning episodes, particularly if the water is cold, due to the protective effect of hypothermia. Children who are unconscious with fixed dilated pupils should therefore be fully resuscitated until their temperature is nearly normal. Immediate management at the waterside is with mouth-to-mouth resuscitation and chest compressions. Heat loss should be prevented by covering and warming. Children who may have inhaled water should be admitted to hospital to be observed for signs of respiratory distress and cardiac arrhythmias. Some children who nearly drown aspirate water and develop pneumonia with secondary infection. Respiratory deterioration can be caused by pulmonary oedema, between 1 and 72 hours after the original incident. This is due to surfactant deficiency. It is now thought that there is no difference in outlook for fresh and salt water drowning.

Choking, suffocation and strangulation

Children may choke on vomit, toys or food. Some children may strangle themselves accidentally on curtain cords, bedding and necklaces. Most are accidents but some such injuries are inflicted deliberately as a form of child abuse. Some adolescents deliberately hang themselves.

In airway obstruction from an aspirated foreign body, the actions outlined in Figures 7.6 and 7.7 should be followed.

Dog bites

One in 100 children present to the A&E department with dog bites. Most dog bites are minor, but severe lacerations, particularly to the face, do occur particularly in the toddler age group. Dog bites usually need only simple wound toilet, but more serious injuries, particularly on the face, may need careful debridement and skilled suturing to avoid unsightly scars. Antibiotics are not usually necessary. Although there has been much publicity about fierce dog breeds, such as Rottweilers, attacking children in parks or public places, most attacks are by dogs known to the child. A tetanus booster may be needed.

Poisoning

Poisoning in children may be:

* accidental – the vast majority
* deliberate self-poisoning in older children
* non-accidental as a form of child abuse
* iatrogenic.

Inhaled foreign body

Airway obstruction from foreign body

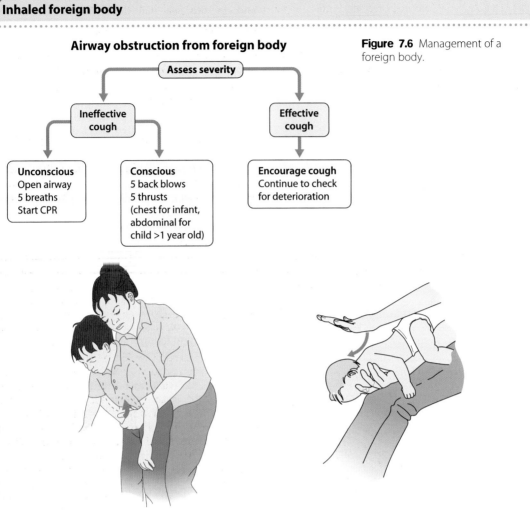

Figure 7.6 Management of a foreign body.

Assess severity

→ Ineffective cough

→ Effective cough

Unconscious
Open airway
5 breaths
Start CPR

Conscious
5 back blows
5 thrusts
(chest for infant, abdominal for child >1 year old)

Encourage cough
Continue to check for deterioration

Figure 7.7a Abdominal thrusts using the Heimlich manoeuvre in older children to expel an inhaled foreign body. One hand is formed into a fist and placed against the child's abdomen above the umbilicus and below the xiphisternum. The other hand is placed over the fist. Both hands are thrust into the abdomen. This is repeated several times. The child can be standing, kneeling, sitting or supine.

Figure 7.7b In infants, back blows and chest thrusts are recommended to expel an inhaled foreign body. Abdominal thrusts are best avoided in infants as they may cause intraabdominal injury.

Accidental poisoning (Tables 7.1 and 7.2)

Although many thousands of young children are rushed to doctors' surgeries or hospital for urgent medical attention following accidental ingestion, most do not develop serious symptoms as they ingest only a small quantity of poison or take relatively non-toxic substances. However, a small percentage of children become seriously ill and a very few children die from poisoning each year.

Most accidental poisoning is in young children, with a peak age of 30 months. Inquisitive toddlers are unaware of the potential danger of taking medicines, household products and eating plants. Most ingestions occur in the child's own home, when supervision is inadequate. Supervision entails not only reacting to a dangerous situation but prevention through anticipation.

The aim of management of poisoning should be to prevent unnecessary admissions to hospital

Table 7.1 Potential toxicity in accidental poisoning in infants and young children, with some examples

Toxicity	Medicines	Household products	Plants
Low	Oral contraceptives, most antibiotics	Chalk and crayons, washing powder	Cyclamen, sweet pea
Intermediate	Paracetamol elixir, salbutamol	Bleach, disinfectants, window cleaners	Fuchsia, holly
High	Alcoholic drinks, digoxin, iron, salicylate, tricyclic antidepressants	Acids, alkalis, petroleum distillates, organophosphorus insecticides	Deadly nightshade, laburnum, yew

while maintaining safety. There has been a marked reduction in the hospital admission rate for poisoning. Reasons for this include:

* the introduction of child-resistant containers – in the UK they must be used for paracetamol and salicylate preparations, and certain household products such as white spirit; an alternative container for tablets is opaque blister packs
* the reduction in the number of tablets per pack
* a reduction in prescriptions of potentially harmful medicines, e.g. aspirin and iron.

Education campaigns have not proved successful in preventing accidental child poisoning.

Management

This is outlined in Figure 7.8.

> ### Summary
>
> **Accidental poisoning in children:**
> * is common in toddlers and young children
> * most do not cause serious illness
> * when an ingestion has occurred, identify the agent and assess its toxicity to plan management
> * potentially harmful poisons in children are alcohol, acids and alkalis, bleach, digoxin, batteries, iron, paracetamol, petroleum distillates, salicylates and tricyclic antidepressants
> * assess the social circumstances behind why it happened.

Deliberate poisoning in older children

These children form one end of the age spectrum of overdose in adults and are more likely to take significant amounts of poison than younger children. Substances that can be regarded as having intermediate toxicity when taken accidentally should be regarded as potentially toxic when taken deliberately. Poisoning in older children should be recognised as a serious symptom and an indication of child and family disturbance, so all children who take poisons deliberately should be assessed by a child or adolescent psychiatrist. Many will also need education or social work assessment.

Chronic poisoning

Children can be poisoned by chronic exposure to chemicals and pollutants. An example from the past is mercury poisoning from teething powders, which used to cause 'pink disease', so called because it resulted in red painful extremities. It also caused anorexia, weight loss and hypotonia. Now the commonest causes are lead ingestion and smoking.

Lead poisoning

Environmental lead levels are now much reduced. In the past, certain paints contained lead. Children are liable to be poisoned from chewing such paintwork or from inhalation when the paint is removed. This is still a problem in parts of the USA. Lead fumes from burning batteries, lead shot for fishing and lead from old water pipes are other potential sources. Children from the Indian subcontinent may be poisoned by surma, the lead-containing eye make-up sometimes used even on young babies. Lead from vehicle exhaust fumes results in higher blood levels in children living in urban compared with rural areas. The change to unleaded petrol was in response to concern about its potential as an environmental hazard.

Children present with pica (compulsive eating of substances other than food), anorexia, colicky abdominal pain, irritability and failure to thrive and pallor from anaemia. Severe lead poisoning may present with neurological symptoms, including drowsiness, convulsions and coma from lead encephalopathy. Raised intracranial pressure with papilloedema may be present. There is increasing evidence that chronic exposure to relatively low lead levels may be harmful to mental development.

The diagnosis is confirmed by elevated blood lead levels. There may be a hypochromic anaemia and basophil stippling of neutrophils. Radiographs of the knee or wrist may show 'lead lines', which are dense metaphyseal bands. The source of lead should be identified and removed. Chelating agents are used to form non-toxic lead compounds. In mild cases, D-penicillamine is given orally, and in severe cases sodium calcium edetate (EDTA) is indicated.

Smoking

The harmful effects of smoking are well documented, with a greatly increased risk of developing chronic bronchitis, lung cancer and cardiovascular disease. Unfortunately, many children become regular smokers while still at school. Children should be given appropriate health education, although its effectiveness is limited by the poor example set by the widespread smoking of adults and the difficulties of health education in secondary

Table 7.2 Potentially harmful poisons

Poison	Adverse effects	Management
Alcohol (accidental experimenting by older children)	Hypoglycaemia Coma Respiratory failure	Monitor blood glucose. Intravenous glucose if necessary. Blood alcohol levels for severity
Acids and alkalis	Inflammation and ulceration of upper gastrointestinal tract leading to stenosis	No emesis/gastric lavage No chemical antidotes as they produce heat Early endoscopy
Digoxin	Arrhythmias, hyperkalaemia	Activated charcoal if <1 h after ingestion. ECG monitoring, serum digoxin concentration
Disc or button batteries	Mild gastrointestinal symptoms Oesophageal stricture with large batteries (>20 mm) Corrosion of gut wall and perforation Break open with release of mercury – rare	Monitor progress with chest and abdominal X-rays – almost all passed within 2 days, no symptoms Remove batteries if in oesophagus or signs of disintegration. Some authorities recommend removal if not passed within 48 h to avoid danger of disintegration
Iron	*Initial*: vomiting, diarrhoea, haematemesis, melaena, acute gastric ulceration *Latent period of improvement* *Hours later*: drowsiness, coma, shock, liver failure with hypoglycaemia and convulsions *Long-term*: gastric strictures	Serious toxicity if >60 mg/kg elemental iron Abdominal X-ray to count the number of tablets Serum iron levels Gastric lavage considered in severe cases if <1 h after ingestion Intravenous desferrioxamine
Paracetamol – large ingestion uncommon in young children as tablets are difficult to swallow and elixir is too sweet	Gastric irritation Liver failure after 3–5 days	Check plasma concentration after 4 h after ingestion. If >150 mg/kg paracetamol is thought to have been taken, or the plasma concentration is high, start intravenous acetylcysteine Monitor prothrombin time, liver function tests and plasma creatinine
Petroleum distillates (paraffin/kerosene, white spirit)	Aspiration causing pneumonitis	Emesis and gastric lavage contraindicated Usually no treatment required
Salicylates	Tinnitus, deafness, nausea, vomiting, dehydration Hyperventilation causing respiratory alkalosis Later, metabolic acidosis Hypoglycaemia Disorientation	Measure plasma salicylate concentration Gastric lavage if <1 h. Give activated charcoal Monitor fluid and electrolyte balance. Correct dehydration, electrolyte imbalance and acidosis. Dialysis
Tricyclic antidepressants	Sinus tachycardia Conduction disorders Dry mouth, blurred vision Agitation, confusion, convulsions, coma Respiratory depression Hypotension	Activated charcoal if within 1 h Cardiac monitoring. Treat arrhythmias conservatively with sodium bicarbonate Correct metabolic acidosis Treat convulsions with diazepam

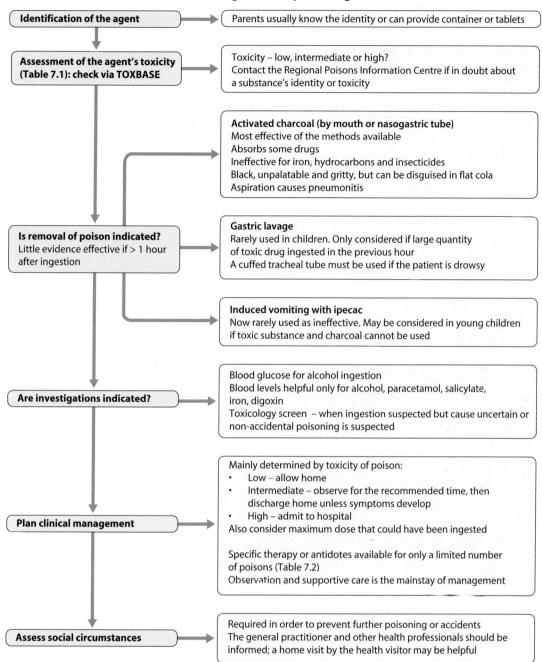

Figure 7.8 Outline of the management of poisoning. TOXBASE is an online database of the National Poisons Information Service for registered users.

The figure contains the following flow chart:

Management of poisoning

Identification of the agent → Parents usually know the identity or can provide container or tablets

Assessment of the agent's toxicity (Table 7.1): check via TOXBASE → Toxicity – low, intermediate or high? Contact the Regional Poisons Information Centre if in doubt about a substance's identity or toxicity

Is removal of poison indicated? Little evidence effective if > 1 hour after ingestion →

- **Activated charcoal (by mouth or nasogastric tube)** Most effective of the methods available. Absorbs some drugs. Ineffective for iron, hydrocarbons and insecticides. Black, unpalatable and gritty, but can be disguised in flat cola. Aspiration causes pneumonitis

- **Gastric lavage** Rarely used in children. Only considered if large quantity of toxic drug ingested in the previous hour. A cuffed tracheal tube must be used if the patient is drowsy

- **Induced vomiting with ipecac** Now rarely used as ineffective. May be considered in young children if toxic substance and charcoal cannot be used

Are investigations indicated? → Blood glucose for alcohol ingestion. Blood levels helpful only for alcohol, paracetamol, salicylate, iron, digoxin. Toxicology screen – when ingestion suspected but cause uncertain or non-accidental poisoning is suspected

Plan clinical management → Mainly determined by toxicity of poison:
- Low – allow home
- Intermediate – observe for the recommended time, then discharge home unless symptoms develop
- High – admit to hospital

Also consider maximum dose that could have been ingested

Specific therapy or antidotes available for only a limited number of poisons (Table 7.2). Observation and supportive care is the mainstay of management

Assess social circumstances → Required in order to prevent further poisoning or accidents. The general practitioner and other health professionals should be informed; a home visit by the health visitor may be helpful

---

school age children. When parents or carers smoke, children have been shown to have a higher incidence of bronchitis, asthma, pneumonia and serous otitis media (glue ear). This particularly applies to babies and young children. Maternal smoking places the infant at increased risk of sudden infant death syndrome (SIDS).

 Parents' smoking adversely affects their children's health.

Child abuse

Children require protection and care. The concept that parents or carers might abuse their children was first recognised as a medical problem only after World War II. Although this caused great concern at the time, child abuse is not a new phenomenon. Children have been physically harmed, neglected and subjected to sexual abuse throughout history. What has changed is that society is no longer prepared to accept that parents or caregivers can do whatever they please to their children. Children are now afforded the right to receive recognised and accepted patterns of child care and rearing. Professionals, whether doctors, health visitors, social workers, teachers or others involved in the care of children, now have duties to ensure this. Recognising potential child abuse has to be weighed against the damage of falsely accusing parents of abusing their children. This requires fine judgement.

Types of child abuse

Initially, attention was focused on the 'battered baby', where severe physical injury was inflicted on babies. We now appreciate that in addition to inflicting physical injuries, adults may harm children in a number of different ways. These can be divided into:

- physical abuse (non-accidental injury, NAI) – bruises, head injury, burns, lacerations, fractures and internal injuries
- neglect
- emotional abuse
- sexual abuse, including the use of children for pornography
- non-accidental poisoning – where children are deliberately poisoned
- fabricated or induced illness (formerly known as Munchausen's syndrome by proxy) – where symptoms or signs of illness in the child are made up or deliberately induced by the carer.

Although children may present with a single type of abuse, it is more common for children to suffer from a combination of several forms; e.g. physically abused children are usually also neglected and emotionally abused. Abuse of all types is very damaging to the emotional development of the child and sexual abuse may also damage the future sexual responses of children. Intervention should aim not only to prevent further injuries but also to provide therapy for any emotional damage inflicted.

Diagnosis

The diagnosis of child abuse is based on assessing the probability that individual injuries or harm have occurred non-accidentally. Serious injuries to children are rarely the initial presentation – they are almost always preceded by minor ones. It is also known that if a particular child in the household has been subjected to abuse, further episodes are more likely to be directed towards the same child. Adults who abuse children do not usually suffer from mental illness, although alcohol, drugs and postnatal depression sometimes contribute. More often, there are personality factors with the abuser who may have experienced poor parenting in childhood. Factors in the child which may predispose to abuse include young age, disability, low birthweight, and a demanding personality.

Physical abuse

Most injuries in children follow genuine accidents and must be differentiated from those which are inflicted deliberately. A full history and examining the whole child is vital. It is essential to try to understand exactly how the injuries occurred and the circumstances surrounding the event. In child abuse there may be:

- a history which is not compatible with the injury
- delay in reporting the injury
- inconsistent histories from caregivers
- inappropriate reaction of parents or caregivers who are vague, elusive, unconcerned or excessively distressed or aggressive
- recurrent injuries
- injuries inconsistent with the child's stage of development.

Presentation of physical abuse

Bruises

These are the commonest mode of presentation (Fig. 7.9a–d). Whereas bruises on the forehead and shins are common in toddlers learning to walk, they are exceptional in non-mobile babies. Bruises on the face, back and buttock are uncommon in genuine accidents. There is little evidence that bruises can be accurately aged. Some patterns of bruising are suggestive of particular injuries. Bruises from fingertips gripping with excessive force are mostly on the trunk, often on either side of the spine, but may also be seen around the mouth from trying to stop a baby crying, or on the arms from shaking. Slap marks resembling handprints may be seen on the face or buttocks. Bruises may outline a particular object, e.g. a hand, belt or flex used in beating.

Non-accidental head injuries

Head injury may follow severe shaking, particularly in children under 6 months. Less often, there are direct blows to the head. Vigorous shaking of babies may rupture the small vessels crossing the subdural space, causing a subdural haemorrhage. There may also be hypoxic-ischaemic damage caused by the apnoea associated with severe shaking. There may be no signs of bruising on the surface of the skull. Retinal haemorrhages are often present in head injuries from non-accidental injury. Clinical features include irritability, poor feeding, increasing head circumference, convulsions, reduced level of consciousness, anaemia and a full fontanelle.

Direct blows to the head are usually less of a diagnostic problem as there is bruising and there may be an underlying skull fracture.

Abdominal injuries

Visceral injuries, particularly to the small bowel, spleen and liver, may follow blows or kicks to the abdomen. They are uncommon and often difficult to diagnose. There may not be any abdominal

Physical injuries that can be caused by child abuse

Bruising

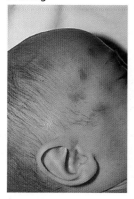

Figure 7.9a Bruising from trauma to a baby's head.

Bruising – unusual sites

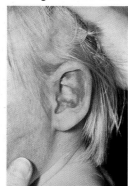

Figure 7.9b Bruising within the pinna is uncommon in accidental injury. Bruising behind the ear may be from blows to the ear.

Torn frenulum

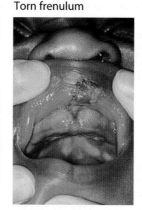

Figure 7.9c A torn frenulum. This may be from trauma to the mouth.

Adult bite

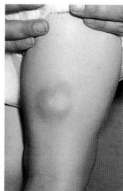

Figure 7.9d A bite mark on an infant's leg. Adult bite marks may be seen in abuse, but bites from other children are not uncommon.

bruising. These injuries are usually in children under 5 years and small bowel injury is more common in abuse than in both road traffic accidents and falls. Non-accidental abdominal trauma carries a high morbidity and mortality.

Burns or scalds

It is often difficult to distinguish burns and scalds inflicted deliberately from those that are accidents. Accidental hot water burns tend to be asymmetrical, spare the flexures and have geographical splash marks. Deliberate bath scalds may scald the back, which is uncommon in accidents. The shape of the injury may be suggestive of its aetiology, e.g. a cigarette burn.

Fractures

Fractures due to child abuse are predominantly a problem of young children under 30 months, particularly babies. The most specific fractures for abuse are those of the ribs, which, if major trauma or bone disease is excluded, have a probability of abuse of 97% (Table 7.3). These rib fractures are due to squeezing and are usually posterior. Anterior Rib Fractures can be caused by abuse but children who have cardiopulmonary resuscitation may rarely have anterior rib fractures.

When assessing fractures, it is the history and the child's age, mobility and development that are the crucial features in distinguishing accidental from non-accidental injuries. In infants accidental fractures of the long bones are uncommon in the non-mobile child. i.e. delete relatively little force needed to produce a linear skull fracture. When considering humeral fractures, the type is

Table 7.3 Likelihood of a fracture being due to non-accidental injury

High	Metaphyseal fractures
	Posterior rib fractures
Moderate	Multiple fractures
	Fractures of different ages
	Complex skull fracture
Low	Clavicular fractures
	Long-bone shaft fractures
	Linear skull fractures

Adapted from Kleinman P K, *Current Concepts: a categorical course in paediatric radiology*, SPR, 1994.

important – only 4% of supracondylar fractures are due to abuse; however, non-supracondylar fractures of the humerus in infants are associated with abuse.

In children over 5 years most long-bone fractures are accidental.

Investigation

Fractures in young children may not be detectable clinically and radiography needs to be undertaken to exclude them in all physically abused children under 30 months. A full radiographic skeletal survey with oblique views of the ribs should be performed in all infants with suspected physical abuse. Some lesions may be inconspicuous initially, but can be identified on a radionuclide bone scan or can become evident on a repeat X-ray 1–2 weeks later (Fig. 7.10a, b). Other medical conditions which

Rib fractures from child abuse

Rib fractures – X-ray

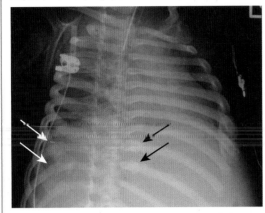

Figure 7.10a Posterior rib fractures are usually from squeezing rather than direct trauma. Anterior and posterior fractures are present. There is a fracture line on the 9th rib on the right; the others are healing with callus formation. The fractures are from different episodes of trauma. (Courtesy of Dr J. Danin.)

Rib fractures – bone scan

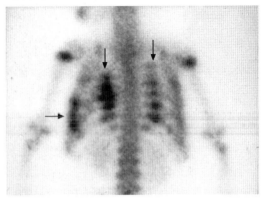

Figure 7.10b A radionuclide bone scan is more sensitive in detecting fractures in the early stages. This scan clearly shows multiple rib fractures. (Courtesy of Dr Cathy Owens.)

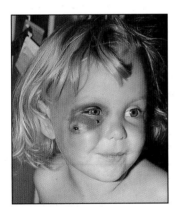

Figure 7.11 A thorough medical assessment is required in all children when non-accidental injury is suspected. This girl's large bruise followed what was said to be a minor bump. Non-accidental injury was suspected, but examination showed multiple bruises and petechiae. She had immune thrombocytopenic purpura (ITP).

need to be considered and excluded in suspected child abuse are:

* Bruising – coagulation disorders (Fig. 7.11).
* Fractures
  – Osteogenesis imperfecta, commonly referred to as brittle bone disease. The type commonly involved with unexplained fractures is type I, which is inherited in a dominant manner, so there may be a family history. Blue sclerae are a key clinical finding and there may be generalised osteoporosis and wormian bones in the skull on skeletal survey.
  – Copper deficiency. Very rarely predisposes to fractures as there is sufficient copper to prevent deficiency in breast milk and all types of milk

formula. It can occur if the infant is preterm or malnourished.
* Scalds and cigarette burns – may be misinterpreted in children with bullous impetigo or scalded skin syndrome.

If there is suspicion that a head injury in a young child is non-accidental, it necessitates:

* an immediate CT scan followed later by a MRI scan
* a skeletal survey to exclude fractures
* an expert ophthalmological examination
* a coagulation screen.

Neglect

Gross neglect of a child's developmental needs may present clinically as:

* failure to thrive
* inadequate hygiene, including severe nappy rash or infestation
* poor development of emotional attachment to the child's caregiver
* delay in development and speech and language
* poor attendance for immunisations and school.

This will improve if the child's environment is changed to provide adequate food, shelter, affection and stimulation.

Emotional abuse

Emotional abuse includes:

* the withdrawal of love by rejecting the child
* malicious criticism, threats and ridicule
* scapegoating.

Children who have been repeatedly emotionally abused usually present with emotional or behavioural disturbances. There may be excessive compliance or aggressive defiance, poor self-esteem, poor ability to enjoy things or sustain self-occupation, or they may exhibit pseudomature behaviour. Emotional abuse is often associated with physical or sexual abuse.

Bullying is being increasingly recognised as an important form of emotional abuse. Every school should have a written bullying policy which needs to be implemented when necessary.

Fictitious or induced illness

In this uncommon variant of physical abuse, illness in the child is fabricated by a parent, usually the mother. Some of the mothers have connections with healthcare services. The abuse appears to be a way in which these disturbed parents obtain satisfaction from close association with hospital care. Examples include:

- putting blood in vomit, stool and urine
- placing sugar in the urine so that a diagnosis of diabetes mellitus is made
- contaminating microbiological specimens.

In non-accidental (induced) poisoning, children are deliberately poisoned by their parents. They present with bizarre symptoms such as:

- hyperventilation after aspirin
- unexplained drowsiness after hypnotics, tranquillisers or alcohol.

A clue may be that the condition only occurs when the parent is present or following a visit. The condition can be extremely difficult to diagnose, but may be suspected if the child has frequent unexplained illnesses and multiple hospital admissions with symptoms that only occur in the mother's presence and are not substantiated by clinical findings. This disorder can be very damaging to the child, as unnecessary investigations and potentially harmful treatment are likely to be given. The child also learns to live with a pattern of illness rather than health. In induced poisoning, the diagnosis is often difficult but can usually be made by identifying the drug in the blood or urine.

Management of suspected child abuse

Abused children may present to doctors in the hospital or to medical or nursing staff in the community. They may also be brought for a medical opinion by social services or the police. In all cases, the procedures of the local safeguarding children committee should be followed. The medical consultation should be the same as for any medical condition, with a full history and full examination. It is usually most productive when this is conducted in a sensitive and concerned way without being accusatory or condemning. Any injuries or medical findings should be carefully noted, measured, recorded and drawn on a body map and photographed (with parental consent). The height, weight and head circumference should be recorded and plotted on a centile chart. The interaction between the child and parents should be noted. All notes must be meticulous, dated, timed and signed. Treatment of specific injuries should be instigated and blood tests and X-rays undertaken.

If abuse is suspected or confirmed, a decision needs to be made as to whether immediate treatment is required and if the child needs immediate protection from further harm. If this is the case, this may be achieved by admission to hospital, which also allows investigations and multidisciplinary assessment. If sympathetically handled, most parents are willing to accept medical advice for hospital admission for observation and investigation. Occasionally this is not possible and legal enforcement is required. The safety of other siblings or children at home needs to be considered. If medical treatment is not necessary but it is felt to be unsafe for the child to return home, a placement may be found in a foster home.

In addition to a detailed medical assessment, evaluation by social workers and other health professionals will be required. A child protection conference will be convened in accordance with local procedures. In the UK, the conference will be chaired by a senior member of the social services department or of the National Society for the Prevention of Cruelty to Children (NSPCC). Members of the conference may include social workers, health visitors, police, general practitioner, paediatricians, teachers and lawyers. Increasingly, parents attend all or part of the case conference. Details of the incident leading to the conference and the family background will be discussed. Good communication and a trusting working relationship between the professionals are vital as it can be extremely difficult to evaluate the likelihood that injuries were inflicted deliberately and the possible outcome of legal proceedings. The conference will decide:

- whether to place the child's name on the Child Protection Register (see Case history 7.1)
- whether there should be an application to the Court to protect the child
- what follow-up is needed.

If the child is placed on the Child Protection Register, the social services department will produce a child protection care plan, which will include medical follow-up in many instances.

In the UK, there have been a number of high profile child protection court cases.

Following the death from abuse of the child Victoria Climbié, the Laming report made recommendations about better communication between the health service, social services and the police, and that the overall responsibility for child protection lies with senior managers as well as junior staff.

Case History
7.1 Child abuse

A 7-month-old boy was noted by a relative to have a large, unexplained bruise over the side of the head. His mother took him to the nearest A&E department where a skeletal survey showed a normal skull X-ray but a metaphyseal fracture (Fig. 7.12). His mother thought that this must have occurred when he had fallen off his parents' bed the previous day. His mother was training to be a nursery school teacher. Her partner had recently been discharged from prison for burglary. Both parents were interviewed by social services and the police. A child protection conference was held, which the mother attended. The findings were suggestive of non-accidental injury, but definite evidence was lacking. The case

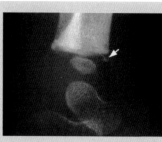

Figure 7.12 A metaphyseal fracture, usually caused by wrenching, is highly suggestive of non-accidental injury.

conference considered the child to be at risk of significant harm and placed him on the Child Protection Register, with close supervision by the health visitor and social services.

In contrast, following the conviction and subsequent acquittal of several mothers accused of murdering their infants, it has been established that:

- parents will not be convicted of child abuse based only on the evidence of expert witnesses
- the evidence base for child abuse needs to be reviewed in a systematic manner.

The approach to dealing with child abuse in all its forms is well-coordinated, ongoing, multi-disciplinary teamwork. The interests of the child should be kept uppermost by all professionals to

prevent them from harm but also to avoid false accusations.

Sexual abuse

A common definition of child sexual abuse is 'involvement of dependent, developmentally immature children and adolescents in sexual activities that they do not fully comprehend, are unable to give informed consent to and that violate social taboos of family roles'. It includes a variety of acts:

- genital exposure
- fondling
- genital, anal or oral sexual activity or intercourse, including rape
- involvement in pornography.

Victims can be of any age and of either sex, but girls outnumber boys, in contrast to other forms of abuse. Risk factors in the family are listed in Box 7.1. Children may be abused by:

- someone in the family
- a trusted adult, such as a baby-sitter
- someone outside the family, but this is much less common.

Male abusers are more common, but female abusers are being recognised with increasing frequency.

Summary

Child abuse:

- is the responsibility of all doctors, and must not be avoided or ignored because it raises difficult issues and possible appearance in Court
- takes various forms – physical abuse (non-accidental injury, NAI), neglect, emotional abuse, sexual abuse, fabricated or induced illness
- is suspected if the history and injury are not consistent or the injury is suggestive, e.g. the pattern of bruises or burns or scalds; presence of subdural haemorrhage or retinal haemorrhages; type of fracture; however, although such injuries are suggestive, they are not diagnostic, and must not be considered in isolation
- if suspected – follow local safeguarding children guidelines. Take a full history and examination, with details and drawings of any injuries. Decide if the child (and siblings) need immediate protection and if investigations are required. Evaluation by social workers and other health professionals will be required and a child protection conference convened.

Box 7.1 Family risk factors for child sexual abuse

Poor parental sexual relationship
Maternal depression or physical illness
Mother sexually abused in childhood
Father/abuser either inadequate or aggressive
Family chaotic, disorganised or socially isolated
Parentified daughter who has taken over mother's role

The assessment of sexual abuse

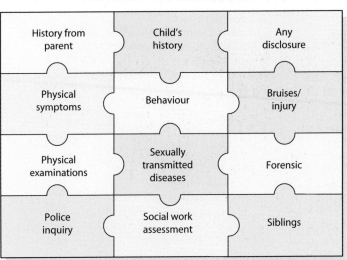

Figure 7.13 The assessment of sexual abuse is like a jigsaw puzzle. Many different pieces of information need to be pieced together to make an informed opinion. (From *Child Protection Companion*, Royal College of Paediatrics and Child Health, 2005.)

Sexual abuse usually presents as an incidental allegation (disclosure) by a child, either spontaneously to a trusted adult or as the result of a crisis, such as running away or taking an overdose. It may also present with:

- genital trauma or infection
- sexually transmitted disease
- highly sexualised behaviour towards adults or children
- unexplained pregnancy
- inexplicable change in behaviour or school work.

When child sexual abuse is suspected, the need for and urgency of a medical examination should be assessed. The examination should be conducted by two doctors skilled in paediatric examination for child sexual abuse or by a single doctor recording the findings photographically by a colposcope. Assessment of growth, behaviour and development should be made. Examination of the genitalia, which is usually only a detailed inspection and not an internal examination, is done as part of the general clinical examination. Forensic swabs and samples should be taken if the alleged abuse is less than 72 hours from the incident. Clinical features include:

- bruising around the thighs, genitalia, anus, perineum, buttocks and lower abdomen
- tears and abrasions to the female genitalia – in particular, the hymen may be torn; however, vulval soreness is common in young girls and is rarely due to abuse
- tears and abrasions to the male genitalia
- anal fissures (may be associated with constipation)
- reflex anal dilatation – this is where the buttocks are parted for 30–45 seconds, and in a positive test the anus opens and the rectum can be seen because of incompetence of the internal sphincter. Reflex anal dilatation and anal fissures in isolation are not reliable signs of child sexual abuse as they may have other causes such as constipation.

The examination should be with the knowledge and agreement of the parent, although it may occasionally be performed at the request of the Court. Adolescent girls must give their consent and all children should be accompanied by a trusted adult. In the case of young children, this is usually a parent. It should be performed in privacy, calmly and in a non-threatening environment. The medical examination is rarely diagnostic and significant physical findings are present in less than 30% of sexually abused children. Physical signs must be interpreted in conjunction with the history. There is considerable variation in the normal appearance of the female genitalia. This is partly age-dependent. A normal examination does not exclude abuse.

If sexual abuse is suspected, the procedures of the local safeguarding children committee should be followed (Fig. 7.13). Further information may be obtained from the child during an interview held jointly by a social worker and police officer experienced in child sexual abuse work. Psychological damage secondary to sexual abuse frequently occurs and may need specialist treatment. Post-traumatic stress disorder is a recognised sequel and can persist into adult life.

 At presentation, less than 30% of sexually abused children have significant clinical abnormalities. Clinical examination must be performed by a specially trained doctor.

Further reading

Hobbs C 1999 Child abuse and neglect: a clinician's handbook, 2nd edn. Churchill Livingstone, London

Hobbs C, Wynne J 2001 Physical signs of child abuse: a colour atlas, 2nd edn. WB Saunders, London

Palmer M M. Dog bites. BMJ 2007: 334; 413–7. Review article

Resuscitation Council (UK) 2005 Resuscitation guidelines

Royal College of Paediatrics and Child Health 2005 Child protection companion. Royal College of Paediatrics and Child Health, London

Internet

Accident prevention:
Children Accident Prevention Trust: www.capt.org.uk
Royal Society for the Prevention of Accidents: www.rospa.org.uk
www.core-info.co.uk Systematic review of physical abuse

Genetics

The Human Genome Project, culminating in the first publication of the human genome sequence in 2001, together with the development of genetic databases has resulted in an explosion of knowledge about the basis of genetic diseases (Fig. 8.1). It is now estimated that the human genome contains 30 000–35 000 genes, although the function of many of these genes remains unknown. Alternative mRNA splicing and post-translational modification of gene products results in a much greater diversity and complexity at the protein level. Access to databases containing DNA sequence and protein structure has greatly enhanced progress in scientific research. Clinical application of these advances is available to families through specialist genetic centres that offer diagnosis, investigation, counselling and antenatal diagnosis for an ever-widening range of disorders. Gene therapy trials are also underway, bringing hope of improved treatment in the future.

Genetic disorders are:

- common, with 2% of live-born babies having a significant congenital malformation and about 5% a genetic disorder
- burdensome to the affected individual, family and society, as many are associated with severe and permanent disability.

Genetically determined diseases include those resulting from:

- chromosomal abnormalities
- the action of a single gene (Mendelian disorders)
- unusual genetic mechanisms
- interaction of genetic and environmental factors (multifactorial or polygenic disorders).

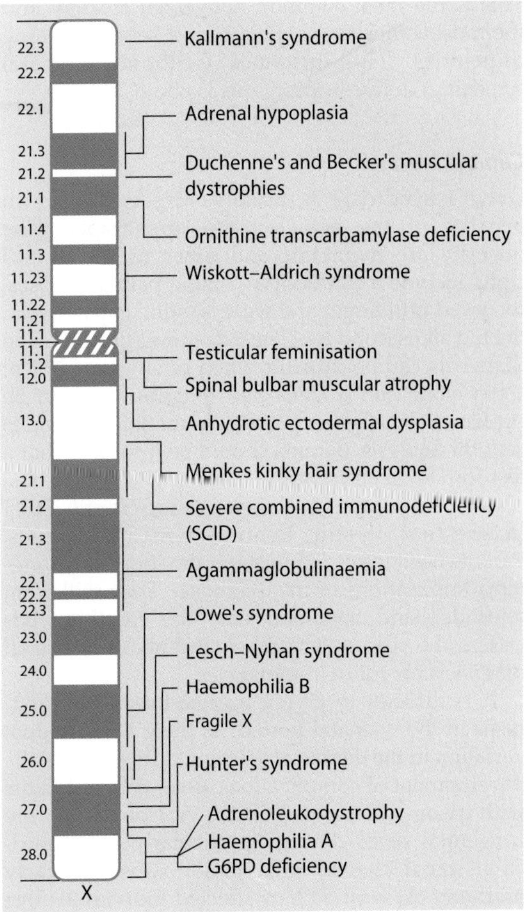

Figure 8.1 Idiogram of the X chromosome, showing some of the many genes for specific disorders located on it.

Chromosomal abnormalities

Genes are composed of DNA that is wound around a core of histone proteins and packaged into a succession of supercoils to form the chromosomes. The human chromosome complement was confirmed as recently as 1956. Following the recognition in 1959 of the chromosomal abnormalities in Down's, Klinefelter's and Turner's syndromes, many hundreds of chromosome defects have now been documented. Chromosomal abnormalities are either numerical or structural. They occur in approximately 10% of spermatozoa and 25% of mature oocytes and are a very common cause of early spontaneous miscarriage. The estimated incidence of chromosomal abnormalities in live-born infants is about 1 in 150 and these usually, but not always, cause multiple congenital anomalies and learning difficulties. Acquired chromosomal changes play a significant role in carcinogenesis and tumour progression.

Down's syndrome (trisomy 21)

This is the most common autosomal trisomy and the most common genetic cause of severe learning difficulties. The incidence (without antenatal screening) in live-born infants is about 1 in 650.

Clinical features

Down's syndrome is usually suspected at birth because of the baby's facial appearance. The majority are hypotonic and other useful clinical signs include a flat occiput, single palmar creases, incurved fifth finger and wide 'sandal' gap between the big and second toe (Fig. 8.2a–c and Box 8.1). The diagnosis can be difficult when relying on clinical signs alone and a suspected diagnosis should be confirmed by a senior paediatrician. Before blood is sent for analysis, parents should be informed that a test for Down's syndrome is being performed. The results may take 1–2 days, using rapid FISH (fluorescent in-situ hybridisation) techniques. Parents need information about the short- and long-term implications of the diagnosis. They will want to understand how and why the condition has arisen, the risk of recurrence and about antenatal diagnosis for future pregnancies.

It is difficult to give a precise long-term prognosis in the neonatal period, as there is individual variation in the degree of learning difficulty and the development of complications. Over 85% of infants with trisomy 21 survive to one year of age. Severe congenital heart disease (particularly atrioventricular canal defect) is a major cause of early mortality. At least 50% of affected individuals live longer than 50 years. Parents also need to know what assistance is available from both professionals and self-help groups. They often find written information valuable, and they can also give it to other family members to read. Counselling may be required to help the family deal with feelings of grief, anger or guilt. It is important to note that parents appreciate it when their baby is referred to, not as a diagnostic category ('a Down's baby'), but as an individual ('a baby with Down's syndrome').

Cytogenetics

The extra chromosome 21 may result from non-disjunction, translocation or mosaicism.

Non-disjunction (94%)

In non-disjunction:

- most cases result from an error at meiosis
- the pair of chromosome 21s fails to separate, so that one gamete has two chromosome 21s and one has none (Fig 8.3)
- fertilisation of the gamete with two chromosome 21s gives rise to a zygote with trisomy 21
- parental chromosomes do not need to be examined.

The incidence of trisomy 21 due to non-disjunction is related to maternal age (Table 8.1). However, as the proportion of pregnancies in older mothers is small, most affected babies are born to younger mothers. All pregnant women are now offered screening tests measuring biochemical markers in blood samples and nuchal thickening on ultrasound (thickening of the fat pad at the back of the neck) to identify an increased risk of Down's syndrome in the fetus. When an increased risk is identified, amniocentesis testing is offered to check the fetal chromosome pattern. Although in most instances a normal chromosome pattern will be identified, the possibility of an abnormal result and the option of termination of pregnancy should be discussed beforehand. Support and counselling needs to be available. After having one child with trisomy 21 due to non-disjunction, the risk of recurrence of Down's syndrome is 1 in 200 for mothers under the age of 35 years, but remains similar to their age-related population risk for those over the age of 35 years.

Table 8.1 Risk of Down's syndrome (live births) with maternal age at delivery, prior to screening in pregnancy

Maternal age (years)	Risk of Down's syndrome
All ages	1 in 650
20	1 in 1530
30	1 in 900
35	1 in 385
37	1 in 240
40	1 in 110
44	1 in 37

Down's syndrome

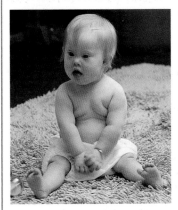

Figure 8.2a Characteristic facies seen in Down's syndrome. Her posture is due to hypotonia.

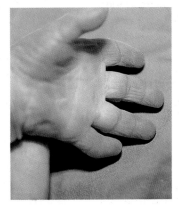

Figure 8.2b Single palmar crease.

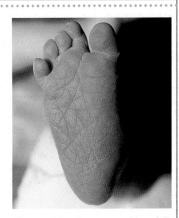

Figure 8.2c Pronounced 'sandal' gap between the big and second toe.

Box 8.1 Characteristic clinical manifestations of Down's syndrome

Typical craniofacial appearance
- Round face and flat nasal bridge
- Upslanted palpebral fissures
- Epicanthic folds (a fold of skin running across the inner edge of the palpebral fissure)
- Brushfield spots in iris (pigmented spots)
- Small mouth and protruding tongue
- Small ears
- Flat occiput and third fontanelle

Other anomalies
- Short neck
- Single palmar creases, incurved fifth finger and wide 'sandal' gap between toes
- Hypotonia
- Congenital heart defects (40%)
- Duodenal atresia
- Hirschsprung's disease

Later medical problems
- Delayed motor milestones
- Moderate to severe learning difficulties
- Small stature
- Increased susceptibility to infections
- Hearing impairment from secretory otitis media
- Visual impairment from cataracts, squints, myopia
- Increased risk of leukaemia and solid tumours
- Risk of atlantoaxial instability
- Hypothyroidism and coeliac disease
- Epilepsy
- Alzheimer's disease

Translocation (5%)

When the extra chromosome 21 is joined onto another chromosome (usually chromosome 14, but occasionally chromosome 15, 22 or 21), this is known as an unbalanced Robertsonian translocation. An affected child has 46 chromosomes, but three copies of chromosome 21 material. In this situation, parental chromosomal analysis is essential since one of the parents carries a balanced translocation in 25% of cases. Translocation carriers have 45 chromosomes, one of which consists of the two joined chromosomes (Fig. 8.4).

In translocation Down's syndrome:

- the risk of recurrence is 10–15% if the mother is the translocation carrier and about 2.5% if the father is the carrier
- if a parent carries the rare 21:21 translocation, all the offspring will have Down's syndrome
- if neither parent carries a translocation (75% of cases), the risk of recurrence is <1%.

Mosaicism (1%)

In mosaicism some of the cells are normal and some have trisomy 21. This usually arises after the formation of the zygote, by non-disjunction at mitosis. The phenotype may be milder in mosaicism.

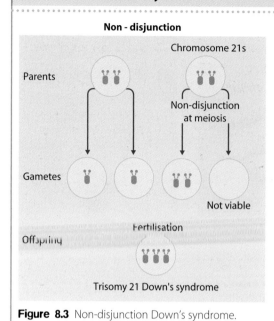

Inheritance of Down's syndrome

Figure 8.3 Non-disjunction Down's syndrome.

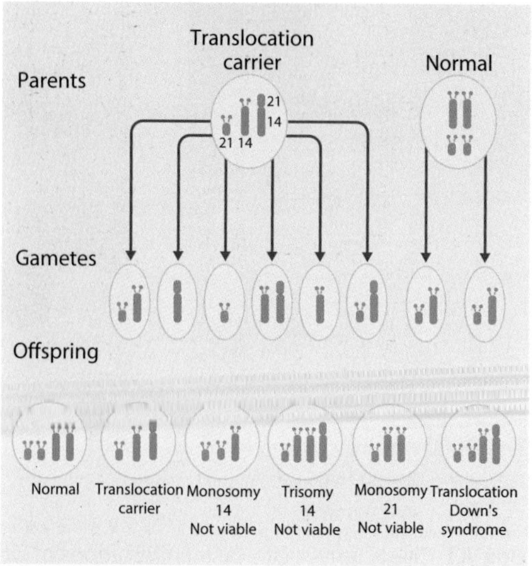

Figure 8.4 Translocation Down's syndrome. There is a translocation between chromosomes 21 and 14 inherited from a parent.

Summary

Down's syndrome (trisomy 21):

- natural incidence 1.5 per 1000 live-born infants
- cytogenetics – non-disjunction (most common, related to maternal age), translocation (parents may carry a balanced translocation) or mosaicism (rare).
- presentation – antenatal ultrasound screening or clinical; confirmed on chromosome analysis
- immediate medical complications – increased risk of duodenal atresia, congenital heart disease
- clinical manifestations – see Box 8.1.

Edwards' syndrome (trisomy 18) and Patau's syndrome (trisomy 13)

Although rarer than Down's syndrome (1 in 8000 and 1 in 14 000 live births, respectively), particular constellations of severe multiple abnormalities suggest the diagnosis at birth and most affected babies die in infancy (Fig. 8.5, Boxes 8.2 and 8.3). The diagnosis is confirmed by chromosome analysis. Many affected fetuses are detected by ultrasound scan during the second trimester of pregnancy and diagnosis can be confirmed antenatally by amniocentesis and chromosome analysis. Recurrence risk is low, except when the trisomy is due to a balanced chromosome rearrangement in one of the parents.

Turner's syndrome (45, X)

Usually (>95%) this results in early miscarriage. Increasingly detected by ultrasound antenatally when fetal oedema of the neck, hands or feet or a cystic hygroma may be identified. In live-born females, the incidence is about 1 in 2500. See Figure 8.6 and Box 8.4 for the clinical features of Turner's syndrome, although short stature may be the only clinical abnormality in children.

Treatment is with:

- growth hormone therapy
- oestrogen replacement for development of secondary sexual characteristics at the time of puberty (but infertility persists).

In about 50% of girls with Turner's syndrome, there are 45 chromosomes, with only one X chromosome. The other cases have a deletion of the short arm of one X chromosome, an isochromosome that has two long arms but no short arm, or a variety of other structural defects of one of the X chromosomes. The incidence does not increase with maternal age and risk of recurrence is very low.

Klinefelter's syndrome (47, XXY)

This disorder occurs in about 1–2 per 1000 live-born males. For clinical features, see Box 8.5. Recurrence risk is also very low.

Reciprocal translocations

An exchange of material between two different chromosomes is called a reciprocal translocation. When this exchange involves no loss or gain of chromosomal material, the translocation is 'balanced' and has no phenotypic effect. Balanced reciprocal translocations are relatively common,

Edwards' and Patau's syndromes

Box 8.2 Clinical features of Edwards' syndrome (trisomy 18)

- Low birthweight
- Prominent occiput
- Small mouth and chin
- Short sternum
- Flexed, overlapping fingers (Fig. 8.5)
- Rocker-bottom feet
- Cardiac and renal malformations

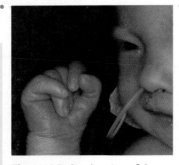

Figure 8.5 Overlapping of the fingers in Edwards' syndrome.

Box 8.3 Clinical features of Patau's syndrome (trisomy 13)

- Structural defect of brain
- Scalp defects
- Small eyes (microphthalmia) and other eye defects
- Cleft lip and palate
- Polydactyly
- Cardiac and renal malformations

Turner's syndrome

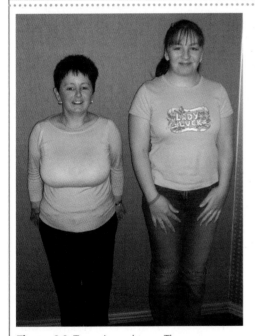

Figure 8.6 Turner's syndrome. The woman on the left has marked short stature but no other clinical features; the adolescent female on the right has neck webbing and has received growth hormone and is 150 cm in height.

Box 8.4 Clinical features of Turner's syndrome

- Lymphoedema of hands and feet in neonate, which may persist
- Spooned shaped nails
- Short stature – cardinal feature
- Neck webbing or thick neck
- Wide carrying angle (cubitus valgus)
- Widely spaced nipples
- Congenital heart defects (particularly coarctation of the aorta)
- Delayed puberty
- Ovarian dysgenesis resulting in infertility, although pregnancy may be possible with in-vitro fertilisation (IVF) with donated ova
- Hypothyroidism
- Renal anomalies
- Pigmented moles
- Recurrent otitis media
- Normal intellectual function in most

occurring in 1 in 500 of the general population. A translocation that appears balanced on conventional chromosome analysis may still involve the loss of a few genes or the disruption of a single gene that results in an abnormal phenotype, often including learning difficulty. Studying the chromosomal breakpoints in such individuals has been one way of identifying the location of specific genes.

Unbalanced reciprocal translocations contain an incorrect amount of chromosomal material and cause a combination of dysmorphic features, congenital malformations, developmental delay and learning difficulties. In a newborn baby, the prognosis is difficult to predict, but the effect is usually severe. The parents' chromosomes should be checked to determine whether the abnormality has arisen de novo, or as a consequence of a parental rearrangement. Finding a balanced translocation in one parent indicates a recurrence risk for future pregnancies and antenatal diagnosis by chorionic villus sampling or amniocentesis should be offered as well as testing of relatives.

Box 8.5 Clinical features of Klinefelter's syndrome

- Infertility – most common presentation
- Hypogonadism with small testes
- Pubertal development apparently normal (some males benefit from testosterone therapy)
- Gynaecomastia in adolescence
- Tall stature
- Intelligence – usually in the normal range, but may have educational and psychological problems

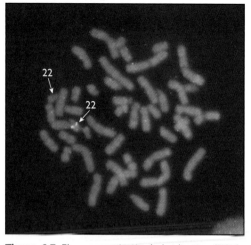

Figure 8.7 Fluorescent in-situ hybridisation (FISH) demonstrating a microdeletion on chromosome 22 associated with DiGeorge's syndrome. Hybridisation signals are seen on one chromosome 22 but not on the other chromosome 22 because of the presence of a deletion. (Courtesy of L. Gaunt, St Mary's Hospital, Manchester.)

Deletions

Deletions are another type of structural abnormality. Loss of part of a chromosome usually results in physical abnormalities and learning difficulties. The deletion may involve loss of the terminal or, less commonly, the interstitial part of a chromosome.

An example of a deletion syndrome involves loss of the tip of the short arm of chromosome 5, hence the name 5p- or monosomy 5p. Because affected babies have a high-pitched mewing cry in early infancy, it is also known as *cri du chat* syndrome. Parental chromosomes should be checked to see if one parent carries a balanced chromosomal rearrangement.

An increasing number of syndromes are now known to be due to chromosome deletions too small to be seen by conventional cytogenetic analysis. These submicroscopic deletions can be detected by FISH (fluorescent in-situ hybridisation) studies using DNA probes specific to particular chromosome regions. DiGeorge's syndrome is due to a deletion of chromosome 22 at band 22q11 (Fig. 8.7). Williams' syndrome is another example of a microdeletion syndrome due to loss of chromosomal material on the long arm of chromosome 7 at band 7q11 (see Fig. 8.18, Box 8.12).

Mendelian inheritance

Disorders with these patterns of inheritance, described by Mendel in 1865, are rare individually, but collectively numerous, with over 15 000 single gene traits or disorders described. For many disorders the Mendelian pattern of inheritance is known. If the diagnosis of a condition is uncertain, its pattern of inheritance may be evident on drawing a family tree (pedigree), which is an essential part of genetic evaluation (Fig. 8.8).

Autosomal dominant inheritance

This is the most common mode of Mendelian inheritance (Box 8.6). An affected individual carries the abnormal gene in the heterozygous state on one of a pair of autosomes (chromosomes 1–22). Male and female offspring each have a 1 in 2 (50%)

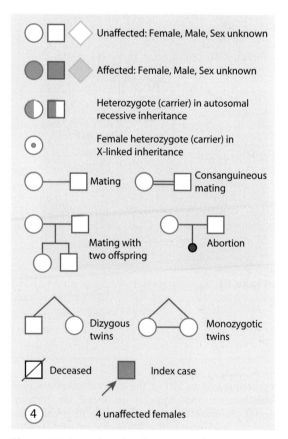

Figure 8.8 Examples of pedigree symbols.

chance of inheriting the abnormal gene from an affected parent (Fig. 8.9a and b). This is straightforward, but complicating factors include the following.

Autosomal dominant inheritance

Box 8.6 Examples of autosomal dominant disorders

- Achondroplasia
- Ehlers–Danlos syndrome
- Familial hyper-cholesterolaemia
- Huntington's disease
- Marfan's syndrome
- Myotonic dystrophy
- Neurofibromatosis
- Noonan's syndrome
- Osteogenesis imperfecta
- Otosclerosis
- Polyposis coli
- Tuberous sclerosis

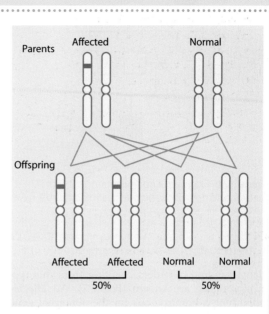

Figure 8.9a Autosomal dominant inheritance.

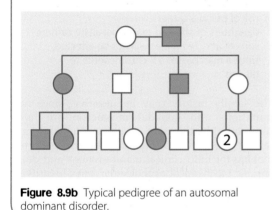

Figure 8.9b Typical pedigree of an autosomal dominant disorder.

Variation in expression

Within a family, some affected individuals may manifest the disorder mildly and others more severely. For example, a parent with tuberous sclerosis may have mild skin abnormalities only, but his or her affected child may have, in addition, epilepsy and learning difficulties.

Non-penetrance

Refers to the lack of clinical signs and symptoms in an individual who must have inherited the abnormal gene. An example of this is otosclerosis, in which only about 40% of gene carriers develop deafness (Fig. 8.10).

No family history of the disorder

May be due to:

- A new mutation in one of the gametes leading to the conception of the affected person. This is the most common reason for absence of a family history in dominant disorders, e.g. >80% of individuals with achondroplasia have normal parents.
- Gonadal mosaicism – very occasionally a healthy parent harbours the mutation only in a number of gametes in the gonad. This can account for

recurrences of autosomal dominant disorders in siblings born to apparently normal parents. It has been described in congenital lethal osteogenesis imperfecta.
- Non-paternity – if the apparent father is not the biological father.

Homozygosity

In the rare situation where both parents are affected by the same autosomal dominant disorder, there is a 1 in 4 risk that a child will be homozygous for the mutant gene.

Summary

Autosomal dominant inheritance:
- most common mode of Mendelian inheritance
- affected individual carries the abnormal gene on one of a pair of autosomes
- 1 in 2 chance of inheriting the abnormal gene from affected parent, but there may be variation in expression, non-penetrance, no family history (new mutation, gonadal mosaicism, non-paternity) or homozygosity (rare).

Mendelian inheritance

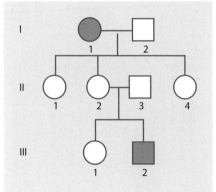

Figure 8.10 Example of non-penetrance. I1 and III2 have otosclerosis. II2 has normal hearing but must have the gene. The gene is non-penetrant in II2.

Autosomal recessive inheritance

Many hundred disorders resulting from this type of inheritance are known (Box 8.7). An affected individual is homozygous for the abnormal gene, having inherited an abnormal allele from each parent, both of whom are unaffected heterozygous carriers. For two carrier parents, the risk of each child, male or female, being affected is 1 in 4 (25%) (Fig. 8.11a and b). All offspring of affected individuals will be carriers.

Consanguinity

It is thought that we all carry at least one abnormal recessive gene. Fortunately, our partners usually carry a different one. Marrying a cousin or other relative increases the chance of both partners carrying the same abnormal autosomal recessive gene, inherited from a common ancestor. A couple who are cousins therefore have a small increase in the risk of having a child with a recessive disorder.

Recessive gene frequencies may vary between racial groups. When the gene occurs sufficiently frequently and the gene or its effect can be detected, population-based carrier testing can be performed and antenatal diagnosis offered for high-risk pregnancies. Disorders that can be screened for in this way include cystic fibrosis in north Europeans, sickle cell disease in black Africans and Americans, thalassaemias in Mediterranean or Asian ethnicity and Tay–Sachs disease in Ashkenazi Jews.

X-linked recessive inheritance

Over 400 disorders have been described in which an abnormal recessive gene is carried on the X chromosome (Box 8.8, Fig. 8.12a and b).

In X-linked recessive inheritance:

- males are affected
- females can be carriers but are usually healthy
- occasionally a female carrier shows mild signs of the disease (manifesting carrier)
- each son of a female carrier has a 1 in 2 (50%) risk of being affected
- each daughter of a female carrier has a 1 in 2 (50%) risk of being a carrier
- daughters of affected males will all be carriers
- sons of affected males will not be affected, since a man passes a Y chromosome to his son.

The family history may be negative, since new mutations and gonadal mosaicism are fairly common. Identification of carrier females in a family requires interpretation of the pedigree, looking for mild clinical manifestations and doing specific biochemical or molecular tests. Identifying carriers is important because a female carrier has a 50% risk of having an affected son regardless of who her partner is, and X-linked recessive disorders are often very severe.

Summary

X-linked recessive inheritance:
- males are affected; females can be carriers but are usually healthy or have mild disease
- family history may be negative - new mutations and gonadal mosaicism
- identifying female carriers is important to be able to provide genetic counselling.

X-linked dominant inheritance

X-linked disorders where the mutation has a dominant effect are rare. Both males and females are affected, e.g. a variant of vitamin D-resistant rickets. In some disorders male lethality is expected and only affected females will be seen, e.g. Rett's syndrome and incontinentia pigmenti.

Y-linked inheritance

Y-linked traits are extremely rare. Y-linked inheritance would result in only males being affected, with transmission from an affected father to all his sons. Y-linked genes determine sexual differentiation and spermatogenesis, and mutations are associated with infertility.

Summary

Autosomal recessive inheritance:
- affected individuals are homozygous for the abnormal gene, each parent is a heterozygous carrier
- 1 in 4 risk of having an affected child for two carrier parents
- risk of these disorders increased by consanguinity and within specific racial groups
- often affect metabolic pathways, whereas autosomal dominant disorders often affect structural proteins.

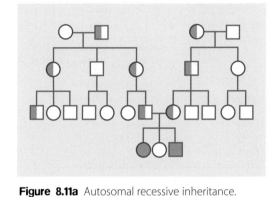

Box 8.7 Examples of autosomal recessive disorders

- Congenital adrenal hyperplasia
- Cystic fibrosis
- Friedreich's ataxia
- Galactosaemia
- Glycogen storage diseases
- Hurler's syndrome
- Oculocutaneous albinism
- Phenylketonuria
- Sickle cell disease
- Tay–Sachs disease
- Thalassaemia
- Werdnig–Hoffmann disease (SMA I)

Figure 8.11a Autosomal recessive inheritance.

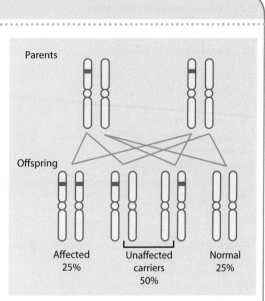

Affected 25%

Unaffected carriers 50%

Normal 25%

Figure 8.11b Pedigree to show autosomal recessive inheritance.

Unusual genetic mechanisms

Trinucleotide repeat expansion mutations

This is a class of unstable mutations caused by expansions of trinucleotide repeat sequences inherited in Mendelian fashion. Fragile X syndrome and myotonic dystrophy were among the first disorders found to be due to such mutations. Other disorders include Huntington's disease, spinocerebellar ataxia and Friedreich's ataxia. These disorders follow different patterns of inheritance but share certain unusual properties due to the nature of the underlying mutation. Clinical anticipation is often seen, with the disorders becoming more severe in successive generations of a family and new mutations being exceedingly rare.

Fragile X syndrome

The prevalence of severe learning difficulties in males due to fragile X syndrome is about 1 in 4000 (Fig. 8.13 and Box 8.9). This condition was initially diagnosed on the basis of the appearance of a gap (fragile site) in the distal part of the long arm of the X chromosome. Diagnosis is now achieved by molecular analysis of the CGG trinucleotide repeat expansion in the relevant gene (*FMR1*).

Although it is inherited as an X-linked recessive disorder, a high proportion of obligate female carriers have learning difficulties (usually mild to moderate) and around one-fifth of males who inherit the mutation are phenotypically normal but may pass the disorder on to their grandsons through their daughters.

These unusual findings are explained by the nature of the mutation, which occurs in 'pre-mutation' and 'full mutation' forms. The normal copy of the gene contains fewer than 50 copies of the CGG trinucleotide repeat sequence and is stable when transmitted to offspring. Genes with the pre-mutation contain 55–199 copies of the repeat sequence. This expansion causes no intellectual disability in male or female carriers, but is unstable and may become larger during transmission through females. Genes with the full mutation contain more than 200 copies of the repeat sequence. This affects gene function, causing the clinical features of fragile X syndrome in virtually all males and around half of the female carriers. These full mutations always arise from expansion of pre-mutations, and never arise directly from normal genes. Hence all mothers of affected males are carriers.

113

X-linked recessive inheritance

Box 8.8 Examples of X-linked recessive disorders

- Colour blindness (red–green)
- Duchenne's and Becker's muscular dystrophies
- Fragile X syndrome
- Glucose-6-phosphate dehydrogenase (G6PD) deficiency
- Haemophilia A and B
- Hunter's syndrome (mucopolysaccharidosis II)

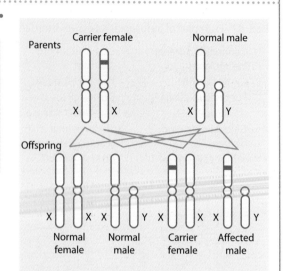

Figure 8.12a X-linked recessive inheritance.

Figure 8.12b (below) Typical pedigree for X-linked recessive inheritance, showing Queen Victoria, a carrier for haemophilia A, and her family. It shows affected males in several generations, related through females, and that affected males do not have affected sons (contrast with autosomal dominant inheritance).

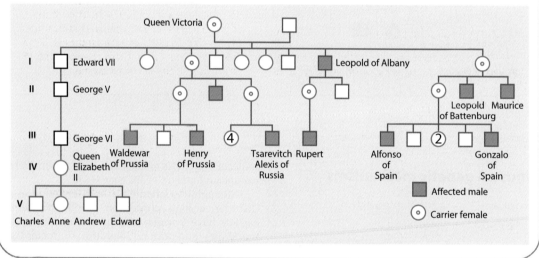

Fragile X

Figure 8.13 A child with fragile X syndrome. At this age, the main physical feature is often the prominent ears.

Box 8.9 Clinical findings in males in fragile X syndrome

- Moderate–severe learning difficulty (IQ 20–80, mean 50)
- Macrocephaly
- Macro-orchidism – postpubertal
- Characteristic facies – long face, large everted ears, prominent mandible and broad forehead, most evident in affected adults.
- Other features – mitral valve prolapse, joint laxity, scoliosis, autism, hyperactivity

> **Fragile X syndrome is the second most common genetic cause of severe learning difficulties after Down's syndrome.**

Mitochondrial or cytoplasmic inheritance

Mitochondria are cytoplasmic organelles that function as major energy producers for the cell and contain their own DNA (mt DNA). Each cell contains thousands of copies of the mitochondrial genome. In mt DNA disorders, the mutation is usually present in only a proportion of the mitochondria, so that cells have a mixture of normal and mutant mt DNA. Mutations in mt DNA cause several disorders such as Leber's hereditary optic neuropathy and various mitochondrial myopathies and encephalopathies. Mitochondrial DNA mutations show only maternal transmission, since only the egg contains cytoplasm and mitochondria. Disorders due to mt DNA deletions are usually not transmitted to offspring. Sperm do not contain mitochondria, so a father with a disorder due to a mitochondrial DNA mutation will not have affected children.

Imprinting and uniparental disomy

In the past, it has been assumed that the activity of a gene is the same regardless of whether it is inherited from the mother or father. It has been shown that some genes are actively expressed only if they have been derived from a parent of a given sex. This phenomenon is called 'imprinting'. An example involves Prader–Willi syndrome (learning difficulties, hypotonia, obesity). The Prader–Willi gene is found in the 15q11–13 region of chromosome 15 (that is, bands 11–13 on the long arm of chromosome 15). Normally, only the paternal copy of the Prader–Willi gene is active. Failure to inherit the active paternal gene will give rise to the syndrome. Failure to inherit the maternal copy of this gene has no effect, since it is inactive. Coincidentally, the gene for Angelman syndrome (severe learning difficulty, ataxia, characteristic facial appearance, epilepsy) is also found in the same chromosome region and is also subject to imprinting. In this case it is the maternal gene that is the active one. Failure to inherit the maternal gene will therefore cause Angelman syndrome. There are two main ways that a child can fail to inherit the active gene for either syndrome:

- De novo *deletion* (Fig. 8.14). Parental chromosomes are normal, and a deletion occurs as a new mutation in the child. If the deletion occurs on the paternal chromosome 15, the child has Prader–Willi syndrome. If the deletion affects the maternal chromosome 15, the child has Angelman syndrome.

Imprinting

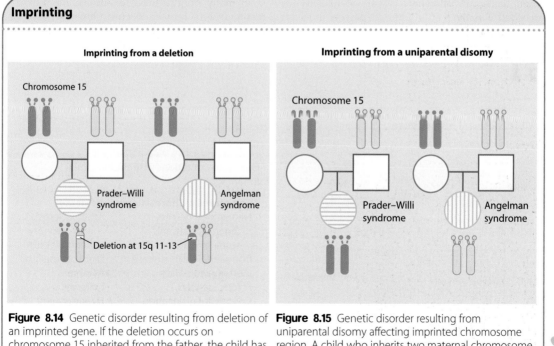

Imprinting from a deletion

Chromosome 15

Prader–Willi syndrome

Angelman syndrome

Deletion at 15q 11-13

Imprinting from a uniparental disomy

Chromosome 15

Prader–Willi syndrome

Angelman syndrome

Figure 8.14 Genetic disorder resulting from deletion of an imprinted gene. If the deletion occurs on chromosome 15 inherited from the father, the child has Prader–Willi syndrome. If the deletion occurs on chromosome 15 from the mother, the child has Angelman syndrome.

Figure 8.15 Genetic disorder resulting from uniparental disomy affecting imprinted chromosome region. A child who inherits two maternal chromosome 15s will have Prader–Willi syndrome. A child who inherits two paternal chromosome 15s will have Angelman syndrome.

- *Uniparental disomy* (Fig. 8.15). This is when a child inherits two copies of a chromosome from one parent and none from the other parent. In Prader–Willi syndrome the affected child has no paternal (but two maternal) copies of chromosome 15q 11–13. In Angelman syndrome the affected child has no maternal (but two paternal) copies of chromosome 15q11–13. This can be detected with DNA analysis.

> Imprinting is the unusual property of some genes to express only the copy derived from a parent of a given sex.

Polygenic or multifactorial inheritance

There is a spectrum in the aetiology of disease, from environmental factors (e.g. trauma) at one end to purely genetic causes (e.g. Mendelian disorders) at the other. Between these two extremes are many disorders which result from the additive effect of several genes (hence the term polygenic) with or without the influence of environmental or other unknown factors (i.e. multifactorial). The two terms are often used interchangeably (Box 8.10).

Normal traits such as height and intelligence are also inherited in this way. These parameters show a Gaussian or normal distribution in the population. Similarly, the liability of an individual to develop a disease of multifactorial or polygenic aetiology also has a normal distribution. The condition occurs when a certain threshold level of liability is exceeded. Relatives of an affected person show an increased liability due to inheritance of genes conferring susceptibility, and so a greater proportion of them than in the general population will fall beyond the threshold and will manifest the disorder (Fig. 8.16).

The risk of recurrence of a polygenic disorder in a family is usually low and is most significant for first-degree relatives. Empirical recurrence risk data are used for genetic counselling. They are derived from family studies that have reported the frequency at which various family members are affected. Factors that increase the risk to relatives are:

- having a more severe form of the disorder, e.g. the risk of recurrence to siblings is greater in bilateral cleft lip and palate than in unilateral cleft lip alone
- close relationship to the affected person, e.g. overall risk to siblings is greater than to more distant relatives
- multiple affected family members, e.g. the more siblings already affected, the greater the risk of recurrence
- sex difference in prevalence, e.g. in Hirschsprung's disease the male to female ratio is 3:1; an affected female must have had a greater genetic predisposition, so the risk to siblings is greater than for an affected male.

The phenotype (clinical picture) of a disorder may have a heterogeneous (mixed) basis in different families; for example, hyperlipidaemia leading to atherosclerosis and coronary heart disease can be due to a single gene disorder such as autosomal dominant hypercholesterolaemia, but some forms of hyperlipidaemia are polygenic and result from an interaction of the effect of genes on various lipoproteins.

In many multifactorial disorders, the 'environmental factors' remain obscure. Obvious exceptions include dietary fat intake and smoking in atherosclerosis, and viral infection in insulin-dependent diabetes mellitus. For neural tube defects, the risk

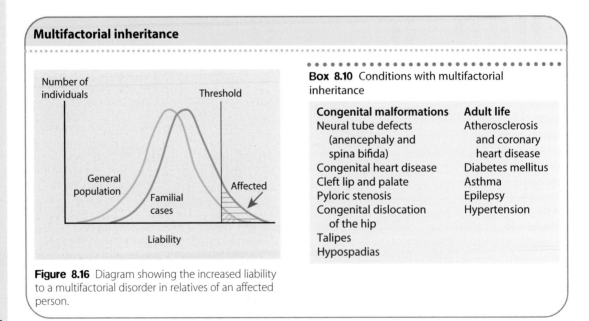

Multifactorial inheritance

Figure 8.16 Diagram showing the increased liability to a multifactorial disorder in relatives of an affected person.

Box 8.10 Conditions with multifactorial inheritance

Congenital malformations	Adult life
Neural tube defects (anencephaly and spina bifida)	Atherosclerosis and coronary heart disease
Congenital heart disease	Diabetes mellitus
Cleft lip and palate	Asthma
Pyloric stenosis	Epilepsy
Congenital dislocation of the hip	Hypertension
Talipes	
Hypospadias	

of recurrence to siblings is lowered from about 4% to 1% or less in future pregnancies if the mother takes folate before conception and in the early weeks of pregnancy.

DNA analysis

New techniques in DNA testing are continually being developed, making more single gene disorders amenable to molecular analysis. Most molecular testing is performed using polymerase chain reaction (PCR). This involves the amplification of specific DNA sequences, enabling rapid analysis of small samples, which is particularly important in antenatal diagnosis.

The main impact of DNA analysis for genetic counselling is:

* confirmation of a clinical diagnosis
* detection of female carriers in X-linked disorders, e.g. Duchenne's and Becker's muscular dystrophies, haemophilia A and B
* carrier detection in autosomal recessive disorders, e.g. cystic fibrosis
* presymptomatic diagnosis in autosomal dominant disorders, e.g. Huntington's disease, myotonic dystrophy
* antenatal diagnosis of an increasing number of Mendelian conditions.

These are accomplished by:

1. Mutation analysis

For an increasing number of disorders, it is possible to directly detect the actual mutation causing the disease. This provides very accurate results for confirmation of diagnosis, and presymptomatic or predictive testing. Identifying the mutation in an affected individual may be very time-consuming, but once this has been done, testing other relatives is usually fairly simple. Examples are:

* Deletions – large deletion mutations are common in a variety of disorders including Duchenne's and Becker's muscular dystrophies, alpha-thalassaemia and 21-hydroxylase deficiency (congenital adrenal hyperplasia). They can be tested for relatively easily.
* Point mutations and small deletions – these can be readily identified if the same mutation causes all cases of the disorder, as in sickle cell disease. For most disorders, however, there is a very diverse spectrum of mutations. About 78% of cystic fibrosis carriers in the UK possess the ΔF508 mutation, but over 900 other mutations have been identified. Most laboratories test for a certain number of the most common mutations in their given population.
* Trinucleotide repeat expansion mutations – these are readily tested for because the mutation in a given disease is always the same. The only difference is the size of the repeat sequence, which can be determined from the size of the DNA fragment containing the repeat.

2. Genetic linkage

If mutation analysis is not available, it may be possible to use DNA sequence variations (markers) located near to, or within, the disease gene to track the inheritance of this gene through a family. This type of analysis requires a suitable family structure and several key members need to be tested to identify appropriate markers before linkage testing can be used predictively.

Presymptomatic testing

In many autosomal dominant disorders, onset is during adolescence or adult life and clinical expression may not be evident at birth. Relatives of affected individuals may request tests to see if they are likely to develop the disorder in question. Examples include myotonic dystrophy, Huntington's disease, autosomal dominant polycystic kidney disease and neurofibromatosis.

Assessment may include:

* careful examination of individuals at risk, e.g. development of café-au-lait patches and axillary freckling in neurofibromatosis
* investigations, e.g. renal ultrasound scans in individuals at risk of autosomal dominant polycystic kidney disease
* DNA analysis using linked markers or mutation analysis.

It is generally accepted that presymptomatic tests (e.g. for Huntington's disease and myotonic dystrophy) and carrier tests (e.g. for cystic fibrosis) should not be performed on healthy children, as these remove the child's future right to choose whether or not to have this information.

> **Presymptomatic testing should not be performed until the individual can give informed consent.**

Gene therapy

The treatment of most genetic disorders is based on conventional therapeutic approaches. These may include health surveillance, supportive measures, medical therapy, surgical procedures, dietary manipulation, replacement of deficient gene products or enzymes and bone marrow transplantation.

Gene therapy involves the repair, suppression or artificial introduction of genes into genetically abnormal cells with the aim of curing the disease and is at an experimental stage for most genetic conditions being studied. There are still many technical and safety issues to be resolved.

Gene therapy has been initiated in adenosine deaminase deficiency (a rare recessive immune disorder), malignant melanoma and cystic fibrosis, and some clinical benefit has been reported in a few patients. At present, it is generally accepted that gene therapy should be limited to somatic (not germ line) cells, so that the risk of adversely affecting future generations is minimised.

Dysmorphology

The term 'dysmorphology' literally means 'the study of abnormal form' and refers to the assessment of birth defects and unusual physical features that have their origin during embryogenesis.

Pathogenic mechanisms

Malformation
A primary structural defect occurring during the development of a tissue or organ, e.g. spina bifida and cleft lip and palate.

Deformation
Implies an abnormal intrauterine mechanical force that distorts a normally formed structure, e.g. joint contractures due to fetal compression caused by severe oligohydramnios.

Disruption
Involves destruction of a fetal part which initially formed normally; e.g. amniotic membrane rupture may lead to amniotic bands which may cause limb reduction defects.

Dysplasia
Refers to abnormal cellular organisation or function of specific tissue types, e.g. skeletal dysplasias and dysplastic kidney disease.

Clinical classification of birth defects

Single-system defects
These include single congenital malformations such as spina bifida and are often multifactorial in nature with fairly low recurrence risks.

Sequence
Refers to a pattern of multiple abnormalities occurring after one initiating defect. Potter's syndrome (fetal compression and pulmonary hypoplasia) is an example of a sequence in which all abnormalities may be traced to one original malformation, renal agenesis.

Association
A group of malformations that occur together more often than expected by chance, but in different combinations from case to case, e.g. VACTERL association (Vertebral anomalies, Anal atresia, Cardiac defects, Tracheo-oEsophageal fistula, Renal anomalies, Limb defects).

Syndrome
When a particular set of multiple anomalies occurs repeatedly in a consistent pattern, this is called a 'syndrome'. Multiple malformation syndromes are often associated with moderate or severe learning difficulties and may be due to:

- chromosomal defects
- a single gene defect (dominant or recessive)
- exposure to teratogens such as alcohol, drugs (especially anticonvulsants such as valproate, carbamazepine and phenytoin) or viral infections during pregnancy
- unknown cause.

Syndrome diagnosis

Although most syndromes are individually rare, recognition of a dysmorphic syndrome may give information regarding:

- risk of recurrence
- prognosis
- likely complications which can be sought and perhaps treated successfully if detected early
- the avoidance of unnecessary investigations
- experience and information which parents can share with other affected families through self-help groups.

Examples of syndromes recognisable by facial appearance are shown in Figures 8.17–8.19 (see also Boxes 8.11–8.13).

> ## Summary
>
> Dysmorphology:
> - comprises birth defects and abnormal clinical features originating during embryogenesis
> - may be a malformation, deformation, disruption or dysplasia
> - may be classified as a single-system defect, sequence, association or syndrome.

Genetic counselling

The main aim of genetic counselling is to give individuals, couples and families information about hereditary disorders so that they understand:

- what it means to have the disorder
- their risk of developing or transmitting it to offspring
- measures to treat or prevent the disorder.

A primary goal of genetic counselling is to provide information to allow for greater autonomy and choice in reproductive decisions. Prevention of genetic disease may also result from genetic counselling, but this is not the main aim. The elements of genetic counselling include:

- Establishing the correct diagnosis. This involves detailed history, examination and appropriate investigations that may include chromosome or DNA analysis, biochemical tests, X-rays and clinical photographs. Despite extensive investigation, the diagnosis may remain unknown, e.g. in children with learning disability and mild or non-specific dysmorphic features.

Syndromes recognised by 'Gestalt' (clinical recognition)

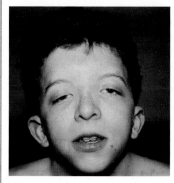

Figure 8.17 Noonan's syndrome affects males and females. There are some similarities to the phenotype in Turner's syndrome, but it is caused by a faulty autosomal dominant gene and the chromosomes are normal.

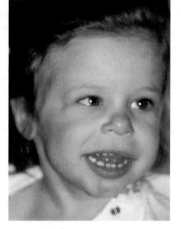

Figure 8.18 Williams' syndrome is usually sporadic.

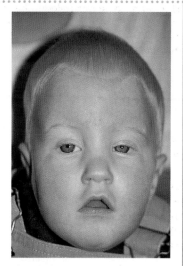

Figure 8.19 Prader–Willi syndrome.

Box 8.11 Clinical features of Noonan's syndrome

- Characteristic facies
- Occasional mild learning difficulties
- Short webbed neck with trident hair line
- Pectus excavatum
- Short stature
- Congenital heart disease (especially pulmonary stenosis, atrial septal defect)

Box 8.12 Clinical features of Williams' syndrome

- Short stature
- Characteristic facies
- Transient neonatal hypercalcaemia (occasionally)
- Congenital heart disease (supravalvular aortic stenosis)
- Mild to moderate learning difficulties

Box 8.13 Clinical features of Prader–Willi syndrome

- Characteristic facies
- Hypotonia
- Neonatal feeding difficulties
- Failure to thrive in infancy
- Obesity in later childhood
- Hypogonadism
- Developmental delay
- Learning difficulties

- Risk estimation. This requires both diagnostic and pedigree information. Drawing a pedigree of three generations is an essential part of genetic counselling. The mode of inheritance may be apparent from the pedigree even when the precise diagnosis is not known. In some cases it may not be possible to define a precise recurrence risk and uncertainty may remain, e.g. conditions that only affect one member of a family and are known to follow autosomal dominant inheritance in some families and autosomal recessive inheritance in others (genetic heterogeneity).
- Communication. Information must be presented in an understandable and unbiased way. Families often find written information very helpful to refer back to and diagrams are often used to explain patterns of inheritance. The impact of saying 'the recurrence risk is 5%' may be different from saying 'the chance of an unaffected child is 95%', and so both should be presented.

- Discussing options for management and prevention. If there appears to be a risk to offspring, all reproductive options should be discussed. These include not having (more) children, reducing intended family size, taking the risk and proceeding with pregnancy or having antenatal diagnosis and selective termination of an affected fetus. For some couples donor insemination or ovum donation may be appropriate and for others achieving a pregnancy through IVF (in-vitro fertilisation) and preimplantation diagnosis may be possible.

Counselling should be non-directive, but should also assist in the decision-making process (Box 8.14). This requires:

- time and possibly several sessions for discussion
- a compassionate approach by the professionals
- awareness by the counsellor of psychological

Box 4.14 Influences on decisions regarding options for genetic counselling

- Magnitude of risk
- Severity of disorder
- Availability of treatment
- Person's experience of the disorder
- Family size
- Availability of a safe and reliable antenatal test
- Parental or cultural ethical values

issues, such as denial, grief and anger, which are often evoked by genetic illness
- awareness by the counsellor of ethnic, social, religious and educational factors
- follow-up consultations to ensure understanding and to offer support – this is an essential part of genetic counselling, particularly when a family is coming to terms with the diagnosis and the implications of a genetic disease, after a termination of pregnancy for fetal abnormality or following the death of an affected child
- provision of information about appropriate lay support groups.

Case History
8.1 Syndrome diagnosis and genetic counselling

Sean, the second child of healthy parents, was born at term by emergency caesarean section for fetal distress. The pregnancy had been uneventful and no abnormalities were detected on antenatal ultrasound scan. He developed respiratory distress and investigation for a cardiac murmur revealed an interrupted aortic arch and ventricular septal defect that required surgical correction in the neonatal period.

The parents asked about recurrence risk for congenital heart disease and were referred to the genetic clinic. At that time, Sean was thriving and early developmental progress appeared normal. On examination there were minor dysmorphic features, including a short philtrum, thin upper lip and prominent ears (Fig. 8.20). There was no family history of congenital heart disease or other significant problems and no abnormalities were detected on examination of the parents.

Because of an association between outflow tract abnormalities of the heart and deletions of chromosome 22, cytogenetic analysis was performed using fluorescent in-situ hybridisation (FISH). A submicroscopic deletion of the long arm of one chromosome 22 (band 22q11) was detected. Other features of DiGeorge syndrome (hypocalcaemia and T-cell deficiency), which occurs with the same chromosome deletion, were excluded by appropriate tests.

Parental chromosome analysis showed no deletion at chromosome 22q11 in either parent, indicating a low recurrence risk for future pregnancies since gonadal mosaicism for this deletion is very rare. The older sibling was also normal on testing. Because the parents had normal karyotypes, their own brothers and sisters did not need to be offered tests.

Identification of a 22q11 deletion indicated that other associated problems were likely. Subsequently, Sean required assessment by a multidisciplinary child

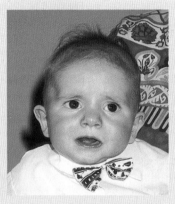

Figure 8.20 Sean's facial appearance showing the short philtrum (vertical groove in the upper lip), thin upper lip and prominent ears.

development team (developmental delay), educational statementing and recommendation for placement in a school for children with special educational needs (learning difficulty), input from a clinical psychologist when behavioural problems appeared (ritualistic behaviour and obsessional tendencies), input from speech therapist and plastic surgeon (indistinct speech due to velopharyngeal incompetence) and audiology review (conductive hearing loss due to recurrent otitis media).

The impact of the diagnosis and its implications was considerable for the family and the parents needed support from a variety of professionals whilst coming to terms with the various problems as they became apparent. Written information and details of the 22q11 support group were given to the parents. Medical care was coordinated by the paediatrician.

There was the additional worry for the family about a subsequent pregnancy. Fetal echocardiography showed no evidence of congenital heart disease, but invasive tests for cytogenetic analysis were declined because of the low recurrence risk. The baby was born unaffected, with chromosome studies performed on a cord blood sample revealing no abnormality.

In the UK all health regions have a clinical genetics centre where specialist genetic services are provided by consultants and other medical staff, genetic counsellors and laboratory scientists. Initiatives to integrate genetic services into primary and secondary care include:

- education of the general public and medical profession about genetic issues
- establishment of comprehensive screening programmes (e.g. for cystic fibrosis) in the community, with facilities for testing and counselling
- extending the role of non-medical genetic counsellors.

Genetic counselling aims to allow parents greater autonomy and choice in reproductive decisions.

Further reading

Baraitser M, Winter R M 1996 Color atlas of congenital malformation syndromes. Mosby-Wolfe, London

Harper P S 2004 Practical genetic counselling, 6th edn. Arnold, London. *Book on clinical genetics and counselling*

Jones K L 2005 Smith's recognisable patterns of human malformation, 5th edn. WB Saunders, Philadephia. *Diagnosing syndromes*

Kingston H M 2002 ABC of clinical genetics, 3rd edn. BMJ Books, London

Read A, Donnai D 2007 New clinical genetics. Scion, Bloxham, Oxfordshire

Strachan T, Read A P 2004 Human molecular genetics, 3rd edn. Garland Publishing, London and New York. *Molecular genetics*

Turnpenny P, Ellard S 2004 Emery's elements of medical genetics, 12th edn. Churchill Livingstone, Edinburgh. *General introduction to medical genetics*

Internet

Contact-a-family: www.cafamily.org.uk (UK family support group alliance)
Information on genetic disorders and testing: www.genetests.org (American website funded by NIH includes review articles on selected genetic disorders)
Omim (Online Mendelian Inheritance in Man): www.ncbi.nlm.nih.gov/omim (has links to other genetic databases)
Your Genes, Your Health: www.ygyh.org (Cold Spring Harbor website giving information on some common genetic disorders and links to DNA tutorials)

Perinatal medicine

The term 'perinatal medicine' refers to medical care of the infant before, during and after birth, acknowledging the continuity of fetal and neonatal life. Using modern technology, such as high-resolution ultrasound and DNA analysis, detailed information about the fetus can now be obtained for a large and increasing number of conditions. Close cooperation is important between the professionals involved in the care of the pregnant mother and fetus and those caring for the newborn infant.

Some definitions

Some definitions used in perinatal medicine are:

- Stillbirth – fetus born with no signs of life ≥24 weeks of pregnancy
- Perinatal mortality rate – stillbirths + deaths within the first week per 1000 live births and stillbirths
- Neonatal mortality rate – deaths of live-born infants within the first 4 weeks of age per 1000 live births
- Neonate – infant ≤28 days old
- Preterm – gestation <37 weeks of pregnancy
- Term – 37–41 weeks of pregnancy
- Post-term – gestation ≥ 42 weeks of pregnancy
- Low birthweight (LBW) – <2500 g
- Very low birthweight (VLBW) – <1500 g
- Extremely low birthweight (ELBW) – <1000 g
- Small for gestational age – birthweight <10th centile for gestational age
- Large for gestational age – birthweight >90th centile for gestational age.

Pre-pregnancy care

The better a mother's state of health and nutrition, and the higher her socioeconomic living standard and the quality of health care she receives, the greater is the chance of a successful outcome to her pregnancy.

Couples planning to have a baby often ask what they should do to optimise their chances of having a healthy child. They can be informed that for the mother:

- *Smoking* reduces birthweight, which may be of critical importance if born preterm. On average, the babies of smokers weigh 170 g less than those of non-smokers, but the reduction in birthweight is related to the number of cigarettes smoked per day. Smoking is also associated with an increased risk of miscarriage and stillbirth. The infant has a greater risk of sudden infant death syndrome (SIDS).
- *Certain medications* such as retinoids or warfarin must be avoided because of teratogenic effects.
- *Excess alcohol* ingestion and *drug abuse* (opiates, cocaine) may damage the fetus.
- *Congenital rubella* is preventable by maternal immunisation before pregnancy.
- *Exposure to toxoplasmosis* should be minimised by avoiding eating undercooked meat and by wearing gloves when handling cat litter.
- *Listeria infection* can be acquired from eating unpasteurised dairy products, soft ripened cheeses, e.g. brie, camembert and blue veined varieties, patés and ready-to-eat poultry unless thoroughly reheated.

- *Eating liver* during pregnancy is best avoided as it contains a high concentration of vitamin A.
- *Pre-pregnancy folic acid* supplements reduce the risk of neural tube defects in the fetus. Low-dose folic acid supplementation is recommended for all women planning a pregnancy, with a higher dose for women with a previously affected fetus.

Any pre-existing maternal medical condition (e.g. hypertension) or obstetric risk factors for complications of pregnancy or delivery (e.g. recurrent miscarriage or previous preterm delivery) should be identified and treated or monitored. Obesity increases the risk of developing gestational diabetes and pregnancy-induced hypertension.

Couples at increased risk of inherited disorders should receive genetic counselling before pregnancy. They can then be fully informed, decide whether or not to proceed, and consider antenatal diagnosis if available. Pregnancies at increased risk of fetal abnormality include those in which:

- the mother is older (if she is >35 years old, the risk of Down's syndrome is >1 in 380)
- there is previous congenital abnormality
- there is a family history of an inherited disorder
- the parents are identified as carriers of an autosomal recessive disorder, e.g. thalassaemia
- a parent carries a chromosomal rearrangement
- a consanguineous relationship exists.

> ✽ **Pre-pregnancy folic acid supplements reduce the risk of neural tube defects in the fetus.**

Antenatal diagnosis

Antenatal diagnosis has become available for an increasing number of disorders. Screening tests performed on maternal blood and ultrasound of the fetus are listed in Box 9.1. The main diagnostic techniques for antenatal diagnosis are detailed ultrasound scanning, amniocentesis and chorionic villus sampling (Fig. 9.1). In addition, preimplantation genetic diagnosis (PGD) allows genetic analysis of cells from a developing embryo before transfer to the uterus, and fetal tissue sampling can be performed. The structural malformations and other lesions which can be identified on ultrasound are listed in Box 9.2, with an example in Figure 9.2.

Antenatal screening for disorders affecting the mother or fetus allows:

- reassurance where disorders are not detected
- optimal obstetric management of the mother and fetus
- therapy to be given for a number of conditions to improve perinatal outcome
- neonatal management to be planned in advance

Box 9.1 Screening tests for antenatal diagnosis

Maternal blood	Blood group and antibodies – for rhesus and other red cell incompatibilities
	Hepatitis B
	Syphilis
	Rubella
	HIV infection
	Neural tube defects – raised maternal serum alphafetoprotein (MSAFP) with spina bifida or anencephaly, but ultrasound alone increasingly used
	Down's syndrome – risk estimate calculated from multiple biochemical markers combined with ultrasound screening for nuchal translucency (back of neck). Aim is to detect >80% with <5% false-positive rate. If high risk, fetal chromosome analysis is offered
Ultrasound screening	Gestational age – can be estimated reliably if early in pregnancy
	Multiple pregnancies – can be identified
	Structural malformation – 30–70% of major congenital malformations can be detected. If a significant abnormality is suspected, a more detailed scan by a specialist is indicated
	Fetal growth – can be monitored by serial measurement of abdominal circumference, head circumference and femur length
	Amniotic fluid volume – oligohydramnios may result from reduced fetal urine production (because of dysplastic or absent kidneys or obstructive uropathy), from prolonged rupture of the membranes or be associated with severe intrauterine growth restriction. It may cause pulmonary hypoplasia and limb and facial deformities from pressure on the fetus (Potter's syndrome)
	Polyhydramnios – is associated with maternal diabetes and gastrointestinal atresia in the fetus

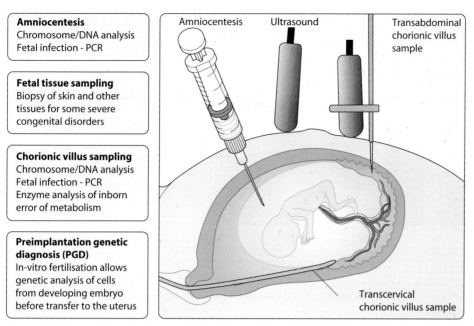

Amniocentesis
Chromosome/DNA analysis
Fetal infection - PCR

Fetal tissue sampling
Biopsy of skin and other tissues for some severe congenital disorders

Chorionic villus sampling
Chromosome/DNA analysis
Fetal infection - PCR
Enzyme analysis of inborn error of metabolism

Preimplantation genetic diagnosis (PGD)
In-vitro fertilisation allows genetic analysis of cells from developing embryo before transfer to the uterus

Amniocentesis   Ultrasound   Transabdominal chorionic villus sample

Transcervical chorionic villus sample

Figure 9.1 Some of the techniques used for antenatal diagnosis.

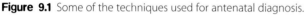

Box 9.2 Main structural malformations and other lesions detectable by ultrasound

CNS	Anencephaly – always detected
	Spina bifida
	Hydrocephalus, microcephaly, encephalocele
Cardiac	About 50% of severe malformations detected on 'routine' screening, about 90% at specialist centres
Intrathoracic	Diaphragmatic hernia
Facial	Cleft lip and palate
Gastrointestinal	Bowel obstruction, e.g. duodenal atresia
	Exomphalos and gastroschisis
Genitourinary	Dysplastic or cystic kidneys
	Obstructive disorders of kidneys or urinary tract (hydronephrosis, distended bladder)
Skeletal	Skeletal dysplasias, e.g. achondroplasia and limb reduction deformities
Hydrops	Oedema of the skin, pleural effusions and ascites
Chromosomal	Down's syndrome – suspected from thickened fat pad at the back of neck (nuchal translucency), duodenal atresia or an atrioventricular canal defect of the heart
	Other chromosomal disorders – from identifying multiple abnormalities

- the option of termination of pregnancy to be offered for severe disorders affecting the fetus (see Case history 9.1) or compromising maternal health.

Parents require accurate medical advice and counselling to help them with these difficult decisions. Many transient or minor structural disorders of the fetus are also detected, which may cause considerable anxiety.

> Antenatal diagnosis allows many congenital malformations which used to be diagnosed at birth or during infancy to be identified before birth.

Fetal medicine

The fetus can sometimes be treated by giving medication to the mother. Examples include:

- *Glucocorticoid therapy* before preterm delivery accelerates lung maturity and surfactant production. This has been tested in over 15 randomised trials and markedly reduces the incidence of respiratory distress syndrome (RDS) (relative risk 0.66), of intraventricular haemorrhage (relative risk 0.54) and neonatal mortality (relative risk 0.69) in preterm infants. For optimal effect, a completed course needs to be given at least 24 hours before delivery.
- *Digoxin or flecainide* can be given to the mother to treat fetal supraventricular tachycardia.

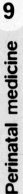

Antenatal diagnosis – gastroschisis

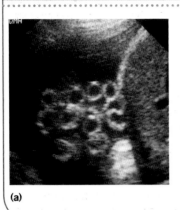

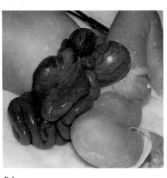

(a)   **(b)**

Figure 9.2 Gastroschisis on antenatal ultrasound showing free loops of small bowel in the amniotic fluid **(a)** and following delivery **(b)**. Antenatal diagnosis allowed the baby to be delivered at a paediatric surgical unit and the parents to be forewarned about the need for surgery. Satisfactory surgical repair was achieved. (Courtesy of Mr Karl Murphy.)

Case History
9.1 Antenatal diagnosis

A routine ultrasound scan at 18 weeks' gestation identified an abnormal 'lemon-shaped' skull (Fig. 9.3). This, together with an abnormal appearance of the cerebellum, is the Arnold–Chiari malformation, which is associated with spina bifida. An extensive spinal defect was confirmed on ultrasound. Dilatation of the cerebral ventricles and talipes already present in this fetus suggested a severe spinal lesion. After counselling, the parents decided to terminate the pregnancy.

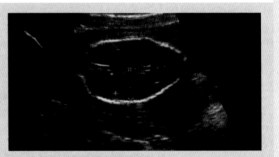

Figure 9.3 Transverse section showing a 'lemon-shaped' skull on ultrasound instead of the normal oval shape. This is associated with spina bifida. (Courtesy of Mr Guy Thorpe-Beeston.)

There are a few conditions where therapy can be given to the fetus directly:

- *Rhesus isoimmunisation.* Severely affected fetuses become anaemic and may develop *hydrops fetalis*, with oedema and ascites. Infants at risk are identified by maternal antibody screening. Regular ultrasound of the fetus is performed to detect fetal hydrops. The development of fetal anaemia is assessed non-invasively using Doppler velocimetry of the fetal middle cerebral artery. Fetal blood transfusion via the umbilical vein may be required regularly from about 20 weeks' gestation. The incidence of rhesus haemolytic disease has fallen markedly since anti-D immunisation of mothers was introduced.
- *Perinatal isoimmune thrombocytopenia.* This condition is analogous to rhesus isoimmunisation but involves maternal anti-platelet antibodies crossing the placenta. It is rare, affecting about 1 in 5000 births. Intracranial haemorrhage secondary to fetal thrombocytopenia occurs in up to 25%. The problem may be anticipated if there was a

previously affected infant, and repeated intrauterine platelet transfusions can then be performed.

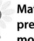 **Maternal glucocorticoid therapy before preterm delivery markedly reduces morbidity and mortality in the neonate.**

Fetal surgery

Fetal surgery is being attempted at a number of centres in the world, but the results have generally been disappointing. Procedures which have been performed include:

- Surgical correction by hysterotomy. This is when the uterus is opened at 22–24 weeks' gestation. It has been performed in a few specialist centres for diaphragmatic hernia and spina bifida but may precipitate preterm delivery and its efficacy remains highly uncertain. Results of fetal surgery to close spina bifida suggest that hydrocephalus may be reduced but does not improve the prognosis of the spinal lesion.

- Catheter shunts inserted under ultrasound guidance. This is to drain fetal pleural effusions (pleuro-amniotic shunts), often from a chylothorax (lymphatic fluid). One end of a looped catheter lies in the chest, the other end in the amniotic cavity.
- Intrauterine shunting for obstruction to urinary outflow as with posterior urethral valves. This has yielded disappointing results to date.
- Intrauterine shunting for hydrocephalus is technically possible but has not been shown to improve outcome.
- Dilatation of stenotic heart valves via a transabdominal catheter inserted under ultrasound guidance into the fetal heart.
- Endotracheal balloon occlusion for congenital diaphragmatic hernia, as tracheal obstruction in utero may promote lung growth.

Careful case selection and follow-up are required to ensure that these novel forms of treatment are of long-term benefit.

Obstetric conditions affecting the fetus

Pre-eclampsia

Mothers with pre-eclampsia may require preterm delivery because of the maternal risks of eclampsia and of cerebrovascular accident or the fetal risks associated with placental insufficiency and growth restriction. Determining the optimal time for preterm delivery requires an evaluation of the risk to the mother and fetus of allowing the pregnancy to continue compared with the neonatal complications associated with preterm birth.

Placental insufficiency and intrauterine growth restriction (IUGR)

Fetal growth may be progressively restricted because of placental insufficiency. Transfer of oxygen and nutrients is reduced. The growth-restricted fetus will need to be monitored closely. This will include assessing fetal size clinically (symphysis to fundal height measurement) and serial ultrasound measurements of fetal growth. Antenatal cardiotocography (CTG) to detect evidence of fetal hypoxia may be combined with an ultrasound assessment of fetal activity, breathing and amniotic fluid volume to form a biophysical profile to identify fetal compromise. Doppler ultrasound is now widely used to obtain a blood flow velocity profile of the uterine artery (maternal circulation to the placental bed) and the umbilical artery (fetal circulation). Absence or reversal of flow velocity in the umbilical artery during diastole carries an increased risk of morbidity from hypoxic damage to the gut or brain, or of intrauterine death. The blood flow velocity waveforms in the fetal descending aorta, cerebral and other arteries give

an indication of fetal circulatory redistribution in response to hypoxia of blood from the gastrointestinal tract and liver, kidney, muscles and subcutaneous tissue to the brain. These measurements assist in deciding the optimal time for delivery of a growth-restricted fetus.

Multiple births

Twins occur naturally in the UK in 1 in 90 deliveries, triplets in 1 in 90^2, i.e. approximately 1 in 8000 and quadruplets in 1 in 90^3, i.e. approximately 1 in every 700 000 deliveries. Over the last decade the number of triplets and higher order births has more than doubled, mainly from assisted reproduction programmes and advancing maternal age. One in 70 births is now a multiple birth, although the number of triplets and higher order births has recently declined.

The main problems for the infant associated with multiple births are:

- *Preterm labour.* The median gestation for twins is 35 weeks, for triplets 32 weeks and for quads 30 weeks. Preterm delivery is the most important cause of the greater perinatal mortality of multiple births, especially for triplets and higher order pregnancies.
- *Intrauterine growth restriction (IUGR).* Fetal growth in one or more fetuses may deteriorate and needs to be monitored regularly.
- *Congenital abnormalities.* These occur twice as frequently as in a singleton, but the risk is increased fourfold in monochorionic twins.
- *Twin–twin blood transfusions in monochorionic twins (shared placenta).* May cause discrepancy in growth.
- *Complicated deliveries*, e.g. due to malpresentation of the second twin at vaginal delivery.

Finding sufficient intensive care cots for preterm multiple births can be problematic.

Although multiple births may look endearing, the families may need additional assistance and support:

- practical – with their care and housework (requires about 200 hours/week for triplets in infancy!)
- emotional and physical exhaustion
- loss of privacy as a couple

Summary

Multiple births:

- have markedly increased in number
- are associated with an increased risk of prematurity, intrauterine growth restriction (IUGR), congenital malformations and twin–twin blood transfusions
- are responsible for 30% of very low birthweight infants (<1.5 kg birthweight)
- provide many additional problems for their parents to care for them.

- additional financial costs
- increased behavioural problems in the infants and their siblings. While being a multiple birth may provide companionship, affection and stimulation between each other, it may also engender domination, dependency and jealousy.

There are local and national support groups for parents of multiple births.

Maternal conditions affecting the fetus

Diabetes

Women with insulin-dependent diabetes find it more difficult to maintain good diabetic control during pregnancy and have an increased insulin requirement. Poorly controlled maternal diabetes is associated with polyhydramnios and pre-eclampsia, increased rate of early fetal loss, congenital malformations and late unexplained intrauterine death. Ketoacidosis carries a high fetal mortality. With meticulous attention to diabetic control, the perinatal mortality rate is now only slightly greater than in non-diabetics.

Fetal problems associated with maternal diabetes are:

- *Congenital malformations.* Overall, there is a 6% risk of congenital malformations, a threefold increase compared with the non-diabetic population. The range of anomalies is similar to that for the general population, apart from an increased incidence of cardiac malformations, sacral agenesis (caudal regression syndrome) and hypoplastic left colon, although the latter two conditions are rare. Studies show that good diabetic control periconceptionally reduces the risk of congenital malformations.
- *Intrauterine growth restriction (IUGR).* There is a threefold increase in growth restriction in mothers with long-standing microvascular disease.
- *Macrosomia* (Fig. 9.4). Maternal hyperglycaemia causes fetal hyperglycaemia as glucose crosses the placenta. As insulin does not cross the placenta, the fetus responds with increased secretion of

insulin which promotes growth by increasing both cell number and size. About 25% of such infants have a birthweight greater than 4 kg compared with 8% of non-diabetics. The macrosomia predisposes to cephalopelvic disproportion, birth asphyxia, shoulder dystocia and brachial plexus injury.

Neonatal problems include:

- *Hypoglycaemia.* Transient hypoglycaemia is common during the first day of life from fetal hyperinsulinism, but can often be prevented by early feeding. The infant's blood glucose should be closely monitored during the first 24 hours and hypoglycaemia treated.
- *Respiratory distress syndrome (RDS).* More common as lung maturation is delayed.
- *Hypertrophic cardiomyopathy.* Hypertrophy of the cardiac septum occurs in some infants. It regresses over several weeks but may cause heart failure from reduced left ventricular function.
- *Polycythaemia* (venous haematocrit >0.65). Makes the infant look plethoric. Treatment with partial exchange transfusion to reduce the haemocrit and normalise viscosity may be required.

Gestational diabetes is when carbohydrate intolerance occurs only during pregnancy. Its definition and method of identification remain controversial. It is more common in women who are obese and in those of Afro-Caribbean and Asian ethnicity. The incidence of macrosomia and its complications is similar to that of the insulin-dependent diabetic mother, but the incidence of congenital malformations is not increased. However, associated with the increase in obesity in the population, there are an increasing number of mothers with type 2 non-insulin dependent diabetes. Their fetuses are also at increased risk of congenital malformations.

> ### SUMMARY
>
> **Maternal diabetes:**
> - meticulous control pre-conceptually and during pregnancy markedly reduces fetal and neonatal morbidity and mortality
> - the fetus may be macrosomic because of fetal hyperglycaemia resulting in hyperinsulinism, or growth-restricted secondary to maternal microvascular disease, and is at increased risk of congenital malformations
> - the macrosomic infant is at increased risk of asphyxia and birth trauma from obstructed labour or delivery
> - the newborn infant is prone to hypoglycaemia and polycythaemia.

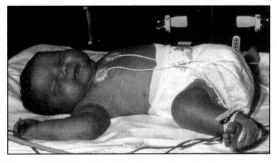

Figure 9.4 Infant of a diabetic mother showing macrosomia and plethora. Born vaginally at 36 weeks' gestation, she weighed 5.5 kg and suffered a right-sided brachial plexus injury.

Hyperthyroidism

One to two per cent of newborn babies whose mothers have had Graves' disease are hyperthyroid, due to circulating thyroid-stimulating antibody which crosses the placenta and stimulates the fetal thyroid. Hyperthyroidism in the fetus is suggested by fetal tachycardia on a CTG trace, and fetal goitre may be evident on ultrasound; in the neonate it is suggested by irritability, weight loss, diarrhoea and exophthalmos lasting several months.

Systemic lupus erythematosus

Systemic lupus erythematosus (SLE) with antiphospholipid syndrome is associated with recurrent miscarriage, intrauterine growth restriction, placental abruption and preterm delivery. Some of the infants born to mothers with antibodies to the Ro (SS-A) or La (SS-B) antigens develop neonatal lupus syndrome, in which there is a self-limiting rash and, rarely, heart block.

Autoimmune thrombocytopenic purpura

In maternal autoimmune thrombocytopenic purpura (AITP), the fetus may become thrombocytopenic because maternal IgG antibodies cross the placenta and damage fetal platelets. Severe fetal thrombocytopenia places the fetus at risk of intracranial haemorrhage from birth trauma. Infants with severe thrombocytopenia or petechiae at birth should be given intravenous immunoglobulin. Platelet transfusions may be required if there is acute bleeding.

Maternal drugs affecting the fetus

Relatively few drugs are known definitely to damage the fetus (Table 9.1), but it is clearly advisable for pregnant women to avoid taking medicines unless it is essential. Whilst the teratogenicity of a drug may be recognised if it causes malformations which are severe and distinctive, as with limb shortening following thalidomide ingestion, milder and less distinctive abnormalities may go unrecognised.

The problem of establishing a link may be compounded by a delay of months or years before any problems present. An example of this is diethylstilbestrol (DES), given in the past for threatened miscarriage, and its subsequent association with vaginal adenosis and carcinoma of the vagina and cervix in female offspring during adolescence or early adult life.

Alcohol and smoking

Excessive alcohol ingestion during pregnancy is sometimes associated with the 'fetal alcohol syndrome'. Its clinical features are growth restriction, characteristic face (Fig. 9.5), developmental delay and cardiac defects (up to 70%). The effects of less severe ingestion and binge-drinking remain uncertain but may affect growth and development.

Maternal cigarette smoking is associated in the fetus with an increased risk of miscarriage and stillbirth, a reduction in birthweight, and intrauterine growth restriction (IUGR). The birthweight reduction is related to the number of cigarettes smoked per day, with an average reduction of 170 g at term.

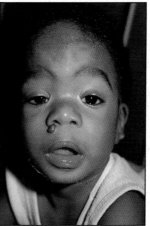

Figure 9.5
Characteristic facies of fetal alcohol syndrome with: a saddle-shaped nose; maxillary hypoplasia; absent philtrum between the nose and upper lip; and short, thin upper lip. This child also has a strawberry naevus below the right nostril.

Table 9.1 Maternal medication which may adversely affect the fetus

Medication	Adverse effect
Anticonvulsant therapy with carbamazepine, valproic acid (sodium valproate) or hydantoins (phenytoin)	Fetal carbamazepine/valproate/hydantoin syndrome – midfacial hypoplasia, CNS, limb and cardiac malformations, developmental delay.
Cytotoxic agents	Congenital malformations
Diethylstilbestrol (DES)	Clear-cell adenocarcinoma of vagina and cervix
Iodides/propylthiouracil	Goitre, hypothyroidism
Lithium	Congenital heart disease
Tetracycline	Enamel hypoplasia of the teeth
Thalidomide	Limb shortening (phocomelia)
Vitamin A and retinoids	Increased spontaneous abortions, abnormal face
Warfarin	Interferes with cartilage formation (nasal hypoplasia and epiphyseal stippling); cerebral haemorrhages and microcephaly

In the infant, maternal smoking associated with an increased risk of sudden infant death syndrome (SIDS) and wheezing in childhood.

Drug abuse

Maternal drug abuse with opiates is associated with an increased risk of prematurity and growth restriction. Many narcotic abusers take multiple drugs. Infants of mothers abusing heroin, methadone and other opiates during pregnancy often show evidence of drug withdrawal, with jitteriness, sneezing, yawning, poor feeding, vomiting, diarrhoea, weight loss and seizures during the first 2 weeks of life. Cocaine abuse is associated with placental abruption and preterm delivery, but rarely with withdrawal in the infant, although it may result in cerebral infarction. Amphetamine abuse is also associated with gastrointestinal and cerebral infarction. Mothers who abuse drugs, and their infants, are also at increased risk of hepatitis B and C and HIV infection.

Infants who develop significant features of drug withdrawal will need treatment. Oral morphine, methadone and diazepam are used at different centres. One of the major problems in managing these infants is that the parents' lifestyle and temperament are often not conducive to the needs of babies and young children. Close supervision or alternative care-givers are often required.

> **If there are unexplained clinical signs in an infant, consider drug withdrawal.**

Drugs given during labour

Potential adverse effects to the fetus of drugs given during labour are:

- *Opioid analgesics/anaesthetic agents.* May suppress respiration at birth.
- *Epidural anaesthesia.* May cause maternal pyrexia during labour. It is often difficult to differentiate this from fever caused by an infection.
- *Sedatives, e.g. diazepam.* May cause sedation, hypothermia and hypotension in the newborn.
- *Oxytocin.* May cause hyperstimulation of the uterus leading to fetal hypoxia. It is also associated with a small increase in bilirubin levels in the neonate.
- *Intravenous fluids.* May cause neonatal hyponatraemia unless they contain an adequate concentration of sodium.

Congenital infections

Intrauterine infection is usually from maternal primary infection during pregnancy. Those that can damage the fetus are:

- rubella
- cytomegalovirus (CMV)
- *Toxoplasma gondii*
- parvovirus
- varicella zoster
- syphilis.

Rubella

The diagnosis of maternal infection must be confirmed serologically as clinical diagnosis is unreliable. The risk and extent of fetal damage are mainly determined by the gestational age at the onset of maternal infection. Infection before 8 weeks' gestation causes deafness, congenital heart disease and cataracts in over 80% (Fig. 9.6a). About 30% of fetuses of mothers infected at 13–16 weeks' gestation have impaired hearing; beyond 18 weeks' gestation the risk to the fetus is minimal. Viraemia after birth continues to damage the infant. Tests used to confirm the diagnosis are shown in Box 9.3. The range of clinical features characteristic of congenital infections is shown in Figure 9.6b

Congenital rubella is preventable. In the UK, it has become rare since the measles/mumps/rubella (MMR) vaccine was introduced into the childhood immunisation programme, but this is dependent on the maintenance of a high vaccine uptake rate.

Cytomegalovirus

CMV is the most common congenital infection, affecting 3–4/1000 live births in the UK, with higher rates reported in parts of the USA. In Europe, 50% of pregnant women are susceptible to CMV. About 1% of susceptible women will have a primary infection during pregnancy, and in about 40% of them the infant becomes infected. The infant may also become infected following recurrent infection in a pregnant woman who is immune, but this is much less likely to damage the fetus.

When an infant is infected:

- 90% are normal at birth and develop normally
- 5% have clinical features at birth, such as hepatosplenomegaly and petechiae (Fig. 9.6b), most of whom will have neurodevelopmental disabilities such as sensorineural hearing loss, cerebral palsy, epilepsy and cognitive impairment
- 5% develop problems later in life, mainly sensorineural hearing loss.

Box 9.3 Diagnosis of congenital rubella, cytomegalovirus (CMV) and *Toxoplasma* infection

Mother	Seroconversion on screening serology
Fetus	Amniocentesis or chorionic villus sample – PCR
Placenta	Microscopy for syphilis, PCR
Urine from infant	Rubella, CMV – culture, PCR
Blood, CSF, other samples from infant	Culture, PCR
Blood serology	Rubella-specific IgM CMV-specific IgM *Toxoplasma*-specific IgM and persistently raised *Toxoplasma* IgG

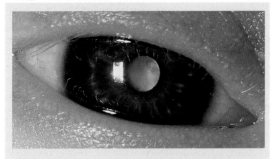

Figure 9.6a Cataract from congenital rubella. Congenital heart disease and deafness are the other common defects.

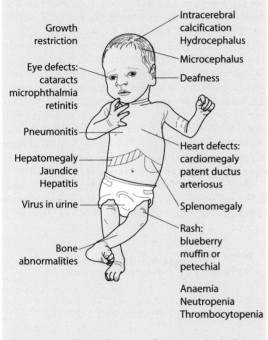

- Growth restriction
- Eye defects: cataracts microphthalmia retinitis
- Pneumonitis
- Hepatomegaly Jaundice Hepatitis
- Virus in urine
- Bone abnormalities
- Intracerebral calcification Hydrocephalus
- Microcephalus
- Deafness
- Heart defects: cardiomegaly patent ductus arteriosus
- Splenomegaly
- Rash: blueberry muffin or petechial

Anaemia
Neutropenia
Thrombocytopenia

Figure 9.6b Clinical features of congenital rubella, cytomegalovirus (CMV), toxoplasmosis and syphilis.

Infection in the pregnant woman is usually asymptomatic or causes a mild non-specific illness. As there is no CMV vaccine and no antiviral therapy which is effective and safe, pregnant women are not screened for CMV.

Toxoplasmosis

Acute infection with *Toxoplasma gondii*, a protozoan parasite, may result from the consumption of raw or undercooked meat and from contact with the faeces of recently infected cats. In the UK, fewer than 20% of pregnant women have had past infection, in contrast to 80% in France and Austria.

Transplacental infection may occur during the parasitaemia of a primary infection, and about 40% of fetuses become infected. In the UK, the incidence of congenital infection is only about 0.1 per 1000 live births. Most infected infants are asymptomatic. About 10% have clinical manifestations (Fig. 9.6b), of which the most common are:

- retinopathy, an acute fundal chorioretinitis which sometimes interferes with vision
- cerebral calcification
- hydrocephalus.

These infants usually have long-term neurological disabilities. Asymptomatic infants remain at risk of developing chorioretinitis into adulthood.

As the specific IgM antibody test has a low sensitivity, serial IgG antibody tests are needed to differentiate passively acquired maternal antibody from fetal infection. In some countries, e.g. France and Austria, pregnant women are screened serologically for *Toxoplasma* infection during pregnancy. Women who show seroconversion can be treated with the antibiotic spiromycin. Confirmation of fetal infection is obtained from amniocentesis and, if positive, treatment with the pyrimethamine and sulfadiazine or termination of pregnancy can be offered. The severely affected fetus may also have evidence on ultrasound of a fetal anomaly, e.g. hydrocephalus or cerebral calcification, but these can only be recognised at advanced gestation. Infected newborn infants are treated for a year. In the UK, in view of the low incidence and the lack of data on the efficacy of treatment, pregnant women are not routinely screened.

Varicella zoster

Fifteen per cent of pregnant women are susceptible to varicella (chickenpox). Usually, the fetus is unaffected but will be at risk if the mother develops chickenpox:

- in the first half of pregnancy (<20 weeks), when there is a <2% risk of the fetus developing severe scarring of the skin and possibly ocular and neurological damage and digital dysplasia
- within 5 days before or 2 days after delivery, when the fetus is unprotected by maternal antibodies and the viral dose is high. About 25% develop a vesicular rash. The illness has a mortality as high as 30%.

Exposed susceptible women can be protected with varicella zoster immune globulin (VZIG) and treated with aciclovir. Infants born in the high-risk period should also receive zoster immune globulin and are often also given aciclovir prophylactically.

> **If a mother develops chickenpox shortly before or after delivery, the infant needs protection from infection.**

Syphilis

Congenital syphilis is rare in the UK. The clinical features are shown in Figure 9.6b. Those specific to congenital syphilis include a characteristic rash on the soles of the feet and hands and bone lesions. If mothers with syphilis identified on antenatal screening are fully treated a month or more before delivery, the infant does not require treatment and has an excellent prognosis. If there is any doubt about the adequacy of maternal treatment, the infant should be treated with penicillin.

Adaptation to extrauterine life

In the fetus, the lungs are filled with fluid and oxygen is supplied by the placenta. The blood vessels that supply and drain the lungs are constricted (high pulmonary vascular resistance), so most blood from the right side of the heart bypasses the lungs and flows through the ductus arteriosus into the aorta, and some flows across the foramen ovale (Fig. 9.7). Shortly before and during labour, lung liquid production is reduced. During descent through the birth canal, the infant's chest is squeezed and lung liquid drained. Multiple stimuli, including thermal, tactile and hormonal (with a particularly dramatic increase in catecholamine levels), initiate breathing. On average, the first breath occurs 6 seconds after delivery. Lung expansion is generated by marked intrathoracic negative pressure and a functional residual capacity is established. The mean time to establish regular breathing is 30 seconds. Once the infant gasps, the remaining lung fluid is absorbed into the lymphatic and pulmonary circulation.

Pulmonary expansion at birth is associated with a rise in the oxygen tension, and with the falling pulmonary vascular resistance the pulmonary blood flow increases. Increased left atrial filling results in a rise in the left atrial pressure with closure of the foramen ovale. The flow of oxygenated blood through the ductus arteriosus causes physiological, and eventual anatomical, ductal closure. After an elective caesarean section, when the mother has not been in labour and the infant's chest has not been squeezed through the birth canal, it may take several hours for the lung fluid to be completely absorbed, causing rapid, laboured breathing (transient tachypnoea of the newborn).

Some infants may fail to adapt to extrauterine life and fail to breathe at birth. The most important cause is 'birth asphyxia' when a fetus has experienced a critical lack of oxygen during labour and delivery. It does not necessarily mean that the brain has been injured but birth asphyxia can lead to brain injury or death. Infants continuously deprived of oxygen at birth will initially gasp before becoming apnoeic (primary apnoea), during which time the heart rate is maintained. This is followed by irregular gasping and then a second period of apnoea (secondary or terminal apnoea), when the heart rate and blood pressure fall. At this stage, the infant will only recover if help with lung expansion is provided, e.g. by positive pressure ventilation by mask or tracheal tube (Fig. 9.8).

The human fetus rarely experiences a continuous asphyxial insult, except after placental abruption or complete occlusion of umbilical blood flow in a

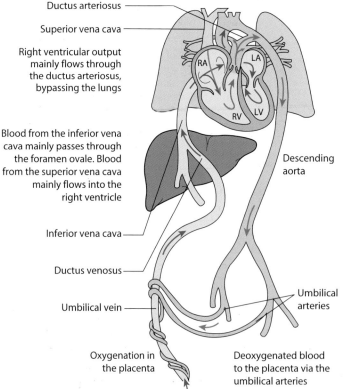

Figure 9.7 The fetal circulation.

Ductus arteriosus

Superior vena cava

Right ventricular output mainly flows through the ductus arteriosus, bypassing the lungs

Blood from the inferior vena cava mainly passes through the foramen ovale. Blood from the superior vena cava mainly flows into the right ventricle

Inferior vena cava

Ductus venosus

Umbilical vein

Oxygenation in the placenta

RA LA

RV LV

Descending aorta

Umbilical arteries

Deoxygenated blood to the placenta via the umbilical arteries

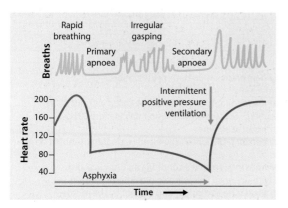

Figure 9.8 Changes in respiration and heart rate with continuous asphyxia. Once the infant has stopped gasping in secondary apnoea, resuscitation with lung expansion is required to establish regular respiration and restore the circulation.

cord prolapse. More commonly, asphyxia which occurs during labour and delivery is intermittent, e.g. from prolonged and frequent uterine contractions. Although birth asphyxia is an important cause of failure to establish breathing, which requires resuscitation at birth, there are other causes, including birth trauma, maternal analgesic or anaesthetic agents, retained lung fluid, preterm delivery or a congenital malformation which interferes with breathing.

The Apgar score is used to describe a baby's condition at 1 and 5 minutes after delivery (Table 9.2). It is also measured at 5-minute intervals thereafter if the infant's condition remains poor. The most important components are the heart rate and respiration.

Neonatal resuscitation

Most infants do not require any resuscitation. Shortly after birth, the baby will gasp or cry, establish normal breathing and become pink. The baby can be handed directly to his or her mother, and covered with a warm towel to avoid becoming cold. However, a newborn infant who does not establish normal respiration directly will need to be transferred to a resuscitation table for further assessment (Fig. 9.9). There should be an overhead radiant heater and the infant should be dried and partially covered and kept warm. The mouth and nose are gently suctioned to remove any fluid or blood if necessary. Vigorous suction of the back of the throat may provoke bradycardia from vagal stimulation and should be avoided. If the infant's breathing in the first minute of life is irregular or shallow, but the heart rate is satisfactory (>100 beats/min), additional oxygen is given and breathing encouraged with gentle tactile stimulation.

If the infant does not start to breathe, or if the heart rate drops below 100 beats/min, airway positioning and breathing by mask ventilation are started (Fig. 9.9b–e). If the baby's condition does not improve promptly with basic resuscitation, or if the infant is clearly in very poor condition at birth, tracheal intubation and artificial ventilation should be performed immediately (Fig. 9.9f). If at any time the heart rate drops below 60 beats/min, external cardiac compression should be given (Fig. 9.9g–i). If the response to ventilation and external cardiac compression remains inadequate, drugs are given (Fig. 9.9j). Evidence for their efficacy is poor.

> **Providing optimal ventilation, evidenced by good chest wall movement, is the key to successful neonatal resuscitation.**

Meconium aspiration

The passage of meconium becomes increasingly common the greater the infant's gestational age. Infants who inhale thick meconium may develop meconium aspiration syndrome. Attempting to aspirate meconium from the nose and mouth while the infant's head is on the perineum is not recommended as it has been shown to be ineffective. If the infant cries at birth and establishes regular respiration, he should be treated as normal and no resuscitation is required. If respiration is not established, the cords should be inspected under direct vision and any meconium present should be aspirated by suctioning with a large-bore suction catheter passed below the cords, or intubated and the tracheal tube aspirated. As much meconium as possible is removed, but if the infant becomes bradycardic, positive pressure ventilation will need to be initiated despite the presence of meconium.

Table 9.2 The Apgar score

	Score		
	0	1	2
Heart rate	Absent	<100 beats/min	>100 beats/min
Respiratory effort	Absent	Gasping or irregular	Regular, strong cry
Muscle tone	Flaccid	Some flexion of limbs	Well flexed, active
Reflex irritability	None	Grimace	Cry, cough
Colour	Pale/blue	Body pink, extremities blue	Pink

Preparation

- All health professionals dealing with newborn infants should be proficient in basic resuscitation; i.e. **A**irway, **B**reathing with mask ventilation, **C**irculation with cardiac compressions
- Additional skilled assistance is needed if the baby does not respond rapidly and should be called without delay
- A person proficient in advanced resuscitation (**A**irway, **B**reathing via tracheal ventilation, **C**irculation, **D**rugs) should be on site and available at short notice in a maternity unit at all times
- The need for resuscitation can usually be anticipated and a person proficient in advanced resuscitation should be in attendance at all high risk deliveries
- A clock should be started at birth for accurate timing of changes in the infant's condition and Apgar scores
- Keep the infant warm. Dry, remove wet towel and replace with dry one. This will also provide stimulation Can place directly on mother's chest and covered if crying, good tone and colour and desired by the mother
- If preterm and <30 weeks' gestation, place under a radiant warmer and cover without drying with plastic wrapping over the head and body, leaving the face exposed
- Assess the infant's condition. Is the baby breathing or crying, good heart rate (120–160 beats/min, best assessed by listening with a stethoscope), good colour and muscle tone?
- If not, commence neonatal resuscitation

Overview

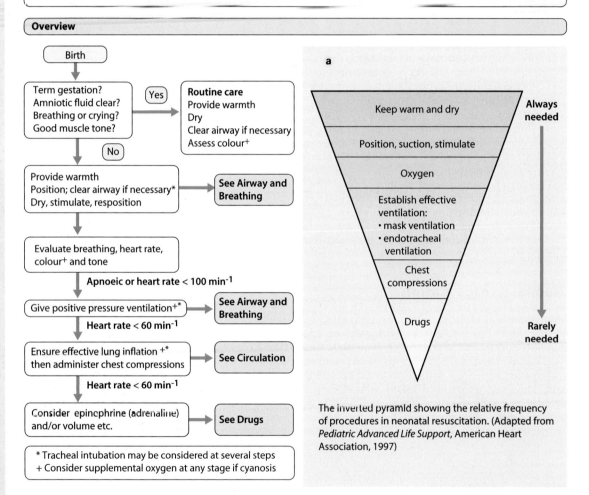

The inverted pyramid showing the relative frequency of procedures in neonatal resuscitation. (Adapted from *Pediatric Advanced Life Support*, American Heart Association, 1997)

Figure 9.9 Neonatal resuscitation.

Naloxone

Infants born to mothers who have received opiate analgesia within a few hours of delivery may occasionally develop respiratory depression which can be reversed by naloxone. It is only given if respiration continues to be depressed following initial resuscitation. As the half-life of naloxone is shorter than that of the maternal opiate, the infant's breathing must be monitored, as further doses of naloxone may be required. With modern obstetric practice, naloxone is rarely needed.

Airway and Breathing

Airway
- Opened by placing the infants's head in a neutral position (**b**)
- Provide chin lift or jaw thrust if necessary (**c**)

Breathing - mask ventilation
- If not breathing adequately by about 90 seconds start mask ventilation
- Mask is placed over mouth and nose (**d**) and connected to flow-controlled pressure-limited circuit (e.g. mechanical ventilator or Neopuff) or self inflating bag (**e**)
- Head in neutral position
- Give 5 inflation breaths, inflation time 2–3 seconds at inspiratory pressure of 30 cm of water in term infants
- If heart rate increases, but breathing does not start , continue with peak inspiratory pressure to achieve chest wall movement (15-25 cm H_2O, 0.5 second inflation time) and rate of 30–40 breaths/min
- Begin ventilatory resuscitation in air to avoid excessive tissue oxygenation; however, increase to 100% oxygen if infant's condition does not rapidly improve. Ideally, use air/oxygen blender to titrate oxygen concentration with oxygen saturation on pulse oximeter, maintaining oxygen saturation 88-95% if preterm, > 95% if term
- Reassess every 30 seconds. If heart rate not responding, check mask position, neck position, is jaw thrust needed, is circuit all right, ensure adequate lung aeration. **Call for help**

Intubation
- If effective ventilation not established, intubate and start mechanical ventilation (**f**)
- If heart rate does not increase and adequate lung inflation not achieved, consider **DOPE**:

Displaced tube (often in oesophagus or right main bronchus)
Obstructed tube (especially meconium)
Patient:
- Lung disorders - lung immaturity/respiratory distress syndrome, pneumothorax, diaphragmatic hernia, lung hypoplasia, pleural effusion
- Shock from blood loss
- Birth asphyxia/trauma
- Upper airways obstruction - choanal atresia

Equipment failure (exhausted gas supply)

b Head position, vital for airway management

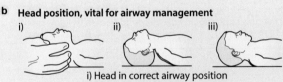

i) Head in correct airway position
ii) Head over-extended - incorrect
iii) Head flexed - incorrect

c

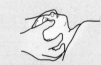

Chin support   Jaw thrust

d Correct size and position of the face mask. It should cover the mouth, nose and chin

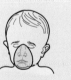

Correct
Covers mouth, nose and chin but not eyes

Incorrect
Too large – covers eyes and extends over chin

Incorrect
Too small – does not cover nose and mouth completely

e Mask ventilation
Pressure limited air/oxygen

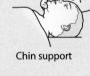

Mask ventilation delivered with pressure-limited circuit via T piece (as shown) or Neopuff or self inflating bag.The head position must be checked – here it is overextended

f Tracheal intubation

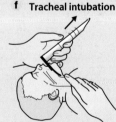

The laryngoscope blade is lifted upwards. Gentle pressure on the trachea helps bring the vocal cords into view

Figure 9.9, *cont'd*

Failure to respond to resuscitation

Poor response to tracheal intubation is usually because the tracheal tube is misplaced or has become blocked with secretions or meconium. Chest wall movement is the best guide to air entry to the lungs. If there is any uncertainty about the adequacy of ventilation and resuscitation continues to be unsuccessful, it is essential to remove the tracheal tube, give mask ventilation and then re-intubate. The decision to stop resuscitation is always difficult and should be made by a senior

Neonatal resuscitation

Circulation

External cardiac compression (g, h and i)
- Start if heart rate < 60 beats/min in spite of effective lung inflation
- Ratio of cardiac compression: lung inflation of 3:1, rate of 90 compressions: 30 breaths/min (120 events/min)
- Recheck heart rate every 30 seconds; stop when heart rate >60 beats/min

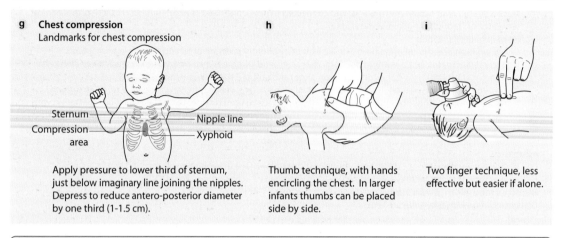

g   Chest compression
Landmarks for chest compression

Sternum — Compression area — Nipple line — Xyphoid

Apply pressure to lower third of sternum, just below imaginary line joining the nipples. Depress to reduce antero-posterior diameter by one third (1-1.5 cm).

h

Thumb technique, with hands encircling the chest. In larger infants thumbs can be placed side by side.

i

Two finger technique, less effective but easier if alone.

Drugs

Consider drugs (j) if heart rate <60 beats/min in spite of adequate ventilation and external cardiac compression, though evidence for their efficacy is lacking
Rarely needed.
Drugs should be given via an umbilical venous catheter, or, if not possible, via an intra-osseous needle.
Drugs given via a peripheral vein are unlikely to reach the heart. Giving standard doses of epinephrine (adrenaline) down the endotracheal tube does not appear to be effective; this route should only be considered whilst intravenous access is being obtained.

j   Drugs used in neonatal resuscitation

Drug	Concentration	Route/dosage	Indications
Epinephrine (adrenaline)	1:10 000	IV: 0.1 ml/kg (10 microgram/kg), then 0.1– 0.3 ml/kg (10–30 microgram/kg) ET: 1ml/kg (100 microgram/kg) i.e. 10 times the IV dose, whilst IV access is obtained	Heart rate <60 beats/min in spite of adequate ventilation and external cardiac compression
Sodium bicarbonate	4.2%	2–4 ml/kg (1–2 mmol/kg)	Severe lactic acidosis
Dextrose	10%	2.5 ml/kg (250 mg/kg)	Hypoglycaemia
Volume expander	Normal saline Blood	10 ml/kg, repeat if necessary	Blood loss

Figure 9.9, *cont'd*

paediatrician. The longer it takes a baby to respond to resuscitation, the less likely is survival. If there is no breathing or cardiac output after 10 minutes of effective resuscitation, further efforts are likely to be fruitless. If prolonged resuscitation has been required, the infant should be transferred to the neonatal unit for assessment and monitoring.

Resuscitation of the preterm infant

Preterm infants are particularly liable to hypothermia, and every effort must be made to keep them warm during resuscitation. Infants of <30 weeks' gestation should, with the exception of the face, be covered completely with plastic wrapping. Excessive tissue oxygenation may potentially cause tissue damage to the lungs and eyes from oxygen free radicals. Ideally, instead of using 100% oxygen, variable oxygen concentration can be administered and is titrated to keep the oxygen saturation between 88 and 95%. Very premature infants often develop respiratory distress syndrome, and early administration of surfactant has been shown to reduce mortality. Resuscitation of infants at the threshold of viability, at 22–24 weeks' gestation, raises particularly difficult ethical and management issues. They should be taken by experienced paediatricians, with as much involvement with the parents as possible.

Size at birth

An infant's gestation and birthweight influence the nature of the medical problems likely to be encountered in the neonatal period. In the UK, 7% of babies are of low birthweight (<2.5 kg). However, they account for about 70% of neonatal deaths.

Definitions

Babies with a birthweight below the 10th centile for their gestational age are called small for gestational age or small-for-dates (Fig. 9.10). The majority of these infants are normal, but small. The incidence of congenital abnormalities and neonatal problems is higher in those whose birthweight falls below the second centile (approximately two standard deviations below the mean), and some authorities restrict the term to this group of babies. An infant's birthweight may also be low because of preterm birth, or because the infant is both preterm and small for gestational age.

Small-for-gestational-age infants may have grown normally but are small, or they may have experienced intrauterine growth restriction (IUGR) i.e. they have failed to reach their full genetically determined growth potential and appear thin and malnourished. Babies with a birthweight above the 10th centile may also be malnourished, e.g. a fetus growing along the 80th centile who develops growth failure and whose weight falls to the 20th centile.

Patterns of growth restriction

Growth restriction in both the fetus and infant has traditionally been classified as symmetrical or asymmetrical. In the more common asymmetrical growth restriction, the weight or abdominal circumference lies on a lower centile than that of the head. This occurs when the placenta fails to provide adequate nutrition late in pregnancy but brain growth is relatively spared at the expense of liver glycogen and skin fat (Fig. 9.11). This form of growth restriction is associated with uteroplacental dysfunction secondary to maternal pre-eclampsia, multiple pregnancy, maternal smoking, or it may be idiopathic. These infants rapidly put on weight after birth.

In symmetrical growth retardation, the head circumference is equally reduced. It suggests a prolonged period of poor intrauterine growth (or that the gestational age is incorrect). It is usually due to a small but normal fetus, but may be due to a fetal chromosomal disorder or syndrome, a congenital infection, maternal drug and alcohol abuse or a chronic medical condition or

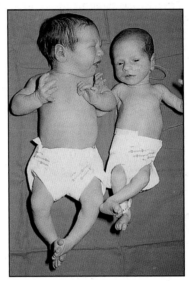

Figure 9.11 Severe intrauterine growth restriction in a twin.

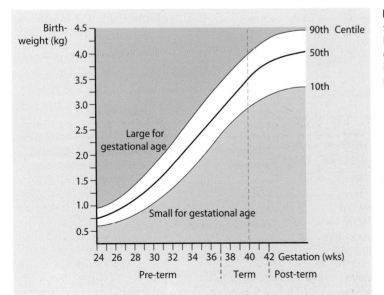

Figure 9.10 The birthweight of small-for-gestational-age infants is below the 10th centile for their gestation. Small-for-gestational-age infants may be preterm, term or post-term.

malnutrition. These infants are more likely to remain small permanently.

In practice, distinction between asymmetrical and symmetrical growth restriction often cannot be made.

Monitoring the growth-restricted fetus

The fetus with IUGR is at risk from:

* intrauterine hypoxia and intrauterine death
* asphyxia during labour and delivery.

The growth-restricted fetus will need to be monitored closely to determine the optimal time for delivery. Progressive uteroplacenta failure results in:

* reduced growth in femur length and abdominal circumference
* abnormal umbilical artery Doppler waveforms – absent or reversed end diastolic flow
* redistribution of blood flow in the fetus – increased to the brain, reduced to gastrointestinal tract, liver, skin and kidneys
* reduced amniotic fluid volume
* reduced fetal movements
* abnormal CTG (cardiotocography)

The growth-restricted infant

After birth, these infants are liable to:

* hypothermia because of their relatively large surface area
* hypoglycaemia from poor fat and glycogen stores
* hypocalcaemia
* polycythaemia (venous haematocrit >0.65).

> ### Summary
>
> **Size at birth:**
> * small for gestational age – birthweight <10th centile
> * intrauterine growth restriction (IUGR) – fails to reach genetically determined growth potential
> * growth restriction – symmetrical or asymmetrical, but often mixed.

Large-for-gestational-age infants

Large-for-gestational-age infants are those above the 90th weight centile for their gestation. Macrosomia is a feature of infants of mothers with diabetes, either permanent or gestational. The problems associated with being large for gestational age are:

* birth asphyxia from a difficult delivery
* birth trauma, especially from shoulder dystocia at delivery (difficulty delivering the shoulders from impaction behind maternal symphysis pubis)
* hypoglycaemia due to hyperinsulinism
* polycythaemia.

Routine examination of the newborn infant

Immediately after a baby is born, parents are naturally anxious to know if their baby is all right and appears normal. To answer this, the midwife (or the paediatrician or obstetrician, if present) will briefly but carefully check that the baby is pink, breathing normally and has no major abnormalities such as cleft lip and palate. If the mother has had polyhydramnios, a feeding tube needs to be passed into the stomach to exclude oesophageal atresia. If a significant problem is identified, an experienced paediatrician needs to explain the situation to the parents. If the baby is markedly preterm, small or ill, admission to a neonatal unit will be required. Should there be any uncertainty about the child's sex, it is important not to guess but to explain to the parents that further tests are necessary. In most hospitals, babies are given vitamin K at birth to prevent haemorrhagic disease of the newborn.

Within 24 hours of birth every baby should have a full and thorough medical examination, the 'routine examination of the newborn infant'. Its purpose is to:

* detect congenital abnormalities not already identified at birth, e.g. congenital heart disease, developmental dysplasia of the hip (DDH)
* check for potential problems arising from maternal disease or familial disorders
* provide an opportunity for the parents to discuss any questions about their baby.

Before approaching the mother and baby, the obstetric and neonatal notes must be checked to identify relevant information. The examination (Fig. 9.12) should be performed with the mother or ideally both parents present. Many findings in the newborn resolve spontaneously (Box 9.4, Fig. 9.13). Common significant abnormalities detectable at birth are listed in Box 9.5 (Fig. 9.14). A serious congenital anomaly is present at birth in about 10–15/1000 live births (Table 9.3). In addition,

Table 9.3 Prevalence of serious congenital anomalies per 1000 live births (England and Wales)

Anomaly	Prevalence
Congenital heart disease	6–8 (0.8 on the first day of life)
Developmental dysplasia of the hip	1.5 (but about 6/1000 have an abnormal initial clinical examination)
Talipes	1.0
Down's syndrome	1.0
Cleft lip and palate	0.8
Urogenital (hypospadias, undescended testes)	1.2
Spina bifida/anencephaly	0.1

Routine examination of the newborn infant

Birthweight, gestational age and birthweight centile are noted (Fig. 9.12b).

General observation of the baby's appearance, posture and movements provides valuable information about many abnormalities. The baby must be fully undressed during the examination.

The head circumference is measured with a paper tape measure and its centile noted. This is a surrogate measure of brain size.

The fontanelle and sutures are palpated. The fontanelle size is very variable. The sagittal suture is often separated and the coronal sutures may be overriding. A tense fontanelle when the baby is not crying may be due to raised intracranial pressure and cranial ultrasound should be performed to check for hydrocephalus. A tense fontanelle is also a late sign of meningitis.

The face is observed. If abnormal, this may represent a syndrome, particularly if other anomalies are present. Down's syndrome is the most common, but there are hundreds of syndromes. When the diagnosis is uncertain, a book or a computer database may be consulted and advice should be sought from a senior paediatrician or geneticist.

If plethoric or pale, the haematocrit should be checked to identify polycythaemia or anaemia. Central cyanosis, which always needs urgent assessment, is best seen on the tongue.

Jaundice within 24 hours of birth requires further evaluation.

The eyes are checked for red reflex with an ophthalmoscope (cataracts, retinoblastoma and corneal opacity).

The palate needs to be inspected, including posteriorly to exclude a posterior cleft palate, and palpated to detect an indentation of the posterior palate from a submucous cleft.

Breathing and chest wall movement are observed for signs of respiratory distress.

On auscultating the heart, the normal rate is 110–160 beats/min in term babies, but may drop to 85 beats/min during sleep.

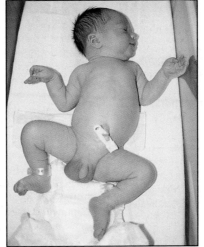

Figure 9.12b Term newborn. Median measurements:
- birthweight 3.5 kg
- head circumference 35 cm
- length 50 cm.

On palpating the abdomen, the liver normally extends 1–2 cm below the costal margin, the spleen tip may be palpable, as may the kidney on the left side. Any intra-abdominal masses, which are usually renal in origin, need further investigation.

The genitalia and anus are inspected on removing the nappy. In boys the presence of testes in the scrotum is confirmed.

The femoral pulses are palpated. Their pulse pressure is:
- reduced in coarctation of the aorta. This can be confirmed by measuring the blood pressure in the arms and legs
- increased if there is a patent ductus arteriosus.

Muscle tone is assessed by observing limb movements and on sitting the baby up while supporting the head. Most babies will support the head briefly when the trunk is held vertically.

The whole of the back and spine is observed, looking for any midline defects of the skin.

The hips are checked for developmental dysplasia of the hips (DDH). This is left until last as the procedure is uncomfortable.

Figure 9.12a Routine examination of the newborn infant.

Lesions in newborn infants which resolve spontaneously

Box 9.4 Lesions in newborn infants which resolve spontaneously

Peripheral cyanosis of the hands and feet – common in the first day.

Traumatic cyanosis from a cord round the baby's neck or from a face or brow presentation – causes blue discoloration of the skin, petechiae over the head and neck or affected part but not the tongue.

Swollen eyelids and distortion of shape of the head from the delivery.

Subconjunctival haemorrhages – occur during delivery.

Small white pearls along the midline of the palate (Epstein's pearls).

Cysts of the gums (epulis) or floor of the mouth (ranula).

Breast enlargement – may occur in newborn babies of either sex (Fig. 9.13a). A small amount of milk may be discharged.

White vaginal discharge or small withdrawal bleed in girls. There may be a prolapse of a ring of vaginal mucosa.

Capillary haemangioma or 'stork bites' – pink macules on the upper eyelids, mid-forehead and nape of the neck are common and arise from distension of the dermal capillaries. Those on the eyelids gradually fade over the first year; those on the neck become covered with hair.

Neonatal urticaria (erythema toxicum) – a common rash appearing at 2–3 days of age, consisting of white pinpoint papules at the centre of an erythematous base (Fig. 9.13b). The fluid contains eosinophils. The lesions are concentrated on the trunk; they come and go at different sites.

Milia – white pimples on the nose and cheeks, from retention of keratin and sebaceous material in the pilaceous follicles (Fig. 9.13c).

Mongolian blue spots – blue/black macular discoloration at the base of the spine and on the buttocks (Fig. 9.13d); occasionally occur on the legs and other parts of the body. Usually but not invariably in Afro-Caribbean or Asian infants. They fade slowly over the first few years. They are of no significance unless misdiagnosed as bruises.

Umbilical hernia – common, particularly in Afro-Caribbean infants. No treatment is indicated as it usually resolves within the first 2–3 years.

Positional talipes – the feet often remain in their in utero position. Unlike true talipes equinovarus, the foot can be fully dorsiflexed to touch the front of the lower leg (Figs 9.13e and 9.13f).

Caput succedaneum (see p. 151).

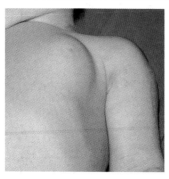

Figure 9.13a Breast enlargement in a newborn infant.

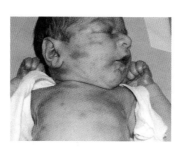

Figure 9.13b Erythema toxicum (neonatal urticaria) often has a raised pale centre. (Courtesy of Dr Nim Subhedar.)

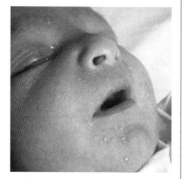

Figure 9.13c Milia. (Courtesy of Dr Rodney Rivers.)

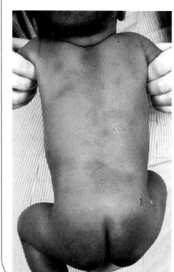

Figure 9.13d Mongolian blue spot.

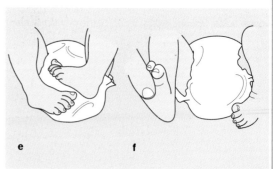

Figure 9.13e Positional talipes.
Figure 9.13f The foot can be fully dorsiflexed to touch the front of the lower leg. In true talipes equinovarus this is not possible.

Box 9.5 Some significant abnormalities detected on routine examination.

Port wine stain (naevus flammeus). Present from birth and usually grows with the infant (Fig. 9.14a). It is due to a vascular malformation of the capillaries in the dermis. Rarely, if along the distribution of the trigeminal nerve, it may be associated with intracranial vascular anomalies (Sturge–Weber syndrome), or severe lesions on the limbs with bone hypertrophy (Klippel–Trenaunay syndrome). Disfiguring lesions can now be improved with laser therapy.

Strawberry naevus (cavernous haemangioma). Not usually present at birth, but appears in the first month of life (Fig. 9.14b). It is more common in preterm infants. It increases in size until 3–9 months old, then gradually regresses. No treatment is indicated unless the lesion interferes with vision or the airway. Ulceration or haemorrhage may occur. Thrombocytopenia may occur with large lesions, when therapy with systemic steroids or interferon-α may be required.

Natal teeth consisting of the front lower incisors – may be present at birth. If loose they should be removed to avoid the risk of aspiration.

Extra digits – are sometimes connected by a thin skin tag but may be completely attached containing bone (Fig 9.14c) and should be removed by a plastic surgeon. Skin tags anterior to the ear and accessory auricles should be removed by a plastic surgeon.

Heart murmur – poses a difficult problem, as most murmurs audible in the first few days of life resolve shortly afterwards. However, some are caused by congenital heart disease. If there are any features of a significant murmur (see Ch. 17), an echocardiogram is indicated. Otherwise, a follow-up examination is arranged and the parents warned to seek medical assistance if their baby feeds poorly, develops laboured breathing or becomes cyanosed.

Midline abnormality over the spine or skull, such as a tuft of hair, swelling or naevus – requires further evaluation as it may indicate an underlying abnormality of the vertebrae, spinal cord or brain.

Palpable and large bladder – if there is urinary outflow obstruction, particularly in boys with a posterior urethral valve. Requires prompt evaluation with ultrasound.

Talipes equinovarus – which cannot be corrected as in positional talipes.

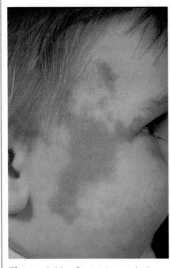

Figure 9.14a Port wine stain in an infant.

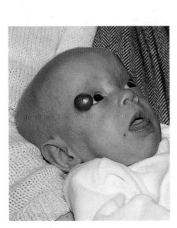

Figure 9.14b Strawberry naevus.

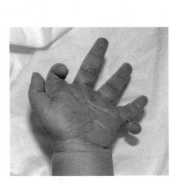

Figure 9.14c Extra digits.

many congenital anomalies, especially of the heart, present clinically at a later age.

Testing for developmental dysplasia of the hip (DDH), also called congenital dislocation of the hip (CDH)

The infant needs to be relaxed, as kicking or crying results in tightening of the muscles around the hip and prevents satisfactory examination. The pelvis is stabilised with one hand. With the other hand, the examiner's middle finger is placed over the greater trochanter and the thumb around the distal medial femur. The hip is held flexed and adducted. The femoral head is gently pushed downwards. If the hip is dislocatable, the femoral head will be pushed posteriorly out of the acetabulum (Fig. 9.15a).

The next part of the examination is to see if the hip can be returned from its dislocated position back into the acetabulum. With the hip abducted, upward leverage is applied (Fig. 9.15b). A dislocated hip will return with a 'clunk' into the acetabulum. Ligamentous clicks without any movement of the head of femur are of no significance. It should also be possible to abduct the hips fully, but this may be restricted if the hip is dislocated. Clinical examination does not identify some infants who have hip dysplasia from lack of development of the acetabular shelf. DDH is more common in girls (sixfold increase), if there is a positive family history (20% of affected infants), if the birth is a breech presentation (30% of affected infants) or if the infant has a neuromuscular disorder.

Early recognition of DDH is important as early splinting in abduction reduces long-term morbidity. A specialist orthopaedic opinion should be sought in the management of this condition. Ultrasound examination of the hip joint is performed increasingly in many hospitals, either following an abnormal examination or to screen babies at increased risk (breech presentation or positive family history). Ultrasound examination can be performed to screen all babies, but is not currently recommended in the UK as it is expensive, requires considerable expertise and there are many false positives. It will, however, identify some babies missed on clinical examination.

Vitamin K therapy

Vitamin K deficiency may result in haemorrhagic disease of the newborn. This disorder can occur early, during the first week of life, or late, from 1 to 8 weeks of age. In most affected infants, the haemorrhage is mild, such as bruising, haematemesis and melaena, or prolonged bleeding of the umbilical stump or after a circumcision. However, some suffer from intracranial haemorrhage, half of whom are permanently disabled or die.

Breast milk is a poor source of vitamin K, whereas infant formula milk has a much higher vitamin K content. Haemorrhagic disease of the newborn may occur in infants who are wholly breast-fed but not if fed with an infant formula. Infants of mothers taking anticonvulsants, which impair the synthesis of vitamin K-dependent clotting factors, are at increased risk of haemorrhagic disease, both during delivery and soon after birth. Infants with liver disease are also at increased risk.

The disease can be prevented if vitamin K is given by intramuscular injection, and in the UK was widely given to all newborn infants immediately after birth. In the early 1990s, one study suggested a possible association between vitamin K given intramuscularly and the development of cancer in childhood, but this has not been found in other, much larger studies. It is still recommended that all newborn infants are given intramuscular vitamin K. However, parents may request oral vitamin K as an alternative. As absorption via the oral route is variable, three doses are needed over the first four weeks of life to achieve adequate liver storage. Mothers on anticonvulsant therapy should receive oral prophylaxis from 36 weeks' gestation and the baby should be given intramuscular vitamin K.

> **Vitamin K should be given to all newborn infants to prevent haemorrhagic disease of the newborn.**

Biochemical screening (Guthrie test)

Biochemical screening is performed on every baby. A blood sample, usually a heel prick, is taken when feeding has been established on day 5–9 of life. In the UK all infants are screened for:

- phenylketonuria
- hypothyroidism
- haemoglobinopathies (sickle cell and thalassaemia)
- cystic fibrosis.

In addition, screening is being introduced for:
- MCAD (medium-chain acyl-CoA dehydrogenase deficiency) – a rare inborn error of mitochondrial

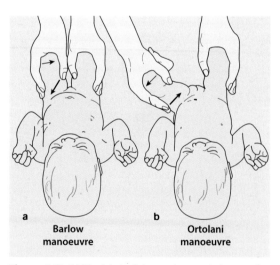

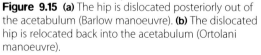

Figure 9.15 (a) The hip is dislocated posteriorly out of the acetabulum (Barlow manoeuvre). **(b)** The dislocated hip is relocated back into the acetabulum (Ortolani manoeuvre).

fatty acid metabolism causing acute illness and hypoglycaemia following fasting, which may also present as an ALTE (acute life-threatening episode).

Screening for cystic fibrosis is performed by measuring the serum immunoreactive trypsin, which is raised if there is pancreatic duct obstruction. If raised, DNA analysis is also performed to reduce the false-positive rate (see Ch. 16).

> In the UK biochemical screening is performed on all babies to identify phenylketonuria, congenital hypothyroidism, haemoglobinopathies, cystic fibrosis and increasingly for MCAD.

Newborn hearing screening

Universal screening has been introduced in the UK to detect severe hearing impairment in newborn infants. Early detection and intervention improves speech and language. Evoked otoacoustic emission (EOAE) testing, when an earpiece is inserted into the ear canal and produces a sound which evokes an echo or emission from the ear if cochlear function is normal, is used as the initial screening test. If a normal test is not achieved, testing with automated auditory brainstem response (AABR) audiometry, using computer analysis of EEG waveforms evoked in response to a series of clicks, is performed with referral to a paediatric audiologist if abnormal (see Ch. 3 for further details).

> Newborn hearing screening is performed on all infants to detect severe hearing impairment.

Further reading

Lissauer T, Fanaroff A 2006 Neonatology at a glance. Blackwell Publishers, Oxford

Rennie J M, 2005 Roberton's textbook of neonatology. Churchill Livingstone, Edinburgh

Resuscitation Council, UK 2005 Newborn life support

Internet

Cochrane Library: www.nelh.nhs.uk/cochrane.asp

Resuscitation Council (UK): www.resus.org.uk

Routine examination of the newborn infant

10

Neonatal medicine

The dramatic reduction in neonatal mortality throughout the developed world has resulted from advances in the management of newborn infants together with improvements in maternal health and obstetric care. Neonatal intensive care became increasingly available in the UK from 1975, and it is since that time that the mortality of very low birthweight infants has fallen (Fig. 10.1).

About 10% of babies born in the UK require special medical and nursing care. This can be provided in special care baby units or in transitional care units on postnatal wards, which have the advantage that they avoid separating mothers from their babies. About 1–3% of babies require intensive care, which is undertaken in neonatal intensive care units, many of which are situated in tertiary referral centres serving a number of maternity departments. Modern technology allows even tiny preterm infants to benefit from the full range of intensive care, anaesthesia and surgery. If it is anticipated during pregnancy that the infant is likely to require long-term intensive care or surgery, it is preferable for the transfer to the tertiary centre to be made in utero. When a baby requires transfer postnatally, transport should be by an experienced team of doctors and nurses. Arrangements should also be made for parents to be close to their infant during this stressful time.

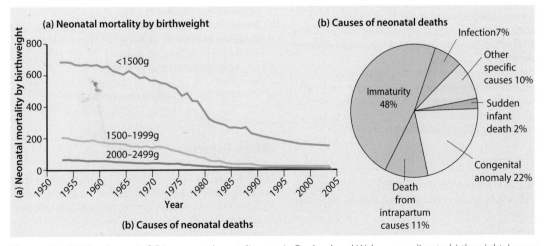

Figure 10.1 (a) The dramatic fall in neonatal mortality rate in England and Wales, according to birthweight. In very low birthweight infants (<1500 g), the marked fall in the mortality rate has been relatively recent. **(b)** Causes of neonatal deaths in England and Wales, 2004. (Adapted from the Audit Commission. Data from OPCS and CEMACH.)

Stabilising the preterm or sick infant

Preterm infants of less than 34 weeks' gestation and newborn infants who become seriously ill require their condition to be stabilised and monitored (Fig. 10.2). Many of them will need respiratory and circulatory support.

Birth asphyxia and hypoxic-ischaemic encephalopathy

Birth asphyxia is characterised by a critical reduction in oxygen delivery to the fetus antenatally, during labour and/or delivery sufficient to produce a lactic acidosis and render the infant in poor condition at birth with delayed respiration. It remains an important cause of brain damage resulting in disability or death and its prevention is one of the key aims of modern obstetric care (Fig. 10.3).

The fetal cardiotocograph (CTG) may be abnormal, but is poor at assessing the severity of asphyxia unless it is profound. However, when normal, the CTG is highly predictive of the absence of asphyxial problems in the neonate. Fetal blood sampling or cord blood analysis may identify a metabolic acidosis, but is also poor at predicting neonatal outcome unless the acidosis is very severe. Low Apgar scores at 1 and 5 minutes, reflecting delayed onset of respiration and circulatory failure at birth, are also poor at predicting outcome, but if the score remains low (5 or less) at 10 minutes of age, the risk of long-term disability or mortality is nearly 50%. Hypoxic-ischaemic encephalopathy (HIE) is the terminology used in the term infant to describe the clinical manifestation of brain injury starting immediately or up to 48 hours after asphyxia, whether antenatal, intrapartum or postnatal. It can be graded as:

- mild – the infant is irritable, responds excessively to stimulation, may have staring of the eyes and hyperventilation and has impaired feeding
- moderate – the infant shows marked abnormalities of tone and movement, cannot feed and may have seizures
- severe – there are no normal spontaneous movements or response to pain; tone in the limbs may fluctuate between hypotonia and hypertonia; seizures are prolonged and often refractory to treatment; multi-organ failure is present.

Management

Skilled resuscitation and stabilisation of sick infants will minimise asphyxial damage. Infants with HIE may need:

- respiratory support
- treatment of clinical seizures with anticonvulsants; continuous amplitude-integrated EEG (cerebral function monitoring) is increasingly used to confirm early encephalopathy and to help with prognosis and interpretation of abnormal movements
- fluid restriction because of transient renal impairment
- treatment of hypotension by volume and inotrope support
- monitoring and treatment of hypoglycaemia and electrolyte imbalance.

Randomised clinical trials have shown that mild hypothermia (cooling by 3–4°C) (Fig. 10.4) can reduce brain damage if started within 6 hours of birth.

Prognosis

When HIE is mild, complete recovery can be expected. Infants with moderate HIE who have recovered fully on clinical neurological examination and are feeding normally by 7 days of age have an excellent long-term prognosis, but if clinical abnormalities persist beyond 10 days, full recovery is unlikely. Severe HIE has a mortality of 30–40%, and, of the survivors, over 80% have neuro-developmental disabilities, particularly cerebral palsy. If magnetic resonance imaging (MRI) at 4–14 days in a term infant shows bilateral abnormalities in the basal ganglia and thalamus and lack of myelin in the posterior limb of the internal capsule, there is a very high risk of later cerebral palsy (Fig. 10.5). In view of the potential medicolegal implications of the term 'birth asphyxia', it has been suggested that infants who fail to breathe at birth or develop seizures or other abnormal neurological signs should be diagnosed as having 'neonatal encephalopathy'. The diagnosis of HIE is made only if there is:

- evidence of hypoxia antenatally (e.g. antepartum haemorrhage) or during labour (e.g. cord prolapse or markedly abnormal CTG trace) or at delivery (e.g. shoulder dystocia)
- resuscitation needed at birth
- features of encephalopathy
- evidence of hypoxic damage to other organs such as liver, kidney, or heart
- no other prenatal or postnatal cause identified
- characteristic findings on neuroimaging.

Birth injuries

Infants may be injured at birth, particularly if they are malpositioned or too large for the pelvic outlet. Injuries may also occur during manual manoeuvres, from forceps blades or at Ventouse deliveries. Fortunately, now that caesarean section is available in every maternity unit, heroic attempts to achieve a vaginal delivery with resultant severe injuries to the infant have become extremely rare.

Stabilising the preterm or sick infant

Airway, breathing
Examination
- Respiratory distress – tachypnoea, laboured breathing with chest wall recession, nasal flaring, expiratory grunting, cyanosis
- Apnoea

Management, as required:
- Clear the airway
- Oxygen
- CPAP (continuous positive airway pressure)
- Mechanical ventilation

Monitoring
- Oxygen saturation (maintain at 88–95% if preterm)
- Heart rate
- Respiratory rate
- Temperature
- Blood pressure
- Blood glucose
- Blood gases
- Weight

Temperature control
Place in plastic bag at birth to keep warm. Perform stabilisation under a radiant warmer or in an incubator to avoid hypothermia, which increases mortality in preterm infants. Avoid hyperthermia, as may increase brain injury.

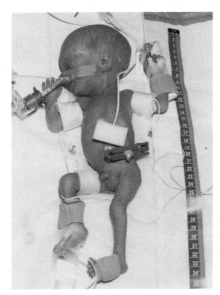

Figure 10.2 Stabilising preterm or sick infants is important to prevent complications. This preterm infant has leads on his limbs for monitoring heart rate and respiratory rate, temperature and oxygen saturation. There are arterial and intravenous cannulae and a nasotracheal tube for artificial ventilation.

Venous and arterial lines
Peripheral intravenous line:
- Required for intravenous fluids, antibiotics, other drugs and may be used for parenteral nutrition.

Umbilical venous catheter:
- May be used for immediate intravenous access to obtain blood samples, or to administer fluids or medications.

Arterial line:
- Inserted if frequent blood gas analysis, blood tests and continuous blood pressure monitoring are required. Usually umbilical artery catheter (UAC), sometimes peripheral cannula if for short period or no umbilical artery catheter possible.
- The arterial oxygen tension is maintained at 8–12 kPa (60–90 mmHg) and the CO_2 tension at 4.5–6.5 kPa (35–50 mmHg). Continuous arterial blood gas monitoring has been developed.

Central venous line for parenteral nutrition, if indicated:
- Inserted peripherally when infant is stable.

Chest X-ray ± abdominal X-ray
Assists in the diagnosis of respiratory disorders and to confirm the position of the tracheal tube and central lines.

Investigations
- Haemoglobin, neutrophil count, platelet count
- Blood urea, creatinine, electrolytes
- Culture – blood ± CSF ± urine
- Blood glucose
- CRP/acute phase reactant
- Coagulation screen if indicated

Antibiotics
Infants requiring intensive care are usually given broad-spectrum antibiotics.

Minimal handling
All procedures, especially painful ones, adversely affect oxygenation and the circulation. Handling the infant is kept to a minimum and done as gently, rapidly and efficiently as possible. Analgesia should be provided to prevent pain.

Parents
Although medical and nursing staff are usually fully occupied stabilising the baby, time must be found for parents and immediate relatives to allow them to see and touch their baby and to be kept fully informed.

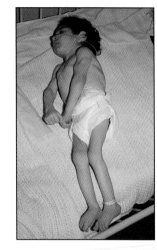

Figure 10.3 Brain damage from severe birth asphyxia at term following a sudden, severe antepartum haemorrhage caused this child to become microcephalic, blind and deaf and to have spastic quadriplegia.

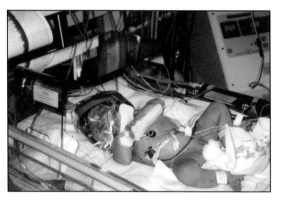

Figure 10.4 An infant with hypoxic-ischaemic encephalopathy (HIE) being monitored with amplitude-integrated EEG and receiving hypothermia via a cooling cap.

Soft tissue injuries

These include:

- Caput succedaneum (Fig. 10.6) – bruising and oedema of the presenting part extending beyond the margins of the skull bones; resolves in a few days.
- Cephalhaematoma (Figs 10.6 and 10.7) – haematoma from bleeding below the periosteum, confined within the margins of the skull sutures. It usually involves the parietal bone. The centre of the haematoma feels soft. It resolves over several weeks. It is occasionally accompanied by a linear skull fracture.
- Chignon (Fig. 10.8) – oedema and bruising from Ventouse delivery.
- Bruising to the face after a face presentation and to the genitalia and buttocks after breech delivery. Preterm infants bruise readily from even mild trauma.
- Abrasions to the skin from scalp electrodes applied during labour or from accidental scalpel incision at caesarean section.
- Forceps marks to face from pressure of blades – transient.
- Subaponeurotic haemorrhage (Fig. 10.6) (very uncommon) – diffuse, boggy swelling of scalp, may be accompanied by serious blood loss leading to hypovolaemic shock.

Nerve palsies

Brachial nerve palsy results from traction to the brachial plexus nerve roots. They may occur at breech deliveries or with shoulder dystocia. Upper nerve root (C5 and C6) injury results in an Erb's palsy (Fig. 10.9). It may be accompanied by phrenic nerve palsy causing an elevated diaphragm. Less often, the lower roots are injured, resulting in

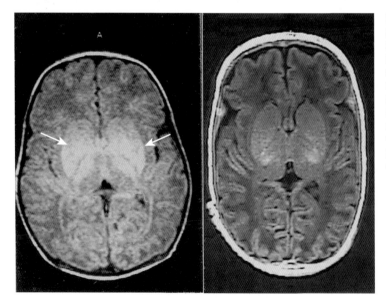

Figure 10.5 Magnetic resonance image of the brain at term. *Left:* Hypoxic-ischaemic encephalopathy (HIE) showing abnormal (white) signal in the basal ganglia and thalami *(arrows)* and absence of signal in the internal capsule bilaterally. *Right:* Normal scan showing grey basal ganglia and a white signal from myelin in the posterior limb of the internal capsule.

Birth injuries

Soft tissue injuries:
- caput succedaneum, cephalhaematoma, chignon, bruises and abrasions
- subaponeurotic haemorrhage

Nerve palsies:
- brachial plexus – Erb's, Klumpke's
- facial nerve

Fractures:
- clavicle, humerus, femur

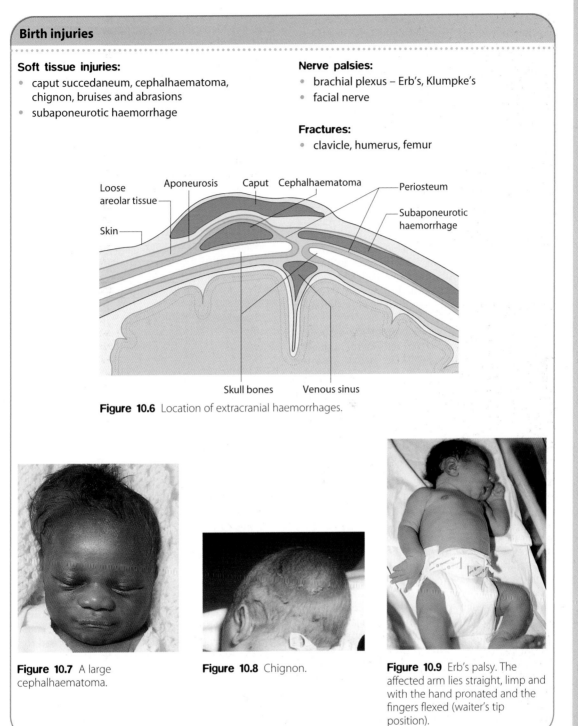

Figure 10.6 Location of extracranial haemorrhages.

Figure 10.7 A large cephalhaematoma.

Figure 10.8 Chignon.

Figure 10.9 Erb's palsy. The affected arm lies straight, limp and with the hand pronated and the fingers flexed (waiter's tip position).

weakness of the wrist extensors and intrinsic muscles of the hand (Klumpke's palsy). Most palsies resolve completely, but should be referred to an orthopaedic surgeon if not resolved by 6 weeks. Ninety per cent recover by 2 years. A facial nerve palsy may result from compression of the facial nerve by forceps blades or against the mother's ischial spine. It is unilateral, and there is facial weakness on crying but the eye remains open. It is usually transient, but methyl cellulose drops may be needed for the eye. Rarely, nerve palsies may be from damage to the cervical spine, when there is lack of movement below the level of the lesion.

Fractures

Clavicle
Usually from shoulder dystocia. A snap may be heard at delivery or the infant may have reduced arm movement on the affected side, or a lump from

callus formation may be noticed over the clavicle at several days of age. The prognosis is excellent.

Humerus/femur

Usually mid-shaft, occurring at breech deliveries, or fracture of the humerus at shoulder dystocia. There is deformity, reduced movement of the limb and pain on movement. They heal rapidly with immobilisation.

The preterm infant

The appearance, the likely clinical course, chances of survival and long-term prognosis depend on the gestational age at birth. The appearance and maturational changes of very preterm infants are shown in Figure 10.10a and Table 10.1. The external appearance and neurological findings can be scored to provide an estimate of an infant's gestational age (see Appendix).

The rate and severity of problems associated with prematurity decline markedly with increasing gestation. Infants born at 23–26 weeks' gestation encounter many problems (Box 10.1), require many weeks of intensive and special care in hospital (Fig. 10.11) and have a high overall mortality. With modern intensive care, the prognosis is excellent after 32 weeks' gestational age. The severity of an infant's respiratory disease and of any episodes of infection largely determine the neonatal course and outcome.

Respiratory distress syndrome

In respiratory distress syndrome (RDS), also called hyaline membrane disease, there is a deficiency of surfactant, the mixture of phospholipids and proteins excreted by the type II pneumocytes of the alveolar epithelium, which lowers surface tension. There is alveolar collapse and inadequate gas exchange. The more preterm the infant, the higher the incidence of RDS; it is common in infants born before 28 weeks' gestation and tends to be more severe in boys than girls. Surfactant deficiency is rare at full term but may occur in infants of diabetic mothers. The term hyaline membrane disease derives from a proteinaceous exudate seen in the airways on histology. Glucocorticoids, given antenatally to the mother, stimulate fetal surfactant production and are used if preterm delivery is anticipated. (See Ch. 9.)

The development of surfactant therapy has been a major advance. The preparations are natural, derived from extracts of calf or pig lung, or synthetic. They are instilled directly into the lung via the tracheal tube. Multinational placebo-controlled trials show that surfactant treatment reduces mortality from RDS by about 40%, without increasing the morbidity rate (Fig. 10.12).

At delivery or within 4 hours of birth, babies with RDS develop clinical signs of:

> **Box 10.1** Medical problems of preterm infants
>
> - Need for resuscitation at birth
> - Respiratory
>   Respiratory distress syndrome (RDS)
>   Pneumothorax
>   Apnoea and bradycardia
> - Hypotension
> - Patent ductus arteriosus
> - Temperature control
> - Metabolic
>   Hypoglycaemia
>   Hypocalcaemia
>   Electrolyte imbalance
>   Osteopenia of prematurity
> - Nutrition
> - Infection
> - Jaundice
> - Intraventricular haemorrhage/periventricular leucomalacia
> - Necrotising enterocolitis
> - Retinopathy of prematurity
> - Anaemia of prematurity
> - Iatrogenic
> - Bronchopulmonary dysplasia (chronic lung disease)
> - Inguinal hernias

- tachypnoea >60 breaths/minute
- laboured breathing with chest wall recession (particularly sternal and subcostal indrawing) and nasal flaring
- expiratory grunting in order to try to create positive airway pressure during expiration and maintain functional residual capacity
- cyanosis.

The characteristic chest X-ray appearance is shown in Figure 10.13. Treatment with raised ambient oxygen is required, which may need to be supplemented with continuous positive airway pressure (delivered via nasal cannulae) or artificial ventilation via a tracheal tube. The ventilatory requirements need to be adjusted according to the infant's oxygenation (which is measured continuously), chest wall movements and blood gas analyses. Artificial ventilation may be synchronised as far as possible with the infant's respiration, or the infant's breathing may be partially or completely suppressed with sedatives and muscle relaxants. Mechanical ventilation may be with intermittent positive pressure ventilation or high-frequency oscillation.

> **Surfactant therapy markedly reduces the mortality of preterm infants with respiratory distress syndrome.**

The preterm infant: maturational changes in appearance and development

Figure 10.10 (a) Preterm infant. **(b)** Term infant.

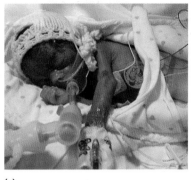

(a)

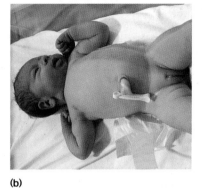

(b)

Table 10.1 The preterm infant

Gestation	23–27 weeks	31–41 weeks
Birthweight (50th centile)	At 24 weeks – male 700 g, female 620 g	At 40 weeks – male 3.55 kg, female 3.4 kg
Skin	Very thin Dark red colour all over body	Thick skin Pale pink colour
Ears	Pinna soft, no recoil	Pinna firm, cartilage to edge, immediate recoil
Breast tissue	No breast tissue palpable	One or both nodules >1 cm
Genitalia	Male – scrotum smooth, no testes in scrotum Female – prominent clitoris, labia majora widely separated, labia minora protruding	Male –scrotum has rugae, testes in scrotum Female – labia minora and clitoris covered
Breathing	Needs respiratory support. Apnoea common	Rarely needs respiratory support. Apnoea rare
Sucking and swallowing	No coordinated sucking	Coordinated after 34–35 weeks' gestation
Feeding	Usually needs TPN (total parenteral nutrition), then tube feeding	Cries when hungry. Feeds on demand
Cry	Faint	Loud
Vision, interaction	Eyelids may be fused. Infrequent eye movements. Not available for interaction	Makes eye contact, alert wakefulness, follows faces
Hearing	Startles to loud noise	Turns head and eyes to sound
Posture	Limbs extended, jerky movements	Flexed posture, smooth movements

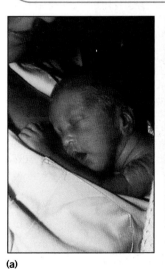

(a)

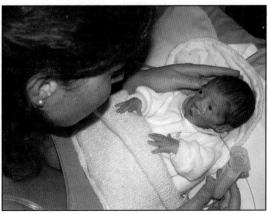

(b)

Figure 10.11 Parental involvement in neonatal care. **(a)** Skin-to-skin contact between infant and parent (Kangaroo care) promotes parental bonding. **(b)** Mother giving her baby expressed breast milk (in syringe) via nasogastric tube, allowing close eye and skin contact between mother and baby.

Respiratory distress syndrome:
* common in very preterm infants
* caused by surfactant deficiency
* antenatal corticosteroids and surfactant therapy markedly reduce morbidity and mortality.

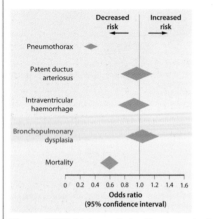

Figure 10.12 Meta-analysis of treatment of preterm infants with natural surfactant, showing a dramatic reduction in pneumothoraces and mortality.

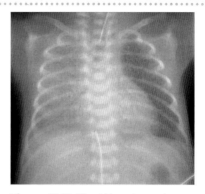

Figure 10.13 Chest X-ray in respiratory distress syndrome showing a diffuse granular or 'ground glass' appearance of the lungs and an air bronchogram, where the larger airways are outlined. The heart border becomes indistinct or obscured completely with severe disease. A tracheal tube and an umbilical artery catheter are present.

Pneumothorax

In respiratory distress syndrome (RDS), air from the overdistended alveoli may track into the interstitium, resulting in pulmonary interstitial emphysema (PIE). In up to 20% of infants ventilated for RDS, air leaks into the pleural cavity and causes a pneumothorax (Fig. 10.14). When this occurs, the infant's oxygen requirement usually increases, the tidal volume decreases and the breath sounds and chest movement on the affected side are reduced, although this can be difficult to detect clinically. A pneumothorax may be readily demonstrated by transillumination with a bright fibreoptic light source applied to the chest wall. A tension pneumothorax is treated by inserting a chest drain. In order to try and prevent pneumothoraces, infants are ventilated with the lowest pressures that provide adequate chest movement and satisfactory blood gases, and ventilation is adjusted to avoid the infant breathing against the ventilator.

Apnoea and bradycardia and desaturation

Episodes of apnoea and bradycardia and desaturation are common in very low birthweight infants until they reach about 32 weeks' gestational age. An episode of bradycardia may occur either when an infant stops breathing for sufficiently long or when the infant continues to breathe but against a closed glottis. An underlying cause (hypoxia,

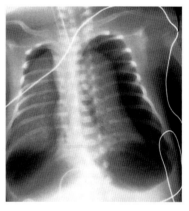

Figure 10.14 Chest X-ray showing bilateral pneumothoraces in a preterm infant with respiratory distress syndrome.

infection, anaemia, electrolyte disturbance, hypoglycaemia, seizures, heart failure or aspiration due to gastro-oesophageal reflux) needs to be excluded, but in many instances no cause is identified. Treatment with a respiratory stimulant such as caffeine often helps. Breathing will usually start again after gentle physical stimulation. Continuous positive airways pressure (CPAP) is often necessary in addition to drug therapy.

Patent ductus arteriosus

The ductus arteriosus remains patent in many preterm infants. Shunting of blood across the ductus, from the left to the right side of the circulation, is most common in infants with RDS. It may produce no symptoms or it may cause apnoea and bradycardia, increased oxygen requirement and difficulty in weaning the infant from artificial ventilation. The pulses are 'bounding' from an increased pulse pressure, the precordial impulse becomes prominent and a systolic murmur may be audible. With increasing circulatory overload, signs of heart failure may develop. More accurate assessment of the infant's circulation can be obtained on echocardiography. If the infant is symptomatic, pharmacological closure with a prostaglandin synthetase inhibitor, indomethacin or ibuprofen, is used. If these measures fail to close a symptomatic duct, surgical ligation will be required.

Temperature control

Hypothermia can cause increased energy consumption resulting in hypoxia and hypoglycaemia, failure to gain weight and increased mortality. Preterm infants are particularly vulnerable to hypothermia as:

- they have a large surface area relative to their mass, so there is greater heat loss (related to surface area) than heat generation (related to mass)
- their skin is thin and heat permeable, so transepidermal water loss is important in the first week of life
- they have little subcutaneous fat for insulation
- they are often nursed naked and cannot conserve heat by curling up or generate heat by shivering.

There is a neutral temperature range in which an infant's energy consumption is lowest. In the very immature baby, the neutral temperature is highest during the first few days of life and subsequently declines. The temperature of these small babies is maintained using incubators (Fig. 10.15) or initially with overhead radiant heaters. Incubators also allow ambient humidity to be provided, which reduces transepidermal heat loss.

Fluid balance

A preterm infant's fluid requirements will vary with gestational and chronological age. On the first day of life, about 60–90 ml/kg is usually required, increasing by 30 ml/kg per day to 150–180 ml/kg per day. This is adjusted according to the infant's clinical condition, plasma electrolytes, urine output and weight change.

Nutrition

Preterm infants have a high nutritional requirement because of their rapid growth. Preterm infants at 28 weeks' gestation double their birthweight in 6 weeks and treble it in 12 weeks, whereas term babies double their weight in only 4.5 months and treble it in a year.

Infants of 35–36 weeks' gestational age are mature enough to suck and swallow milk. Less mature infants will need to be fed via an oro- or nasogastric tube. Even in very preterm infants, enteral feeds, preferably breast milk, are introduced as soon as possible. In infants under 1500 g, breast milk always needs to be supplemented with

---

Temperature control

Prevention of heat loss in newborn infants
1. Convection:
   - raise temperature of ambient air in incubator
   - clothe, including covering head
   - avoid draughts
2. Radiation:
   - cover baby
   - double walls for incubators
3. Evaporation:
   - dry and wrap at birth
   - humidify incubator
4. Conduction:
   - nurse on mattress

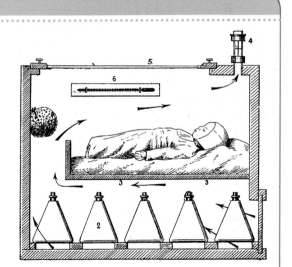

Figure 10.15 The importance of avoiding hypothermia in newborn infants has long been recognised. This incubator was used in the late 19th century to keep newborn infants warm. The sponge is to increase ambient humidity.

phosphate and in selected cases supplementation with protein, calories and calcium is needed. There are also special infant formulas designed to meet the increased requirements of preterm infants but, in contrast to breast milk, do not provide protection against infection. In the very immature or sick infant, parenteral nutrition is often required. This is usually given through a central venous catheter, inserted peripherally (PICC lines, peripherally inserted central catheters), paying strict attention to aseptic technique both during insertion and when fluids are changed. However, PICC lines carry a significant risk of septicaemia; other risks include thrombosis of a major vein. For this reason, parenteral nutrition may be given via a peripheral vein, but extravasation may cause skin damage with scarring. Because of the significant risk of septicaemia from parenteral nutrition and the increased risk of necrotising enterocolitis with cow's milk based formula, mothers should be encouraged and supported to provide breast milk.

Poor bone mineralisation (osteopenia of prematurity) was previously common but is prevented by provision of adequate phosphate, calcium and vitamin D. Because iron is mostly transferred to the fetus during the last trimester, preterm babies have low iron stores and are at a risk of iron deficiency. This is in addition to loss of blood from sampling and an inadequate erythropoietin response. Iron supplements are continued after discharge home.

Infection

Preterm infants are at increased risk of infection, as IgG is mostly transferred across the placenta in the last trimester and no IgA or IgM is transferred. In addition, infection in or around the cervix is often a reason for preterm labour and may cause infection shortly after birth. Most infections in preterm infants occur after several days of age and are nosocomial (hospital-derived); they are often associated with indwelling catheters or artificial ventilation.

> **Infection in preterm infants is a major cause of death and contributes to bronchopulmonary dysplasia (chronic lung disease), white matter injury in the brain and later disability.**

Preterm brain injury

Haemorrhages in the brain occur in 25% of very low birthweight infants and are easily recognised on cranial ultrasound scans (Fig. 10.16). Typically, they occur in the germinal matrix above the caudate nucleus, which contains a fragile network of blood vessels. Most haemorrhages occur within the first 72 hours of life. They are more common following perinatal asphyxia and in infants with severe RDS. Pneumothorax is a significant risk factor. Small haemorrhages confined to the germinal matrix do not increase the risk of cerebral palsy. Haemorrhage may occur in the ventricles; large intraventricular haemorrhages have a 25–30% risk of cerebral palsy. The most severe haemorrhage is unilateral haemorrhagic infarction involving the parenchyma of the brain; this usually results in hemiplegia (Fig. 10.16b).

A large intraventricular haemorrhage may impair the drainage and reabsorption of cerebrospinal fluid (CSF), thus allowing CSF to build up under pressure. This dilatation (Fig. 10.16c) may resolve spontaneously or progress to hydrocephalus, which may cause the sutures to separate, the head circumference to increase rapidly and the anterior fontanelle to become tense. A ventriculoperitoneal shunt may be required, but initially symptomatic relief may be provided by removal of CSF by lumbar puncture or ventricular tap. About half of infants with progressive post-haemorrhagic ventricular dilatation have cerebral palsy, a higher proportion if parenchymal infarction is also present.

Periventricular white injury may occur following ischaemia or inflammation and may occur in the absence of haemorrhage. It is more difficult to detect by cranial ultrasound. Initially there may be an echodense area or 'flare' within the brain parenchyma. This may resolve within a week (in which case the risk of cerebral palsy is not increased), but if cystic lesions become visible on ultrasound 2–4 weeks later, there is definite loss of white matter. Bilateral multiple cysts, also called periventricular leukomalacia (PVL), have an 80–90% risk of spastic diplegia if posteriorly sited (Fig. 10.16d). Intraventricular haemorrhage and periventricular leucomalacia may occur in the absence of abnormal clinical features.

Necrotising enterocolitis

Necrotising enterocolitis is a serious illness mainly affecting preterm infants in the first few weeks of life. It is caused by bacterial invasion of ischaemic bowel wall and may be accelerated by feeding with milk. Preterm infants fed cow's milk formula are six times more likely to develop this condition than if they are fed only breast milk. The infant stops tolerating feeds, milk is aspirated from the stomach and there may be vomiting, which may be bile-stained. The abdomen becomes distended (Fig. 10.17a) and the stool sometimes contains fresh blood. The infant may rapidly become shocked and require artificial ventilation because of abdominal distension and pain. The characteristic X-ray features are distended loops of bowel and thickening of the bowel wall with intramural gas, and there may be gas in the portal tract (Fig. 10.17b). The disease may progress to bowel perforation, which can be detected by X-ray or by transillumination of the abdomen.

Treatment is to stop oral feeding and give broad-spectrum antibiotics to cover both aerobic and anaerobic organisms. Parenteral nutrition is always needed and artificial ventilation and circulatory

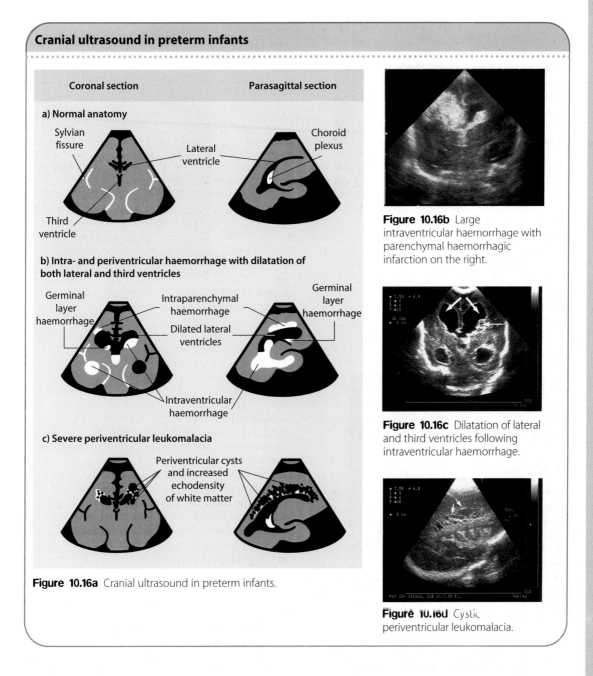

Cranial ultrasound in preterm infants

Coronal section **Parasagittal section**

a) Normal anatomy

Sylvian fissure

Lateral ventricle

Choroid plexus

Third ventricle

b) Intra- and periventricular haemorrhage with dilatation of both lateral and third ventricles

Germinal layer haemorrhage

Intraparenchymal haemorrhage

Germinal layer haemorrhage

Dilated lateral ventricles

Intraventricular haemorrhage

c) Severe periventricular leukomalacia

Periventricular cysts and increased echodensity of white matter

Figure 10.16a Cranial ultrasound in preterm infants.

Figure 10.16b Large intraventricular haemorrhage with parenchymal haemorrhagic infarction on the right.

Figure 10.16c Dilatation of lateral and third ventricles following intraventricular haemorrhage.

Figure 10.16d Cystic periventricular leukomalacia.

support are often needed. Surgery is performed for bowel perforation. The disease has significant morbidity and a mortality of about 20%. Long-term sequelae include the development of strictures and malabsorption if extensive bowel resection has been necessary.

Retinopathy of prematurity

Retinopathy of prematurity (ROP) affects developing blood vessels at the junction of the vascular and non-vascularised retina. There is vascular proliferation which may progress to retinal detachment, fibrosis and blindness. It was initially recognised that the risk is increased by uncontrolled use of high concentrations of oxygen. Now, even with careful monitoring of the infant's oxygenation, retinopathy of prematurity is still found in about 20% of all very low birthweight infants. As laser therapy reduces visual impairment, the eyes of susceptible preterm infants (<1500 g birthweight or <32 weeks' gestation) are screened by an ophthalmologist. Severe bilateral visual impairment occurs in about 1% of very low birthweight infants, mostly in infants of less than 28 weeks' gestation.

Bronchopulmonary dysplasia

Infants who still have an oxygen requirement at a post-menstrual age of 36 weeks are described as having bronchopulmonary dysplasia (BPD) or chronic lung disease. The lung damage comes from pressure and volume trauma from artificial ventilation, oxygen toxicity and infection. The chest

Necrotising enterocolitis

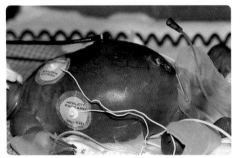

Figure 10.17a Necrotising enterocolitis showing gross abdominal distension and tense and shiny skin over the abdomen.

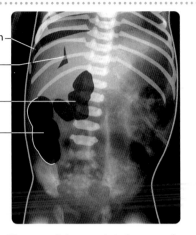

Air under diaphragm from bowel perforation

Air in portal tract

Distended bowel loops

Intramural air

Figure 10.17b Diagram of characteristic features of necrotising enterocolitis on abdominal X-ray.

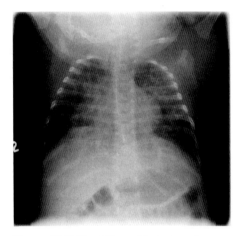

Figure 10.18 Chest X-ray of bronchopulmonary dysplasia (BPD) showing fibrosis and lung collapse, cystic changes and overdistension of the lungs.

X-ray characteristically shows widespread areas of opacification, sometimes with cystic changes (Fig. 10.18). Some infants need prolonged artificial ventilation, but most are weaned onto continuous positive airways pressure (CPAP) followed by additional ambient oxygen, sometimes over several months. Corticosteroid therapy may facilitate earlier weaning from the ventilator and often reduces the infant's oxygen requirements, but concern about adverse effects on the immature brain limits use to those at highest risk and only short courses are given. Some babies go home while still receiving additional oxygen. A few infants with severe disease may die of intercurrent infection or pulmonary hypertension. Subsequent pertussis and RSV (respiratory syncytial virus) infection may cause respiratory failure necessitating intensive care.

Problems following discharge

Iron supplementation should be continued until 6 months corrected age, when iron becomes available from solid foods. Multivitamins are also recommended. Readmission to hospital during the first year of life is increased approximately fourfold in very low birthweight infants. Those with bronchopulmonary dysplasia (chronic lung disease of prematurity) are more susceptible to recurrent wheezing, bronchiolitis and chest infections. A monoclonal antibody to RSV, the commonest cause of bronchiolitis, is now available (palivizumab, given monthly by intramuscular injection); its use reduces the hospital admission rate of preterm infants, but its high cost limits its use. The standard immunisations, including against pertussis, should be given. Inguinal hernias, usually in boys, may appear in the first few months of life.

Very low birthweight infants are at increased risk of a wide range of neurodevelopmental problems. Cerebral palsy occurs in 5–10% and many of these can be predicted on the basis of cranial ultrasound. Even with normal cranial ultrasound, very low birthweight infants are prone to learning difficulties, particularly delayed language development, poor attention span and difficulty with fine motor skills, and have more behavioural problems than siblings born at term. The risk of developing these problems increases markedly if born at very early gestational age (<26 weeks' gestation) (Fig. 10.19a and b). Sensorineural hearing loss and visual impairment are also more common. At school age, many have problems with abstract reasoning, e.g. mathematics, and in performing several tasks simultaneously. All very low birthweight infants should have their developmental progress monitored to allow early detection and treatment of any problems.

◎ Summary

Summary of problems of very lows birthweight infants

Respiratory

Respiratory distress syndrome (surfactant deficiency)(74%)
- respiratory distress within 4 hours of birth
- antenatal corticosteroids and surfactant therapy reduce morbidity and mortality
- oxygen therapy, but excess may damage the retina
- nasal CPAP (continuous positive airway pressure (65%) and mechanical ventilation (68%) - often required to expand lungs and prevent lung collapse

Pneumothorax (5%)

Apnoea and bradycardia and desaturations

Bronchopulmonary dysplasia (chronic lung disease) – O_2 requirement at 36 weeks post-menstrual age (37%)

Circulation

Hypotension – may require volume support, intropes or corticosteroids

Patent ductus arteriosus – needing medical treatment (34%) or surgical ligation (8%)

Temperature control

Avoid hypothermia
Nurse in neutral thermal environment
Nurse in incubator or under radiant warmer
Clothe if possible
Humidity reduces evaporative heat loss

Nutrition

Nasogastric tube feeding – until 35–36 weeks post-menstrual age

Feeding intolerance - TPN (total parenteral nutrition) often required

Infection

Common and potentially serious (25%)
Increased risk of early onset infection – Group B streptococcus
Main problem is nosocomial infection – mainly coagulase negative staphylococcus, also fungal and otherinfections

Gastrointestinal

Necrotising enterocolitis (6%) – serious, management is medical or surgery for bowel necrosis or perforation

Jaundice – common, low treatment threshold

Metabolic

Hypoglycaemia – common
Electrolyte disturbances
Osteopaenia of prematurity from phosphate deficiency

Anaemia
Often need blood transfusions

Brain injury

Haemorrhage (27%) - germinal layer, intraventricular, parenchymal

Ventricular dilatation – may need ventriculo-peritoneal shunt

Periventricular leucomalacia (3%) – ischaemic white matter injury

Hearing

Checked before discharge

Eyes

Retinopathy of prematurity – may need laser therapy (5%)

Following discharge

Specialist community nursing support helpful, if available
Increased risk of respiratory infection and wheezing - especially from bronchiolitis (caused by respiratory syncitial virus, RSV) and pertussis; may need intensive care
Consider prophylaxis against RSV infection
Increased rehospitalisation - respiratory disorders, inguinal hernias
Monitor growth, development (for learning disorders, co-ordination, cerebral palsy), behaviour, attention, vision, hearing – increased risk of impairment

The preterm infant

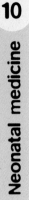

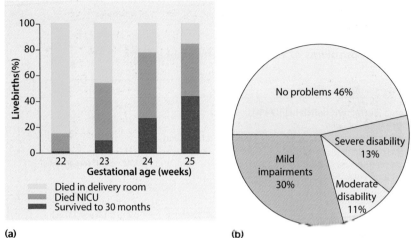

(a)   (b)

Figure 10.19 EPICure study, a population-based study of mortality and disability in the UK and Ireland in 1995 of all infants born alive at 22 to 25 weeks of gestation. **(a)** Survival. (Adapted from Wood N S et al. Neurologic and developmental disability after extremely preterm birth. *New England Journal of Medicine* 2000; 343:378–384). **(b)** Proportion of survivors with disability at 6 years of age. (Adapted from Marlow N et al. Neurologic and developmental disability at six years of age after extremely preterm birth. *New England Journal of Medicine* 2005; 352:9–19).

Jaundice

Over 60% of all newborn infants become visibly jaundiced. This is because:

- there is marked physiological release of haemoglobin from the breakdown of red cells because of the high Hb concentration at birth (Fig. 10.20)
- the red cell life span of newborn infants (70 days) is markedly shorter than that of adults (120 days)
- hepatic bilirubin metabolism is less efficient in the first few days of life.

Neonatal jaundice is important as:

- it may be a sign of another disorder, e.g. haemolytic anaemia, infection, metabolic disease
- unconjugated bilirubin can be deposited in the brain, particularly in the basal ganglia, causing kernicterus.

Kernicterus

This is the encephalopathy resulting from the deposition of unconjugated bilirubin in the basal ganglia and brainstem nuclei (Fig. 10.21). It may occur when the level of unconjugated bilirubin exceeds the albumin-binding capacity of bilirubin of the blood. As this free bilirubin is fat-soluble, it can cross the blood–brain barrier. The neurotoxic effects vary in severity from transient disturbance to catastrophic damage and death. Acute manifestations are lethargy and poor feeding. In severe cases, there is irritability, increased muscle tone causing the baby to lie with an arched back (opisthotonos), seizures and coma. Infants who survive may develop choreoathetoid cerebral palsy

(due to damage to the basal ganglia), learning difficulties and sensorineural deafness. Kernicterus used to be an important cause of brain damage in infants with severe rhesus haemolytic disease, but has become rare since the introduction of prophylactic anti-D immunoglobulin for rhesus-negative mothers.

Clinical evaluation

Babies become clinically jaundiced when the bilirubin level reaches 80–120 µmol/L. Management varies according to the infant's gestational age, age at onset, bilirubin level and rate of rise, and the overall clinical condition.

1. Age at onset

The age of onset is a useful guide to the likely cause of the jaundice (Table 10.2).

Jaundice <24 hours of age

Jaundice starting within 24 hours of birth usually results from haemolysis. This is particularly important to identify as the bilirubin is unconjugated and can rise very rapidly and reach extremely high levels.

Haemolytic disorders

Rhesus haemolytic disease Affected infants are usually identified antenatally and monitored and treated if necessary (see Ch. 9). The birth of a severely affected infant, with anaemia, hydrops and hepatosplenomegaly with rapidly developing, severe jaundice, has become rare. Antibodies may develop to rhesus antigens other than D and to the

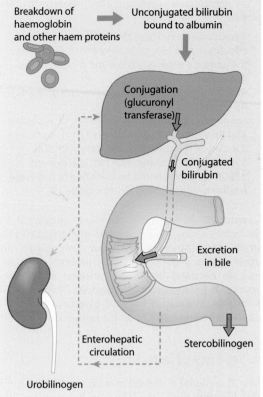

Figure 10.20 The initial breakdown product of haemoglobin is unconjugated bilirubin (indirect bilirubin) which is insoluble in water but soluble in lipids. It is carried in the blood bound to albumin. It is taken up by the liver and conjugated by the enzyme glucuronyl transferase to conjugated bilirubin (direct bilirubin), which is water-soluble and excreted in bile into the gut and is detectable in urine when blood levels rise. Reabsorption of bilirubin from the gut (enterohepatic circulation) is increased when milk intake is low.

Table 10.2 Causes of neonatal jaundice

Jaundice starting at <24 h of age	Haemolytic disorders: Rhesus incompatibility ABO incompatibility G6PD deficiency Spherocytosis, pyruvate kinase deficiency Congenital infection
Jaundice at 24 h to 3 weeks of age	Physiological jaundice Breast milk jaundice Infection, e.g. urinary tract infection Haemolysis, e.g. G6PD deficiency, ABO incompatibility Bruising Polycythaemia Crigler–Najjar syndrome
Jaundice at >3 weeks of age	*Unconjugated:* Physiological or breast milk jaundice Infection (particularly urinary tract) Hypothyroidism Haemolytic anaemia, e.g. G6PD deficiency High gastrointestinal obstruction *Conjugated (>20% of total bilirubin):* Bile duct obstruction Neonatal hepatitis

Kell and Duffy blood groups, but haemolysis is usually much less severe.

ABO incompatibility This is now more common than rhesus haemolytic disease. Most ABO antibodies are IgM and do not cross the placenta, but some group O women have an IgG anti A haemolysin in the blood which can cross the placenta and haemolyse the red cells of a group A infant. Occasionally group B infants are affected by anti-B haemolysins. Haemolysis can cause severe jaundice but it is usually less severe than in rhesus disease. The infant's haemoglobin level is usually normal or only slightly reduced and, in contrast to rhesus disease, hepatosplenomegaly is absent. The direct antibody test (Coombs' test), which demonstrates antibody on the surface of red cells, is positive. The jaundice usually peaks in the first 12–72 hours.

G6PD deficiency The Mediterranean and Middle- and Far-Eastern and African American variants may cause neonatal jaundice (see Ch. 22). Parents of affected infants should be given a list of drugs to be avoided as they may precipitate haemolysis.

Spherocytosis This is considerably less common than G6PD deficiency (see Ch. 22). There is often,

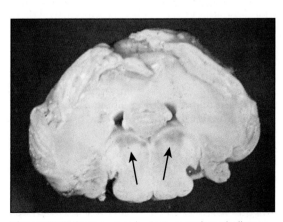

Figure 10.21 Postmortem brainstem and cerebellum showing kernicterus with yellow bilirubin staining of brain stem nuclei (*arrows*).

but not always, a family history. The disorder can be identified by recognising spherocytes on the blood film.

Congenital infection

Jaundice at birth can also be from congenital infection. In this case the bilirubin is conjugated and the infants have other abnormal clinical signs.

Jaundice at 2 days to 3 weeks of age

Physiological jaundice

Most babies who become mildly or moderately jaundiced during this period have no underlying cause and the bilirubin has risen as the infant is adapting to the transition from fetal life. The term 'physiological jaundice' can only be used after other causes have been considered.

Breast milk jaundice

This does not mean that breast milk contains toxins. It is, however, an epidemiological observation that jaundice is more common and more prolonged in breast-fed infants. The hyperbilirubinaemia is unconjugated. The cause is multifactorial but may involve increased enterohepatic circulation of bilirubin. In some infants the jaundice appears to be exacerbated if milk intake is poor from delay in establishing breast-feeding and the infant becomes dehydrated. Weight loss will indicate the extent of dehydration. Breast-feeding should be continued, although the bilirubin level will fall if it is interrupted. In some infants intravenous fluids are needed to correct dehydration.

Infection

An infected baby may develop an unconjugated hyperbilirubinaemia from poor fluid intake, haemolysis, reduced hepatic function and an increase in the enterohepatic circulation. If infection is suspected, appropriate investigations and treatment should be instigated. In particular, urinary tract infection may present in this way.

Other causes

Although jaundice from haemolysis usually presents in the first day of life, it may occur during the first week. Bruising and polycythaemia (venous haematocrit is >0.65) will exacerbate the infant's jaundice. The very rare Crigler–Najjar syndrome, when the enzyme glucuronyl transferase is deficient or absent, may result in extremely high levels of unconjugated bilirubin.

Jaundice at >3 weeks of age (persistent neonatal jaundice)

Jaundice in babies more than 3 weeks old is called persistent or prolonged neonatal jaundice. In most infants the hyperbilirubinaemia will still be unconjugated, but this needs to be confirmed on laboratory testing.

In prolonged unconjugated hyperbilirubinaemia:

- 'breast milk jaundice' is the most common cause, affecting up to 15% of healthy breast-fed infants; the jaundice gradually fades and disappears by 4–5 weeks of age
- infection, particularly of the urinary tract, needs to be considered
- congenital hypothyroidism needs to be excluded as it may present with prolonged jaundice before the clinical features of coarse facies, dry skin, hypotonia and constipation become evident. Affected infants should be identified on neonatal biochemical screening (Guthrie test).

Conjugated hyperbilirubinaemia is suggested by the baby passing dark urine and unpigmented pale stools. Hepatomegaly and poor weight gain are other clinical signs that may be present. Its causes include neonatal hepatitis syndrome and biliary atresia. It is important to diagnose biliary atresia promptly, as delay in surgical treatment adversely affects outcome (see Ch. 20 for further details).

2. Severity of jaundice

Jaundice can be observed most easily by blanching the skin with the finger. The jaundice tends to start on the head and face and then spreads down the trunk and limbs. A transcutaneous jaundice meter is used in some centres, but if the jaundice appears clinically significant or there is any doubt about its severity, a bilirubin level should be checked on a blood sample. It is easy to underestimate jaundice in Afro-Caribbean, Asian and preterm babies, and a low threshold should be adopted for measuring the bilirubin of these infants. Enlargement of the spleen or liver indicates that the jaundice is not physiological.

3. Rate of change

The rate of rise tends to be linear until a plateau is reached, so serial measurements can be plotted on a chart and used to anticipate the need for treatment before it rises to a dangerous level.

4. Gestation

Preterm infants are more susceptible to damage from raised bilirubin (lower albumin levels) so the intervention threshold is lower.

5. Clinical condition

Infants who experience severe hypoxia, hypothermia or any serious illness may be more susceptible to damage from severe jaundice. Drugs which may displace bilirubin from albumin, e.g. sulphonamides and diazepam, are rarely used in newborn infants.

Management

Poor milk intake and dehydration will exacerbate jaundice and should be corrected, but studies have failed to show that routinely supplementing breast-fed infants with water or dextrose solution reduces jaundice. Phototherapy is the most widely used therapy, with exchange transfusion for severe cases.

Phototherapy

Light (wavelength 450 nm) from the blue-green band of the visible spectrum converts unconjugated bilirubin by photodegradation into a harmless water-soluble pigment. It is delivered with an overhead light source placed the optimal distance above the infant to achieve high irradiance. Although no long-term sequelae of phototherapy from overhead light have been reported, it is disruptive to normal nursing of the infant and should not be used indiscriminately. The infant's eyes are covered, as bright light is uncomfortable. Phototherapy can result in temperature instability as the infant is undressed, a macular rash and bronze discoloration of the skin if the jaundice is conjugated.

Phototherapy can also be provided by a fibre-optic blanket applied directly to the skin. For maximal phototherapy, both an overhead light with a high irradiance together with lying on a fibreoptic blanket can be used simultaneously, and is often called intensive (double) phototherapy.

Exchange transfusion

Exchange transfusion is required if the bilirubin rises to levels which are considered potentially dangerous, particularly if there is associated anaemia from haemolysis or the serum albumin is low. Exchange transfusions have been performed traditionally via an umbilical venous catheter by alternately withdrawing 10–20 ml aliquots of the baby's blood and replacing them with donor blood. The procedure can be performed more efficiently, and avoiding the complications associated with umbilical vein cannulation, by infusing the blood via a peripheral vein while extracting blood from an arterial line. Twice the infant's blood volume (2 × 80 ml/kg) is exchanged. Donor blood should be as fresh as possible and screened to exclude CMV, hepatitis B and C and HIV infection. The procedure does carry some risk of morbidity and mortality.

There are no bilirubin levels which are known to be safe or which will definitely cause kernicterus. In rhesus haemolytic disease, it was found that kernicterus could be prevented if the bilirubin was kept below 340 mmol/L (20 mg/dl). As there is no consensus among paediatricians in the UK on the bilirubin levels at which phototherapy and exchange transfusion should be performed, each department should have clear guidelines for the management of jaundice. Phototherapy has been very successful in reducing the need for exchange transfusion. In infants with rhesus haemolytic disease unresponsive to intensive phototherapy, intravenous immunoglobulin reduces the need for exchange transfusion. Severely jaundiced infants with low serum albumin, e.g. preterm, may be given intravenous albumin, although its efficacy is uncertain.

Respiratory distress in term infants

Newborn infants with respiratory problems develop the following signs of respiratory distress:

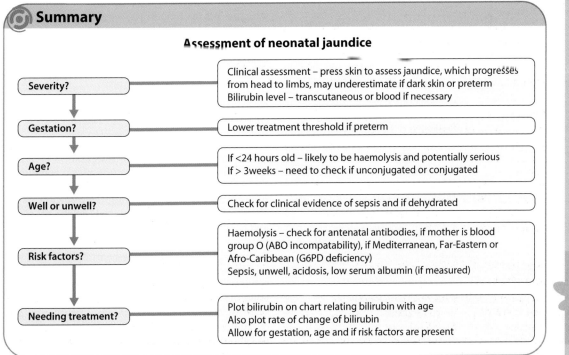

Summary

Assessment of neonatal jaundice

Severity?	Clinical assessment – press skin to assess jaundice, which progresses from head to limbs, may underestimate if dark skin or preterm Bilirubin level – transcutaneous or blood if necessary
Gestation?	Lower treatment threshold if preterm
Age?	If <24 hours old – likely to be haemolysis and potentially serious If > 3weeks – need to check if unconjugated or conjugated
Well or unwell?	Check for clinical evidence of sepsis and if dehydrated
Risk factors?	Haemolysis – check for antenatal antibodies, if mother is blood group O (ABO incompatability), if Mediterranean, Far-Eastern or Afro-Caribbean (G6PD deficiency) Sepsis, unwell, acidosis, low serum albumin (if measured)
Needing treatment?	Plot bilirubin on chart relating bilirubin with age Also plot rate of change of bilirubin Allow for gestation, age and if risk factors are present

- tachypnoea (>60 breaths/min)
- laboured breathing, with chest wall recession (particularly sternal and subcostal indrawing) and nasal flaring
- expiratory grunting
- cyanosis if severe.

The causes in term infants are listed in Table 10.3.

Affected infants should be admitted to the neonatal unit for monitoring of heart and respiratory rates, oxygenation and circulation. A chest X-ray will be required to help identify the cause, especially those causes which may need immediate treatment, e.g. pneumothorax or diaphragmatic hernia. Additional ambient oxygen, mechanical ventilation and circulatory support are given as required.

Transient tachypnoea of the newborn

This is by far the commonest cause of respiratory distress in term infants. It is caused by delay in the resorption of lung liquid and is more common after birth by caesarean section. The chest X-ray may show fluid in the horizontal fissure. Additional ambient oxygen may be required. The condition usually settles within the first day of life but can take several days to resolve completely. This is a diagnosis made after consideration and exclusion of other causes.

Meconium aspiration

Meconium is passed before birth by 8–20% of babies. It is rarely passed by preterm infants, and occurs increasingly the greater the gestational age, affecting 20–25% of deliveries by 42 weeks. It may be passed in response to fetal hypoxia. At birth these infants may inhale thick meconium. Asphy-

Table 10.3 Causes of respiratory distress in term infants

Pulmonary	
Common	Transient tachypnoea of the newborn
Less common	Meconium aspiration
	Pneumonia
	Respiratory distress syndrome
	Pneumothorax
	Persistent pulmonary hypertension of the newborn
	Milk aspiration
Rare	Diaphragmatic hernia
	Tracheo-oesophageal fistula (TOF)
	Pulmonary hypoplasia
	Airways obstruction, e.g. choanal atresia
	Pulmonary haemorrhage
Non-pulmonary	Congenital heart disease
	Intracranial birth trauma/ encephalopathy
	Severe anaemia
	Metabolic acidosis

xiated infants may start gasping and aspirate meconium before delivery. Meconium is a lung irritant and results in both mechanical obstruction and a chemical pneumonitis, as well as predisposing to infection. In meconium aspiration the lungs are over-inflated, accompanied by patches of collapse and consolidation. There is a high incidence of air leak, leading to pneumothorax and pneumomediastinum. Artificial ventilation is often required. Infants with meconium aspiration may develop persistent pulmonary hypertension of the newborn which may make it difficult to achieve adequate oxygenation despite high pressure ventilation (see below for management). Severe meconium aspiration is associated with significant morbidity and mortality.

Pneumonia

Prolonged rupture of the membranes, chorioamnionitis and low birthweight predispose to pneumonia. Infants with respiratory distress will usually require investigation to identify any infection. Broad-spectrum antibiotics are started early until the results of the infection screen are available.

Pneumothorax

A pneumothorax may occur spontaneously in up to 2% of deliveries. It is usually asymptomatic but may cause respiratory distress. Pneumothoraces also occur secondary to meconium aspiration, RDS or as a complication of ventilation. Management is described on page 154.

Milk aspiration

This occurs more frequently in preterm infants and those with respiratory distress or neurological damage. Babies with bronchopulmonary dysplasia often have gastro-oesophageal reflux, which predisposes to aspiration. Infants with a cleft palate are prone to aspirate respiratory secretions or milk.

Persistent pulmonary hypertension of the newborn

This life-threatening condition is usually associated with birth asphyxia, meconium aspiration, septicaemia or respiratory distress syndrome. It sometimes occurs as a primary disorder. As a result of the high pulmonary vascular resistance, there is right-to-left shunting within the lungs and at atrial and ductal levels. Cyanosis occurs soon after birth. Heart murmurs and signs of heart failure are often absent. A chest X-ray shows that the heart is of normal size and there may be pulmonary oligaemia. An urgent echocardiogram is required to establish that the child does not have congenital heart disease.

Most infants require mechanical ventilation and circulatory support in order to achieve adequate oxygenation. Inhaled nitric oxide, a potent vasodilator, is often beneficial. Another vasodilator, sildenafil, has been introduced more recently. High-frequency or oscillatory ventilation is sometimes helpful. Extracorporeal membrane oxygenation (ECMO), where the infant is placed on heart and lung bypass for several days, is indicated for severe cases, but is only performed in a few specialist centres.

Diaphragmatic hernia

This occurs in about 1 in 4000 births. Many are now diagnosed on antenatal ultrasound screening. In the newborn period, it usually presents with failure to respond to resuscitation or as respiratory distress. In most cases there is a left-sided herniation of abdominal contents through the posterolateral foramen of the diaphragm. The apex beat and heart sounds will then be displaced to the right side of the chest, with poor air entry in the left chest. Vigorous resuscitation may cause a pneumothorax in the normal lung, thereby aggravating the situation. The diagnosis is confirmed by X-ray of the chest and abdomen (Fig. 10.22). Once the diagnosis is suspected, a large nasogastric tube is passed and suction is applied to prevent distension of the intrathoracic bowel. After stabilisation, the diaphragmatic hernia is repaired surgically, but in most infants with this condition the main problem is pulmonary hypoplasia – where compression by the herniated viscera throughout pregnancy has prevented development of the lung in the fetus. If the lungs are hypoplastic, mortality is high. ECMO has been used pre- and postoperatively to provide respiratory support.

Other causes

Other causes of respiratory distress are listed in Table 10.3. When due to heart failure, abnormal heart sounds and/or heart murmurs may be present on auscultation. An enlarged liver from venous congestion is a helpful sign. The femoral arteries must be palpated in all infants with respiratory distress, as coarctation of the aorta and interrupted aortic arch are important causes of heart failure in newborn infants.

Infection

Early-onset infection (<48 hours)

Infants are exposed to a wide range of potential pathogens from the birth canal. The risk of infection is increased if there has been prolonged rupture of the membranes, especially if chorioamnionitis has developed, if the mother develops a fever and if the infant is preterm. The route of infection is usually ascending from the cervix to the membranes, amniotic fluid and into the fetal respiratory tract. Thus the presentation is usually with respiratory distress, apnoea and temperature instability (Box 10.2). A chest X-ray is performed, together with a septic screen comprising a full blood count to detect neutropenia and blood cultures. An acute-phase reactant (C-reactive protein) is helpful but takes 12–24 hours to rise, so one normal result does not exclude infection but two consecutive normal values are strong evidence against infection. Antibiotics are started immediately without waiting for culture results. Intravenous antibiotics are given to cover group B streptococci, *Listeria monocytogenes* and other Gram-positive organisms (usually benzylpenicillin or amoxicillin), combined with cover for Gram-negative organisms (usually an aminoglycoside such as gentamicin). If cultures and CRP are negative and the infant has recovered clinically, antibiotics can be stopped after 48 hours. If the blood culture is positive or if there are any neurological signs, CSF must be examined and cultured.

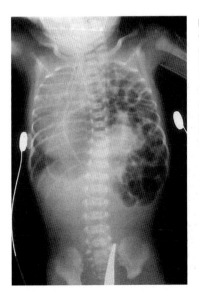

Figure 10.22 Chest X-ray in diaphragmatic hernia showing loops of bowel in the left chest and displacement of the mediastinum.

• •

Box 10.2 Clinical features of neonatal sepsis

- Fever or temperature instability or hypothermia
- Poor feeding
- Vomiting
- Apnoea and bradycardia
- Respiratory distress
- Abdominal distension
- Jaundice
- Neutropenia
- Hypo-/hyperglycaemia
- Shock
- Irritability
- Seizures
- Lethargy, drowsiness
- *In meningitis:*
- Tense or bulging fontanelle
- Head retraction (opisthotonos)

Late-onset infection (>72 hours)

After 72 hours, the source of infection is usually the infant's environment. The presentation is usually non-specific (Box 10.2). Nosocomially acquired infections are an inherent risk in a neonatal unit or postnatal ward. All staff must adhere strictly to effective handwashing to prevent cross-infection. In intensive care, the other main sources of infection are indwelling catheters for parenteral nutrition or arterial blood gas sampling, tracheal tubes and invasive procedures which break the protective barrier of the skin. Coagulase-negative staphylococcus (*Staph. epidermidis*) is the most common pathogen in this situation, but the range of organisms is broad, and includes *Staph. aureus*, *Escherichia coli*, *Pseudomonas* species, and fungal infections e.g. *Candida*. Initial therapy (e.g. with flucloxacillin and gentamicin) is aimed to cover most staphylococci and Gram-negative bacilli. If the organism is resistant to these antibiotics or the infant's condition does not improve, more powerful antibiotics (e.g. vancomycin) may be needed. Serial measurements of an acute-phase reactant (CRP) are useful to monitor response to therapy.

Neonatal meningitis, although uncommon, has a mortality of 20–50%, with one-third of survivors having serious sequelae. Presentation is the same as for other forms of neonatal sepsis. A bulging fontanelle and hyperextension of neck and back (opisthotonos) are late signs. If meningitis is thought likely, ampicillin or penicillin and a third-generation cephalosporin (e.g. cefotaxime which has CSF penetration) are given. Complications include cerebral abscess, ventriculitis, hydrocephalus, hearing loss and neurodevelopmental impairment.

Some specific infections

Group B streptococcal infection

Fifteen to thirty per cent of pregnant women have faecal or vaginal carriage of group B streptococci. Transmission from mother to infant occurs during delivery or by ascending infection shortly before birth. Up to half of the infants born to these mothers carry the organism on their mucous membranes or skin, but only 1% of them become ill. The incidence of disease varies widely between countries, from 1 to 5 per 1000 live births. Preterm infants are at increased risk. Early-onset disease typically presents on day 1 with pneumonia, septicaemia and, occasionally, meningitis. Mortality is up to 10%. Late-onset disease, from 3 days to 3 months of age, is less common. It usually causes meningitis but may present with focal infections such as osteomyelitis or septic arthritis. Preterm infants are at increased risk.

Maternal colonisation with group B streptococci may be identified by universal screening at 35–38 weeks' gestation, as is practised in the USA, Australia and several other countries, and positive mothers are given prophylactic intrapartum anti-biotics. The neonatal infection rate in these countries has fallen markedly. The UK appears to have a lower infection rate than initially experienced in the USA and Australia, and selective screening of mothers at increased risk (previous baby with group B streptococcal infection, preterm labour, prolonged rupture of the membranes, fever in labour >38°C) is recommended, with intrapartum antibiotics given if positive.

Listeria monocytogenes infection

Perinatal and neonatal *Listeria* infection is uncommon but serious. It is transmitted to the mother in food, such as unpasteurised milk, soft cheeses and undercooked poultry. It can cause a mild, influenza-like illness in the mother, or there may be asymptomatic faecal and vaginal carriage. Infection in pregnancy may cause spontaneous abortion, preterm delivery or fetal infection. The fetus usually acquires infection transplacentally, but also by ascending infection from the genital tract or at delivery. A characteristic feature of *Listeria* infection, even in preterm infants, is meconium staining of the liquor, which is otherwise unusual at an early gestation. In early-onset disease, presentation is at delivery or within the first few hours of life with septicaemia and pneumonia, a widespread rash and meningitis. The mortality is 30%. In late-onset disease, presentation is at 1–8 weeks of age, most often with meningitis, and has a better prognosis.

Gram-negative infections

Escherichia coli and other Gram-negative organisms, which are present in faeces and carried vaginally, used to be the most common cause of early-onset sepsis in the newborn. In the UK and the USA, group B streptococcal infection is now more common.

Conjunctivitis

Sticky eyes are common in the neonatal period, starting on the third or fourth day of life. Cleaning with saline or water is all that is required and the condition resolves spontaneously. A more troublesome discharge may be due to staphylococcal or streptococcal infection and can be treated with a topical antibiotic eye ointment, e.g. neomycin.

Purulent discharge with swelling of the eyelids within the first 48 hours of life may be due to gonococcal infection. The discharge should be Gram-stained urgently, as well as cultured, and treatment started immediately as permanent loss of vision can occur. In countries such as the UK and the USA where penicillin resistance is a problem, a third-generation cephalosporin is given intravenously. The eye needs to be cleansed frequently.

Chlamydia trachomatis eye infection usually presents with a purulent discharge, together with swelling of the eyelids (Fig. 10.23) at 1–2 weeks of age, but may also present shortly after birth. The organism can be identified with immunofluorescent staining. Treatment is with oral erythromycin for 2

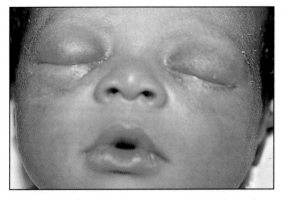

Figure 10.23 Purulent discharge together with swollen eyelids in an 8-day-old infant. This is the characteristic presentation of conjunctivitis from *Chlamydia trachomatis*. *Neisseria gonorrhoeae* was absent.

weeks. The mother and partner also need to be checked and treated.

Umbilical infection

The umbilicus dries and separates during the first few days of life. If the skin surrounding the umbilicus becomes inflamed, systemic antibiotics are indicated. Sometimes the umbilicus continues to be sticky, as it is prevented from involuting by an umbilical granuloma. This can be removed by applying silver nitrate while protecting the surrounding skin to avoid chemical burns, or by applying a ligature around the base of the exposed stump.

Herpes simplex virus (HSV) infections

Neonatal HSV infection is uncommon, occurring in 1 in 3000 to 1 in 20 000 live births. HSV infection is usually transmitted during passage through an infected birth canal or by ascending infection. Most infections are caused by HSV-2. The risk to an infant born to a mother with a primary genital infection is high, about 40%, while the risk from recurrent maternal infection is less than 3%. In most infants who develop HSV infection, the condition is un-expected as the mother's primary infection is asymptomatic or causes a non-specific illness.

The infection is more common in preterm infants. Presentation is at any time up to 4 weeks of age, with localised herpetic lesions on the skin or eye, or with encephalitis or disseminated disease. Mortality due to localised disease is low, but, even with aciclovir treatment, disseminated disease has a high mortality with considerable morbidity after encephalitis. If the mother is recognised as having primary disease or develops genital herpetic lesions at the time of delivery, elective caesarean section is indicated. Women with a history of recurrent genital infection can be delivered vaginally as the risk of neonatal infection is very low and maternal treatment before delivery minimises the presence of virus at delivery. Aciclovir can be given prophyl-actically to the baby during the at-risk period, but its efficacy is unproven.

Hepatitis B

Infants of mothers who are hepatitis B surface antigen (HBsAg)-positive should receive hepatitis B vaccination shortly after birth to prevent vertical transmission. The vaccination course needs to be completed during infancy and antibody response checked. Babies are at highest risk of becoming chronic carriers when their mothers are 'e' antigen-positive but have no 'e' antibodies. Infants of 'e' antigen-positive mothers should also be given passive immunisation with hepatitis B immuno-globulin within 24 hours of birth.

> Infants of HBsAg-positive mothers should be vaccinated against hepatitis B.

Neonatal seizures

Many babies startle or have tremors when stim-ulated or make strange jerks during active sleep. Seizures, on the other hand, are unstimulated. Typically, there are repetitive, rhythmic (clonic) movements of the limbs which persist despite restraint and are often accompanied by eye move-ments and changes in respiration. Many neonatal units now use continuous single channel EEG (amplified integrated EEG, also called a cerebral function monitor) to be able to confirm changes in electrical discharges in the brain. The causes of seizures are listed in Box 10.3.

Whenever seizures are observed, hypoglycaemia and meningitis need to be excluded or treated urgently. A cerebral ultrasound is performed to identify haemorrhage or cerebral malformation. Identification of cerebral ischaemic lesions or some cerebral malformations may require MRI imaging of the brain. Treatment is directed at the cause whenever possible. Ongoing or repeated seizures are treated with an anticonvulsant, although their efficacy in suppressing seizures is much poorer

Box 10.3 Causes of neonatal seizures

- Hypoxic-ischaemic encephalopathy
- Cerebral infarction
- Septicaemia/meningitis
- Metabolic
    Hypoglycaemia
    Hypo-/hypernatraemia
    Hypocalcaemia
    Hypomagnesaemia
    Inborn errors of metabolism
    Pyridoxine dependency
- Intracranial haemorrhage
- Cerebral malformations
- Drug withdrawal, e.g. maternal opiates
- Congenital infection
- Kernicterus

than in older children. The prognosis depends on the underlying cause.

Cerebral infarction (neonatal stroke)

Infarction in the territory of the middle cerebral artery may present with seizures at 12–48 hours in a term infant. The seizures may be focal or generalised. In contrast to infants with hypoxic-ischaemic encephalopathy, there are no other abnormal clinical features. The diagnosis is confirmed by MRI imaging (Fig. 10.24). The mechanism is thought to be thrombotic, either thromboembolism from placental vessels or sometimes secondary to inherited thrombophilia. In spite of pronounced abnormalities on the MRI images, the prognosis is relatively good, with only 20% having hemiparesis or epilepsy presenting later in infancy or early childhood.

Hypoglycaemia

Hypoglycaemia is particularly likely to occur in the first 24 hours of life in babies who had intrauterine growth restriction, who are preterm, born to mothers with diabetes mellitus, are large-for-dates, hypothermic, polycythaemic or ill for any reason. Growth-restricted and preterm infants have poor glycogen stores, whereas the infants of a diabetic mother have sufficient glycogen stores, but hyperplasia of the islet cells in the pancreas causes high insulin levels. Symptoms are jitteriness, irritability, apnoea, lethargy, drowsiness and seizures.

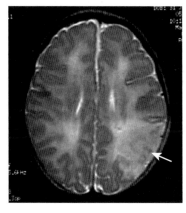

Figure 10.24 MRI scan showing infarction in the territory of a branch of the left middle cerebral artery.

There is no agreed definition of hypoglycaemia in the newborn. Many babies tolerate low blood glucose levels in the first few days of life, as they are able to utilise lactate and ketones as energy stores. Recent evidence suggests that blood glucose levels above 2.6 mmol/L are desirable for optimal neurodevelopmental outcome, although during the first 24 hours after birth many asymptomatic infants transiently have blood glucose levels below this level. There is good evidence that prolonged, symptomatic hypoglycaemia can cause permanent neurological disability.

Hypoglycaemia can usually be prevented by early and frequent milk feeding. In infants at increased risk of hypoglycaemia, blood glucose is regularly monitored at the bedside. If an asymptomatic infant has two low glucose values (i.e. below 2.6 mmol/L) in spite of adequate feeding or one very low value (<1.6 mmol/L) or becomes symptomatic, glucose is given by intravenous infusion aiming to maintain the glucose >2.6 mmol/L. The concentration of the intravenous dextrose may need to be increased from 10% to 15% or even 20%. Abnormal blood glucose results should be confirmed in the laboratory. High concentration intravenous infusions of glucose should be given via a central venous catheter to avoid extravasation into the tissues, which may cause skin necrosis and reactive hypoglycaemia. If there is difficulty or delay in starting the infusion, or a satisfactory response is not achieved, glucagon or hydrocortisone can be given.

Craniofacial disorders

Cleft lip and palate

A cleft lip (Fig. 10.25a) may be unilateral or bilateral. It results from failure of fusion of the frontonasal and maxillary processes. In bilateral cases the premaxilla is anteverted. Cleft palate results from failure of fusion of the palatine processes and the nasal septum. Cleft lip and palate affect about 0.8 per 1000 babies. Most are inherited polygenically, but they may be part of a syndrome of multiple abnormalities, e.g. chromosomal defects. Some are associated with maternal anticonvulsant therapy. They may be detected on antenatal ultrasound scanning.

Surgical repair of the lip (Fig. 10.25b) may be performed within the first week of life for cosmetic

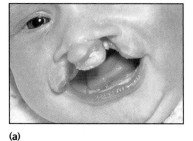

(a)

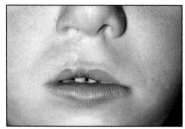

(b)

Figure 10.25 Before **(a)** and after **(b)** operation for cleft lip. Photographs showing the impressive results of surgery help many patients cope with the initial distress at having an affected infant. (Courtesy of Mr N. Waterhouse.)

reasons, although some surgeons feel that better results are obtained if surgery is delayed. The palate is usually repaired at several months of age. A cleft palate may make feeding more difficult, but some affected infants can still be breast-fed successfully. In bottle-fed babies, if milk enters the nose and causes choking, special teats and feeding devices may be helpful. Orthodontic advice and a dental prosthesis may help with feeding. Secretory otitis media is relatively common and should be sought on follow-up. Infants are also prone to acute otitis media. Adenoidectomy is best avoided, as the resultant gap between the abnormal palate and nasopharynx will exacerbate feeding problems and the nasal quality of speech. A multidisciplinary team approach is required, involving plastic and ENT surgeons, paediatrician, orthodontist, audiologist and speech therapist. Parent support groups can provide valuable support and advice for families (Cleft Lip and Palate Association, CLAPA).

Pierre Robin sequence

The Pierre Robin sequence is an association of micrognathia (Fig. 10.26), posterior displacement of the tongue (glossoptosis) and midline cleft of the soft palate. There may be difficulty feeding and, as the tongue falls back, there is obstruction to the upper airways which may result in cyanotic episodes. The infant is at risk of failure to thrive during the first few months. If there is upper airways obstruction, the infant may need to lie prone, allowing the tongue and small mandible to fall forward. Persistent obstruction can be treated using a nasopharyngeal airway. Eventually the mandible grows and these problems resolve. The cleft palate can then be repaired.

Gastrointestinal disorders

Oesophageal atresia

Oesophageal atresia is usually associated with a tracheo-oesophageal fistula (Fig. 10.27). It occurs in 1 in 3500 live births and is associated with polyhydramnios during pregnancy. If suspected, a wide-calibre feeding tube is passed and checked to see if it reaches the stomach. If not diagnosed at birth, clinical presentation is with persistent salivation and drooling from the mouth after birth, associated with choking and cyanotic episodes. If the diagnosis is not made at this stage, the infant will cough and choke when fed. There may be aspiration into the lungs of saliva (or milk) from the upper airways and acid secretions from the stomach. Almost half of the babies have other congenital malformation, e.g. as part of the VACTERL association (Vertebral, Anorectal, Cardiac, Tracheo-oEsophageal, Renal and Radial Limb anomalies). In oesophageal atresia, a chest X-ray will confirm that a wide-calibre feeding tube has failed to reach the stomach. Continuous suction is applied to the tube to reduce aspiration of saliva and secretions pending transfer to a neonatal surgical unit.

Small bowel obstruction

This may be recognised antenatally on ultrasound scanning. Otherwise, small bowel obstruction

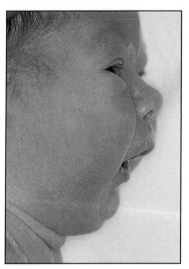

Figure 10.26 Micrognathia in Pierre Robin sequence.

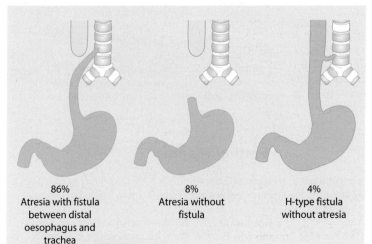

Figure 10.27 Oesophageal atresia and tracheo-oesophageal fistula.

86%
Atresia with fistula between distal oesophagus and trachea

8%
Atresia without fistula

4%
H-type fistula without atresia

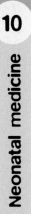

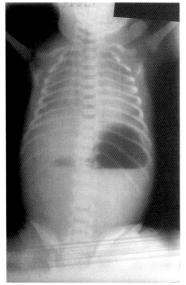

Figure 10.28
Abdominal X-ray in duodenal atresia showing a 'double bubble' from distension of the stomach and duodenal cap. There is absence of air distally.

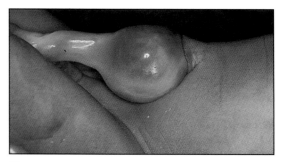

Figure 10.29 Small exomphalos with loops of bowel confined to the umbilicus. Care needs to be taken not to put a cord clamp across these lesions.

presents with persistent vomiting, which is bile-stained unless the obstruction is above the ampulla of Vater. Meconium may initially be passed, but subsequently its passage is usually delayed or absent. Abdominal distension becomes increasingly prominent the more distal the bowel obstruction. High lesions will present soon after birth, but lower obstruction may not present for some days.

Small bowel obstruction may be caused by:

- atresia or stenosis of the duodenum (Fig. 10.28) – a third have Down's syndrome and it is also associated with other congenital malformations
- atresia or stenosis of the jejunum or ileum – there may be multiple atretic segments of bowel
- malrotation with volvulus – a dangerous condition as it may lead to infarction of the entire midgut
- meconium ileus – thick inspissated meconium, of putty-like consistency, becomes packed into the lower ileum; almost all affected neonates have cystic fibrosis
- meconium plug – a plug of inspissated meconium causes lower intestinal obstruction.

The diagnosis is made on clinical features and abdominal X-ray showing intestinal obstruction. Atresia or stenosis of the bowel and malrotation are treated surgically, after correction of fluid and electrolyte depletion. A meconium plug will usually pass spontaneously. Meconium ileus may be dislodged using Gastrografin contrast medium.

Large bowel obstruction

This may be caused by:

- *Hirschsprung's disease.* Absence of the myenteric nerve plexus in the rectum which may extend along the colon. The baby often does not pass meconium within 48 hours of birth and subsequently the abdomen distends. About 15% present as an acute enterocolitis (see Ch. 13).

- *Rectal atresia.* Absence of the anus at the normal site. Lesions are high or low, depending whether the bowel ends above or below the levator ani muscle. In high lesions there is a fistula to the bladder or urethra in boys, or the vagina or bladder in girls. Treatment is surgical.

> Bile-stained vomiting is from intestinal obstruction until proved otherwise.

Exomphalos/gastroschisis

These lesions are often diagnosed antenatally (see Ch. 9). In exomphalos (also called omphalocele), the abdominal contents protrude through the umbilical ring, covered with a transparent sac formed by the amniotic membrane and peritoneum (Fig. 10.29). It is often associated with other major congenital abnormalities. In gastroschisis the bowel protrudes through a defect in the anterior abdominal wall, adjacent to the umbilicus, and there is no covering sac (see Fig. 9.2). It is not associated with other congenital abnormalities.

Gastroschisis carries a much greater risk of dehydration and protein loss, so the abdomen of affected infants should be wrapped in several layers of clingfilm to minimise fluid and heat loss. A nasogastric tube is passed and aspirated frequently and an intravenous infusion of dextrose established. Colloid support is often required to replace protein loss. Many lesions can be repaired by primary closure of the abdomen. With large lesions, the intestine is enclosed in a silastic sac sutured to the edges of the abdominal wall and the contents gradually returned into the peritoneal cavity.

Further reading

Lissauer T, Fanaroff A A 2006 Neonatology at a glance. Blackwell Science, Oxford. *Short, illustrated textbook*

Rennie J M 2005 Roberton's textbook of neonatology, 4th edn. Elsevier Churchill Livingstone. *Comprehensive textbook*

Growth and puberty

There are four phases of human growth (Fig. 11.1).

Fetal

This is the fastest period of growth, accounting for about 30% of eventual height. Size at birth is determined by the size of the mother and by placental nutrient supply, which in turn modulates fetal growth factors (IGF-2, human placental lactogen and insulin). Severe intrauterine growth restriction and extreme prematurity can result in permanent short stature.

The infantile phase

Growth during infancy to around 18 months of age is also largely dependent on adequate nutrition. Good health and normal thyroid function are also necessary. This phase is characterised by a rapid but decelerating growth rate, and accounts for about 15% of eventual height. By the end of this phase, children have changed from their fetal length, largely determined by the uterine environment, to their genetically determined height. An inadequate rate of weight gain during this period is called 'failure to thrive'.

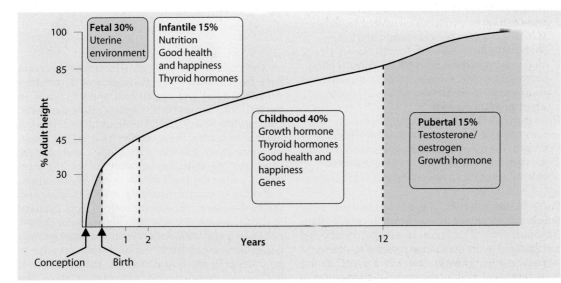

Figure 11.1 Diagrammatic representation of the phases of growth in childhood. The fetal and infantile phases are mainly dependent on adequate nutrition, whereas the childhood and pubertal phases are dependent on growth hormone and other hormones.

Childhood phase

This is a slow, steady but prolonged period of growth which contributes 40% of final height. Pituitary growth hormone (GH) secretion acting to produce insulin-like growth factor 1 (IGF-1) at the epiphyses is the main determinant of a child's rate of growth, provided there is adequate nutrition and good health. Thyroid hormone, vitamin D and steroids also affect cartilage cell division and bone formation. Profound chronic unhappiness can decrease GH secretion and accounts for psycho-social short stature.

Pubertal growth spurt

Sex hormones, mainly testosterone and oestradiol, cause the back to lengthen and boost GH secretion. This adds 15% to final height. The same sex steroids cause fusion of the epiphyseal growth plates and a cessation of growth. If puberty is early, which is not uncommon in girls, the final height is reduced because of early fusion of the epiphyses.

Measurement

Growth must be measured accurately, with attention to correct technique and accurate plotting of the data:

- Weight – readily and accurately determined with electronic scales but must be performed on a naked infant or a child dressed only in underclothing as an entire month's or year's weight gain can be represented by a wet nappy or heavy jeans, respectively.
- Height – the equipment must be regularly calibrated and maintained. In children over 2 years of age, the standing height is measured as illustrated (Fig. 11.2). In children under 2 years, length is measured lying horizontally (Fig. 11.3), using the mother to assist. Accurate length measurement in infants can be difficult to obtain, as the legs need to be held straight and infants often dislike being held still. For this reason, routine measurement of length in infancy is often omitted from child surveillance, but it should always be performed whenever there is doubt about an infant's growth.
- Head circumference – the occipitofrontal circumference is a measure of head and brain growth. The mean of three measurements is used. It is of particular importance in developmental delay or suspected hydrocephalus.

These measurements should be plotted as a simple dot on an appropriate growth centile chart. Standards for a population should be constructed and updated every generation to allow for the trend towards earlier puberty and taller adult stature from improved childhood nutrition. Height in a population is normally distributed and the deviation from the mean can be measured as a centile or standard deviation (Fig. 11.4). The bands

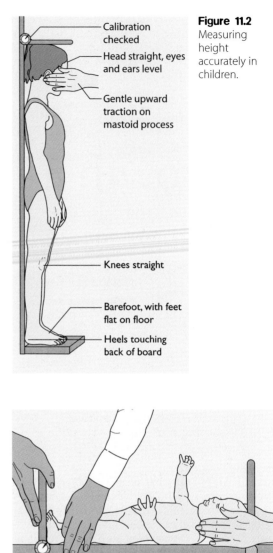

Figure 11.2 Measuring height accurately in children.

Calibration checked

Head straight, eyes and ears level

Gentle upward traction on mastoid process

Knees straight

Barefoot, with feet flat on floor

Heels touching back of board

Figure 11.3 Measuring length in infants and young children. An assistant is required to hold the legs straight.

on the current UK 1990 growth reference charts have been chosen to be two-thirds of a standard deviation apart and correspond approximately to the 25th, 9th, 2nd and 0.4th centiles below the mean, and the 75th, 91st, 98th and 99.6th centiles above the mean. The further these centiles lie from the mean, the more likely it is that a child has a pathological cause for his short or tall stature. For instance, values below the 0.4th or above the 99.6th centile will occur by chance in only 4 per 1000 children and can be used as a criterion for referral from primary to specialist care. A single growth parameter should not be assessed in isolation from the other growth parameters; e.g. a child's low weight may be in proportion to the height if short, but abnormal if tall. Serial measurements are used to show the pattern and determine the rate of growth. This is helpful in diagnosing or monitoring many paediatric conditions.

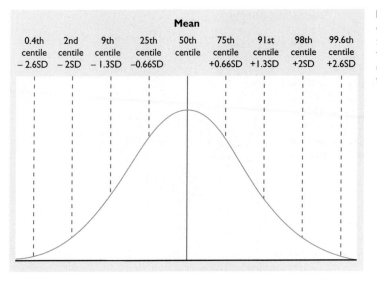

				Mean				
0.4th centile −2.6SD	2nd centile −2SD	9th centile −1.3SD	25th centile −0.66SD	50th centile	75th centile +0.66SD	91st centile +1.3SD	98th centile +2SD	99.6th centile +2.6SD

Figure 11.4 Interpretation of the UK growth reference charts. The lines show the mean and bands which are two-thirds of a standard deviation (SD) apart. The centiles are shown in the diagram.

Summary

Regarding measurement of children:
- must be accurate for meaningful monitoring of growth
- growth parameters should be plotted on charts
- significant abnormalities of height are:
  - measurements outside the 2nd or 98th centiles if the mid-parental height is not short or tall
  - if markedly discrepant from weight
  - serial measurements cross growth centile lines after the first year of life.

Puberty

Puberty follows a well defined sequence of changes that may be assigned stages as shown in Figures 11.5 and 11.6.

In *females* the features of puberty are:

- breast development – the first sign, usually starting between 8.5 and 12.5 years
- pubic hair growth and a rapid height spurt – occur almost immediately after breast development
- menarche – occurs on average 2.5 years after the start of puberty and signals the end of growth (only around 5 cm height gain remaining).

In *males*:

- testicular enlargement to greater than 4 ml volume measured using an orchidometer (Fig. 11.7) – the first sign of puberty
- pubic hair growth – follows testicular enlargement, usually between 10 and 14 years of age
- height spurt – when the testicular volume is 12–15 ml, after a delay of around 18 months.

The height spurt in males occurs later and is of greater magnitude than in females, accounting for the greater final average height of males than females.

In *both sexes* there will be development of acne, axillary hair, body odour and mood changes.

If puberty is abnormally early or late, it can be further assessed:

- bone age measurement from a hand and wrist X-ray to determine skeletal maturation (Fig. 11.8)
- in females – pelvic ultrasound to assess uterine size and endometrial thickness.

Summary

Regarding puberty:
- the first sign in females is breast development; in males it is testicular enlargement
- in females the height spurt occurs shortly after breast development; in males it starts almost 18 months after the first signs of puberty.

Short stature

Short stature is usually defined as a height below the second (i.e. two standard deviations below the mean) or 0.4th centile (−2.6 SD). Only 1 in 50 children will be shorter than the second centile and 1 in 250 shorter than the 0.4th centile. Most such children will be normal, though short, but the further the child is below these centiles, the more likely it is that there will be a pathological cause. However, the rate of growth may be pathological long before a child's height falls below these values. This growth failure can be identified from the child's height falling across centile lines plotted on a growth chart. This allows growth failure to be identified even though the child's height is still above the second centile.

Measuring height velocity is a sensitive indicator of growth failure. Two *accurate* measurements at

Stages of puberty

a Female breast changes

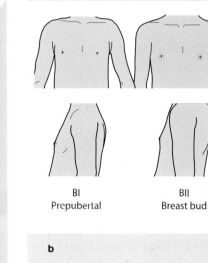

| BI Prepubertal | BII Breast bud | BIII Juvenile smooth contour | BIV Areola and papilla project above breast | BV Adult |

b Pubic hair changes–female and male

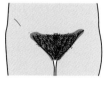

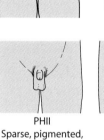

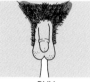

| PHI Pre-adolescent No sexual hair | PHII Sparse, pigmented, long, straight, mainly along labia or at base of penis | PHIII Dark, coarser, curlier | PHIV Filling out towards adult distribution | PHV Adult in quantity and type with spread to medial thighs in male |

c Male genital stages

| GI Preadolescent | GII Lengthening of penis | GIII Further growth in length and circumference | GIV Development of glans penis, darkening of scrotal skin | GV Adult genitalia |

Figure 11.5 Schematic drawings of male and female stages of puberty. Pubertal changes are shown according to the Tanner stages of puberty.

least 6 months but preferably a year apart allow calculation of height velocity in cm/year (Fig. 11.9). This is plotted at the midpoint in time on a height/velocity chart. A height velocity persistently below the 25th centile is abnormal and that child will eventually become short. (A tall child with a height on the 98th centile will grow at approximately the 75th velocity centile; a short child with a height on the second centile will grow at approximately the 25th velocity centile – hence the boundaries of a normal growth rate approximate to the 25th–75th centile.) A disadvantage of using height velocity calculations is that they are highly dependent on the accuracy of the height measurements and so tend not to be used outside specialist growth units.

The height centile of a child must be compared with the weight centile and an estimate of their genetic target centile and range calculated from the height of their parents (See Appendix).

Timing of puberty

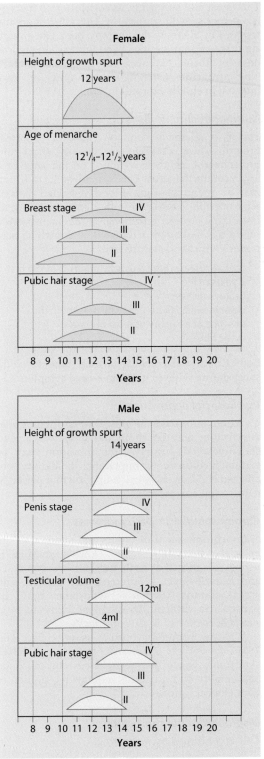

Figure 11.6 Timing of puberty. Pubertal changes are shown according to the Tanner stages of puberty. (Diagrams based on Zitelli B J, Davis H W *Atlas of Pediatric Physical Diagnosis*, 2nd edn, Lippincott, Philadelphia, 1992 and Johnson T R, Moore W M, Jeffries J E *Children are Different*, 2nd edn, Ross Laboratories, Division of Abbot Laboratories, Columbus, OH, 1978.)

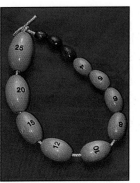

Figure 11.7 Orchidometer to assess testicular volume (in ml). (From Wales J K H, Rogol A D, Wit J M, *Pediatric Endocrinology and Growth*, Mosby-Wolfe, London, 2003, with permission.)

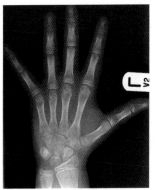

Figure 11.8 An X-ray of the left wrist and hand to determine bone age. It allows assessment of skeletal maturation from the time of appearance or maturity of the epiphyseal centres, using a standardised rating system. The child's height can be compared with skeletal maturation and an adult height prediction made.

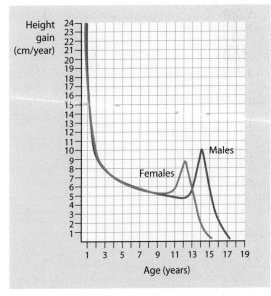

Figure 11.9 Male and female height velocity charts (50th centile) showing that adult males are taller than females as they have a longer childhood growth phase, their peak height velocity is higher and their growth ceases later.

Most short children are psychologically well adjusted to their size. However, there may be problems from being teased or bullied at school, poor self-esteem and they are at a considerable disadvantage in most competitive sport. They are also assumed by adults to be younger than their true age and may be treated inappropriately.

Causes (Fig. 11.10)

Familial

Most short children have short parents and fall within the centile target range allowing for mid-parental height. Care needs to be taken, though, that both the child and a parent do not have an inherited growth disorder.

Intrauterine growth restriction (IUGR) and extreme prematurity

About one-third of children born with severe intra-uterine growth restriction or who were extremely premature remain short.

Constitutional delay of growth and puberty

These children have delayed puberty, which is often familial, usually having occurred in the parent of the same sex. It is commoner in males. It is a variation of the normal timing of puberty rather than an abnormal condition. It may also be induced by dieting or excessive physical training. An affected child will not show the same sexual changes as his peers, and bone age would show moderate delay. The legs will be long in comparison to the back. Eventually the target height will be reached. The condition may cause psychological upset. The onset of puberty can be induced with androgens or oestrogens.

Endocrine

Hypothyroidism, growth hormone (GH) deficiency and steroid excess are uncommon causes of short stature. They are associated with children being relatively overweight, i.e. their weight on a higher centile than their height.

Hypothyroidism

This is usually caused by autoimmune thyroiditis during childhood. Congenital hypothyroidism (see Ch. 25) is diagnosed soon after birth by screening and so does not result in any abnormality of growth.

Growth hormone deficiency

This may be an isolated defect or secondary to panhypopituitarism. Pituitary function may be abnormal in congenital mid-facial defects or as a result of a craniopharyngioma (a tumour affecting the pituitary region), a hypothalamic tumour or trauma such as head injury, meningitis and cranial irradiation. Craniopharyngioma usually presents in late childhood and may result in abnormal visual fields (characteristically a bitemporal hemianopia as it impinges on the optic chiasm), optic atrophy or papilloedema on fundoscopy. In GH deficiency, the bone age is markedly delayed.

Corticosteroid excess

This is usually iatrogenic, as corticosteroid therapy is a potent growth suppressor. This effect is greatly reduced by alternate day therapy, but some growth suppression may be seen even with relatively low doses of inhaled steroids in susceptible individuals. Non-iatrogenic Cushing's syndrome is very unusual in childhood (see Ch. 25).

Nutritional/chronic illness

This is a relatively common cause of abnormal growth. These children are usually short and underweight; i.e. their weight is on the same or a lower centile than their height. Inadequate nutrition may be due to insufficient food, restricted diets or poor appetite associated with a chronic illness, or from the increased nutritional requirement from a raised metabolic rate. Chronic illnesses which may present with short stature include:

* coeliac disease, which usually presents in the first 2 years of life
* Crohn's disease
* chronic renal failure – may be present in the absence of a history of renal disease
* cystic fibrosis.

Both Crohn's and coeliac disease may result in short stature without gastrointestinal symptoms.

Psychosocial deprivation

Children subjected to physical and emotional deprivation may be short and underweight and show delayed puberty. This condition may be extremely difficult or impossible to identify, but affected children show catch-up growth if placed in a nurturing environment.

Chromosomal disorder/syndromes

Many chromosomal disorders and syndromes are associated with short stature. Down's syndrome is usually diagnosed at birth, but Turner's, Noonan's and Russell–Silver syndromes may present with short stature. Turner's syndrome may be particularly difficult to diagnose clinically and *should be considered in all short females.*

Whereas Turner's syndrome is associated with 45XO karyotype, Noonan's and Russell–Silver syndromes have no recognised chromosomal abnormality and diagnosis requires recognition of their clinical features.

Disproportionate short stature

This is confirmed by measuring:

* sitting height – base of spine to top of head
* subischial leg length – subtraction of sitting height from total height.

Charts exist to assess the normality of body proportions. These conditions are rare and may be caused by disorders of the formation of bone. They include achondroplasia and other short-limbed dysplasias. If the legs are extremely short, treatment

Table 11.1 Investigation of short stature

Investigation	Significance
X-ray of wrist and hand for bone age	Some delay in constitutional delay of growth and puberty
	Marked delay for hypothyroidism or growth hormone deficiency or other endocrine causes
Full blood count	Anaemia in coeliac or Crohn's disease
Creatine and electrolytes	Creatinine raised in chronic renal failure
Thyroid-stimulating hormone (TSH)	Raised in hypothyroidism
Karyotype in females	Turner's syndrome shows 45XO
Endomysial and gliadin antibodies	Usually present in coeliac disease
CRP (acute-phase reactant)	Raised in Crohn's disease
Growth hormone provocation tests (using insulin, glucagon or arginine in specialist centres)	Growth hormone deficiency
MRI scan if neurological symptoms/signs	Craniopharyngioma or intracranial tumour

by surgical leg lengthening may be appropriate. The back may be short from severe scoliosis or some storage disorders, such as the mucopolysaccharidoses.

Examination and investigation

Plotting present and previous heights and weights on appropriate growth charts, together with the clinical features, usually allows the cause to be identified without any investigations. Previous height and weight measurements should be available from the parent-held personal child health record. The bone age may be helpful as it is markedly delayed in some endocrine disorders, e.g. hypothyroidism and GH deficiency, and is used to estimate adult height potential. Investigations which may be indicated are shown in Table 11.1.

Summary

Assessment of a child with short stature

Examination of the growth chart:
- Following growth centile lines?
  Consider familial, low birthweight, constitutional delay of growth and puberty, syndromes and skeletal dysplasias
- Growth failure with crossing of centile lines?
  Consider endocrine (including therapeutic corticosteroids), nutrition/chronic illness, psychosocial deprivation

Determine the mid-parental height
- For genetic predisposition

History
- Family history of constitutional delay of growth and puberty?
- Features of chronic illness, endocrine causes, e.g. hypothyroidism, pituitary tumour, Cushing's or psychosocial deprivation?
- Medications e.g. corticosteroids?

Examination
- Chromosome/syndrome present? (But in Turner's syndrome other stigmata may be absent)
- Chronic illness, e.g. Crohn's, cystic fibrosis, coeliac disease?
- Evidence of endocrine causes?
- Disproportionate short stature from skeletal dysplasia?

Diagnosis
Cause can usually be determined from the above and no tests are required

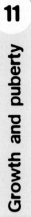

Causes & evaluation of short stature

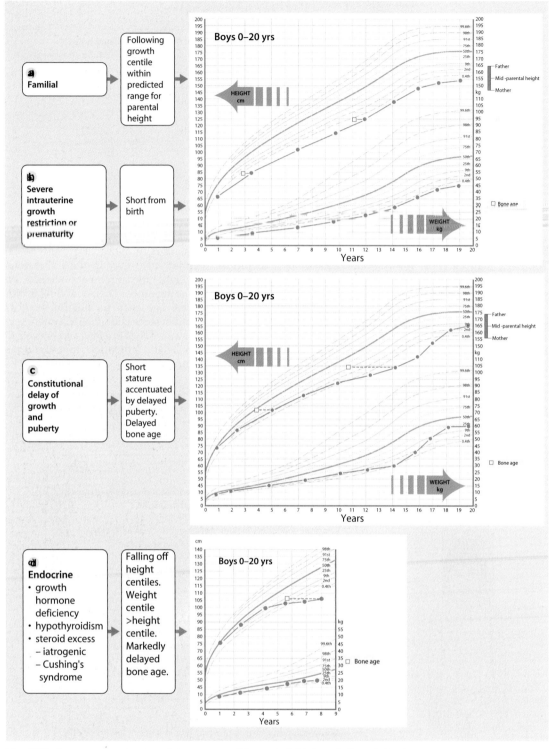

a) Familial → Following growth centile within predicted range for parental height

b) Severe intrauterine growth restriction or prematurity → Short from birth

c) Constitutional delay of growth and puberty → Short stature accentuated by delayed puberty. Delayed bone age

d) Endocrine
- growth hormone deficiency
- hypothyroidism
- steroid excess
  – iatrogenic
  – Cushing's syndrome

→ Falling off height centiles. Weight centile >height centile. Markedly delayed bone age.

Fig. 11.10 Causes and evaluation of short stature. (Charts © Child Growth Foundation.)

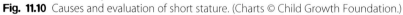

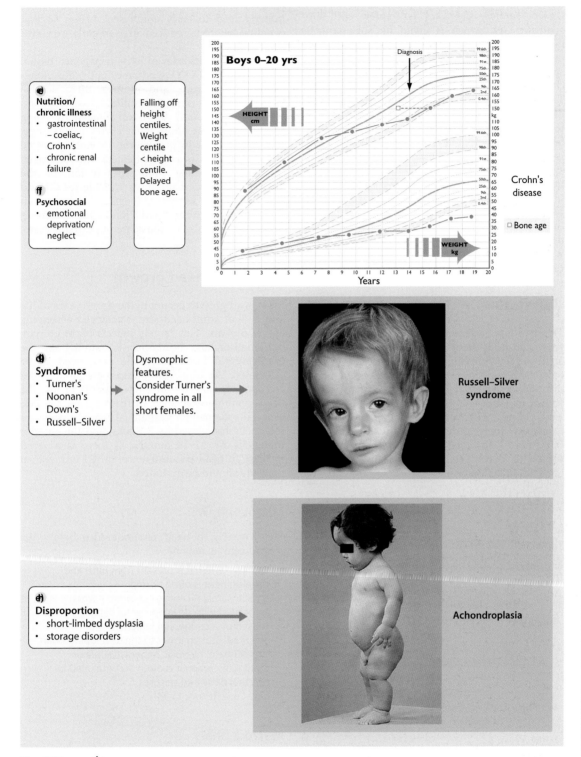

e)
Nutrition/chronic illness
- gastrointestinal – coeliac, Crohn's
- chronic renal failure

f)
Psychosocial
- emotional deprivation/neglect

Falling off height centiles. Weight centile < height centile. Delayed bone age.

Boys 0–20 yrs

Diagnosis

HEIGHT cm

WEIGHT kg

Years

Crohn's disease

□ Bone age

d)
Syndromes
- Turner's
- Noonan's
- Down's
- Russell–Silver

Dysmorphic features. Consider Turner's syndrome in all short females.

Russell–Silver syndrome

e)
Disproportion
- short-limbed dysplasia
- storage disorders

Achondroplasia

Fig. 11.10, *cont'd.*

Treatment of endocrine causes

Growth hormone deficiency is treated with bio-synthetic GH, which is given by subcutaneous injection, usually daily. GH is expensive and the management of GH deficiency is undertaken at specialist centres. The best response is seen in children with the most severe hormone deficiency. There is no longer a risk of transmission of prion diseases, e.g. Creutzfeldt–Jakob disease, which unfortunately occurred in a number of instances before 1985 when cadaveric GH was used. Other indications for GH therapy include Turner's syndrome, Prader–Willi syndrome, chronic renal failure and intrauterine growth restriction (IUGR).

Congenital hypothyroidism is treated with thyroxine replacement therapy from detection, usually by the end of the second week of life, and growth is then normal. *Acquired hypothyroidism* is also treated with thyroxine although short stature may still result if the diagnosis has been delayed.

Tall stature

This is a less common presenting complaint than short stature, as many parents are proud that their child is tall. However, some adolescents (mainly females) become concerned about excessive height during their pubertal growth spurt. The causes are shown in Table 11.2. Most tall stature is inherited from tall parents. Overeating in childhood leading to obesity 'fuels' early growth and may result in tall stature; however, because puberty is often somewhat earlier than average, final height is usually not excessive.

Table 11.2 Causes of excessive growth or tall stature

Familial	Most common cause
Obesity	Puberty is advanced so final height centile is less than in childhood
Secondary	Hyperthyroidism Excess sex steroids – precocious puberty from whatever cause Excess adrenal androgen steroids – congenital adrenal hyperplasia True gigantism (excess GH secretion)
Syndromes	Long-legged tall stature: – Marfan's syndrome – homocystinuria – Klinefelter's syndrome (47 XXY and XXY karyotype) Proportionate tall stature at birth: – maternal diabetes – primary hyperinsulinism – Beckwith syndrome Sotos syndrome – associated with large head, characteristic facial features and learning difficulties

Secondary endocrine causes are rare. Both congenital adrenal hyperplasia and precocious puberty lead to early epiphyseal fusion so that eventual height is reduced after an early excessive growth rate.

Marfan's (a disorder of loose connective tissue) and Klinefelter (XXY) syndromes both cause long-legged tall stature, and in XXY there is also infertility and learning difficulties.

Tall children may be disadvantaged by being treated as older than their chronological age. Excessive height in prepubertal or early pubertal adolescent females can be treated with oestrogen therapy to induce premature fusion of the epiphyses, but as it produces variable results and has potentially serious side-effects it is seldom undertaken. Surgical destruction of the epiphyses in the legs may also be considered in extreme cases.

Abnormal head growth

Most head growth occurs in the first 2 years of life and 80% of adult head size is achieved before the age of 5 years. This largely reflects brain growth, but small or large heads may be familial and the mid-parental head percentile may need to be calculated. At birth, the sutures and fontanelles are open. During the first few months of life, the head circumference may increase across centiles, especially if small for gestational age. The posterior fontanelle has closed by 8 weeks, and the anterior fontanelle by 12–18 months. If there is a rapid increase in head circumference, raised intracranial pressure should be excluded.

Microcephaly

Microcephaly, a head circumference below the second centile, may be:

- familial – when it is present from birth and development is often normal
- an autosomal recessive condition – when it is associated with developmental delay
- caused by a congenital infection
- acquired after an insult to the developing brain, e.g. perinatal hypoxia, hypoglycaemia or meningitis, when it is often accompanied by cerebral palsy and seizures.
  (See Case History 11.1.)

Macrocephaly

Macrocephaly is a head circumference above the 98th centile. The causes of a large head are listed in Box 11.1. Most are normal children and often the parents have large heads. A rapidly increasing head circumference, even if the head circumference is still below the 98th centile, suggests raised intracranial pressure and may be due to hydrocephalus, subdural haematoma or brain tumour. It must be investigated promptly by intracranial ultrasound

Case History
11.1 Microcephaly

Figure 11.11 shows the head circumference chart of Tim, who was healthy and was developing normally. At 9 months of age, he was rushed to hospital as he was unrousable from profound hypoglycaemia secondary to the deliberate administration of insulin by his mother, who had diabetes. Although Tim was taken into care and had no further hypo-glycaemic episodes, his head circumference shows cessation of growth. He has developed moderate learning difficulties and mild cerebral palsy.

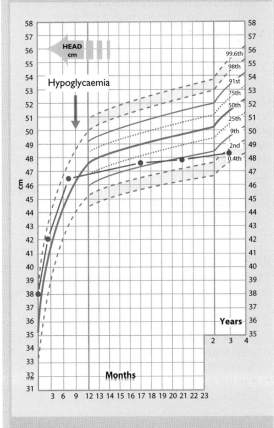

Figure 11.11 Tim's head circumference chart. (Chart © Child Growth Foundation.)

Box 11.1 Causes of a large head

- Tall stature
- Familial macrocephaly
- Raised intracranial pressure
- Hydrocephalus – progressive or arrested
- Chronic subdural haematoma
- Cerebral tumour
- Neurofibromatosis
- Cerebral gigantism (Sotos syndrome)
- CNS storage disorders, e.g. mucopolysaccharidosis (Hurler's syndrome)

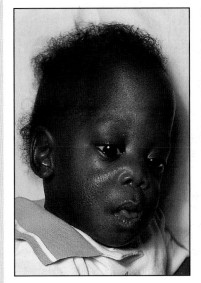

Figure 11.12 Long flat head of a preterm infant. This can be avoided by lying preterm infants on a soft surface and regularly changing their head position.

that babies should sleep lying on their back. It improves with time as the infant becomes more mobile. Plagiocephaly is also seen in infants with hypotonia, e.g. preterm infants may develop long, flat heads from lying on their sides for long periods on the hard surface of incubators (Fig. 11.12). Under these circumstances, it is not associated with abnormal development.

Craniosynostosis

The sutures of the skull bones do not finally fuse until about 12 years of age. Premature fusion of a suture (craniosynostosis) may lead to distortion of the head shape (Box 11.2). The craniosynostosis may be a feature of a syndrome or may be an isolated finding. The fused suture may be felt or seen as a palpable ridge and confirmed on skull X-ray or cranial CT scan. If necessary, the condition can be treated surgically because of raised intracranial pressure or for cosmetic reasons. Such operations are performed in specialist centres for craniofacial reconstructive surgery (Fig. 11.13).

if the anterior fontanelle is still open, otherwise by CT or MRI scan.

Asymmetric heads

Skull asymmetry may result from an imbalance of the growth rate at the coronal, sagittal or lambdoid sutures, although the head circumference increases normally. Occipital plagiocephaly, a parallelogram-shaped head with flattening of the back of the skull, is seen with increased frequency since the advice

Localised
- Coronal suture only – asymmetrical skull
- Sagittal suture only – a long narrow skull

Generalised
- Multiple sutures resulting in microcephaly and developmental delay
- Genetic syndromes, e.g. with syndactyly in Apert's syndrome, with exophthalmos in Crouzon's syndrome.

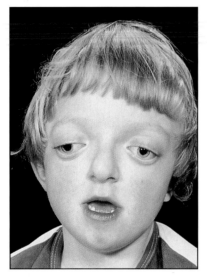

Figure 11.13 Crouzon's syndrome showing the typical shallow orbits and exophthalmos. Craniofacial reconstructive surgery is required to prevent visual loss and cerebral damage from raised intracranial pressure.

> If an infant's head circumference is enlarging and crossing centile lines – check for raised intracranial pressure

Premature sexual development

The development of secondary sexual characteristics before 8 years old in females and 9 years old in males is outside the normal range. It may be due to:

- precocious puberty when it is accompanied by a growth spurt
- premature breast development (thelarche)
- premature pubic hair development (pubarche).

Precocious puberty

Precocious puberty (PP) may be categorised according to the levels of the pituitary-derived gonado-tropins, follicle-stimulating hormone (FSH) and luteinising hormone (LH), (Fig. 11.14) as:

- gonadotropin-dependent (central, 'true' PP) from premature activation of the hypothalamic–pituitary–gonadal axis
- gonadotropin-independent (pseudo, 'false' PP) from excess sex steroids.

Females

This is usually idiopathic or familial and follows the normal sequence of puberty. Organic causes are rare and are associated with:

- dissonance, when the sequence of pubertal changes is abnormal, e.g. isolated pubic hair with virilisation of the genitalia, suggesting excess androgens from either congenital adrenal hyperplasia or an androgen-secreting tumour
- rapid onset
- neurological symptoms and signs, e.g. neurofibromatosis.

Ultrasound examination of the ovaries and uterus is helpful in establishing the cause of precocious puberty. In the premature onset of normal puberty, multicystic ovaries and an enlarging uterus will be identified.

> Precocious puberty in females is usually due to the premature onset of normal puberty.

Males (see Case history 11.2)
This is uncommon and usually has an organic cause, particularly intracranial tumours. Examination of the testes may be helpful:

- bilateral enlargement suggests gonadotropin release, usually from an intracranial lesion
- small testes suggest an adrenal cause (e.g. a tumour or adrenal hyperplasia)
- a unilateral enlarged testis suggests a gonadal tumour.

Tumours in the hypothalamic region are best investigated by cranial MRI scan.

> Central precocious puberty in males usually has an organic cause.

Management

The management of precocious puberty is directed towards:

- Detection and treatment of any underlying pathology, e.g. intracranial tumour in males, reducing the rate of skeletal maturation if necessary. Skeletal maturation is assessed by bone age. An early growth spurt may result in early cessation of growth and a reduction in adult height.
- Addressing psychological/behavioural difficulties associated with early progression through puberty.

Causes of precocious puberty

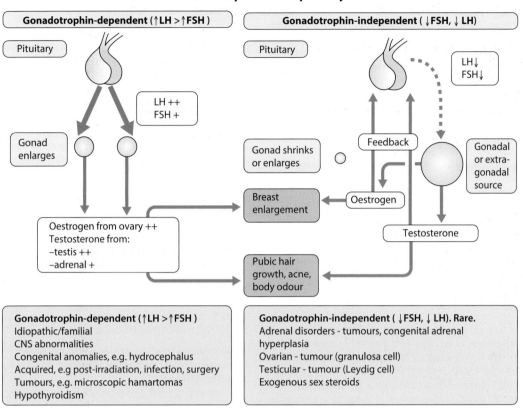

Figure 11.14 Causes of precocious puberty. (Courtesy of Dr Emma Rhodes.)

Case History
11.2 Precocious puberty in a boy

This 6-year-old boy presented with precocious puberty (Fig. 11.15a and b). He was noted to have multiple café-au-lait spots consistent with a diagnosis of neurofibromatosis type 1. An MRI scan showed a mass in the hypothalamus which proved to be an optic glioma. He was treated with radiotherapy, although full remission was not possible to achieve. The site of injection of gonadotropin superagonist treatment to suppress his sexual development is covered by the plaster.

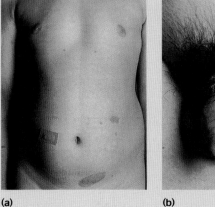

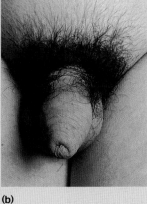

Figure 11.15 (a) He has multiple café-au-lait spots. Neurofibromatosis type 1 was diagnosed. **(b)** Genitalia showing stage 3 genitalia and pubic hair with 12 ml testicles bilaterally. He also had adult body odour. (From Wales J K H, Rogol A D, Wit J M, *Pediatric Endocrinology and Growth*, Saunders, London, 2003, with permission.)

(a)   (b)

Deciding whether to treat a girl who is simply going through puberty early needs consideration of all these factors. If treatment is required for gonadotropin-dependent disease, gonadotropin-releasing hormone (GnRH) analogues are the treatment of choice. In gonadotropin-independent cases, the source of excess sex steroids needs to be identified. Inhibitors of androgen or oestrogen production or action (e.g. medroxyprogesterone acetate, cyproterone acetate, testolactone, ketoconazole) may be used.

Premature breast development (thelarche)

This usually affects females between 6 months and 2 years of age. The breast enlargement may be asymmetrical. It is differentiated from precocious puberty by the absence of axillary and pubic hair and of a growth spurt. It is non-progressive and self-limiting. Investigations are not usually required (see Case history 11.3).

Premature pubarche

This occurs when pubic hair develops before 8 years of age in females and before 9 years in males but with no other signs of sexual development. It is most commonly caused by an accentuation of the normal maturation of androgen production by the adrenal gland (adrenarche). It is more common in Asian and Afro-Caribbean children. There may be a slight increase in growth rate. It is usually self-limiting. An ultrasound scan of the ovaries and uterus and a bone age should be obtained to exclude central precocious puberty. A more aggressive course of virilisation would suggest late-onset congenital adrenal hyperplasia or an adrenal tumour.

Delayed puberty

Delayed puberty is often defined as the absence of pubertal development by 14 years of age in females and 15 years in males. The causes of delayed puberty are listed in Box 11.3. In contrast to precocious puberty, the problem is common in males, in whom it is mostly due to constitutional delay. Affected males are short during childhood and have delayed skeletal maturity on bone age. There is often a family history of delayed puberty in the boy's father. Eventually puberty will occur and near predicted height attained, as he will continue to grow for longer than his peers. The boys may suffer from teasing, poor self-esteem and do badly in competitive sports. Assessment in boys includes:

- pubertal staging, especially testicular volume
- identification of chronic systemic disorders.

In girls, karyotype should be performed to identify Turner's syndrome, and thyroid and sex steroid hormones should be measured.

The aims of management are to:

- identify and treat any underlying pathology
- ensure normal psychological adaptation to puberty and adulthood
- accelerate growth and promote entry into puberty if necessary.

Following reassurance that puberty will occur, treatment is often not required. Should treatment be wanted, oral oxandrolone can be used in young males. This weakly androgenic anabolic steroid will induce some catch-up growth but not secondary sexual characteristics. In older boys, low-dose testosterone will accelerate growth as well as

---

Case History
11.3 Premature thelarche

This 18-month-old female developed enlargement of both breasts (Fig. 11.16). There was no pubic hair growth, sweatiness or body odour and her height was in the mid-parental range. Her bone age was only mildly advanced (21 months) and a pelvic ultrasound showed a prepubertal uterus, small volume ovaries with two cysts in the left ovary. Her subsequent growth rate was normal. A diagnosis of premature thelarche was made.

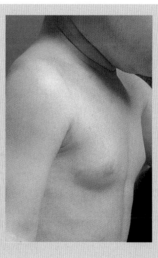

Figure 11.16
Premature breast development in an 18-month-old girl. The absence of a growth spurt and axillary and pubic hair differentiates it from precocious puberty. It is self-limiting and often resolves. (From Wales J K H, Rogol A D, Wit J M, *Pediatric Endocrinology and Growth*, Saunders, London, 2003, with permission.)

Box 11.3 Causes of delayed puberty

Box 11.3 Causes of delayed puberty

Constitutional delay of growth and puberty/ familial

By far the commonest

Low gonadotropin secretion

- Systemic disease
  Cystic fibrosis, severe asthma, Crohn's disease, organ failure, anorexia nervosa, starvation, excess physical training
- Hypothalamopituitary disorders
  Panhypopituitarism
  Isolated gonadotropin or growth hormone deficiency
  Intracranial tumours (including craniopharyngioma)
  Kallmann syndrome (LHRH deficiency and inability to smell)
- Acquired hypothyroidism

High gonadotropin secretion

- Chromosomal abnormalities
  Klinefelter's syndrome (47 XXY)
  Turner's syndrome (45 XO)
- Steroid hormone enzyme deficiencies
- Acquired gonadal damage
  Post-surgery, chemotherapy, radiotherapy, trauma, torsion of the testis, autoimmune disorder

inducing secondary sexual characteristics. Females may be treated with oestradiol.

Disorders of sexual differentiation

The fetal gonad is initially bipotential (Fig. 11.17) In the male, a testis-determining gene on the Y chromosome (SRY) is responsible for the differentiation of the gonad into a testis. The production of testosterone and its metabolite, dihydrotestosterone, results in the development of male genitalia. In the absence of SRY, the gonads become ovaries and the genitalia female.

Rarely, newborn infants may be born with ambiguous genitalia and there may be uncertainty about the infant's sex. Ambiguous external genitalia may be secondary to:

- excessive androgens producing virilisation in a female – the commonest cause of this is congenital adrenal hyperplasia
- inadequate androgen action, producing undervirilisation in a male – this can result from inability to respond to androgens (a receptor problem – androgen insensitivity syndrome, which may be complete or partial) or to convert testosterone to dihydrotestosterone (5α-reductase deficiency) or abnormalities of the synthesis of androgens from cholesterol

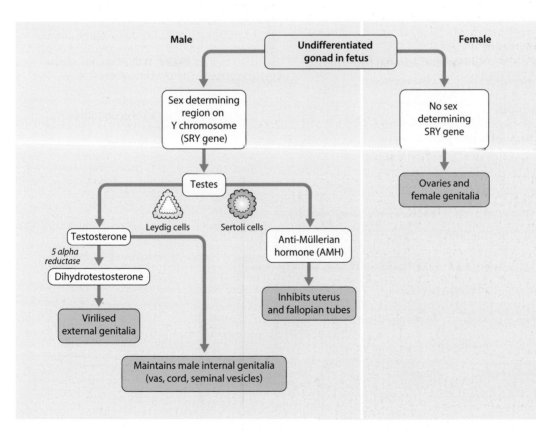

Figure 11.17 Sexual differentiation in the fetus.

- gonadotropin insufficiency, also seen in several syndromes such as Prader–Willi syndrome and congenital hypopituitarism, which results in a small penis and cryptorchidism
- true hermaphroditism, caused by both XX- and Y-containing cells being present in the fetus leading to both testicular and ovarian tissue being present and a complex external phenotype; this is rare.

All parents and their relatives are desperate to know the sex of their newborn baby. However, if the genitalia are ambiguous, the infant's sex must not be assigned until detailed assessment by medical, surgical and psychological specialists has been performed followed by full discussion with the parents. Birth registration must be delayed until this has been completed. Incorrect assignment of sex may have lifelong medical and legal consequences.

Sexuality is complex and depends on more than the phenotype, chromosomes and hormone levels. Before the most appropriate sex of rearing is decided upon, the karyotype needs to be determined, adrenal and sex hormone levels measured, and ultrasound of the internal structures and gonads performed. Sometimes laparoscopic imaging and biopsy of internal structures are necessary. In many intersex conditions, it has been usual to raise the child as a female, as it is easier to fashion female external genitalia, whereas it is not possible surgically to create an adequately

functioning penis. However, it may be impossible to predict the sexual identity of the child in eventual adult life and further support or gender reassignment may be required. For this reason there is a move toward delaying definitive surgery to allow the affected individual to give informed consent to any reconstructive procedures. This is a controversial area and is best managed by experienced multidisciplinary teams.

If the genitalia at birth are ambiguous:
- **do not guess the infant's gender**
- **the most common cause is female virilisation from congenital adrenal hyperplasia.**

Congenital adrenal hyperplasia

A number of autosomal recessive disorders of adrenal steroid biosynthesis result in congenital adrenal hyperplasia. Its incidence is about 1 in 5000 births, and it is commoner in the offspring of consanguineous marriages. Over 90% have a deficiency of the enzyme 21-hydroxylase which is needed for cortisol biosynthesis; 80% of cases are also unable to produce aldosterone (Fig. 11.18). In the fetus, the resulting cortisol deficiency stimulates the pituitary to produce adrenocorticotropic hormone (ACTH), which drives overproduction of adrenal androgens.

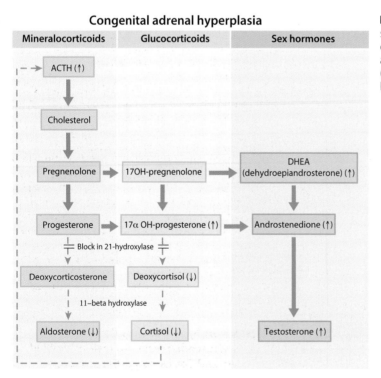

Congenital adrenal hyperplasia

Mineralocorticoids	Glucocorticoids	Sex hormones

ACTH (↑)
→ Cholesterol
→ Pregnenolone → 17OH-pregnenolone → DHEA (dehydroepiandrosterone) (↑)
Pregnenolone → Progesterone
17OH-pregnenolone → 17α OH-progesterone (↑)
DHEA → Androstenedione (↑)
Block in 21-hydroxylase
Progesterone → Deoxycorticosterone
17α OH-progesterone → Deoxycortisol (↓)
11–beta hydroxylase
Deoxycorticosterone → Aldosterone (↓)
Deoxycortisol → Cortisol (↓)
Androstenedione → Testosterone (↑)

Figure 11.18 Abnormal adrenal steroid biosynthesis is the commonest form of congenital adrenal hyperplasia. (ACTH, adrenocorticotropic hormone).

Presentation:

- virilisation of the external genitalia in female infants, with clitoral hypertrophy and variable fusion of the labia (see Case history 11.4)
- in the infant male, the penis may be enlarged and the scrotum pigmented, but these changes are seldom identified
- a salt-losing adrenal crisis in the 80% of males who are salt losers; this occurs at 1–3 weeks of age, presenting with vomiting and weight loss, floppiness and circulatory collapse
- tall stature in the 20% of male non-salt losers; both male and female non-salt losers also develop a muscular build, adult body odour, pubic hair and acne from excess androgen production, leading to precocious pubarche.

There may be a family history of neonatal death if a salt-losing crisis had not been recognised and treated.

Diagnosis

This is made by finding markedly raised levels of the metabolic precursor 17α-hydroxyprogesterone in the blood. In salt losers, the biochemical abnormalities are:

- low plasma sodium
- high plasma potassium

- metabolic acidosis
- hypoglycaemia

Management

Affected females will require corrective surgery to their external genitalia, but as they have a uterus and ovaries they should usually be reared as girls and are able to have children. Males in a salt-losing crisis require saline, dextrose and hydrocortisone intravenously.

The long-term management of both sexes is with:

- lifelong glucocorticoids to suppress ACTH levels (and hence testosterone) to allow normal growth and maturation
- mineralocorticoids (fludrocortisone) if there is salt loss; before weaning, infants may need added sodium chloride
- monitoring of growth, skeletal maturity and plasma androgens and 17α-hydroxyprogesterone – insufficient hormone replacement results in increased ACTH secretion and androgen excess, which will cause rapid initial growth and skeletal maturation at the expense of final height; excessive hormonal replacement will result in skeletal delay and slow growth
- additional hormone replacement to cover illness or surgery, as they are unable to mount a cortisol response.

Case History
11.4 Ambiguous genitalia at birth

The appearance of this newborn infant's genitalia is shown in Figure 11.19.

Investigation revealed:

- a normal female karyotype, 46XX
- the presence of a uterus on ultrasound examination
- a markedly raised plasma 17α-hydroxy-progesterone concentration, confirming congenital adrenal hyperplasia.

Plasma electrolytes were checked every few days for the first 4 weeks to check for salt loss, which was absent. After detailed explanation with her parents, she was started on oral hydrocortisone replacement therapy. Surgery was performed at 9 months of age to reduce clitoral size and separate the labia. Her growth, biochemistry and bone age were monitored frequently at follow-up and she attained normal adult height. Psychological counselling and support were offered around puberty and further genital surgery was needed before she became sexually active.

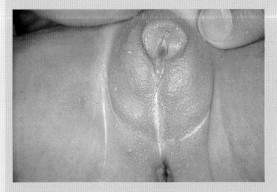

Figure 11.19 Ambiguous genitalia at birth. Investigation established that this was a female infant with congenital adrenal hyperplasia causing clitoral hypertrophy with fusion of the labia.

> Severe hypospadias and bilateral undescended testes – a male or virilised female? The karyotype is required.

Death can occur from adrenal crisis at the time of illness or injury. Females require surgery to reduce clitoromegaly and a vaginoplasty before sexual intercourse is attempted. Females often experience psychosexual problems, which may relate to the high androgen levels experienced in utero prior to diagnosis.

Prenatal diagnosis and treatment are possible when a couple have had a previously affected child. Dexamethasone may be given to the mother around the time of conception, and continued if the fetus is found to be female, in order to reduce fetal ACTH drive and hence the virilisation.

Summary

Congenital adrenal hyperplasia:
- autosomal recessive disorder of adrenal steroid biosynthesis
- females present with virilisation of the external genitalia
- males present with salt loss (80%) or tall stature and precocious puberty (20%)
- long-term medical management with lifelong glucocorticoids, mineralocorticoids/sodium chloride if salt loss
- additional corticosteroids to cover illness or surgery
- salt-losing adrenal crisis needs urgent treatment with hydrocortisone, saline and glucose given intravenously
- monitor growth, skeletal maturity, plasma androgens and 17α-hydroxyprogesterone
- surgery for females.

Further reading

Brook C, Clayton P, Brown R 2005 Brook's clinical paediatric endocrinology. Blackwell, Oxford

Lifshitz F (ed.) 2002. Pediatric endocrinology, 4th edn. Marcel Dekker, New York.

Wales J K H, Rogol A D, Wit J M 2003 Pediatric endocrinology and growth. Saunders, London

Nutrition

Children need food of appropriate quantity and quality for optimal growth and development. If their nutritional intake is inadequate they will fail to gain weight or lose it and will subsequently fail to grow in height. Prolonged or severe nutritional deficiency will result in malnutrition.

The nutritional vulnerability of infants and children

Infants and children are more vulnerable to poor nutrition than are adults. There are a number of reasons for this.

Low nutritional stores
Newborn infants, particularly those born before term, have poor stores of fat and protein (Fig. 12.1). The smaller the child, the less the calorie reserve and the shorter the period the child will be able to withstand starvation (Fig. 12.2).

High nutritional demands for growth
The nourishment children require, per unit body size, is greatest in infancy (Table 12.1), because of their rapid growth during this period. At 4 months of age, 30% of an infant's energy intake is used for growth, but by 1 year of age this falls to 5%, and by 3 years to 2%. The risk of growth failure from restricted energy intake is therefore greater in the first 6 months of life than in later childhood. Even small but recurrent deficits in early childhood will lead to a cumulative deficit in weight and height.

Rapid neuronal development
The brain grows rapidly during the last trimester of pregnancy and throughout the first 2 years of life. The complexity of interneuronal connections also increases substantially during this time. This process appears to be sensitive to undernutrition. Even modest energy deprivation during periods of rapid brain growth and differentiation is thought to lead to an increased risk of adverse neurodevelopmental outcome. This is not surprising when one

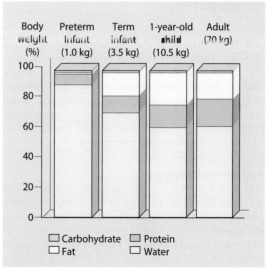

Figure 12.1 Body composition of preterm and term infants, children and adults. Newborn infants, particularly the preterm, have poor stores of fat and protein.

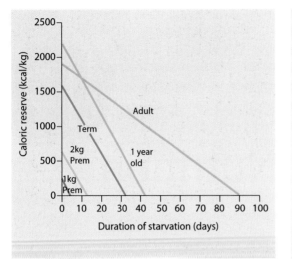

Figure 12.2 Reduced ability of children to withstand starvation from lack of food but not fluid compared to adults. (After Heird et al, *Journal of Pediatrics*, 1972; 80: 351–372.)

Table 12.1 Reference values for energy and protein requirements

Age	Energy (kcal/kg per 24 h)	Protein (g/kg per 24 h)
0–6 months	115	2.2
6–12 months	95	2.0
1–3 years	95	1.8
4–6 years	90	1.5
7–10 years	75	1.2
Adolescence	(male/female)	
11–14 years	65/55	1.0
15–18 years	60/40	0.8

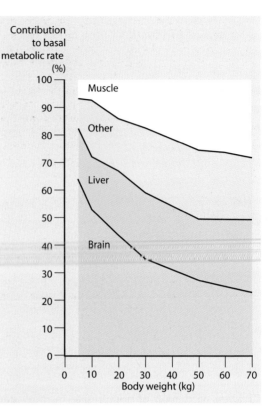

Figure 12.3 The relative contribution to basal metabolic rate derived from brain, liver and muscle changes with growth. Whereas the brain accounts for two-thirds of the basal metabolic rate at birth, this falls to 25% in adults. (Adapted from Halliday M A 1971 *Pediatrics* 47(1) Suppl 2: 169.)

considers that at birth the brain accounts for approximately two-thirds of basal metabolic rate, and at 1 year for about 50% (Fig. 12.3). Many studies have drawn attention to the delayed development seen in children suffering from protein-energy malnutrition due to inadequate food intake, although inadequate psychosocial stimulation may also contribute.

Acute illness or surgery

A child's nutrition may be compromised following an acute illness or surgery. After a brief anabolic phase, catecholamine secretion is increased causing the metabolic rate and energy requirement to increase. Urinary nitrogen losses may become so great that it is impossible to achieve a positive nitrogen balance and weight is lost. After uncomplicated surgery this phase may last for a week, but it can last several weeks after extensive burns, complicated surgery or severe sepsis. Thereafter, previously lost tissue is replaced and a positive energy and nitrogen balance can be achieved.

However, infants may not show catch-up growth unless their energy intake is as high as 150–200 kcal/kg per day.

Long-term outcome of early nutritional deficiency

Linear growth of populations

Growth and nutrition are closely related, such that the mean height of a population reflects its nutritional status. Thus, in the developed world, people have become taller. Height is adversely affected by lower socioeconomic status and increasing number of children in families. Children's size increases amongst populations emigrating from poor to more affluent countries.

Disease in adult life

Evidence suggests that undernutrition in utero resulting in growth restriction is associated with an increased incidence of coronary heart disease, stroke, non-insulin-dependent diabetes, hypertension and metabolic syndrome in later life (Fig. 12.4). There is also a similar but weaker association with low weight at 1 year of age. For example, there is a twofold reduction in death rates from coronary heart disease and stroke between the lower and upper ends of birthweight distribution, and coronary heart disease doubles in men who weighed less than 8 kg at 1 year compared with those over 12.2 kg. The mechanism is unclear, but it is recognised that fetal undernutrition leads to redistribution of blood flow and changes in fetal hormones, such as insulin-like growth factors and cortisol. Alternatively, it may be the rapid, post-natal growth (catch-up) seen in babies suffering from intra-uterine growth restriction that is the causal factor.

⦿ Summary

Nutritional vulnerability
Infants are more vulnerable to poor nutrition because of:
- poor stores of fat and protein
- extra nutritional demands for growth – the weight of a term infant doubles by 4 months and trebles by 1 year.
- more frequent intercurrent illnesses that reduce food intake and increase nutritional demands.

Infant feeding

Breast-feeding

There can be no doubt that breast milk is the best diet for babies, although the popularity of breast-feeding has frequently reflected the whim of fashion.

Advantages (Box 12.1)

In developing countries, where the environment is often highly contaminated, breast-feeding dramatically improves survival during infancy as a result of reduced gastrointestinal infection. Consequently, breast-feeding is one of the four most important World Health Organization strategies for improving infant and child survival. The superiority of breast milk over modern adapted cow's milk formulae is less easy to prove in developed countries. This is partly because it is impossible to conduct randomised studies and partly because of confounders such as social class, education and smoking.

However, there is convincing evidence that gastrointestinal infection is less common in breast-fed infants even in developed countries. There is also evidence that human milk feeds reduce the incidence of necrotising enterocolitis in preterm infants.

Many mothers who breast-feed find that it helps them establish an intimate, loving relationship with their baby. However, establishing breast-feeding is not always straightforward, and many mothers need help and encouragement.

Breast-feeding may confer an advantage in cognitive development in children although there

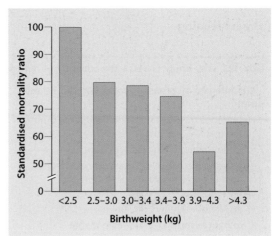

Figure 12.4 Death rates from coronary heart disease according to birthweight. (After Barker D J, *Fetal Origins of Adult Disease*. In: *Growing up in Britain: Ensuring the Healthy Future for our Children. A Study of 4–5 year olds*, BMJ Books, London, 1999.)

are many confounding variables in this relationship. Potential nutrients in breast milk that confer this advantage are probably long-chain polyunsaturated fatty acids. These are now added to formula feeds.

Breast-feeding is associated with a reduced incidence of obesity and hypertension in later life, and may lead to reduced inflammatory bowel disease and diabetes mellitus in children when they grow up. There is also a reduction in breast cancer in mothers who breast-feed. Claims that breast-feeding reduces the incidence of allergic disorders and sudden infant death have not been substantiated.

❀ **Exclusive breast-feeding in early infancy is life-saving in developing countries.**

Disadvantages (Box 12.2)

As one cannot readily tell how much milk a baby is taking from the breast, the baby's weight should be checked regularly, every few days in the first couple of weeks, then weekly until feeding is well established. Successful breast-feeding of twins can be achieved, but is more difficult (Fig. 12.5). It is rarely possible to totally breast-feed triplets and higher-order births. Preterm infants can be breast-fed, but the milk will need to be expressed from the breast until the infant can suck. Maintaining the supply of milk can be a problem for mothers of preterm babies.

Whilst two-thirds of mothers in the UK initially breast-feed, this proportion rapidly declines during the first few months (Fig. 12.6). Nearly 90% of social class I mothers start breast-feeding, but only 60% of mothers from social class V. Breast-feeding is restrictive for the mother as others cannot take charge of her baby for any length of time. This is particularly important if she goes to work. Facilities for breast-feeding in public places are still limited.

Breast-feeding

Box 12.1 Why breast is best – the advantages of breast milk

Advantages of breast-feeding for the infant are:

- provides the ideal nutrition for infants during the first 4–6 months of life
- is life-saving in developing countries
- reduces the risk of gastrointestinal infection, and, in preterm infants, of necrotising enterocolitis
- improves cognitive development
- enhances mother–child relationship
- reduces risk of insulin-dependent diabetes, inflammatory bowel, sudden infant death syndrome (unproven) in later life

Advantages for the mother:

- promotes close attachment between mother and baby
- contraceptive – although not a reliable contraceptive, increases the time interval between children, which is important in reducing birth rate in developing countries
- possible reduction in premenopausal breast cancer

Scientific explanation of some of the properties of breast milk

Anti-infective properties

Humoral

Secretory IgA	Comprises 90% of immunoglobulin in human milk. Provides mucosal protection, but of uncertain benefit
Bifidus factor	Promotes growth of *Lactobacillus bifidus*, which metabolises lactose to lactic and acetic acids. The resulting low pH may inhibit growth of gastrointestinal pathogens
Lysozyme	Bacteriolytic enzyme
Lactoferrin	Iron binding protein. Inhibits growth of *Escherichia coli*
Interferon	Antiviral agent

Cellular

Macrophages	Phagocytic. Synthesise lysozyme, lactoferrin, C3, C4
Lymphocytes	T cells may transfer delayed hypersensitivity responses to infant. B cells synthesise IgA

Nutritional properties

Protein quality	More easily digested curd (60 : 40 whey : casein ratio)
Hypoallergenic	May reduce subsequent atopic disease. Conflicting evidence
Lipid quality	Rich in oleic acid (with palmitate in C-2 position). Improved digestibility and fat absorption
Breast milk lipase	Enhanced lipolysis
Calcium : phosphorus ratio of 2 : 1	Prevents hypocalcaemic tetany and improves calcium absorption
Low renal solute load	
Iron content	Bioavailable (40–50% absorption)
Long-chain polyunsaturated fatty acids	Structural lipids, important in retinal development

Box 12.2 Disadvantages of breast-feeding

Unknown intake	Volume of milk intake not known
Transmission of infection	Maternal CMV, hepatitis B and HIV – increases risk of transmission to the baby
Breast milk jaundice	Mild, self-limiting, unconjugated hyperbilirubinaemia; continue breast-feeding
Transmission of drugs	Antimetabolites
Nutrient inadequacies	Breast-feeding beyond 6 months without timely introduction of appropriate solids may lead to poor weight gain and rickets
Vitamin K deficiency	There is insufficient vitamin K in breast milk to prevent haemorrhagic disease of the newborn
Potential transmission of environmental contaminants	Nicotine, alcohol, caffeine, etc.
Less flexible	Other family members cannot help or take part. More difficult in public places
Emotional upset	If difficulties or lack of success can be upsetting

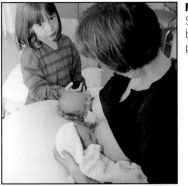

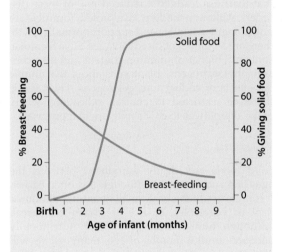

Figure 12.6 Prevalence of breast-feeding and proportion of infants given solid feeds during the first 9 months of life in the UK (2000).

Although breast-feeding avoids the preparation needed for infant formulae, it is not necessarily cheaper for the family if it delays a mother returning to work.

Establishing breast-feeding

Colostrum, rather than milk, is produced for the first few days. Colostrum differs from mature milk in that the content of protein and immunoglobulin is much higher. Volumes are low but water or formula supplements are not required whilst the supply of breast milk is becoming established.

The first breast-feed should take place as soon as possible after birth. Subsequently, frequent suckling is beneficial as it enhances the secretion of the hormones initiating and promoting lactation (Fig. 12.7).

Primates probably do not breast-feed instinctively. Monkeys bred in captivity in zoos have to be taught how to breast-feed by their keepers. It is therefore important that breast-feeding should have as high a public profile as possible. Women who have never seen an infant being breast-fed are less likely to want to breast-feed themselves. Education in schools and during pregnancy about the advantages of breast-feeding is advantageous. Advice and support from other women who have breast-fed may be important in dealing with early problems such as engorgement or cracked nipples.

'Bonding', a critical period shortly after birth in establishing a mother–infant relationship, is seen in many animals. In humans, there is no evidence for a similar critical period and there is considerable flexibility in the timing and manner in which this close relationship develops.

Physiology of breast feeding

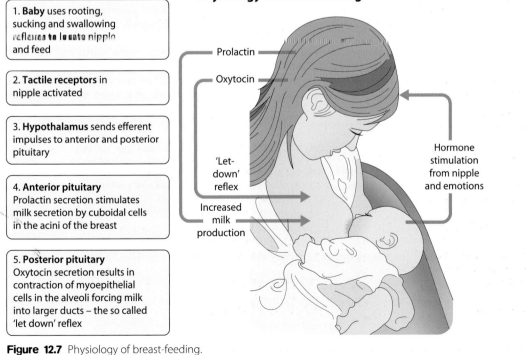

1. **Baby** uses rooting, sucking and swallowing reflexes to locate nipple and feed

2. **Tactile receptors** in nipple activated

3. **Hypothalamus** sends efferent impulses to anterior and posterior pituitary

4. **Anterior pituitary**
Prolactin secretion stimulates milk secretion by cuboidal cells in the acini of the breast

5. **Posterior pituitary**
Oxytocin secretion results in contraction of myoepithelial cells in the alveoli forcing milk into larger ducts – the so called 'let down' reflex

Figure 12.7 Physiology of breast-feeding.

🌼 Newborn infants of mothers planning to breast-feed should ideally not be given any formula feeds.

◎ **Summary**

Formula feeding:
- infant formula, not unmodified cow's milk, should be used in the first year of life.

Formula feeding

Infants who are not breast-fed require a formula feed based on cow's milk. Unmodified cow's milk is unsuitable for feeding in infancy as it contains too much protein and electrolyte and inadequate iron and vitamins. Even after considerable modification, differences remain between formula feeds and breast milk (Table 12.2).

Most modern cow's milk-based formulae may be divided into two types, depending upon whether or not the casein to non-casein ratio has been modified by the addition of demineralised whey (soluble protein). A casein : whey ratio of 40 : 60 forms a smaller curd and provides an amino acid profile more like breast milk than a higher casein milk.

All milks currently available in the UK have been modified to make their mineral content and renal solute load comparable with that of mature human milk. Since these changes were introduced in the UK (in the 1970s), there has been an impressive reduction in the incidence of hypernatraemic dehydration in infants with gastroenteritis. There is no evidence that any one of the many brands is superior to any other.

Introduction of whole, pasteurised cow's milk

Breast or formula feeding is recommended until the age of 12 months, and there are advantages in continuing to 18 months of age. Pasteurised cow's milk is deficient in vitamins A, C and D and in iron, and if introduced in the first year will require supplements unless the infant is having a good diet of mixed solids. Alternatively, 'follow-on' formulae can be used from 6 months of age. They contain more protein and sodium than infant formulae and, in contrast to cow's milk, are fortified with iron and vitamins.

Soya formulae

Soya formulae have been widely used instead of cow's milk formulae in the belief that they may help prevent atopic manifestations such as eczema or asthma. However, there is no compelling evidence that their use leads to a reduced risk of these disorders. Although modern soya protein formulae are nutritionally adequate and support normal growth, there are a number of disadvantages. Soya formulae contain a higher aluminium content and also contain phytoestrogens, plant substances that mimic the effects of endogenous oestrogens. Their use is therefore restricted to clinical indications where other alternatives to cow's milk are inappropriate.

Weaning

Solid foods are ideally introduced between the ages of 4 and 6 months, although it is often earlier. It is done gradually, with small quantities of pureed fruit or vegetables, or rice or gluten-free cereal. Although human milk should be nutritionally adequate until 6 months of age, many babies will exhibit behavioural changes from 3 to 4 months, such as increased crying and poor sleeping, which may represent hunger and a need for solid food. After 6 months of age, breast milk becomes increasingly nutritionally inadequate as a sole feed, leading to deficiencies in energy, vitamins and iron.

Breast- or formula-fed infants obtain about half their energy from fat. After 1 year of age, whole cow's milk still provides a major contribution to the diet of most children. Some nutritionists have suggested that dietary fat intake should be reduced to supply less than 35% of energy requirements and fibre intake increased. The later introduction of solids, more breast-feeding and the fact that many

Table 12.2 A comparison of human milk, cow's milk and infant formula (per 100 ml)

	Mature breast milk	Cow's milk	Infant formula (modified cow's milk)
Energy (kcal)	62	67	60–65
Protein (g)	1.3	3.5	1.5–1.9
Carbohydrate (g)	6.7	4.9	7.0–8.6
Casein : whey	40 : 60	63 : 37	40 : 60 to 63 : 37
Fat (g)	3.0	3.6	2.6–3.8
Sodium (mmol)	0.65	2.3	0.65–1.1
Calcium (mmol)	0.88	3.0	0.88–2.1
Phosphorus (mmol)	0.46	3.2	0.9–1.8
Iron (μmol)	1.36	0.9	8–12.5

weaning foods are gluten-free may be responsible for the reduction in the incidence of coeliac disease in infancy. A lower incidence of gastroenteritis may also be a factor.

Failure to thrive

The term 'failure to thrive' is used to describe suboptimal weight gain in infants and toddlers. It is also called weight or growth faltering in case parents consider the term pejorative. Recognition of the entity depends upon demonstration of inadequate weight gain when plotted on a centile chart, with mild failure to thrive being a fall across two centile lines and severe being a fall across three centile lines. Between 6 weeks and 1 year of age, only 5% of children will cross two lines, and only 1% will cross three. The weight of a child with 'failure to thrive' may fall within the normal range, but most are below the 2nd centile when identified. Repeated observations are therefore essential and are usually available in the child's personal child health record. A single observation of weight is difficult to interpret unless markedly discrepant from the head circumference or length, although the further the weight is below the 2nd centile, the more likely the child is 'failing to thrive'. A weight below the 0.4th centile should always trigger an evaluation.

Differentiating the infant who is failing to thrive from a normal but small or thin baby is often a problem (Fig. 12.8). Normal but short infants have no symptoms, are alert, responsive and happy, and their development is satisfactory. The parents may be short (low mid-parental height) or the infant may have been extremely preterm or growth-restricted at birth. Any intercurrent illness will be accompanied by a temporary failure to gain weight.

An additional diagnostic problem is 'catch-down' (as opposed to 'catch-up') weight. This is when an infant's weight falls from the birth centile, which is affected by the intrauterine environment, to a lower, genetically determined growth centile. These infants need only close monitoring of their growth over a few months.

Children with recent onset failure to thrive usually maintain their height, which is compromised only by prolonged, severe, illness. The child's developmental progress may be adversely affected.

Causes

The causes of failure to thrive are usually classified as organic and non-organic (Fig. 12.9). Non-organic failure to thrive is traditionally believed to be associated with a broad spectrum of psychosocial and environmental deprivation. It is estimated that 5–10% of children with failure to thrive will be on a child protection register or be subjected to abuse or neglect, while a somewhat larger proportion will have socioeconomic deprivation as an important factor.

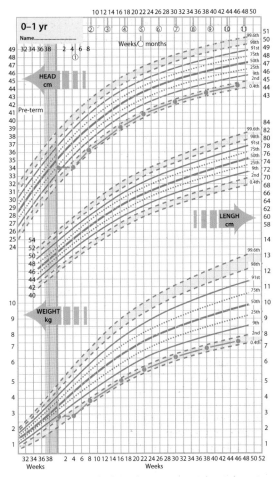

Figure 12.8 Growth chart showing normal weight gain and growth in a constitutionally small infant. The further below the 2nd, and especially the 0.4th, centile, the more likely it is that there will be an organic cause. (Chart © Child Growth Foundation.)

The mother may be depressed, have an eating disorder herself or have poor understanding of her baby's needs. There may be poor housing, poverty, inadequate social support and lack of an extended family, which make good child care even more difficult. However, some studies suggest that failure to thrive is not more common in deprived than in non-deprived communities, and that identification of deprivation leads to the inappropriate application of that diagnostic label. Undernutrition is the final common pathway for poor weight gain in most cases of organic and non-organic failure to thrive, and in many cases both organic and environmental factors are present.

Organic causes are listed in Figure 12.9. Less than 5% of children with 'failure to thrive' will be found to have an organic cause. The commonest are gastro-oesophageal reflux, coeliac disease, cystic fibrosis, cardiac disease and renal failure.

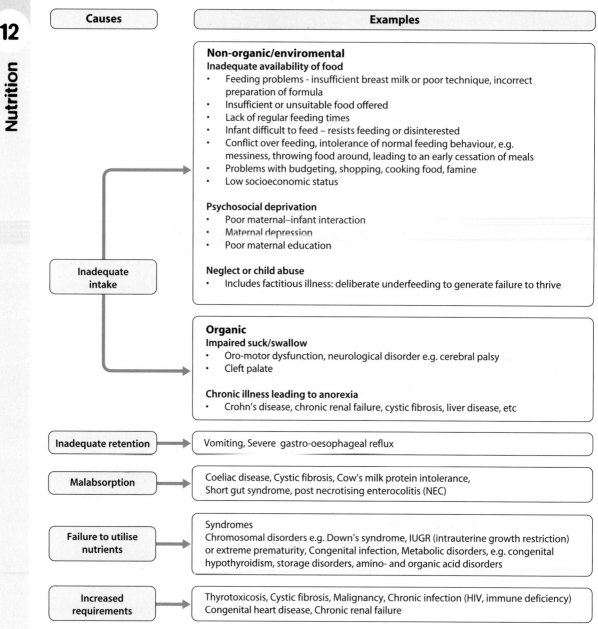

Causes of failure to thrive

Causes	Examples
Inadequate intake	**Non-organic/enviromental** **Inadequate availability of food** • Feeding problems - insufficient breast milk or poor technique, incorrect preparation of formula • Insufficient or unsuitable food offered • Lack of regular feeding times • Infant difficult to feed – resists feeding or disinterested • Conflict over feeding, intolerance of normal feeding behaviour, e.g. messiness, throwing food around, leading to an early cessation of meals • Problems with budgeting, shopping, cooking food, famine • Low socioeconomic status **Psychosocial deprivation** • Poor maternal–infant interaction • Maternal depression • Poor maternal education **Neglect or child abuse** • Includes factitious illness: deliberate underfeeding to generate failure to thrive
	Organic **Impaired suck/swallow** • Oro-motor dysfunction, neurological disorder e.g. cerebral palsy • Cleft palate **Chronic illness leading to anorexia** • Crohn's disease, chronic renal failure, cystic fibrosis, liver disease, etc
Inadequate retention	Vomiting, Severe gastro-oesophageal reflux
Malabsorption	Coeliac disease, Cystic fibrosis, Cow's milk protein intolerance, Short gut syndrome, post necrotising enterocolitis (NEC)
Failure to utilise nutrients	Syndromes Chromosomal disorders e.g. Down's syndrome, IUGR (intrauterine growth restriction) or extreme prematurity, Congenital infection, Metabolic disorders, e.g. congenital hypothyroidism, storage disorders, amino- and organic acid disorders
Increased requirements	Thyrotoxicosis, Cystic fibrosis, Malignancy, Chronic infection (HIV, immune deficiency) Congenital heart disease, Chronic renal failure

Figure 12.9 The main causes of failure to thrive.

Clinical features and investigation

Studying the growth chart in combination with the history and examination of the child is the key to its evaluation. The history should focus on:

• a detailed dietary history; a food diary over a few days can be informative
• feeding, including details of exactly what happens at mealtimes
• if the child is well and has lots of energy or has other symptoms such as diarrhoea, vomiting, cough, lethargy

• if the child was premature or had intrauterine growth restriction at birth or any significant medical problems
• the growth of other family members and any illnesses in the family
• if the child's development is normal
• if there are psychosocial problems at home.

Examination focuses on identifying whether there is any evidence of organic disease – dysmorphic features, distended abdomen, thin buttocks and

Box 12.3 Investigations to be considered in failure to thrive

Investigation	Significance of an abnormality
Full blood count and differential	Anaemia, infection, inflammation, immune deficiency
Plasma creatinine and electrolytes	Renal failure, renal tubular acidosis, metabolic disorders
Liver function tests	Liver disease, malabsorption, metabolic disorders
Thyroid function tests	Congenital hypothyroidism
Acute-phase reactant	Inflammation, e.g. Crohn's disease
Ferritin	Iron deficiency anaemia
Immunoglobulins	Immune deficiency
Anti-endomysial and anti-gliadin antibodies	Coeliac disease
Urine microscopy and culture and dipsticks	Urinary tract infection, renal disease
Stool microscopy and culture	Intestinal infection, parasites
Karyotype in girls	Turner's syndrome
Chest X-ray and sweat test	Cystic fibrosis

irritability in coeliac disease, respiratory signs and malabsorption in cystic fibrosis, evidence of nutritional deficiencies or evidence of chronic illness.

Further information about the child and family from the health visitor, general practitioner or other professionals involved with the family can be particularly helpful. Investigations to be considered are listed in Box 12.3. They should be selected according to the likely diagnosis. In some children who are failing to thrive a full blood count and serum ferritin may be helpful to identify iron deficiency anaemia. This is common secondary to inadequate iron intake in children with failure to thrive and correcting it may improve appetite. However, in most instances no investigations are required.

Management

The management of most non-organic failure to thrive is multidisciplinary and is carried out in primary care. The health visitor is well placed to make home visits to assess eating behaviour and provide support. Direct practical advice following observation may well be beneficial. A paediatric dietician may be helpful in assessing the quantity and composition of food intake, and recommending strategies for increasing energy intake and a speech and language therapist has specialist skills with feeding disorders. Input from a clinical psychologist and from social services may also be appropriate. Nursery placement may be helpful in alleviating stress at home and assist with feeding.

Hospital admission may occasionally be necessary for a period of assessment and observation of the child and family, or when detailed investigations are required.

Outcome

Follow-up studies suggest that children with non-organic failure to thrive continue to under-eat (see Case history 12.1). Although there is usually a gradual improvement in the preschool years, a lasting deficit is common and these children tend to remain underweight. In contrast, impairment of development is only short term.

Prevention of failure to thrive is an essential part of the management of any child whose condition severely affects sucking and swallowing, such as prematurity, cleft palate, oesophageal malformation and cerebral palsy when a gastrostomy may be required to maintain reasonable nutrition. In children who are unable to tolerate gastric feeding because of severe illness or multiple bowel operations, total parenteral nutrition (TPN) is needed to prevent malnutrition, but is accompanied by increased risk of infection.

Summary

Failure to thrive:
- is a description, not a diagnosis
- weights of infants are only helpful if accurate and plotted on a centile chart
- is present if an infant's weight falls across two centile lines
- is likely to be present the further the weight is below the 2nd centile
- is mostly due to inadequate food intake
- is accompanied by abnormal symptoms or signs if there is organic disease
- most affected infants and toddlers do not require any investigations and are managed in primary care by increasing energy intake by dietary and behavioural modification and monitoring growth.

Malnutrition

Worldwide, malnutrition is common and is responsible directly or indirectly for about half of all deaths of children under 5 years of age. Primary malnutrition also continues to occur in developed countries as a result of poverty, parental neglect or poor education. Specific nutritional deficiencies, particularly of iron, remain common in developed countries. Restrictive diets may be iatrogenic as a result of exclusion diets or parental food fads, or may be self-inflicted.

Case History
12.1 Non-organic failure to thrive

Jamie, aged 11 months, was causing concern to his health visitor as he was not putting on any weight (Fig. 12.10). She arranged for him to be assessed by his general practitioner, who found that he was otherwise well. His mother was a single parent who left school at 16 years and had Jamie at the age of 18.

They lived in a high rise flat and Jamie's mother received income support. Her own mother lived on the other side of the city.

On visiting the home, the health visitor found Jamie's mother to be tense and anxious. In particular, she was worried about making ends meet. She fed Jamie the same food as she ate herself, together with pasteurised milk which she had started at 6 months of age. The meals were chaotic. After a few mouthfuls, Jamie stopped eating and his mother did not coax him but became frustrated and angry.

Jamie's health visitor suggested strategies for increasing Jamie's food intake (Box 12.4). She continued to provide support and encouragement to his mother and arranged a nursery placement for Jamie. By 2 years of age he had caught up by one centile line, but still ate erratically.

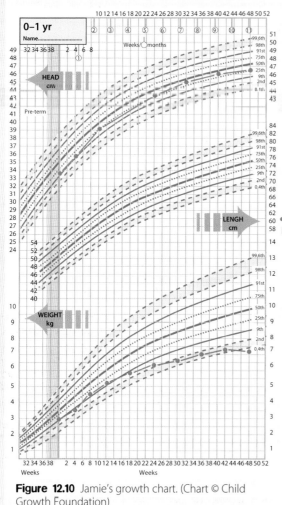

Figure 12.10 Jamie's growth chart. (Chart © Child Growth Foundation)

Box 12.4 Strategies for increasing energy intake

Dietary
- Three meals and two snacks each day
- Increase number and variety of foods offered
- Increase energy density of usual foods (e.g. add cheese, margarine and cream)
- Decrease fluid intake, particularly squash

Behavioural
- Have meals at regular times, eaten with other family members
- Praise when food is eaten
- Gently encourage child to eat, but avoid conflict
- Never force-feed

After Wright C M (2000) Identification and management of failure to thrive: a community perspective. *Archives of Disease in Childhood* 82:5–9.

Malnutrition is far from rare in hospital, affecting 20–40% of patients in a children's hospital. The chronically ill are at particular risk, especially preterm infants and those children with congenital heart disease or chronic gut or respiratory disorders. In these children, malnutrition may result from a combination of anorexia, malabsorption and increased requirements because of infection or inflammation. Anorexia nervosa and other feeding disorders cause malnutrition in older children and adolescents. The diencephalic syndrome, which is extremely rare, comprises severe protein-energy malnutrition in association with a cerebral tumour, usually of the hypothalamus. Food intake is often high, suggesting a possible defect in energy metabolism.

Assessment of nutritional status

Malnutrition must be recognised and accurately defined for rational decisions to be made about refeeding. Evaluation is divided into assessment of past and present dietary intake, anthropometry and laboratory assessments (Fig. 12.11).

Nutritional assessment

Nutritional assessment

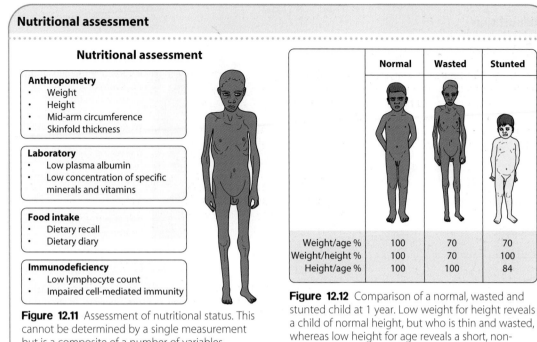

Anthropometry
- Weight
- Height
- Mid-arm circumference
- Skinfold thickness

Laboratory
- Low plasma albumin
- Low concentration of specific minerals and vitamins

Food intake
- Dietary recall
- Dietary diary

Immunodeficiency
- Low lymphocyte count
- Impaired cell-mediated immunity

Figure 12.11 Assessment of nutritional status. This cannot be determined by a single measurement but is a composite of a number of variables.

	Normal	Wasted	Stunted
Weight/age %	100	70	70
Weight/height %	100	70	100
Height/age %	100	100	84

Figure 12.12 Comparison of a normal, wasted and stunted child at 1 year. Low weight for height reveals a child of normal height, but who is thin and wasted, whereas low height for age reveals a short, non-wasted child.

Dietary assessment

Parents are asked to record as best they can all food the child eats during several days. This gives a reasonably accurate assessment of habitual food intake. Children under 12 years are likely to give unreliable information if questioned directly.

Anthropometry

Regular growth measurements are valuable as a fall-off of a growth parameter is one of the earliest indicators of incipient malnutrition. Height, weight, triceps skinfold thickness and mid-arm circumference are basic measures which permit a reasonably accurate assessment of nutritional status. The World Health Organization recommends that nutritional status is expressed as:

- height for age – a measure of stunting and an index of chronic malnutrition
- weight for height – a measure of wasting and an index of acute malnutrition (Fig. 12.12).

Subcutaneous fat stores can be assessed by measuring skinfold thickness, whilst upper arm circumference in conjunction with triceps skinfold thickness is an indication of skeletal muscle mass. However, it is difficult to measure skinfold thickness accurately in young children, so this reduces its use in reflecting short-term changes in body composition.

Laboratory investigations

These are useful in the detection of early physiological adaptation to malnutrition, but clinical history, examination and anthropometry are of greater value than any single biochemical or immunological measurement.

Consequences of malnutrition

Malnutrition is a multisystem disorder. When severe, immunity is impaired, wound healing is delayed and operative morbidity and mortality increased. Malnutrition worsens the outcome of illness, e.g. respiratory muscle dysfunction may delay a child being weaned from mechanical ventilation. Malnourished children are less active, less exploratory and more apathetic. These behavioural abnormalities are rapidly reversed with proper feeding, but prolonged and profound malnutrition probably does cause some permanent delay in intellectual development.

The role of intensive nutritional support

Malnutrition from many childhood disorders is due to inadequate nutrient intake and responds to tube feeding nasogastrically or by gastrostomy. Thus malnourished children with cystic fibrosis, malignancy, inflammatory bowel disease, advanced liver disease, congenital heart disease, cerebral palsy and chronic renal failure will all grow if given supplementary enteral feeds. Other than for Crohn's disease, whether such nutritional support alters prognosis or quality of life remains uncertain.

Marasmus and kwashiorkor

Severe protein-energy malnutrition in children usually leads to marasmus, with a weight less than 60% of the mean for age, and a wasted, wizened

Malnutrition

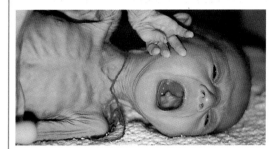

Figure 12.13 Marasmus in a 3-month-old baby who was unable to establish breast-feeding because of a cleft palate.

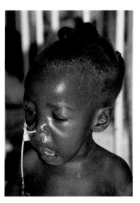

Figure 12.14 Kwashiorkor, a particular manifestation of severe protein-energy malnutrition in some developing countries where infants are weaned late from the breast and the young child's diet is high in starch. There is oedema, hyperkeratosis and depigmentation of the skin and redness of the hair. (Courtesy of Dr Sharon Taylor.)

appearance (Fig. 12.13). Oedema is not present. Skinfold thickness and mid-arm circumference are markedly reduced, and affected children are often withdrawn and apathetic.

Kwashiorkor is another manifestation of severe protein malnutrition (Fig. 12.14), in which body weight is 60–80% of expected and generalised oedema is present. In addition, there may be:

- a 'flaky-paint' skin rash with hyperkeratosis (thickened skin) and desquamation
- a distended abdomen and enlarged liver (usually due to fatty infiltration)
- angular stomatitis
- hair which is sparse and depigmented
- diarrhoea, hypothermia, bradycardia and hypotension
- low plasma albumin, potassium, glucose and magnesium.

It is unclear why some children with protein-energy malnutrition develop kwashiorkor and others develop marasmus. Kwashiorkor is a feature of children reared in traditional, polygamous societies, where infants are not weaned from the breast until about 12 months of age. The subsequent diet tends to be relatively high in starch. Kwashiorkor often develops after an acute inter-current infection, such as measles or gastroenteritis. There is some evidence that kwashiorkor is a manifestation of primary protein deficiency with energy intake relatively well maintained or, alternatively, that it results from excess generation of free radicals.

Management

Urgent treatment for severe malnutrition involves correcting dehydration, acid–base disturbance and hypocalcaemia and treating infection. Hypothermia is common and children require careful wrapping, particularly at night. Children with severe malnutrition are deficient in potassium and magnesium and these should be supplemented. Diarrhoea is a frequent complication of refeeding, but parenteral nutrition is not usually required. Overzealous

treatment with fluids may lead to cardiac failure. In kwashiorkor, severe hypoglycaemia is frequently associated with coma, hypothermia and infection and carries a high mortality. Feeding 2- to 4-hourly, including during the night, has reduced the frequency of hypoglycaemia and the mortality. The overall mortality of severe malnutrition among children treated in hospital is about 30%.

Summary

Malnutrition:
- worldwide – contributes to about half of all childhood deaths; often a consequence of war and social disruption as well as natural disasters
- in developed countries – results from poverty, parental neglect or poor education, restrictive diets, children with feeding disorders or chronic illness and anorexia nervosa
- can be identified by anthropometric measurement; laboratory tests are not usually required
- marasmus – weight <60% mean for age, wasted, wizened appearance
- kwashiorkor – 60–80% expected weight, sparse and depigmented hair, skin rash, generalised oedema, angular stomatitis, distended abdomen and enlarged liver, diarrhoea

Vitamin D deficiency

Vitamin D deficiency usually results from deficient intake or defective metabolism of vitamin D causing a low serum calcium (Fig. 12.15). This triggers the secretion of parathyroid hormone and normalises the serum calcium but demineralises the bone. Parathyroid hormone causes renal losses of phosphate and consequently low serum phosphate levels, further reducing the potential for bone calcification.

Vitamin D deficiency usually presents with bony deformity and the classical picture of rickets. It

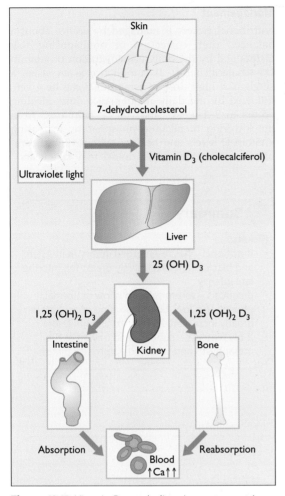

Figure 12.15 Vitamin D metabolism. In most countries, sunlight is the most important source of vitamin D. Vitamin D is not abundant naturally in food except in fish liver oil, fatty fish and egg yolk. Vitamin D_2 (ergocalciferol) is the form used to fortify food such as margarine. Vitamin D_3 is hydroxylated in the liver and again in the kidney to produce 1,25-dihydroxyvitamin D $(1,25(OH)_2D_3)$, the most active form of the vitamin. It is produced following parathormone secretion in response to a low plasma calcium.

Box 12.5 Causes of rickets

Nutritional (primary) rickets – risk factors

- Living in northern latitudes
- Dark-skinned people
- Decreased exposure to sunlight, e.g. in some Asian children living in the UK
- Maternal vitamin D deficiency
- Diets low in calcium, phosphorus and vitamin D, e.g. exclusive breast-feeding into late infancy or, rarely, toddlers on unsupervised 'dairy-free' diets
- Macrobiotic, strict vegan diets
- High phytic acid diet, e.g. chapattis
- Prolonged parenteral nutrition in infancy with an inadequate supply of parenteral calcium and phosphate

Intestinal malabsorption

- Defective production of $25(OH)D_3$ – liver disease
- Increased metabolism of $25(OH)D_3$ – enzyme induction by anticonvulsants

Defective production of $1,25(OH)_2D_3$

- Hereditary type I vitamin D-resistant (or dependent) rickets (mutation which abolishes activity of renal hydroxylase)
- Familial (X-linked) hypophosphataemic rickets (renal tubular defect in phosphate transport)
- Chronic renal disease
- Fanconi syndrome (renal loss of phosphate)

Target organ resistance to $1,25(OH)_2D_3$

- Hereditary vitamin D-dependent rickets type II (due to mutations in vitamin D receptor gene)

can also present without bone abnormalities but with symptoms of hypocalcaemia; i.e. seizures, neuromuscular irritability (tetany), apnoea, stridor. This presentation is more common before 2 years of age and in adolescence, when a high demand for calcium in rapidly growing bone results in hypocalcaemia before rickets develops.

Rickets

Rickets signifies a failure in mineralisation of the growing bone or osteoid tissue. Failure of mature bone to mineralise is osteomalacia.

Aetiology

The predominant cause of rickets during the early 20th century was nutritional vitamin D deficiency due to inadequate intake or insufficient exposure to direct sunlight. In developed countries nutritional rickets has become rare, as formula milk and many foods such as breakfast cereals are supplemented with vitamin D. However, nutritional rickets has re-emerged in developed countries in black or Asian infants totally breast-fed in late infancy. It is also seen in extremely preterm infants from dietary deficiency of phosphorus, together with low stores of calcium and phosphorus. Nutritional rickets still remains the major cause in developing countries.

In developed countries, rickets now mainly results from impaired metabolic conversion or activation of vitamin D.

Children with malabsorptive conditions such as cystic fibrosis, coeliac disease and pancreatic insufficiency can develop rickets due to deficient absorption of vitamin D, calcium or both. Drugs, especially anticonvulsants such as phenobarbital and phenytoin, interfere with the metabolism of vitamin D and may also cause rickets. The causes of rickets are listed in Box 12.5.

Clinical manifestations

The earliest sign of rickets is a ping-pong ball sensation of the skull (craniotabes) elicited by pressing firmly over the occipital or posterior parietal bones. The costochondral junctions may be palpable (rachitic rosary), wrists (especially in crawling infants) and ankles (especially in walking infants) may be widened and there may be a horizontal depression on the lower chest corresponding to attachment of the softened ribs and with the diaphragm (Harrison's sulcus) (Figs 12.16 and 12.17). The legs may become bowed (see Fig. 12.16). The clinical features are listed in Box 12.6 (see also Case history 12.2).

Diagnosis

This is made from:

- dietary history for vitamin and calcium intake
- blood tests – serum calcium is low or normal, phosphorus low, plasma alkaline phosphatase activity greatly increased, and 25-hydroxyvitamin D may be low
- X-ray of the wrist joint – shows cupping and fraying of the metaphyses and a widened epiphyseal plate.

Management

Nutritional rickets is managed by advice about a balanced diet, correction of predisposing risk factors and by the daily administration of vitamin D3 (cholecalciferol). If compliance is an issue, a single oral high dose of vitamin D3 can be given, followed by the daily maintenance dose. Healing occurs in 2–4 weeks and can be monitored from the lowering of alkaline phosphatase, increasing vitamin D levels and healing on X-rays, but complete reversal of bony deformities may take years.

> ### ⊙ Summary
>
> **Rickets:**
> - nutritional – has re-emerged in the UK in Asian and black infants exclusively breast-fed into the late infancy
> - diagnosis – serum calcium is low or normal, phosphorus low, plasma alkaline phosphatase greatly increased, 25-hydroxyvitamin D low
> - X-ray features – cupping and fraying of the metaphyses and widened epiphyseal plate.

Rickets

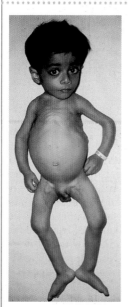

Figure 12.16 Rickets in a 3-year-old boy secondary to coeliac disease. He has frontal bossing, a Harrison's sulcus and bow legs.

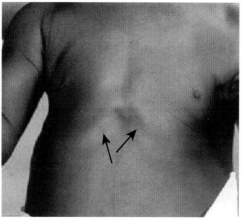

Figure 12.17 Harrison's sulcus, indentation of the softened lower rib cage at the site of attachment of the diaphragm. (Courtesy of Dr Nick Shaw.)

Box 12.6 Clinical features of rickets

- Misery
- Failure to thrive/short stature
- Frontal bossing of skull
- Craniotabes
- Delayed closure of anterior fontanelle
- Delayed dentition
- Rickety rosary

- Harrison's sulcus (Fig. 12.17)
- Expansion of metaphyses (especially wrist)
- Bowing of weight-bearing bones
- Hypotonia
- Seizures (late)

Case History
12.2 Seizures and rickets

Mohammed, a 13-month-old Somalian boy, was admitted to the A&E department with a generalised afebrile seizure. This was initially controlled with per rectum diazepam. Twenty minutes later he had another generalised seizure and needed intravenous anticonvulsants.

His mother said that he was a healthy child. He was born at term, birthweight 3.1 kg, and was still breast-fed. Some weaning foods were started at 7–8 months, but he preferred feeding at the breast. He had only recently begun to sit without support.

His weight and head circumference were on the 2nd–9th centile. He had marked frontal bossing, widened wrist (Fig. 12.18) and other epiphyses, Harrison's sulci, wide anterior fontanelle, craniotabes and a rachitic rosary. He would not take his weight on standing.

Investigations showed a low calcium and phosphate level, a high alkaline phosphatase and parathormone level and a very low vitamin D level, confirming rickets. Liver and renal function tests were normal and coeliac screen was negative. His wrist X-ray showed characteristic features (Fig. 12.19) such as cupping. A detailed dietetic history revealed a diet deficient in calcium and vitamin D, confirming nutritional rickets as the cause.

Dietetic input was provided. He was started on oral vitamin D and his solid food intake was increased to ensure that he was receiving sufficient calcium and vitamin D in his diet. His rickets resolved.

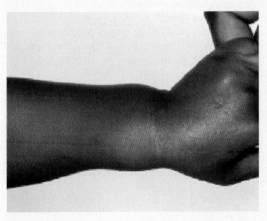

Figure 12.18 Wrist expansion from rickets. (Courtesy of Dr Nick Shaw.)

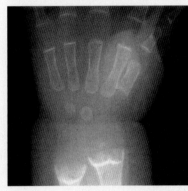

Figure 12.19 X-ray of the child's wrist showing rickets. The ends of the radius and ulna are expanded, rarefied and cup-shaped and the bones are poorly mineralised.

Vitamin A deficiency

In developed countries, biochemical vitamin A deficiency is seen as a complication of fat malabsorption when supplementation has been inadequate. Clinical manifestations under these circumstances are rare, except for impaired dark adaptation. Vitamin A deficiency is common in many developing countries, where it causes eye damage from corneal scarring and acceleration of malnutrition from impairment of mucosal function and immunity. A number of community-based trials of supplementation have shown a marked reduction in mortality by reducing the incidence of infection.

Obesity

Obesity is now the most common disorder affecting children and adolescents, reflecting the current epidemic. It is associated with a constellation of immediate and late adverse effects (Box 12.7). Precise causes of this marked increase in prevalence are unclear, but result from both increased intake of energy-dense food and reduced exercise. Although household energy intakes in the UK have been falling since the 1970s, there is a link between obesity and the intake of high-fat, energy-rich food such as fast foods. Energy expenditure has fallen as a result of an increase in sedentary behaviour. Less sport is played in schools and fewer children walk to school and are able to play outside. There has been an increase in the use of computers, the telephone and watching television. Obesity is more common in children from low socioeconomic homes.

Exogenous causes of obesity are rare. They are hypothyroidism, Cushing's syndrome and some genetic syndromes. As overnutrition accelerates growth and the onset of puberty, most obese children are also above the 50th centile for height. This makes the differentiation from hypothyroidism or Cushing's syndrome easier as these conditions are associated with short stature from a decline in growth velocity. An uncommon syndrome associated with obesity is Prader–Willi syndrome (poor linear growth, developmental delay, dysmorphic facial features, hypotonia and undescended testicles in males).

Emotional disturbance is seen in some affected children and unhappiness may lead to further excessive eating. The child or teenager may be teased and develop a poor self-image, adversely affecting self-confidence, particularly in establishing relationships with the opposite sex. Psychological support may be required.

Definitions

Body mass index (BMI = weight in kg/height in metres^2) is the best single index of obesity (Fig. 12.20). It is easy to measure, centile charts are available, and a BMI >95th centile predicts both an increased risk of persistence of obesity into adult life and abnormalities in blood lipids and blood pressure.

For clinical use, obese children are those with a BMI above the 98th centile of the UK 1990 reference chart for age and sex. Overweight is defined as a BMI above the 91st centile.

By definition, only 5% and 2% of children should be above the 95th and 98th centiles respectively.

Overall, in England the prevalence of obesity in boys (5–10 years) increased from 1.2% in 1984 to 3.4% in 1996–97 and to 6.0% in 2002–03. In girls (5–10 years), obesity increased from 1.8% in 1984 to 4.5% in 1996–97 and to 6.6% in 2002–03.

Complications

These are shown in Box 12.7.

Prevention

There are few randomised controlled trials in this area and most involve a complex package of interventions. These include a reduction in television viewing, increased physical activity, decreased fat intake, increased fruit and vegetables and education. Of these, a reduction in television viewing appears to be the most effective single factor.

Management

There is no good evidence-base on which to base treatments and no evidence at all on drug therapy, surgery or residential treatments in children. There is also a body of opinion which supports the view that childhood obesity is a societal problem and one which it is unrealistic to expect individual families to solve.

In the absence of evidence from randomised controlled trials, a pragmatic approach in any

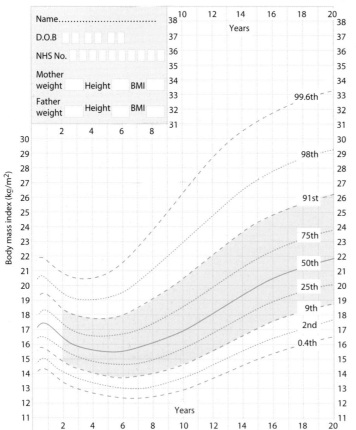

Figure 12.20 Body mass index (BMI) centile chart (Child Growth Foundation).

- Orthopaedic
  - Slipped upper femoral epiphysis
  - Tibia vara (bow legs)
  - Abnormal foot structure and function
- Benign intracranial hypertension (headaches, blurred optic disc margins)
- Hypoventilation syndrome (daytime somnolence; sleep apnoea; snoring; hypercapnia; heart failure)
- Gall bladder disease
- Polycystic ovary disease
- Hyperinsulinaemia and non-insulin-dependent diabetes mellitus
- Hypertension
- Abnormal blood lipids
- Other medical sequelae
  - Asthma
- Psychological sequelae
  - Low self-esteem
  - Teasing
  - Depression
  - Body dissatisfaction

Box 12.8 Main messages for patients and parents about obesity

- Obesity in children is becoming more common
- Obesity is due to an imbalance between energy consumption and energy expenditure. Obese children do not have low energy needs. They have high energy needs to support their high body weight
- Obesity is a health concern in itself and also increases the risk of other serious health problems such as high blood pressure, diabetes and psychological distress
- An obese child tends to become an obese adult
- There is no evidence that any drug treatment is effective in treating obesity in children
- Obesity in children may be prevented and treated by increasing physical activity/decreasing physical inactivity (e.g. TV watching) and encouraging a well-balanced and healthy diet
- Lifestyle changes involve making small gradual changes to behaviour
- Family support is necessary for treatment to succeed
- Generally the aim of treatment is to help children maintain their weight (so that they can 'grow into it')
- Most children are not obese because of an underlying medical problem but as a result of their lifestyle

Adapted from Scottish Intercollegiate Guidelines Network, SIGN.

individual child based on consensus criteria has to be adopted (Box 12.8). Treatment should be considered where the child is above the 98th centile for BMI and the family are willing to make the necessary lifestyle changes. Weight maintenance is a more realistic goal than weight reduction. It can only be achieved by sustained changes in lifestyle:

- healthier eating
- an increase in habitual physical activity to 30 to 60 minutes of moderate or vigorous physical activity per day
- reduction in physical inactivity (e.g. watching TV) during leisure time to less than an average of 2 hours per day.

Maintenance of baseline weight will result over time in a demonstrable fall in BMI on the centile chart as height increases.

Most obese children can be managed in primary care but those children who have serious obesity-related morbidity that requires active weight loss (benign intracranial hypertension, sleep apnoea, obesity hypoventilation syndrome, orthopaedic problems and psychological morbidity), children with a suspected underlying medical cause for their obesity, all children under 24 months of age who are severely obese and all children with a BMI above the 99.6 centile should be referred to a paediatrician.

⊚ Summary

Obesity:
- has become a major health issue for children, predisposing them to a wide range of medical and psychological problems in childhood and adult life, especially non-insulin-dependent diabetes mellitus and hypertension
- is defined as a BMI >98th centile of the UK 1990 reference chart for age and sex; overweight is BMI >91st centile
- exogenous causes (hypothyroidism and Cushing's syndrome) of obesity are rare, and more likely in a child who is also short from falling height velocity; there are also some rare genetic syndromes
- successful management requires sustained changes in lifestyle, with healthier eating, increased physical activity and reduction in physical inactivity
- success is more likely if there is family support and participation
- lifestyle changes are difficult to achieve and even harder to maintain
- is resulting in cultural change in our society, e.g. removal of 'tuck shops' and vending machines with unhealthy food and drinks from schools.

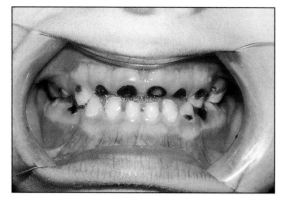

Figure 12.21 Dental caries. Prop feeding infants when put to sleep with a bottle containing milk or other fermentable liquids places them at high risk of severe dental caries and should be discouraged.

Dental caries

Dental caries occurs as a result of exposure to organic acids produced by bacterial fermentation of carbohydrate, particularly sucrose (Fig. 12.21). Prevalence is now rising in young children. It is strongly related to socioeconomic deprivation.

Prevention involves:

- a reduction in plaque bacteria (brushing and flossing)
- less frequent ingestion of carbohydrates
- regular inspection by a dentist
- an optimal intake of fluoride up to puberty to improve the resistance of the tooth to damage; water fluoridation is one of the most effective ways of achieving this.

Incorporation of fluoride in enamel by ionic substitution leads to replacement of calcium hydroxyapatite with calcium fluorapatite, which is less soluble in organic acids. In areas where drinking water contains a low concentration of fluoride, supplementation with fluoride drops or tablets is needed. Additionally, topical fluoride in toothpaste or mouthwashes is also advisable. Excess fluoride administration, before enamel has formed, may lead to mottled enamel (dental fluorosis).

Infants and children who are put to bed with a bottle containing fermentable liquid (milk or a sucrose-containing fruit juice) are at particular risk of developing severe dental caries. Characteristically, fluid collects around the upper anterior and posterior teeth, which become extensively damaged. Because of reduced salivation and swallowing during sleep, clearance and neutralisation of organic acids are also reduced. So called 'prop feeding' should therefore be energetically discouraged.

Further reading

Walker W A, Watkins J B, Duggan C 2003 Nutrition in pediatrics. Basic science and clinical applications, 3rd edn. B C Decker

Internet

http://www.babyfriendly.org.uk/parents/byb.asp
(Practical information on breast-feeding)
www.nice.org.uk
Obesity Guidance on the prevention, identification, assessment and management of overweight and obesity in adults and children
(NICE guideline, 2006)
www.ic.nhs.uk/pubs/breastfeed2005
Infant feeding survey 2005
www.who.int
Management of the child with a serious infection or severe malnutrition. Guidelines for care at the first-referral level in developing countries

Gastroenterology

Few children reach adulthood without experiencing gastrointestinal disorders such as vomiting, gastroenteritis, episodes of abdominal pain or constipation. In most instances, the symptoms are mild and transient, but serious causes need to be excluded. Chronic gastrointestinal disorders are a potent cause of weight loss and poor growth in spite of the enormous reserve capacity of the gut.

Vomiting

Posseting and *regurgitation* are terms used to describe the non-forceful return of milk, but differ in degree. Posseting describes the small amounts of milk which often accompany the return of swallowed air ('wind'), whereas regurgitation describes larger, more frequent losses. Posseting occurs in nearly all babies from time to time, whereas regurgitation usually indicates the presence of gastro-oesophageal reflux.

Vomiting is the forceful ejection of gastric contents. It is a common problem in infancy and childhood (Fig. 13.1 and Box 13.1). It is usually benign and is often caused by feeding disorders or mild gastro-oesophageal reflux or gastroenteritis. Potentially serious disorders need to be excluded if the vomiting is bilious or prolonged, or if the child is systemically unwell or failing to thrive. In infants, vomiting may be associated with infection outside the gastro-intestinal tract, especially in the urinary tract and central nervous system. In intestinal obstruction, the more proximal the obstruction, the more prominent the vomiting and the sooner it becomes bile-stained (unless the obstruction is proximal to the ampulla of Vater). With lower intestinal obstruction the abdomen becomes distended.

Summary

Vomiting in infants:
- common chronic causes are gastro-oesophageal reflux and feeding problems, e.g. force-feeding or overfeeding
- if transient, with other symptoms, e.g. fever, diarrhoea or runny nose and cough, most likely to be gastroenteritis or respiratory tract infection, but consider urine infection and meningitis
- if projectile at 2–7 weeks of age, exclude pyloric stenosis
- if bile stained, exclude intestinal obstruction, especially intussusception, malrotation and a strangulated inguinal hernia
- assess for dehydration and shock.

Box 13.1 Diagnostic clues in a vomiting infant

- Bile-stained vomit – intestinal obstruction must be excluded
- Blood in the vomit – suggests oesophagitis or peptic ulceration or oral/nasal bleeding or malrotation
- Projectile vomiting in the first few weeks of life – is it pyloric stenosis?
- Are there symptoms to suggest urinary tract, central nervous system or gastrointestinal infection?
- Vomiting at the end of paroxysmal coughing – is it whooping cough (pertussis)?
- Is the infant dehydrated or in shock?
- Abdominal distension – is there lower intestinal obstruction? Check for a strangulated inguinal hernia.

Causes of vomiting

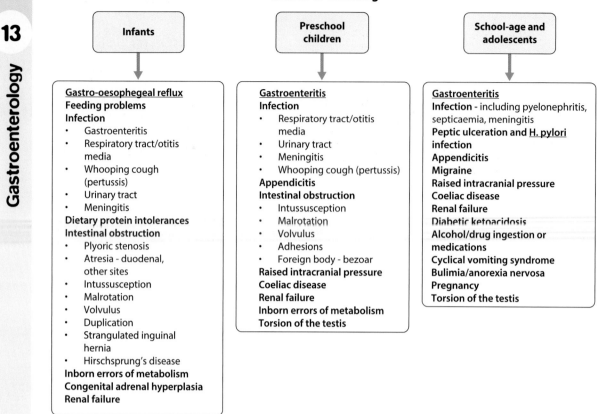

Infants	Preschool children	School-age and adolescents
Gastro-oesophegeal reflux **Feeding problems** **Infection** • Gastroenteritis • Respiratory tract/otitis media • Whooping cough (pertussis) • Urinary tract • Meningitis **Dietary protein intolerances** **Intestinal obstruction** • Plyoric stenosis • Atresia - duodenal, other sites • Intussusception • Malrotation • Volvulus • Duplication • Strangulated inguinal hernia • Hirschsprung's disease **Inborn errors of metabolism** **Congenital adrenal hyperplasia** **Renal failure**	**Gastroenteritis** **Infection** • Respiratory tract/otitis media • Urinary tract • Meningitis • Whooping cough (pertussis) **Appendicitis** **Intestinal obstruction** • Intussusception • Malrotation • Volvulus • Adhesions • Foreign body - bezoar **Raised intracranial pressure** **Coeliac disease** **Renal failure** **Inborn errors of metabolism** **Torsion of the testis**	**Gastroenteritis** **Infection** - including pyelonephritis, septicaemia, meningitis **Peptic ulceration and H. pylori infection** **Appendicitis** **Migraine** **Raised intracranial pressure** **Coeliac disease** **Renal failure** **Diabetic ketoacidosis** **Alcohol/drug ingestion or medications** **Cyclical vomiting syndrome** **Bulimia/anorexia nervosa** **Pregnancy** **Torsion of the testis**

Figure 13.1 Causes of regurgitation/vomiting.

Gastro-oesophageal reflux

Physiological, asymptomatic reflux may occur in any child or adult but it is infrequent. Measurement of lower oesophageal pH shows that in normal individuals there is acidity from reflux of stomach contents for less than 4% of a 24-hour period. Reflux occurring more frequently than this results from functional immaturity of the lower oesophageal sphincter leading to episodes of inappropriate relaxation. A short intra-abdominal length of oesophagus probably also contributes. It is common in the first year of life. By 12 months of age, nearly all symptomatic reflux will have resolved spontaneously, presumably due to a combination of maturation of the lower oesophageal sphincter, assumption of an upright posture and more solids in the diet. A sliding hiatus hernia is present in some symptomatic infants, but many children with a hiatus hernia are symptom-free.

Severe reflux is uncommon, but may be associated with potentially serious complications (Box 13.2). Reflux is often problematic:

• in children with cerebral palsy or other neurodevelopmental disorders, when energetic management, surgical if necessary, may transform the child's quality of life

Box 13.2 Complications of gastro-oesophageal reflux

• Pain, bleeding, iron deficiency
• Pulmonary aspiration leading to 'bronchitis' or pneumonia
• Peptic stricture – associated with oesophagitis
• Dystonic movements of head and neck (Sandifer's syndrome)
• Apnoea in preterm infants
• Apparent life-threatening events (ALTEs) or sudden infant death syndrome (SIDS) – controversial

• in preterm infants who develop bronchopulmonary dysplasia (chronic lung disease of prematurity)
• following surgery for oesophageal atresia or diaphragmatic hernia.

Management

Patients with mild, uncomplicated reflux can be diagnosed clinically and treated without further investigation. However, when the history is atypical or when complications are present, further investigation is indicated (Case history 13.1). The best diagnostic test is 24-hour oesophageal pH

13.1 Severe gastro-oesophageal reflux

This infant (Fig. 13.2a) had a history of frequent regurgitation from the first few days of life. He developed two chest infections. Some of the vomits contained altered blood. A 24-hour oesophageal pH study showed severe gastro-oesophageal reflux (Figs 13.2b and c). Endoscopy showed oesophagitis. He had probably had episodes of aspiration pneumonia. Symptoms resolved on treatment with feed thickeners and omeprazole. His parents also commented on how much better he slept at night. Treatment was reduced from 14 months of age and symptoms did not recur.

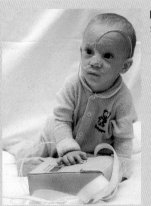

Figure 13.2a The pH study in progress.

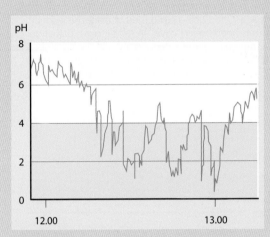

Figure 13.2b Part of the 24-hour oesophageal pH study showing severe reflux, with frequent drops in pH below 4.

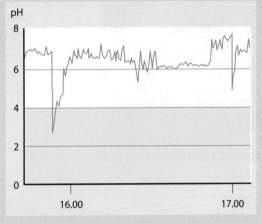

Figure 13.2c Part of a normal oesophageal pH study. The lower oesophageal pH is above 4 for most of the time.

monitoring. Contrast studies of the upper gastro-intestinal tract may be required to exclude underlying anatomical abnormalities in the oesophagus, stomach and duodenum, and malrotation. Endoscopy and oesophageal biopsy are performed in some centres if oesophagitis is suspected.

It is worthwhile treating all infants with symptomatic reflux; repeated regurgitation is smelly and unpopular with the family. Mild reflux responds well to the addition of inert thickening agents to feeds (e.g. Nestargel, Carobel), and positioning in a 30° head-up prone position after feeds. Drugs which enhance gastric emptying (e.g. domperidone) may be useful in more severe forms of reflux, as are proton pump inhibitors (e.g. omeprazole) to reduce oesophagitis. Surgery, called fundoplication, in which the fundus of the stomach is wrapped around the intra-abdominal oesophagus, is reserved for those patients with complications failing to respond to intensive medical treatment, oesophageal stricture or recurrent respiratory symptoms, especially aspiration.

Summary

Gastro-oesophageal reflux:
- occurs in otherwise normal infants, but risk is increased if neuromuscular problems or surgery to the oesophagus or diaphragm
- is treated if troublesome with upright positioning, feed thickening, medication and sometimes fundoplication
- investigations are performed if complications are suspected.

Pyloric stenosis

In pyloric stenosis, there is hypertrophy of the pylorus causing gastric outlet obstruction. It presents at between 2 and 7 weeks of age, irrespective of gestational age. It is more common in boys (4 : 1), particularly first-borns, and there may be a family history, especially on the maternal side.

Vomiting

Pyloric stenosis

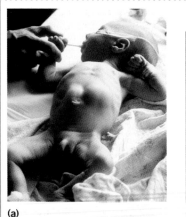

(a)

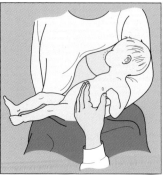

(b)

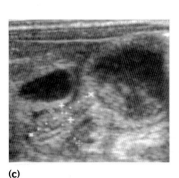

(c)

(d)

Figure 13.3 **(a)** Visible gastric peristalsis in an infant with pyloric stenosis. **(b)** Diagram showing a test feed being performed to diagnose pyloric stenosis. The pyloric mass feels like an 'olive' on gentle, deep palpation halfway between the midpoint of the anterior margin of the right ribcage and the umbilicus. **(c)** Ultrasound examination showing pyloric stenosis. **(d)** Pyloric stenosis at operation showing pale, thick pyloric muscle and pyloromyotomy incision.

Clinical features are:

- projectile vomiting (not bile-stained), which increases in frequency and severity with time
- constant hunger even after vomiting; only when markedly dehydrated do they refuse to feed
- a hypochloraemic alkalosis with a low plasma potassium from vomiting acid stomach contents
- weight loss or poor weight gain if presentation is delayed.

Diagnosis

Unless immediate fluid resuscitation is required, a test feed is performed. The baby is given a milk feed, which will calm the hungry infant, allowing examination. Gastric peristalsis may be seen as a wave moving from left to right across the abdomen (Fig. 13.3a). The pyloric mass or 'olive' is usually palpable in the right upper quadrant (Fig. 13.3b). If the stomach is overdistended with air, it will need to be emptied by a nasogastric tube to allow palpation. Ultrasound examination is used to confirm the diagnosis (Fig. 13.3c) if no mass is felt. A barium meal is only performed when the diagnosis remains in doubt.

Management

Initial management is to correct any fluid and electrolyte disturbance with intravenous fluids. The chloride and potassium deficits should be replaced. Treatment is by pyloromyotomy, when the muscle but not the mucosa of the pylorus is cut (Fig. 13.3d). The operation can be performed through a variety of incisions, including through the umbilicus or laparoscopically. Postoperatively the child can be fed the next day and is usually discharged within 2–3 days of surgery.

Summary

Pyloric stenosis:

- is more common in boys and those with a maternal family history
- signs are visible gastric peristalsis, palpable abdominal mass on test feed and possible dehydration
- is associated with a hypochloraemic alkalosis
- diagnosis is confirmed on ultrasound
- is treated by surgery after rehydration and correction of electrolyte imbalance.

Crying

Excessive crying in infants is distressing for all concerned. Advice on appropriate feeding, wrapping and reassurance will usually suffice. The emotional climate within a home is readily transmitted to a baby, and tense, anxious or irritable care-givers are likely to have similar babies. Organic causes should not be overlooked. Crying of sudden onset may be due to a urinary tract, middle ear or meningeal infection, to pain from an unrecognised fracture, oesophagitis or torsion of the testis. Severe nappy rash, constipation or coeliac disease may produce a miserable, crying infant. The complaint that a baby is 'always crying' may be a pointer to potential or actual non-accidental injury. On the basis of countless reports of parents, there seems little doubt that the eruption of teeth is painful in some infants. However, teething does not cause vomiting, diarrhoea, high fever or convulsions.

Infant 'colic'

The term 'colic' is used to describe a common symptom complex which occurs during the first few months of life. Paroxysmal, inconsolable crying or screaming accompanied by drawing up of the knees takes place several times a day, particularly in the evening. There is no firm evidence that the cause is intestinal, but this is often suspected. The condition usually resolves by 4 months of age. Occasionally, cow's milk protein intolerance or gastro-oesophageal reflux may be responsible. Sympathetic advice is helpful. The condition is essentially benign, although it may precipitate non-accidental injury in infants already at risk. Therapies such as gripe water are of unproven benefit. In severe, persistent cases an empirical 2-week trial of a cow's milk-free diet followed by a trial of anti-reflux treatment may be worthwhile.

Acute abdominal pain

Managing acute abdominal pain in children requires considerable skill. In nearly half the children admitted to hospital, the pain resolves undiagnosed. In young children it is essential not to delay the diagnosis and treatment of acute appendicitis, as progression to perforation can be rapid. It is easy to belittle the clinical signs of abdominal tenderness in young children. Of the surgical causes, appendicitis is by far the most common. It needs to be differentiated from non specific abdominal pain and the other surgical and medical conditions listed in Figure 13.4. The testes, hernial orifices and hip joints must always be checked. It is noteworthy that:

- Lower lobe pneumonia may cause pain referred to the abdomen.
- Primary peritonitis is seen in patients with ascites from nephrotic syndrome or liver disease.
- Diabetic ketoacidosis may cause severe abdominal pain.
- Urinary tract infection, including acute pyelonephritis, is a relatively uncommon cause of acute abdominal pain, but must not be missed. It is important to test a urine sample in order to identify not only diabetes mellitus but also conditions affecting the liver and urinary tract.

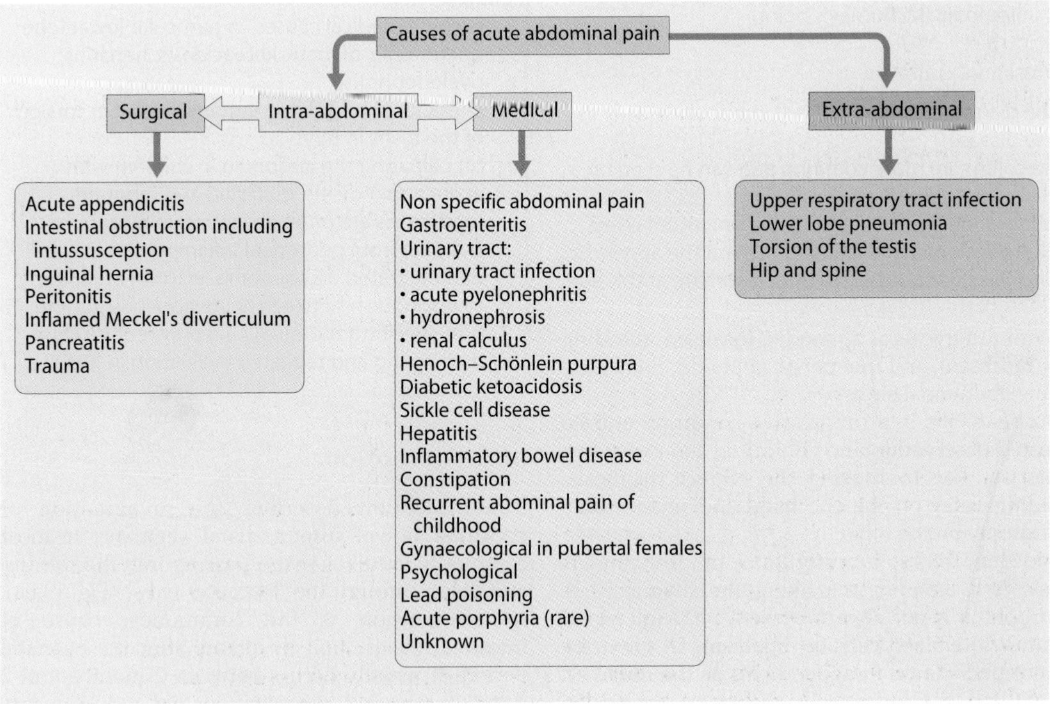

Figure 13.4 Causes of acute abdominal pain.

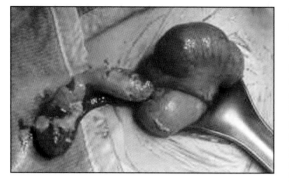

Figure 13.5 Appendicitis at operation showing a perforated acutely inflamed appendix covered in fibrin.

Acute appendicitis

Acute appendicitis is the commonest cause of abdominal pain in childhood requiring surgical intervention (Fig. 13.5). Although it may occur at any age, it is very uncommon in children less than 3 years old. The clinical features of acute uncomplicated appendicitis are:

- Symptoms
  - anorexia
  - vomiting (usually only a few times)
  - abdominal pain, initially central and colicky (appendicular midgut colic) but then localising to the right iliac fossa (from localised peritoneal inflammation)
- Signs
  - flushed face with oral fetor
  - low-grade fever 37.2–38°C
  - abdominal pain aggravated by movement
  - persistent tenderness with guarding in the right iliac fossa (McBurney's point).

In preschool children:

- the diagnosis is more difficult, particularly early in the disease
- faecoliths are more common and can be seen on a plain abdominal X-ray
- perforation may be rapid, as the omentum is less well developed and fails to surround the appendix, and the signs are easy to underestimate at this age.

With a retrocaecal appendix, localised guarding may be absent, and in a pelvic appendix there may be few abdominal signs.

Appendicitis is a progressive condition and so repeated observation and clinical review every few hours are key to making the correct diagnosis, avoiding delay on the one hand and unnecessary laparotomy on the other.

No laboratory investigation or imaging is consistently helpful in making the diagnosis. A neutrophilia is not always present on a full blood count. White blood cells or organisms in the urine are not uncommon in appendicitis as the inflamed appendix may be adjacent to the ureter or bladder. In some centres, laparoscopy is available to see whether or not the appendix is inflamed. Appendicectomy is straightforward in uncomplicated appendicitis.

Complicated appendicitis includes the presence of an appendix mass, an abscess or perforation. If there is generalised guarding consistent with perforation, fluid resuscitation and intravenous antibiotics are given prior to laparotomy. If there is a palpable mass in the right iliac fossa and there are no signs of generalised peritonitis, it may be reasonable to elect for conservative management with intravenous antibiotics, with appendicectomy being performed after several weeks. If symptoms progress, laparotomy is indicated. If an abscess is confirmed on abdominal ultrasound, operative drainage and appendicectomy will be required.

Non-specific abdominal pain and mesenteric adenitis

Non-specific abdominal pain (NSAP) is abdominal pain which resolves in 24–48 hours. The pain is less severe than in appendicitis, and tenderness in the right iliac fossa is variable. It is often accompanied by an upper respiratory tract infection with cervical lymphadenopathy. In some of these children, the abdominal signs do not resolve and an appendicectomy is performed. The diagnosis of mesenteric adenitis can only be made definitively in those children in whom large mesenteric nodes are seen at laparotomy or laparoscopy and whose appendix is normal.

Summary

Acute abdominal pain in older children and adolescents:

- exclude medical causes, in particular lower lobe pneumonia, diabetic ketoacidosis, hepatitis, pyelonephritis
- check for strangulated inguinal hernia or torsion of the testis in boys
- on palpating the abdomen in children with acute appendicitis, guarding and rebound tenderness are often absent or unimpressive, but pain from peritoneal inflammation may be demonstrated on coughing, walking or jumping
- to distinguish between acute appendicitis and non-specific abdominal pain may require close monitoring and repeated evaluation in hospital.

Intussusception

Intussusception describes the invagination of proximal bowel into a distal segment. It most commonly involves ileum passing into the caecum and colon through the ileocaecal valve (Fig. 13.6a). Intussusception is the commonest cause of intestinal obstruction in infants after the neonatal period. It usually occurs between 2 months and 2 years of age and resuscitation and reduction are urgent.

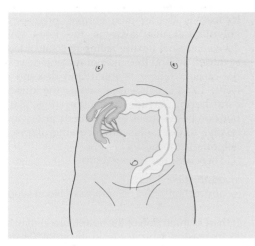

Figure 13.6a Intussusception, showing why the blood supply to the gut rapidly becomes compromised, making relief of this form of obstruction urgent.

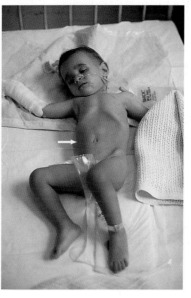

Figure 13.6b A child with an intussusception. The mass can be seen in the upper abdomen. The child has become shocked.

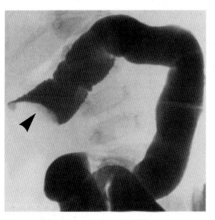

Figure 13.6c An abdominal X-ray demonstrating an intussusception (see arrow), taken during reduction by air insufflated per rectum.

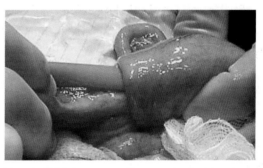

Figure 13.6d Intussusception at operation showing the ileum entering the caecum. The surgeon is squeezing the colon to reduce the intussusception.

Presentation is with:

- paroxysmal, severe colicky pain and pallor – during episodes of pain, the child becomes pale, especially around the mouth, and draws up his legs
- a sausage-shaped mass – often palpable in the abdomen (Fig. 13.6b)
- passage of a characteristic redcurrant jelly stool comprising blood-stained mucus – this is a characteristic sign but tends to occur later in the illness and may be first seen after a rectal examination
- abdominal distension and shock.

Usually, no underlying intestinal cause for the intussusception is found, although there is some evidence that viral infection leading to enlargement of Peyer's patches may form the lead point of the intussusception. An identifiable lead point such as a Meckel's diverticulum or polyp is more likely to be present in children over 2 years old. Intravenous volume expansion is likely to be required immediately as there is often pooling of fluid in the gut, which may lead to hypovolaemic shock.

An X-ray of the abdomen may show distended small bowel and absence of gas in the distal colon or rectum. Sometimes the outline of the intussusception itself can be visualised. Unless there are signs of peritonitis, reduction of the intussusception by rectal air insufflation is usually attempted (Fig. 13.6c). Abdominal ultrasound is helpful in both diagnosis and checking response to insufflation. The success rate of this procedure is about 75%. The remaining 25% require operative reduction (Fig. 13.6d). Recurrence of the intussusception occurs in less than 5% but is more frequent after hydrostatic reduction.

Summary

Intussusception:

- usually occurs between 2 months and 2 years of age.
- clinical features are paroxysmal, colicky pain with pallor, abdominal mass, redcurrant jelly stool
- shock is an important complication and requires urgent treatment
- reduction is attempted by rectal air insufflation unless peritonitis is present
- surgery is required if reduction with air is unsuccessful or for peritonitis.

Meckel's diverticulum

Two per cent of individuals have an ileal remnant of the vitellointestinal duct, in the form of a Meckel's diverticulum, which contains ectopic gastric mucosa or pancreatic tissue. Most are asymptomatic but they may present with severe rectal bleeding which is neither bright red nor true melaena. Other forms of presentation include intussusception, volvulus around a band, or diverticulitis which mimics appendicitis. A technetium scan will demonstrate increased uptake by ectopic gastric mucosa in 70% of cases (Fig. 13.7). Treatment is by surgical resection.

Malrotation

If the small bowel mesentery is not fixed at the duodenojejunal flexure or in the ileocaecal region, its base is shorter than normal, predisposing to volvulus. It may arise in the fetus from the duodenojejunal flexure failing to rotate adequately to the left around the superior mesenteric vessels or the caecum failing to rotate and descend on the right. Ladd's bands may cross the duodenum, contributing to an obstruction (Fig. 13.8). The position of the superior mesenteric artery and vein relative to each other on abdominal ultrasound is helpful diagnostically.

There are two presentations:

- obstruction
- obstruction with a compromised blood supply.

If there is infarction of the bowel, blood may be seen in the gastric aspirates or in the stool. Obstruction with bilious vomiting usually presents in the first few days of life but can be seen at a later age. Any child with dark green vomiting needs an upper gastrointestinal contrast study to assess intestinal rotation, unless signs of vascular compromise are present, when an urgent laparotomy is needed.

At operation, the volvulus is untwisted, the duodenum mobilised and the bowel placed in the non-rotated position with the duodenojejunal flexure on the right and the caecum and appendix on the left. The malrotation is not 'corrected', but the mesentery broadened. The appendix may be removed to avoid later diagnostic confusion in the event of appendicitis.

Meckel's diverticulum

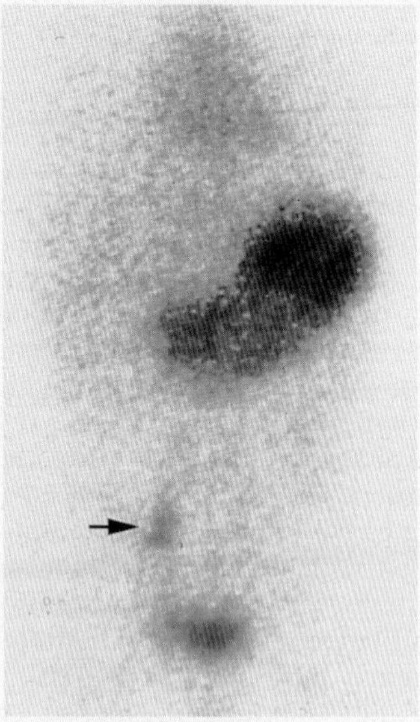

Figure 13.7 A technetium scan showing uptake by ectopic gastric mucosa in a Meckel's diverticulum in the right iliac fossa.

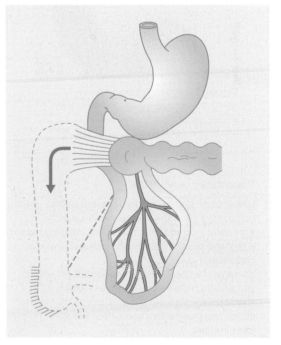

Figure 13.8 The commonest form of malrotation, with the caecum remaining high and fixed to the posterior abdominal wall. There are Ladd's bands obstructing the duodenum. *Dotted lines* show normal anatomy.

Summary

Malrotation:

- usually presents in the first 1–3 days of life with intestinal obstruction from Ladd's bands obstructing the duodenum or volvulus
- may present at any age with volvulus causing obstruction and ischaemic bowel
- clinical features are bile- or blood-stained vomiting, abdominal pain and tenderness from peritonitis or ischaemic bowel
- an urgent upper gastrointestinal contrast study is indicated whenever there is bile- or blood-stained vomiting
- treatment is urgent surgical correction.

Recurrent abdominal pain

Recurrent pain, sufficient to interrupt normal activities and lasting for at least 3 months, occurs in 10% of school-age children. Less than 10% of these children will have a definable organic cause. The widely held belief that the remainder have psychogenic pain is without foundation. A number of studies have failed to show a difference between such children and their families and controls. However, in some children, it may be a manifestation of stress (see p. 395) or it may become part of a vicious cycle of anxiety and escalating pain leading to family distress and demands for increasingly invasive investigations. There is evidence that anxiety may lead to altered motility, which may be perceived by the child as pain.

Over 90% of children with recurrent abdominal pain have no structural or mucosal abnormality in the gastrointestinal tract. Their pain is characteristically central, around the umbilicus, and the children are otherwise entirely well. It is increasingly recognised, however, that most have one of three distinct symptom constellations resulting from functional abnormalities of gut motility or enteral neurons – irritable bowel syndrome (usually), non-ulcer dyspepsia or abdominal migraine.

Irritable bowel syndrome

This disorder, also common in adults, is associated with altered gastrointestinal motility and an abnormal sensation of intra-abdominal events. Studies of pressure changes within the small intestine of children with irritable bowel syndrome suggest that abnormally forceful contractions occur. It has also been shown that affected adults experience pain from the inflation of balloons in the intestine at substantially lower volumes than do controls. There is therefore an interplay between these two factors, both of which are modulated by psychosocial factors such as stress and anxiety.

There is often a positive family history and a characteristic set of symptoms, although not all patients experience every symptom:

- abdominal pain, often worse before or relieved by defecation
- mucousy stools
- bloating
- feeling of incomplete defecation
- constipation, often alternating with normal or loose stools.

Non-ulcer dyspepsia

Some children with abdominal pain have symptoms suggesting an upper gastrointestinal disorder:

- epigastric pain
- postprandial vomiting
- belching
- bloating
- early satiety
- heartburn.

If present, *Helicobacter pylori* infection should be excluded. Endoscopy fails to reveal an ulcer or other mucosal disease in the stomach or duodenum. However, gastric motility is abnormal.

Abdominal migraine

Classical cranial migraine is often associated with abdominal pain in addition to headaches, and in some children the abdominal pain predominates. The attacks of pain are midline, paroxysmal, stereotypic and associated with facial pallor. There is usually a personal or family history of migraine. Pizotifen, a serotonin receptor antagonist, is a helpful prophylactic agent in those children with frequent, severe symptoms.

Management of recurrent abdominal pain

It is important that a full history and examination are not only done, but seen to be done, otherwise reassurance will be unconvincing. It will also establish that the child is growing normally and that there are no abnormalities on examination. In children with irritable bowel syndrome and non-ulcer dyspepsia, it can be helpful to explain to both the child and parents that 'sometimes the insides of the intestine become so sensitive that some children can feel the food going round the bends'. It is also necessary to make a distinction between 'serious' and 'dangerous'. These disorders can be serious, if, for example, they lead to substantial loss of schooling, but they are not dangerous.

Investigations should be guided by the clinical features. Although there are many potential organic causes, most are rare and investigations are only performed if indicated. A urine microscopy and culture is mandatory as urinary tract infections may cause pain in the absence of other symptoms or signs.

The long-term prognosis is:

- about half of affected children rapidly become free of symptoms

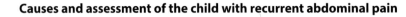

⊙ Summary

Causes and assessment of the child with recurrent abdominal pain

> **>90% no structural cause identified**

Gastrointestinal
- Irritable bowel syndrome
- Constipation
- Non-ulcer dyspepsia
- Abdominal migraine
- Gastritis and peptic ulceration
- Inflammatory bowel disease
- Malrotation

Gynaecological
- Dysmenorrhoea
- Ovarian cysts
- Pelvic inflammatory disease

Psychosocial - bullying, abuse, stress etc - a small proportion

Liver
- Hepatitis

Pancreatitis

Urinary tract infection

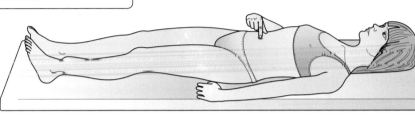

Symptoms and signs that suggest organic disease:
- Epigastric pain at night, haematemesis (duodenal ulcer)
- Diarrhoea, weight loss, growth failure, blood in stools (inflammatory bowel disease)
- Vomiting (pancreatitis)
- Jaundice (liver disease)
- Dysuria, secondary enuresis (urinary tract infection)
- Vomiting and abdominal distension (malrotation)

- in one-quarter, the symptoms take some months to resolve
- in one-quarter, symptoms continue or return in adulthood as irritable bowel syndrome, non-ulcer dyspepsia or cranial migraine.

Gastritis and peptic ulceration

The greater use of endoscopy in children and the identification of the Gram-negative organism *Helicobacter pylori* in association with antral gastritis have focused attention on it as a potential cause of abdominal pain in children. In adults, there is substantial evidence that *H. pylori* is a strong predisposing factor to duodenal ulcers. This association in children is much less clear. Duodenal ulcers are uncommon in children but should be sought in those with night pain, particularly if it wakes them, or when there is a history of peptic ulceration in a first-degree relative.

H. pylori causes a nodular antral gastritis which may be associated with abdominal pain and nausea. It is usually identified in gastric antral biopsies, but may also be present on micro-aerophilic culture. The organism produces urease, which forms the basis for a laboratory test on biopsies, and the ^{13}C breath test following the administration of ^{13}C-labelled urea by mouth.

Serological tests are unreliable in children. Treatment regimens vary but often consist of triple therapy with, for example, amoxicillin, metronidazole and clarithromycin.

Gastroenteritis

Infective diarrhoea and vomiting remain an important cause of morbidity in developed countries, although mortality is very low. In developing countries, gastroenteritis still claims the lives of 1.8 million children under the age of 5 each year.

The commonest cause of gastroenteritis in developed countries is rotavirus infection, which accounts for up to 60% of cases in children less than 2 years of age, particularly during the winter months. An effective vaccine against rotavirus is now available. Other viruses, particularly adenovirus, calicivirus, coronavirus and astrovirus, have been implicated in outbreaks but are much less common and their role as pathogens is less clear.

Bacterial causes are less common in developed countries, and are suggested by the presence of blood in the stools. *Campylobacter jejuni* infection, usually the commonest of the bacterial infections in developed countries, is often also associated with severe abdominal pain. *Shigella* and some salmonellae produce a dysenteric type of infection, with blood and pus in the stool, pain and tenesmus. *Shigella* may be accompanied by high fever causing a febrile convulsion. Cholera and enterotoxigenic *E. coli* infection are associated with profuse, rapidly dehydrating diarrhoea. However, clinical features act as a poor guide to the pathogen.

A number of disorders may masquerade as gastroenteritis (Box 13.3) and, when in doubt, hospital referral is essential. Dehydration and its complications are the usual cause of death in gastroenteritis, and its correction is the fundamental aim of treatment. Accurate clinical assessment of dehydration is important but difficult (Fig. 13.9 and Table 13.1).

Infants are at particular risk of dehydration because of their:

- greater surface area to weight ratio, leading to greater insensible water losses (300 ml/m² per day, equivalent in infants to 15–17 ml/kg per day)

Box 13.3 Conditions which can mimic gastroenteritis

Systemic infection	Septicaemia, meningitis
Local infections	Respiratory tract infection, otitis media, hepatitis A, urinary tract infection
Surgical disorders	Pyloric stenosis, intussusception, acute appendicitis, necrotising enterocolitis, Hirschsprung's disease
Metabolic disorder	Diabetic ketoacidosis
Renal disorder	Haemolytic uraemic syndrome
Other	Coeliac disease, cow's milk protein intolerance, adrenal insufficiency

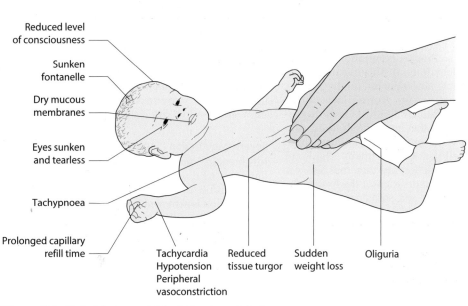

Reduced level of consciousness
Sunken fontanelle
Dry mucous membranes
Eyes sunken and tearless
Tachypnoea
Prolonged capillary refill time
Tachycardia Hypotension Peripheral vasoconstriction
Reduced tissue turgor
Sudden weight loss
Oliguria

Figure 13.9 Clinical features of dehydration in an infant.

Table 13.1 Clinical assessment of dehydration

	Moderate dehydration	Severe dehydration
Body weight loss	5–10%	>10%
General appearance	Thirsty, drowsy	Drowsy, limp, cold, sweaty, cyanotic extremities
Respiration*	Deep, may be rapid	Deep and rapid
Eyes	Sunken	Grossly sunken
Tears	Reduced/absent	Absent
Mucous membranes	Dry	Very dry
Capillary refill time*	Prolonged (> 2 seconds)	Prolonged (>2 seconds)
Tissue turgor*	Retracts slowly	Retracts very slowly
Blood pressure	Normal or low	Low
Radial pulse	Rapid and weak	Rapid, thready, may be impalpable
Anterior fontanelle	Sunken	Very sunken
Urine output	Reduced	Marked oliguria

*Most helpful and reliable signs.

Gastroenteritis

- inability to gain access to fluids when thirsty
- higher basal fluid requirements (100–120 ml/kg per day, i.e. 10–12% of body weight)
- immature renal tubular reabsorption processes.

Isonatraemic and hyponatraemic dehydration

In dehydration, there is a total body deficit of sodium and water. In most instances, the losses of sodium and water are proportional and plasma sodium remains within the normal range (isonatraemic dehydration). When sodium losses exceed those of water, plasma sodium falls (hyponatraemic dehydration) and this is associated with a shift of water from extra- to intracellular compartments. The increase in intracellular volume leads to an increase in brain volume, sometimes resulting in convulsions, whereas the marked extracellular depletion leads to a greater degree of shock per unit of water loss. This form of dehydration is more common in poorly nourished infants in developing countries.

Hypernatraemic dehydration

Infrequently, water loss exceeds the relative sodium loss and plasma sodium concentration increases (hypernatraemic dehydration). This usually results from high insensible water losses (high fever or hot, dry environment) or from profuse, low-sodium diarrhoea. The extracellular fluid becomes hypertonic with respect to the intracellular fluid and there is a shift of water into the extracellular space from the intracellular compartment. Signs of extracellular fluid depletion are therefore less per unit of fluid loss, and depression of the fontanelle, reduced tissue elasticity and sunken eyes are less obvious. This makes this form of dehydration more difficult to recognise clinically, particularly in an obese infant. It is a particularly dangerous form of dehydration as water is drawn out of the brain and cerebral shrinkage within a rigid skull may lead to multiple, small cerebral haemorrhages and convulsions. Transient hyperglycaemia occurs in some patients with hypernatraemic dehydration; it is self-correcting and does not require insulin.

Management

Mild dehydration (<5% body weight loss)

In most cases of gastroenteritis in infants and toddlers in developed countries, dehydration is mild, with less than 5% loss of body weight, and there are few, if any, clinical signs of dehydration. It can usually be managed by short-term substitution of normal feeds with a maintenance type of glucose–electrolyte solution (Table 13.2). The glucose or sucrose is present in oral rehydration solutions to enhance sodium and water absorption, not as a calorie source. Rehydration solutions may be rice-based. The solution is given until vomiting and profuse diarrhoea subside. This usually lasts less than 24 hours and a normal diet can then be introduced immediately. Contrary to previous teaching, there is no need to reintroduce milk gradually or to avoid milk or milk-containing foods.

Table 13.2 Composition (mmol/L) of oral rehydration solutions

	European solution	WHO/UNICEF
Sodium	60	90
Potassium	20	20
Chloride	50	80
Citrate	10	10
Glucose	75–110	110

The WHO/UNICEF solution is designed principally for use in developing countries in children with moderate to severe dehydration. The sodium concentration is too high for routine use in developed countries.

> Throughout the world, oral rehydration solution saves the lives of millions of children each year.

Moderate dehydration (5–10% body weight loss)

These children have clinical signs of dehydration. A 6-hour trial of oral rehydration can be instituted, aiming to give 100 ml/kg over this period (orally or by nasogastric tube). If there is no improvement in the child's symptoms and state of hydration, intravenous rehydration should be given.

Severe dehydration (>10% body weight loss)

Intravenous rehydration is always indicated. Patients who are shocked require immediate resuscitation with normal saline (Fig. 13.10a). Rehydration is achieved by replacement of the fluid deficit, whilst allowing for maintenance fluid requirement and any ongoing fluid losses (Figs 13.10b and c). Fluid balance needs to be closely monitored by clinical reassessment, including the child's weight and measurement of plasma electrolytes. Acute renal failure may rarely complicate severe dehydration. Failure to recognise continuing oliguria leads to overhydration and pulmonary oedema.

Hypernatraemic dehydration

The management of hypernatraemic dehydration is particularly difficult. Once circulation has been restored, a too rapid reduction in plasma sodium concentration and osmolality will lead to a shift of water into cerebral cells, resulting in cerebral oedema and possible convulsions. The reduction in plasma sodium should therefore be slow, over 48 hours, in order not to exceed a reduction in plasma sodium of 10 mmol/L per 24 hours.

Anti-diarrhoea drugs (e.g. loperamide, Lomotil) and anti-emetics

There is no place for medications for the vomiting or diarrhoea of gastroenteritis as they:

- are ineffective
- may prolong the excretion of bacteria in stools

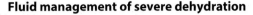

Fluid management of severe dehydration

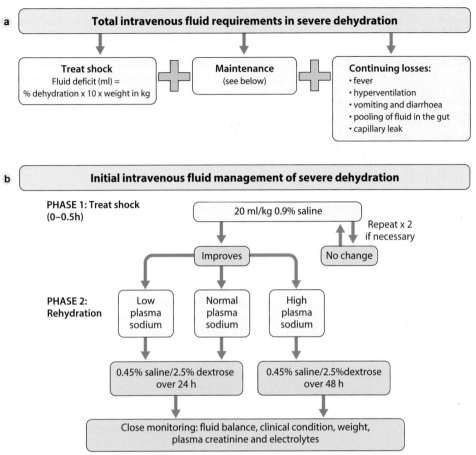

a | **Total intravenous fluid requirements in severe dehydration**

Treat shock
Fluid deficit (ml) =
% dehydration x 10 x weight in kg

+

Maintenance
(see below)

+

Continuing losses:
• fever
• hyperventilation
• vomiting and diarrhoea
• pooling of fluid in the gut
• capillary leak

b | **Initial intravenous fluid management of severe dehydration**

PHASE 1: Treat shock
(0–0.5h)

20 ml/kg 0.9% saline

Improves → No change

Repeat x 2
if necessary

PHASE 2:
Rehydration

Low plasma sodium | Normal plasma sodium | High plasma sodium

0.45% saline/2.5% dextrose over 24 h

0.45% saline/2.5%dextrose over 48 h

Close monitoring: fluid balance, clinical condition, weight, plasma creatinine and electrolytes

c | **Maintenance intravenous fluid requirements**

Body weight	Fluid (ml/kg/24h)	Sodium (mmol/kg/24 h)	Potassium (mmol/kg/24 h)
First 10 kg	100	2–4	1.5–2.5
Second 10 kg	50	1–2	0.5–1.5
Subsequent kg	20	0.5–1	0.2–0.7

For example, the maintenance fluid requirements of a 24 kg child are:
1000 + 500 + 80 = 1580 ml/24 h.

Figure 13.10 Fluid management of severe dehydration.

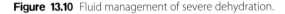

• can be associated with side-effects
• add unnecessarily to cost
• focus attention away from oral rehydration.

Antibiotics are indicated only for specific bacterial or protozoal infections (e.g. cholera, shigellosis, giardiasis).

> **Death in gastroenteritis is caused by dehydration. Its correction is the mainstay of treatment.**

Post-gastroenteritis syndrome

Infrequently, following an episode of gastro-enteritis, the introduction of a normal diet results in a return of watery diarrhoea. Temporary lactose intolerance may have developed, which can be confirmed by the presence of non-absorbed sugar in the stools giving a positive Clinitest result. In such circumstances, a return to an oral rehydration solution for 24 hours, followed by a further introduction of a normal diet, is usually successful.

Rarely, multiple dietary intolerances may result, such that specialist dietary management is required

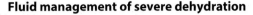

in the implementation of a diet which excludes cow's milk, disaccharides and gluten. In very severe cases, a period of parenteral nutrition is required to enable the injured small intestinal mucosa to recover sufficiently to absorb luminal nutrients.

Post-infective irritable bowel syndrome

Following an episode of gastroenteritis, particularly with a bacterial cause, a substantial proportion of children will develop symptoms of irritable bowel syndrome which may persist for some years. Characteristically, intermittent diarrhoea and abdominal pain (often relieved by defecation) occur, sometimes interspersed with constipation. In between episodes of pain and diarrhoea, affected children are symptom-free, have good general health and grow normally. The condition usually resolves spontaneously. No medication has been shown to be effective, except loperamide for diarrhoea.

Summary

Gastroenteritis
Gastroenteritis in developing countries:
- results in death from dehydration of millions of children worldwide
- is mostly bacterial from contaminated drinking water and food
- can usually be effectively treated with oral rehydration solution

Gastroenteritis in developed countries:
- is mostly viral, but it can be caused by *Campylobacter*, *Shigella* and *Salmonella*
- infants are particularly susceptible to dehydration.
- dehydration is assessed as a mild (<5%), moderate (5–10%) or severe (>10%), according to history and examination, but clinical assessment of severity is problematic
- oral rehydration solution is effective in most, but intravenous fluid is required for severe dehydration, or moderate dehydration with ongoing vomiting or inadequate fluid intake.

Malabsorption

Disorders affecting the digestion or absorption of nutrients manifest as:

- abnormal stools
- failure to thrive or poor growth in most but not all cases
- specific nutrient deficiencies, either singly or in combination.

In general, parents know when their children's stools have become abnormal. The true malabsorp-

tion stool is difficult to flush down the toilet and has an odour which pervades the whole house. In general, colour is a poor guide to abnormality. Reliable dietetic assessment is important. It is inappropriate to investigate children for malabsorption as a cause of their failure to thrive when dietary energy intake is demonstrably low and other symptoms are absent. Some disorders affecting the small intestinal mucosa or pancreas may lead to the malabsorption of many nutrients (pan-malabsorption), whereas others are highly specific, e.g. zinc malabsorption in *acrodermatitis enteropathica*.

Coeliac disease

Coeliac disease is an enteropathy in which the gliadin fraction of gluten provokes a damaging immunological response in the proximal small intestinal mucosa. As a result, the rate of migration of absorptive cells moving up the villi (enterocytes) from the crypts is massively increased but is insufficient to compensate for increased cell loss from the villous tips. Villi become progressively shorter and then absent, leaving a flat mucosa.

The incidence of coeliac disease, diagnosed in childhood on the basis of characteristic clinical symptoms, has been about 1 in 3000 in Europe, including the UK. The age at presentation is partly influenced by the age of introduction of gluten into the diet.

Classically, children present in the first few years of life with failure to thrive following the introduction of gluten in cereals. General irritability, abnormal stools, abdominal distension and buttock wasting are the usual symptoms (see Case history 13.2). Increasingly, children may present in later childhood with anaemia (iron and/or folate deficiency) or growth failure, with little or no gastrointestinal symptoms.

The introduction of highly sensitive and specific serological screening tests (tissue transglutaminase antibodies and anti-endomysial antibodies) has provided evidence that coeliac disease is more common than previously thought and as many as 1 in 100 UK school-age children may be antibody positive. Many children are now identified on screening of children with type 1 diabetes mellitus, in whom the incidence is about 5%.

Diagnosis

Although the diagnosis is strongly suggested by positive serology, confirmation depends upon the demonstration of a flat mucosa on jejunal biopsy followed by the resolution of symptoms and catch-up growth upon gluten withdrawal. There is no place for the empirical use of a gluten-free diet as a diagnostic test for coeliac disease in the absence of a jejunal biopsy. Serological tests such as tissue transglutaminase antibodies and anti-endomysial antibodies are not currently considered sufficiently sensitive and specific to replace jejunal biopsy, particularly as the diet is lifelong.

Case History
13.2 'Classic' coeliac disease

This 2-year-old (Fig. 13.11a) had a history of poor growth from 12 months of age (Fig. 13.11b). His parents had noticed that he tended to be crotchety and had three or four foul-smelling stools a day. A jejunal biopsy at 2 years of age showed subtotal villous atrophy (Fig. 13.11c and d) and he was started on a gluten-free diet. Within a few days, his parents commented that his mood had improved and within a month he was a 'different child'. He subsequently exhibited good catch-up growth.

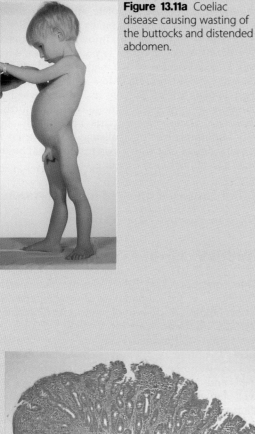

Figure 13.11a Coeliac disease causing wasting of the buttocks and distended abdomen.

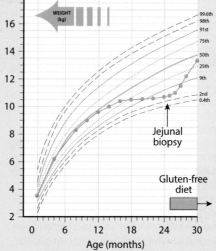

Figure 13.11b Growth chart showing failure to thrive and response to a gluten-free diet. (Adapted from chart © Child Growth Foundation.)

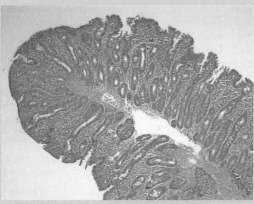

Figure 13.11c Histology of a jejunal biopsy showing lymphocytic infiltration and villous atrophy confirming coeliac disease. (Courtesy of Dr Marie-Anne Brundler.)

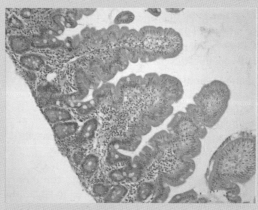

Figure 13.11d Normal jejunal histology is shown for comparison. (Courtesy of Dr Marie-Anne Brundler.)

Management

All products containing wheat, rye and barley are removed from the diet and this results in resolution of symptoms. Supervision by a dietician is essential. In children in whom the initial biopsy or the response to gluten withdrawal is doubtful, or when the disease presents before the age of 2, a gluten challenge is required in later childhood to demonstrate continuing susceptibility of the jejunal mucosa to damage by gluten. The gluten-free diet should be adhered to for life. The incidence of small bowel malignancy in adulthood is increased in coeliac disease although a gluten-free diet probably reduces the risk to normal.

Summary

Coeliac disease:
- is a gluten-sensitive enteropathy
- classical presentation is at 8–24 months with abnormal stools, failure to thrive, abdominal distension and wasted buttocks, and irritability
- other modes of presentation – short stature, anaemia, screening, e.g. children with diabetes mellitus
- diagnosis – positive serology (tissue transglutaminase and anti-endomysial antibodies), flat mucosa on jejunal biopsy and resolution of symptoms and catch-up growth upon gluten withdrawal
- treatment – gluten-free diet for life.

Transient dietary protein intolerances

In contrast to coeliac disease, which requires life-long gluten withdrawal, there are a number of transient intolerances to dietary proteins. These usually manifest as:

- diarrhoea and/or vomiting with failure to thrive
- eczema
- acute colitis
- migraine
- occasionally, an acute anaphylactic reaction with urticaria, stridor, bronchospasm and shock.

Cow's milk protein is the most commonly incriminated antigen, but intolerances to soya and less frequently to wheat, fish, egg, chicken and rice are also described. When an acute reaction occurs immediately after ingestion, the diagnosis can be readily established. When the reaction is delayed, diagnosis is difficult. Intolerances occur more commonly in infants with IgA deficiency or with a strong family history of atopy.

Although no single laboratory test is diagnostic, affected children may have:

- eosinophilia in the peripheral blood
- positive antibody tests to specific food proteins (RAST tests)
- a high IgE concentration in plasma.

Those children who present with failure to thrive and protracted diarrhoea may require a jejunal biopsy to establish the diagnosis, in particular to differentiate it from coeliac disease. In cow's milk protein intolerance, there is a patchy enteropathy in the jejunal mucosa, usually with prominent eosinophils in the lamina propria. Elimination of the offending antigen results in rapid resolution of symptoms and this, together with their return upon challenge, is the only diagnostic test. The advice of an experienced dietician is essential in the supervision of all exclusion diets in infancy and childhood, to ensure complete antigen exclusion whilst maintaining a nutritionally adequate diet.

In cow's milk protein intolerance, a casein hydrolysate-based formula is preferred to a soya-based feed because of the high phyto-oestrogen content of soy formula. Most children outgrow their intolerance by the age of 2 years, which is therefore an appropriate time to conduct a further challenge. Anaphylaxis occurs infrequently, but it is important that the challenge is conducted in hospital, beginning with a skin test followed by the ingestion of increasing amounts of antigen.

Other causes of nutrient malabsorption

These are shown in Figure 13.12.

Toddler diarrhoea

This condition, also called chronic non-specific diarrhoea, is the commonest cause of persistent loose stools in preschool children. Characteristically, the stools are of varying consistency, sometimes well formed, sometimes explosive and loose. The presence of undigested vegetables in the stools is common, giving rise to the alternative title 'peas and carrots syndrome'. Affected children are well and thriving and there are no precipitating dietary factors.

Toddler diarrhoea probably results from an underlying maturational delay in intestinal motility. Most children have grown out of their symptoms by 5 years of age but achieving faecal continence may be significantly delayed.

Summary

Chronic diarrhoea:
- in an infant with failure to thrive, consider cow's milk protein intolerance and coeliac disease
- following gastroenteritis, consider post-gastroenteritis syndrome, usually temporary lactose intolerance
- following bowel resection, cholestatic liver disease or exocrine pancreatic dysfunction, consider malabsorption
- in an otherwise well toddler with undigested vegetables in the stool, consider toddler diarrhoea.

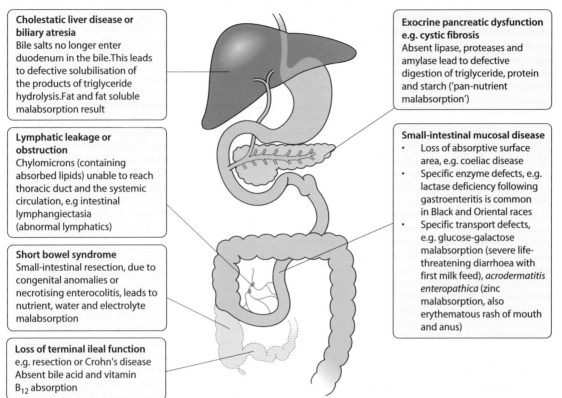

Causes of nutrient malabsorption

Cholestatic liver disease or biliary atresia
Bile salts no longer enter duodenum in the bile. This leads to defective solubilisation of the products of triglyceride hydrolysis. Fat and fat soluble malabsorption result

Lymphatic leakage or obstruction
Chylomicrons (containing absorbed lipids) unable to reach thoracic duct and the systemic circulation, e.g intestinal lymphangiectasia (abnormal lymphatics)

Short bowel syndrome
Small-intestinal resection, due to congenital anomalies or necrotising enterocolitis, leads to nutrient, water and electrolyte malabsorption

Loss of terminal ileal function
e.g. resection or Crohn's disease
Absent bile acid and vitamin B_{12} absorption

Exocrine pancreatic dysfunction e.g. cystic fibrosis
Absent lipase, proteases and amylase lead to defective digestion of triglyceride, protein and starch ('pan-nutrient malabsorption')

Small-intestinal mucosal disease
- Loss of absorptive surface area, e.g. coeliac disease
- Specific enzyme defects, e.g. lactase deficiency following gastroenteritis is common in Black and Oriental races
- Specific transport defects, e.g. glucose-galactose malabsorption (severe life-threatening diarrhoea with first milk feed), *acrodermatitis enteropathica* (zinc malabsorption, also erythematous rash of mouth and anus)

Figure 13.12 Causes of nutrient malabsorption. They are uncommon.

No treatment is usually required. Loperamide used cautiously may be helpful in children with socially disruptive symptoms.

Inflammatory bowel disease

Crohn's disease

Since the 1950s, there has been a marked increase in the incidence of Crohn's disease in all age groups. It becomes progressively more common throughout childhood. In northern Europe and North America, the overall incidence is about 4 per 100 000. About a quarter of patients with Crohn's disease present in childhood or adolescence.

Crohn's disease is a transmural, focal, subacute or chronic inflammatory disease. It affects any part of the gastrointestinal tract from the mouth to the anus, but most commonly the distal ileum and proximal colon. The affected intestine is thickened and adhesions between affected loops are common. Perianal skin tags, fissures and fistulae are also common. The histological hallmark is the presence of non-caseating epithelioid cell granulomata.

Abdominal pain, diarrhoea and growth failure with pubertal delay are the most common presenting features. There may be oral and perianal ulcers. The disease may be insidious in onset, and extraintestinal symptoms such as growth failure, intermittent fever, arthritis, uveitis and erythema nodosum may be present with few or no pointers towards gastrointestinal disease. Some adolescents may present with a clinical picture virtually indistinguishable from anorexia nervosa.

Diagnosis rests upon the demonstration of characteristic abnormalities on barium follow-through (narrowing, fissuring, mucosal irregularities and mural thickening), and at colonoscopy and on histology of a biopsy. Acute phase reactants, e.g. C-reactive protein and ESR, are usually raised and can be useful in monitoring disease severity. The aims of treatment are to induce remission by suppressing inflammation by treatment with steroids or by using an elemental diet for about 6 weeks. Recurrence is common but azathioprine may be helpful in maintaining remission. Anti tumour necrosis factor α (infliximab) may be needed as a third-line agent when conventional treatments have failed. Overnight enteral feeding may be helpful in correcting growth failure. Surgery is necessary for complications of Crohn's disease – obstruction, fistulae, failed medical treatment, growth failure or abscess formation. In general, the long-term prognosis for Crohn's disease beginning in childhood is good and most patients lead normal lives despite occasional recurrent disease.

Growth failure and delayed puberty are features of Crohn's disease in children

Ulcerative colitis

Ulcerative colitis is a recurrent, inflammatory and ulcerating disease involving the mucous membrane of the colon. Characteristically, the disease presents with rectal bleeding, diarrhoea, colicky pain and weight loss.

The diagnosis is made on the characteristic appearance at colonoscopy and on the histological features, after exclusion of infective causes of colitis. Extraintestinal complications include erythema nodosum, pyoderma gangrenosum, arthritis and spondylitis. There is an increased incidence of adenocarcinoma of the colon in adults (1 in 200 risk for each year of disease between 10 and 20 years from diagnosis).

Mild attacks are managed with topical steroids when the disease is confined to the rectum and sigmoid colon, or sulfasalazine for more extensive disease. More severe disease requires systemic steroids. Severe fulminating disease is a medical emergency and requires treatment with broad-spectrum antibiotics, intravenous fluids and steroids. One-third of patients require colectomy during the course of their disease. Colectomy is performed for chronic poorly controlled disease, to prevent malignancy in long-standing disease or for severe fulminating disease, sometimes complicated by a toxic megacolon, which fails to respond to intensive medical treatment.

Constipation

In healthy infants there is a wide range in bowel frequency. Breast-fed infants may not pass stools for several days and be entirely healthy. In young children, constipation, which is the painful passage of hard, infrequent stools, is common. It often follows an acute febrile illness or a transient superficial anal fissure. The problem usually resolves with mild laxatives and extra fluids. Occasionally, following such events, or perhaps in association with forceful potty training, the use of uncomfortable lavatories on holiday or at school, or psychological family stress, more protracted constipation results. Children may refrain from defecation for fear of the associated pain. The rectum becomes full and overdistended, and with time the capacity of the rectum increases and the sensation of needing to defecate is lost. Involuntary soiling usually follows as contractions of the full rectum inhibit the internal sphincter leading to overflow. Children of school age are frequently teased as a result and secondary behavioural problems are common. At this stage, the use of stimulant laxatives without first emptying the rectum completely is likely to make soiling worse.

Examination often reveals an abdominal mass and, on rectal examination, stool is present down to the anal margin. Organic causes of constipation are uncommon, but hypothyroidism, hypercalcaemia, a urinary concentrating defect or Hirschsprung's disease should be considered.

It should be explained to the child and the parents that soiling is involuntary and that recovery of normal rectal size and sensation may take a long time.

For mild cases, where faeces are not palpable per abdomen, dietary fluid and fibre should be increased. Stool softeners (lactulose or docusate) and stimulant laxatives (sodium picosulfate or senna) may be required.

For more severe cases, when the faeces are palpable per abdomen, the first aim of management is to evacuate the overloaded rectum completely. Following 1–2 weeks of stool softeners (macrogol (Movicol), lactulose or docusate), large doses of powerful oral laxatives (sodium picosulfate or senna) and high volumes of oral macrogol solutions (Movicol) are given daily until the stools are liquid. Advice about improving the dietary fluid and food intake is given. This is followed by daily evening doses of a stimulant laxative (e.g. senna), combined with regular postprandial visits to the lavatory, and a star chart may be introduced to record and reward progress.

Encouragement by family and health professionals is essential, as relapse is common and psychological support is sometimes required. Occasionally the faecal retention is so severe that evacuation is only possible using enemas or by manual evacuation under an anaesthetic. Care must be taken to avoid distress if enemas or washouts are used. The management of constipation is summarised in Figure 13.13.

Hirschsprung's disease

The absence of ganglion cells from the myenteric and submucosal plexuses of part of the large bowel results in a narrow, contracted segment. The abnormal bowel extends from the rectum for a variable distance proximally, ending in a normally innervated, dilated colon. In 75% of cases, the lesion is confined to the rectosigmoid, but in 10% the entire colon is involved. Presentation is usually in the neonatal period with intestinal obstruction heralded by failure to pass meconium within the first 24 hours of life. Abdominal distension and later bile-stained vomiting develop (Fig. 13.14). Rectal examination may reveal a narrowed segment and withdrawal of the examining finger often releases a gush of liquid stool and flatus. Temporary improvement in the obstruction following the dilatation caused by the rectal examination can lead to a delay in diagnosis.

Occasionally infants present with severe, life-threatening Hirschsprung's enterocolitis during the first few weeks of life, sometimes due to *Clostridium difficile* infection. In later childhood, presentation is with chronic constipation, usually profound, and associated with abdominal distension but usually without soiling. Growth failure may also be present.

Diagnosis is made by demonstrating the absence of ganglion cells together with the presence of large, acetylcholinesterase-positive nerve trunks

Constipation management algorithm

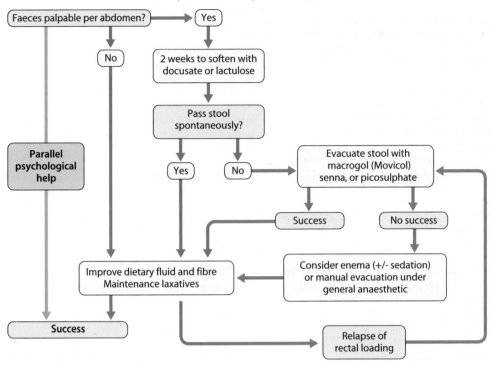

Figure 13.13 Summary of the management of constipation.

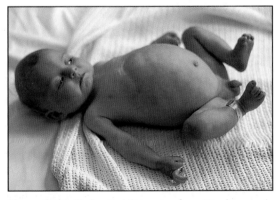

Figure 13.14 Abdominal distension from Hirschsprung's disease.

on a suction rectal biopsy. Anorectal manometry or barium studies may be useful in giving the surgeon an idea of the length of the aganglionic segment but are unreliable for diagnostic purposes. Management is surgical and usually involves an initial colostomy followed by anastomosing normally innervated bowel to the anus.

Summary

Hirschsprung's disease:
- absence of myenteric plexuses of rectum and variable distance of colon
- presentation – usually intestinal obstruction in the newborn period following delay in passing meconium. In later childhood – with profound chronic constipation, abdominal distension and growth failure
- diagnosis – suction rectal biopsy.

Further reading

Walker W A, Goulet O V, Kleinman R E, Sherman P M, Schneider B L, Sanderson I R (eds) 2004 Pediatric gastrointestinal disease, 4th edn. Decker, Ontario. *Comprehensive 2-volume textbook*

Constipation

14

Infection

At birth, infants possess all the essential components of the immune system, although these are immature. Circulating immunoglobulins are derived transplacentally from the mother (Fig. 14.1) and decrease during the first few months of life, leaving them susceptible to the common infections.

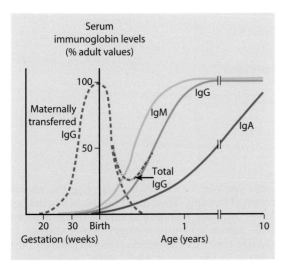

Figure 14.1 Serum immunoglobulin levels in the fetus and infant. When maternal immunoglobulin levels decline, infants become susceptible to viral infections.

Infections are the most common cause of acute illness in children. Worldwide, acute respiratory infections, diarrhoea, malaria, measles and HIV infection, often accompanied by malnutrition, are major causes of death (Fig. 14.2). It has been estimated that each year they are responsible for the deaths of about 7 million children under the age of 5 years.

In developed countries, with improved nutrition, living conditions, sanitation, immunisations, antibiotic therapy and modern medical care, morbidity from infections has declined dramatically, and deaths from infectious diseases are uncommon. However, some infections remain a major problem, e.g. meningococcal septicaemia, meningitis, malaria and HIV. Some have re-emerged, e.g. tuberculosis. Children with immuno-deficiency, whether congenital or acquired, are also vulnerable to a range of unusual or opportunist pathogens. To facilitate the control of communicable diseases within the community, certain diseases must be notified by doctors to the local public health specialist.

Many of the common childhood infections present with both a rash and fever. Figure 14.3 shows the different types of rash and the infections associated with them. The incubation period and length of time affected children should be kept away from nursery or school are shown in Table 14.1.

Worldwide causes of death in children < 5 years old

Each year, 7 million children die before 5 years of age from infections

Figure 14.2 Worldwide causes of death in children <5 years old (www.WHO.int, 2005).

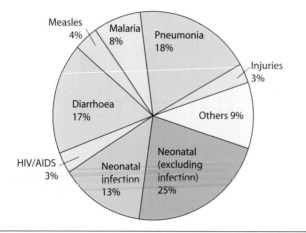

Figure 14.2 Worldwide causes of death in children <5 years old (www.WHO.int, 2005).

Malaria
- Deaths mostly from cerebral malaria from *Plasmodium falciparum* in Sub-Saharan Africa
- Antimalarial therapy must be started promptly, on clinical suspicion
- Drug resistance is problematic

Diarrhoea
- Most <2 years old
- Often bacterial
- Results in undernutrition, poor growth, death
- Usually treated with oral rehydration solution, continuing to breast-feed
- Antibiotics only for cholera, dysentry, giardiasis, amoebiasis

HIV
- > 2million children infected
- 14 million children orphaned through infection of parent

Tuberculosis
- Increasing incidence, especially with HIV infection
- > 150 000 deaths/year, from meningitis and disseminated miliary tuberculosis
- Usually acquired from infected adults in household

Pneumonia
- Risk factors – low birthweight, young age, not breast-fed, vitamin A deficiency, overcrowding
- Predominantly bacterial
- Mortality reduced by WHO guidelines for diagnosis (tachypnoea, cough, fever, head nodding and chest recession) and treatment with an antibiotic

Measles
- Preventable by immunisation

Common viral infections

Measles

Since the introduction of an effective vaccine in 1968, the incidence of measles in England and Wales has declined dramatically, from a peak of 800 000 cases per year in the early 1960s to 3000 cases per year in the 1990s. Following the widely reported but unjustified public health scares linking MMR (measles, mumps and rubella immunisation) with autism and inflammatory bowel disease in the late 1990s, immunisation rates declined and the disease incidence has risen again, appearing in clusters in unvaccinated populations. In un-vaccinated individuals, older children tend to have more severe disease than the very young. For

Rashes caused by childhood infections

Type of lesion	Infection
Macular/papular/maculopapular Macules – red/pink discrete flat areas, blanch on pressure Papules – solid raised hemispherical lesions, usually tiny, also blanch on pressure	Rubella (macular only), measles, HHV6/7, enterovirus Uncommon: scarlet fever, Kawasaki's disease (but remember drug rashes)
Purpuric/petechial Non-blanching red/purple spots, test with a glass	Meningococcal, Henoch–Schönlein purpura, enterovirus, thrombocytopenia
Vesicular Raised hemispherical lesions, <0.5 cm diameter, contain clear fluid	Chickenpox, shingles, herpes simplex, hand, foot and mouth disease
Pustular/bullous Raised hemispherical lesions, >0.5 cm diameter, contain clear or purulent fluid	Impetigo, scalded skin syndrome
Desquamation Dry and flaky loss of surface epidermis, often peripheries	Post-scarlet fever, Kawasaki's disease

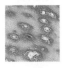

Figure 14.3 Rashes caused by childhood infections.

Table 14.1 Incubation and school exclusion period of common childhood infections

Illness	Incubation (days)	Period of infectiousness	School/nursery exclusion
Chickenpox (varicella)	10–23 (median 14)	-2 to +5 days	Until all lesions have crusted
Enterovirus (non-polio; non hand, foot and mouth)	2–7	NK	Only with viral meningitis outbreak
Gastroenteritis (viral)	1–10	NK	24 hours from last episode of diarrhoea
Gastroenteritis (bacterial)	1–10 depending on organism	1–3 weeks depending on organism	24 hours from last episode of diarrhoea except for E. Coli – 2 negative stools
Hand, foot and mouth (Coxsackie)	3–5	<7 days	None
Herpes simplex stomatitis	3–5	NK	Until lesions have crusted or been treated
HHV6/7	10–15	NK	None
Impetigo	2–15	NK	Until lesions are dry
Measles	6–19 (median 13)	1–2 days prior to rash to 6 days after	5 days from onset of rash
Mumps	15–24 (median 19)	NK	7 days from onset of parotitis
Parvovirus	13–18	NK	None
Rubella	15–20 (median 17)	Most infectious in prodrome	5 days from onset of rash
Tuberculosis	1–12 months	NK	If sputum positive: for 2 weeks after treatment starts; culture negative: none

NK: not known.
Source: Richardson et al (2001) *Pediatric Infectious Disease Journal* 20(4):380–391.

Clinical features and complications of measles

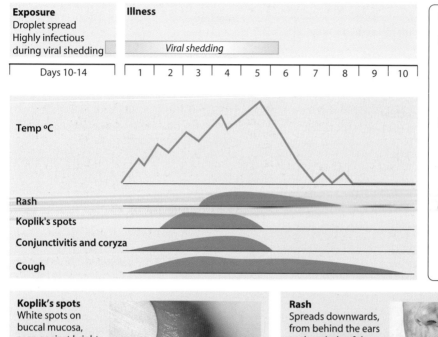

Complications
Respiratory
Pneumonia
Secondary bacterial infection and otitis media
Tracheitis
Neurological
Febrile convulsions
EEG abnormalities
Encephalitis
Subacute sclerosing panencephalitis (SSPE)
Other
Diarrhoea
Hepatitis
Appendicitis
Corneal ulceration
Myocarditis

Koplik's spots
White spots on buccal mucosa, seen against bright red background. Pathognomonic, but difficult to see.

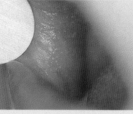

Rash
Spreads downwards, from behind the ears to the whole of the body. Discrete, maculopapular rash initially, becomes blotchy and confluent. May desquamate in second week.

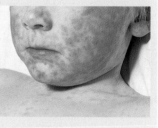

Figure 14.4 Clinical features and complications of measles.

epidemiological tracking of infection, serological confirmation of clinical cases of measles should be undertaken by testing either blood or saliva.

Clinical features

These are shown in Figure 14.4. There are a number of serious complications which can occur in previously healthy children:

- *Encephalitis* – occurs in only 1 in 5000, about 8 days after the onset of the illness. Initial symptoms are headache, lethargy and irritability, proceeding to convulsions and ultimately coma. Mortality is 15%. Serious long-term sequelae include seizures, deafness, hemiplegia and severe learning difficulties affecting up to 40% of survivors.
- *Subacute sclerosing panencephalitis (SSPE)* – a rare but devastating illness manifesting, on average, 7 years after measles infection in about 1 in 100 000 cases. Most children who develop SSPE had primary measles infection before 2 years of age. SSPE is caused by a variant of the measles virus which persists in the central nervous system. The disorder presents with loss of neurological function, which progresses over several years to dementia and death. The diagnosis is essentially clinical, supported by finding high levels of measles antibody in both blood and cerebrospinal

fluid and by characteristic EEG abnormalities. Since the introduction of measles immunisation, it has become extremely rare.

In developing countries, where malnutrition and particularly vitamin A deficiency lead to impaired cell-mediated immunity, measles often follows a protracted course with severe complications. The rash may progress to a dark red/violet colour followed by desquamation and depigmentation, which may last weeks or months. Pre-existing malnutrition is further exacerbated by oral infections and diarrhoea.

Lack of an effective T-lymphocyte response in immunocompromised patients makes measles a dangerous illness. A measles interstitial pneumonitis, known as 'giant cell pneumonia', may be fatal in children with malignant disease, even when in remission. These children are also susceptible to a measles encephalopathy.

Treatment

Treatment for measles is symptomatic. Children who are admitted to hospital should be isolated. In immunocompromised patients, the antiviral drug ribavirin may be used. Vitamin A, which may modulate the immune response, should be given in developing countries.

Prevention

Prevention by immunisation is the most successful strategy for reducing the morbidity and mortality of measles. There is a 10% vaccine failure rate from primary vaccination with MMR (measles, mumps, rubella vaccine) at 12–18 months of age, but immunisation coverage of school-age children in the UK has been improved by the introduction of a preschool booster of MMR.

❀ **Measles remains a major cause of death in childhood in developing countries.**

⊙ Summary

Measles:
- incidence has declined dramatically since immunisation was introduced; recent small increase from fall in immunisation uptake
- clinical features – fever, cough, runny nose, conjunctivitis, marked malaise, Koplik's spots, maculopapular rash
- complications – common if malnourished or immunocompromised; major cause of death in developing countries.

Mumps

Mumps occurs worldwide, but its incidence has declined dramatically because of the mumps component of the MMR vaccine. Following the decrease in the uptake of the MMR immunisation in the late 1990s, there has been a rise in unimmunised children and unvaccinated young adults. Mumps usually occurs in the winter and spring months. It is spread by droplet infection to the respiratory tract where the virus replicates within epithelial cells. The virus gains access to the parotid glands before further dissemination to other tissues.

Clinical features

The incubation period is 15–24 days. Onset of the illness is with fever, malaise and parotitis, but in up to 30% of cases the infection is subclinical. Only one side may be swollen initially, but bilateral involvement usually occurs over the next few days. The parotitis is uncomfortable and children may complain of earache or pain on eating or drinking. Examination of the parotid duct may show redness and swelling. Occasionally, parotid swelling may be absent. The fever usually disappears within 3–4 days. Plasma amylase levels are often elevated and, when associated with abdominal pain, may be evidence of pancreatic involvement. Infectivity is for up to 7 days after the onset of parotid swelling. The illness is generally mild and self-limiting. Although hearing loss can follow mumps, it is usually unilateral and transient.

Viral meningitis and encephalitis

Lymphocytes are seen in the CSF in about 50%, meningeal signs are only seen in 10% and encephalitis in about 1 in 5000. The common clinical features are headache, photophobia, vomiting and neck stiffness.

Orchitis

This is the most feared complication, although it is uncommon in prepubertal males. When it does occur, it is usually unilateral. Although there is some evidence of a reduction in sperm count, infertility is actually extremely unusual. Rarely, oophoritis, mastitis and arthritis may occur.

Rubella (German measles)

Rubella is generally a mild disease in childhood. It occurs in winter and spring. It is an important infection as it can cause severe damage to the fetus (see Ch. 9). The incubation period is 15–20 days. It is spread by the respiratory route, frequently from a known contact. The prodrome is usually mild with a low-grade fever or none at all. The maculopapular rash is often the first sign of infection, appearing initially on the face and then spreading centrifugally to cover the whole body. It fades in 3–5 days. Unlike in adults, the rash is not itchy. Lymphadenopathy, particularly the suboccipital and postauricular nodes, is prominent. Complications are rare in childhood but include arthritis, encephalitis, thrombocytopenia and myocarditis. Clinical differentiation from other viral infections is unreliable. The diagnosis should be confirmed serologically if there is any risk of exposure of a non-immune pregnant woman. There is no effective antiviral treatment. Prevention therefore lies in immunisation.

⊙ Summary

Rubella
- importance – congenital infection.

The human herpesviruses

There are currently eight known human herpesviruses (herpes simplex virus 1 and 2, varicella zoster virus, cytomegalovirus, Epstein–Barr virus, and human herpesviruses 6, 7 and 8). The hallmark of the herpesviruses is that, after primary infection, latency is established and there is long-term persistence of the virus within the host, usually in a dormant state. After certain stimuli, reactivation of infection may occur.

1. Herpes simplex infections

Herpes simplex virus (HSV) usually enters the body through the mucous membranes or skin. The incubation period for primary infection is 3–5 days. After the neonatal period, HSV1 infections

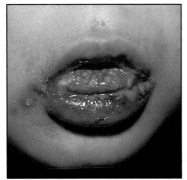

Figure 14.5
Vesicles with ulceration in gingivostomatitis.

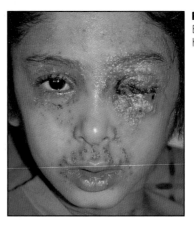

Figure 14.6
Eczema herpeticum.

predominate. The prevalence of HSV2 increases in early adulthood. HSV1 is transmitted in body fluids such as saliva, while HSV2 is mainly transmitted through the transfer of genital secretions. The wide variety of clinical manifestations are described below. Treatment is with aciclovir, a viral DNA polymerase inhibitor, which may be used to treat severe symptomatic skin, ophthalmic, cerebral and systemic infections.

Asymptomatic

Herpes simplex infections are very common and are mostly asymptomatic.

Gingivostomatitis

This is the most common form of primary HSV illness in children. It usually occurs from 10 months to 3 years of age. There are vesicular lesions on the lips, gums and anterior surfaces of the tongue and hard palate, which often progress to extensive, painful ulceration with bleeding (Fig. 14.5). There is a high fever and the child is very miserable. The illness may persist for up to 2 weeks. Eating and drinking are painful, which may lead to dehydration. Management is symptomatic, but severe disease may necessitate intravenous fluids and aciclovir.

Skin manifestations

Mucocutaneous junctions and damaged skin are particularly prone to infection. 'Cold sores' are recurrent HSV1 lesions on the lip margin.

Eczema herpeticum In this serious condition, widespread vesicular lesions develop on eczematous skin (Fig. 14.6). This may be complicated by secondary bacterial infection, which may result in septicaemia.

Herpetic whitlows These are painful, erythematous, oedematous white pustules on the site of broken skin on the fingers. Spread is by autoinoculation from gingivostomatitis and infected adults kissing their children's fingers. In sexually active adolescents, HSV2 may be the cause.

Eye disease

Eye disease may cause a blepharitis or conjunctivitis. It may extend to involve the cornea,

producing dendritic ulceration. This can lead to corneal scarring and ultimately loss of vision. Any child with herpetic lesions near or involving the eye requires ophthalmic investigation of the cornea by slit lamp examination.

Central nervous system infection

Aseptic meningitis This is rare in children, but may occur in sexually active adolescents. It is usually a complication of HSV2 infection, occurring within 10 days of a primary infection. It resolves without sequelae.

Encephalitis By contrast, this is a very serious condition with a mortality of more than 70% if untreated. It may follow either primary or recurrent infection. The clinical features and management are described on p. 243.

Neonatal infection (see Ch. 10) The infection may be focal, affecting the skin or eyes, may cause encephalitis or may be widely disseminated. Its morbidity and mortality are high.

Infection in the immunocompromised host Infection is severe. Cutaneous lesions may spread to involve adjacent sites, e.g. oesophagitis and proctitis. Pneumonia and disseminated infections involving multiple organs are serious complications.

2. Varicella zoster

Chickenpox

Varicella zoster virus (VZV) shares many features with HSV, as both produce a vesicular rash. In contrast to HSV, however, varicella zoster is spread by the respiratory route, progressing via the blood and lymphatics to cause vesicular lesions in the skin. More than 90% of primary VZV infections are clinically symptomatic with a vesicular rash.

Clinical features These are shown in Figure 14.7. There are a number of rare but serious complications which can occur in previously healthy children:

- *Secondary bacterial infection* with staphylococci, streptococci or other organisms. May lead to

Clinical features and complications of chickenpox

Exposure
Spread by respiratory droplets
Highly infectious during viral shedding

Illness

Viral shedding

Days: incubation
10–23 (median 14) −2 −1 0 1 2 3 4 5 6 7

Temp (°C): 40°C — 37°C

Papules
Vesicles
Pustules
Crusts

Rash comes in crops for 3–5 days

Complications

Bacterial superinfection
Staphylococcal
Streptococcal
May lead to toxic shock syndrome or necrotising fasciitis

Central nervous system
Cerebellitis
Generalised encephalitis
Aseptic meningitis

Immunocompromised
Haemorrhagic lesions
Pneumonitis
Progressive and disseminated infection
Disseminated intravascular coagulation

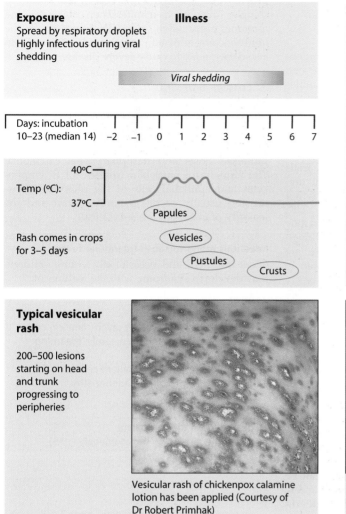

Typical vesicular rash

200–500 lesions starting on head and trunk progressing to peripheries

Vesicular rash of chickenpox calamine lotion has been applied (Courtesy of Dr Robert Primhak)

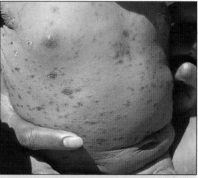

Haemorrhagic chickenpox seen in malnourished or immunodeficient children (Courtesy of Dr Sam Walters)

Figure 14.7 Clinical features and complications of chickenpox.

further complications such as toxic shock syndrome or necrotising fasciitis. Secondary bacterial infection should be considered where there is onset of a new fever or persistent high fever after the first few days.

- *Encephalitis*. This may be generalised, usually occurring early during the illness. In contrast to the encephalitis caused by HSV, the prognosis is good. Most characteristic is a VZV-associated cerebellitis. This usually occurs within a week of the onset of rash. The child is ataxic with cerebellar signs. It usually resolves over a few days.
- *Purpura fulminans*. This is the consequence of vasculitis in the skin and subcutaneous tissues. It is best known in relation to meningococcal disease and can lead to loss of large areas of skin by necrosis. It may rarely occur after VZV infection due to production of antiviral antibodies which cross-react and inactivate the coagulation factor protein S. There is subsequent dysregulation of fibrinolysis and an increased risk of clotting, most often manifest in the skin.

- *Strokes*. Although very rare, there is an increased incidence of strokes in children after VZV infection, due to either vasculitis or protein S deficiency.

In the immunocompromised, primary varicella infection may result in severe progressive disseminated disease, which has a mortality of up to 20%. The vesicular eruptions persist and frequently become haemorrhagic (see Fig. 14.7). The disease in the neonatal period is described in Chapter 10.

Treatment and prevention Human varicella zoster immunoglobulin (ZIG) is recommended for high-risk immunosuppressed individuals with deficient T-lymphocyte function, following contact with chickenpox. They include:

- bone marrow transplant recipients
- patients with congenital or acquired immune deficiency affecting T cell function
- patients on high doses of steroids or other immunosuppressive drugs within the previous 3 months

- neonates whose mothers develop varicella within 5 days before or 2 days after delivery
- neonates born at less than 30 weeks' gestation who have been exposed to varicella.

Protection from infection with zoster immuno-globulin is not absolute, and depends on how soon after contact with chickenpox it is given. Families should be warned that after zoster immuno-globulin, onset of chickenpox may be delayed and the lesions may be atypical, so they should seek urgent medical attention if any rash appears. Intravenous aciclovir should be given in severe chickenpox and in the immunocompromised. Trials in the USA have shown some benefit from oral aciclovir in normal children, but the drug is not currently recommended for this in the UK. Adolescents should be treated with aciclovir as they are more likely to develop severe disease. Although an effective varicella vaccine exists, there are concerns that adults may become susceptible to infection when immunity wanes. It is not currently part of the routine immunisation schedule in the UK, although it is in the USA and many other countries.

> ❀ **Beware of admitting a chickenpox contact to a clinical area with immunocompromised children.**

Shingles (herpes zoster)

Latent varicella zoster can reactivate, causing a vesicular eruption in the distribution of sensory nerves (shingles). It occurs most commonly in the thoracic region, although any dermatome can be affected (Fig. 14.8). Children, unlike adults, rarely suffer neuralgic pain with shingles. Shingles in

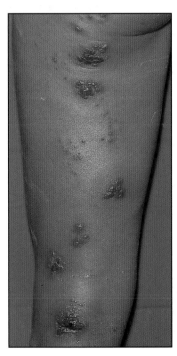

Figure 14.8
Herpes zoster (shingles) in a child. Distribution is along the S1 dermatome.

childhood is more common in those who had primary infection in the first year of life. Recurrent shingles may be a manifestation of underlying immune suppression, e.g. HIV infection. In the immunocompromised, reactivated infection can also disseminate to cause severe disease.

3. Epstein–Barr virus

Epstein–Barr virus (EBV) is the major cause of the infectious mononucleosis syndrome, but it is also involved in the pathogenesis of Burkitt's lymph-oma, lymphoproliferative disease in immunocom-promised hosts and nasopharyngeal carcinoma. The virus has a particular tropism for B lympho-cytes and epithelial cells of the pharynx. Trans-mission usually occurs by oral contact and the majority of infections are subclinical.

Infectious mononucleosis (glandular fever)

Older children, and occasionally young children, may develop a syndrome with the features of:

- fever
- malaise
- tonsillopharyngitis – often severe, limiting oral ingestion of fluids and food; rarely, breathing may be compromised
- lymphadenopathy – prominent cervical lymph nodes, often with diffuse adenopathy.

Other features include:

- petechiae on the soft palate
- splenomegaly (50%), hepatomegaly (10%)
- a maculopapular rash (5%)
- jaundice.

Diagnosis is supported by:

- atypical lymphocytes (numerous large T cells seen on blood film)
- a positive Monospot test (the presence of heterophil antibodies, i.e. antibodies that agglutinate sheep or horse erythrocytes but which are not absorbed by guinea pig kidney extracts – this test is often negative in young children with the disease)
- seroconversion with production of IgM and IgG to Epstein–Barr virus antigens.

Symptoms may persist for 1–3 months but ultimately resolve. They are caused by the host immune response to the infection, rather than the virus itself.

Treatment is symptomatic. When the airway is severely compromised, corticosteroids may be considered. In 5% of infected individuals, group A *Streptococcus* is grown from the tonsils. This should be treated with penicillin. Ampicillin or amoxicillin may cause a florid maculopapular rash in children infected with EBV and should be avoided.

4. Cytomegalovirus (CMV)

Cytomegalovirus is usually transmitted via saliva, genital secretions or breast milk, and more rarely via blood products, organ transplants and transplacentally. The virus causes mild or subclinical infection in normal hosts. In developed countries, about half of the adult population show serological evidence of past infection. In developing countries, most children have been infected by 2 years of age, often via breast milk. In the immunocompromised and the fetus, CMV is an important pathogen.

As with EBV, CMV may cause a mononucleosis syndrome. Pharyngitis and lymphadenopathy are not usually as prominent as in EBV infections. Patients may have atypical lymphocytes on the blood film but are heterophile antibody-negative. Maternal CMV infection may result in congenital infection (see Ch. 9), which may be present at birth or develop when older. In the immunocompromised host, CMV can cause retinitis, pneumonitis, bone marrow failure, encephalitis, hepatitis, colitis and oesophagitis. It is a very important pathogen following organ transplantation. Organ recipients are closely monitored for evidence of CMV activation by sensitive tests such as polymerase chain reaction (PCR). Interventions used to reduce the risk of transmission of CMV disease are CMV-negative blood for transfusions and anti-CMV drug prophylaxis; also, if possible, CMV-positive organs are not transplanted into CMV-negative recipients.

CMV disease may be treated with ganciclovir or foscarnet, but both have serious side-effects.

5. Human herpesvirus 6 (HHV6)

Most children are infected with HHV6 by the age of 2, usually from the oral secretions of a family member. The classic infectious syndrome associated with HHV6 is exanthem subitum (also known as roseola infantum) where there is a high fever with malaise lasting a few days, followed by a generalised macular rash which appears as the fever wanes. Many children have a febrile illness without rash, and some have a subclinical infection. Exanthem subitum is frequently clinically misdiagnosed as measles or rubella; these more significant infections should be confirmed serologically. Another frequent clinical consequence of primary HHV6 infection is that infants seen by a doctor during the febrile stage may be prescribed antibiotics, and then, when the rash appears, it is erroneously attributed to an 'allergic' reaction to the drug. Primary HHV6 infection is a common cause of febrile convulsions. It is associated with up to a third of febrile convulsions in the first year of life. HHV6 has rarely been associated with aseptic meningitis, encephalitis, hepatitis, infectious mononucleosis-like syndrome and haematological malignancies.

6. Human herpesvirus 7 (HHV7)

This virus is very closely related to HHV6, causing similar clinical disease, including exanthem subitum and febrile convulsions. Again, most children are infected with HHV7 in the first few years of life.

Summary

Herpesvirus infections

Herpes simplex infections:
- most asymptomatic
- gingivostomatitis – may necessitate intravenous fluids and aciclovir
- skin manifestations – mucocutaneous junctions, e.g. lips and damaged skin
- eczema herpeticum – may result in secondary bacterial infection and septicaemia
- herpetic whitlows – painful pustules on the fingers
- eye disease – blepharitis, conjunctivitis, corneal ulceration and scarring
- CNS – aseptic meningitis, encephalitis
- pneumonia and disseminated infection in the immunocompromised

Chickenpox:
- clinical features – fever and itchy, vesicular rash which crops
- complications – secondary bacterial infection, encephalitis; disseminated disease in the immunocompromised
- human varicella zoster immunoglobulin (ZIG) – if immunosuppressed and in contact with chickenpox or if maternal chickenpox shortly before or after delivery
- treatment is symptomatic; aciclovir for severe chickenpox or immunocompromised.

7. Human herpesvirus 8 (HHV8)

This virus is associated with Kaposi's sarcoma (KS), a tumour which occurs in immunosuppressed patients as well as certain populations in Africa and around the Mediterranean. HHV8 does not appear to be associated with disease in otherwise healthy children. Primary HHV8 infection may be associated with a mild febrile illness, and infection is usually transmitted from saliva. Up to 40% of African teenagers have antibodies to HHV8, whereas <5% are seropositive in the UK.

Parvovirus B19

Parvovirus B19 causes erythema infectiosum or fifth disease (so-named because it was the fifth disease to be described of a group of illnesses with similar rashes), also called slapped cheek syndrome. Infections can occur at any time of the year, although outbreaks are most common during the spring months. Transmission is via respiratory secretions from viraemic patients, by vertical transmission from mother to fetus and by transfusion of contaminated blood products. Parvovirus B19 infects the erythroblastoid red cell precursors in the bone marrow.

Parvovirus causes a range of clinical syndromes:

- asymptomatic infection – common; about 5–10% of preschool children and 65% of adults have antibodies

- erythema infectiosum – the most common illness, with a viraemic phase of fever, malaise, headache and myalgia followed by a characteristic rash a week later on the face ('slapped cheek'), progressing to a maculopapular, 'lace'-like rash on the trunk and limbs; complications are rare in children, although arthralgia or arthritis is common in adults
- aplastic crisis – the most serious consequence of parvovirus infection; it occurs in children with chronic haemolytic anaemias, where there is an increased rate of red cell turnover (e.g. sickle cell disease or thalassaemia); and in immunodeficient children (e.g. malignancy) who are unable to produce an antibody response to neutralise the infection
- fetal disease – transmission of maternal parvovirus infection may lead to fetal hydrops and death due to severe anaemia, although the majority of infected fetuses will recover.

Summary

Parvovirus:
- usually asymptomatic or erythema infectiosum
- can cause aplastic crisis in haemolytic anaemias (e.g. sickle cell) or the fetus (causes hydrops).

Enteroviruses

Human enteroviruses, of which there are many (including the coxsackie viruses, echoviruses and polio viruses), are a common cause of childhood infection. Transmission is primarily by the faecal–oral route. Following replication in the pharynx and gut, the virus spreads to infect other organs. Infections occur most commonly in the summer and autumn. Over 90% of infections are asymptomatic or cause a non-specific febrile illness, but characteristic clinical syndromes exist and are listed below. An effective vaccine is available against the polioviruses.

The following may be caused by enteroviruses:

Asymptomatic or non-specific febrile illness
Over 90% of infections.

Herpangina
Vesicular and ulcerated lesions on the soft palate and uvula causing anorexia, pain on swallowing and fever.

Hand, foot and mouth disease
Painful vesicular lesions on the hands, feet, mouth and tongue. Systemic features are mild. The disease subsides within a few days.

Meningitis/encephalitis
Aseptic meningitis is caused by many of the enteroviruses. There may be a skin rash, which can

be petechial and therefore difficult to differentiate clinically from meningococcal infection. Complete recovery can be expected.

Pleurodynia (Bornholm's disease)
An acute illness with fever, pleuritic chest pain and muscle tenderness. There may be a pleural rub but examination is otherwise normal. Recovery is within a few days.

Myocarditis and pericarditis
Heart failure associated with a febrile illness and ECG evidence of myocarditis.

Poliovirus infection
Clinical disease is now very rare, due to successful immunisation programmes. It falls into four main categories:

- >90% are asymptomatic
- 5% have a poliomyelitis 'minor illness' – fever, headache, malaise, sore throat and vomiting occur within 4 days of exposure and recovery is uneventful
- 2% of patients progress to central nervous system involvement with aseptic meningitis; there is stiffness of the back, neck and hamstrings from meningeal irritation
- in <1% of cases, classical paralytic polio occurs about 4 days after the minor illness has subsided – involvement of the anterior horn cells and cerebral cortex leads to varying degrees of paralysis which may recover completely or be permanent; involvement of the muscles of respiration may call for long-term respiratory support or be fatal.

Infection in the immunocompromised host
Enteroviruses can cause severe disease in immunocompromised individuals. Echovirus can cause a persistent and sometimes fatal central nervous system infection in agammaglobulinaemic patients.

Summary

Enterovirus infections:
- mostly asymptomatic but can cause herpangina, hand, foot and mouth disease, meningitis/encephalitis.

Common bacterial infections

Staphylococcal and Group A streptococcal infections

Staphylococcal and streptococcal infections are usually caused by direct invasion of the organisms. They may also cause disease by releasing toxins which act as superantigens. Whereas conventional antigens stimulate only a small subset of T cells which have a specific receptor, superantigens bind

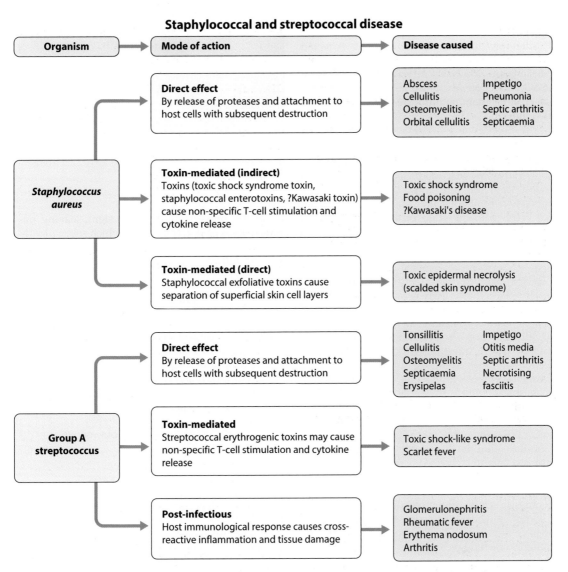

Staphylococcal and streptococcal disease

Organism	Mode of action	Disease caused

Staphylococcus aureus

Direct effect
By release of proteases and attachment to host cells with subsequent destruction

Abscess	Impetigo
Cellulitis	Pneumonia
Osteomyelitis	Septic arthritis
Orbital cellulitis	Septicaemia

Toxin-mediated (indirect)
Toxins (toxic shock syndrome toxin, staphylococcal enterotoxins, ?Kawasaki toxin) cause non-specific T-cell stimulation and cytokine release

Toxic shock syndrome
Food poisoning
?Kawasaki's disease

Toxin-mediated (direct)
Staphylococcal exfoliative toxins cause separation of superficial skin cell layers

Toxic epidermal necrolysis (scalded skin syndrome)

Group A streptococcus

Direct effect
By release of proteases and attachment to host cells with subsequent destruction

Tonsillitis	Impetigo
Cellulitis	Otitis media
Osteomyelitis	Septic arthritis
Septicaemia	Necrotising
Erysipelas	fasciitis

Toxin-mediated
Streptococcal erythrogenic toxins may cause non-specific T-cell stimulation and cytokine release

Toxic shock-like syndrome
Scarlet fever

Post-infectious
Host immunological response causes cross-reactive inflammation and tissue damage

Glomerulonephritis
Rheumatic fever
Erythema nodosum
Arthritis

Figure 14.9 Staphylococcal and streptococcal disease caused by direct invasion or by the release of toxins. Immune-mediated disease may also follow streptococcal infections.

to a part of the T-cell receptor which is shared by many T cells and therefore stimulates massive T-cell proliferation and cytokine release. Other diseases following staphylococcal and streptococcal infections are immune-mediated. The wide range of diseases caused by these organisms is shown in Figure 14.9.

Impetigo

This is a localised, highly contagious, staphylococcal and/or streptococcal skin infection, most common in infants and young children. It is more common where there is pre-existing skin disease, e.g. atopic eczema. Lesions are usually on the face, neck and hands and begin as erythematous macules which become vesicular (Fig. 14.10). Rupture of the vesicles with exudation of fluid leads to the characteristic confluent honey-coloured crusted lesions. The lesions are sometimes bullous. Infection is readily spread to adjacent areas and

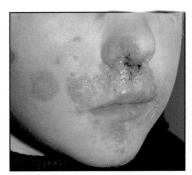

Figure 14.10 Impetigo showing characteristic confluent honey-coloured crusted lesions. (Courtesy of Dr Paul Hutchins.)

other parts of the body by autoinoculation of the infected exudate. Topical antibiotics (e.g. mupirocin) are sometimes effective for mild cases. Narrow-spectrum systemic antibiotics (e.g. flucloxacillin or erythromycin) are needed for more severe infections, although more broad-spectrum antibiotics such as co-amoxiclav or cefaclor have

Common bacterial infections

235

simpler oral administration regimens, taste better and therefore have better adherence. Affected children should not go to nursery or school until the lesions are dry. Nasal carriage is an important source of infection which can be eradicated with a nasal cream containing mupirocin or chlorhexidine and neomycin.

Boils

These are infections of hair follicles or sweat glands, usually caused by *Staphylococcus aureus*. Treatment is with systemic antibiotics and occasionally surgery. Recurrent boils are usually from persistent nasal carriage in the child or family acting as a reservoir for reinfection. Only rarely are they a manifestation of immune deficiency.

Periorbital cellulitis

In periorbital cellulitis there is fever with erythema, tenderness and oedema of the eyelid (Fig. 14.11). It is almost always unilateral. In young, unimmunised children it may also be caused by a *Haemophilus influenzae* type b infection, which may also cause infection at other sites, e.g. meningitis. It may follow local trauma to the skin. In older children, it may spread from a paranasal sinus infection or dental abscess. Periorbital cellulitis should be treated promptly with intravenous antibiotics to prevent posterior spread of the infection to become an orbital cellulitis. In orbital cellulitis, there is proptosis, painful or limited ocular movement and reduced visual acuity. It may be complicated by abscess formation, meningitis or cavernous sinus thrombosis. Where orbital cellulitis is suspected, a CT scan should be performed to assess the posterior spread of infection and a lumbar puncture may be required to exclude meningitis.

Scalded skin syndrome

This is caused by an exfoliative staphylococcal toxin which causes separation of the epidermal skin through the granular cell layers. It affects infants and young children, who develop fever and malaise and may have a purulent, crusting, localised infection around the eyes, nose and mouth with subsequent widespread erythema and tenderness of the skin. Areas of epidermis separate

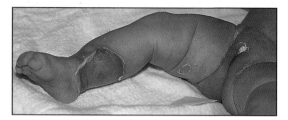

Figure 14.12 Staphylococcal scalded skin syndrome. Its appearance must not be mistaken for a scald from non-accidental injury.

on gentle pressure (Nikolsky's sign), leaving denuded areas of skin (Fig. 14.12) which subsequently dry and heal without scarring. Management is with an intravenous anti-staphylococcal antibiotic, analgesia and monitoring of fluid balance.

Summary

Staphylococcal and streptococcal infections:
- symptoms are caused by direct invasion of bacteria or by release of toxins
- impetigo is highly contagious
- periorbital cellulitis should be treated aggressively to prevent spread to the orbit or brain
- scalded skin syndrome is rare but serious.

Pneumococcal infections

Streptococcus pneumoniae is often present for long periods in the nasopharynx of healthy children. Asymptomatic carriage is particularly prevalent among young children and may be responsible for the transmission of pneumococcal disease to other individuals by respiratory droplets. The organism may cause pharyngitis, otitis media, conjunctivitis, sinusitis as well as 'invasive' disease (pneumonia, bacterial sepsis and meningitis). Invasive disease, which carries a high burden of morbidity and mortality, mainly occurs in young infants as their immune system responds poorly to encapsulated pathogens such as pneumococcus. With the inclusion of pneumococcal vaccine into the standard immunisation schedule in the UK, the incidence of invasive disease should decline. Children at increased risk, e.g. from hyposplenism, should also be given daily prophylactic penicillin.

Summary

Pneumococcal infection:
- causes not only minor infections such as otitis media but also invasive disease
- susceptibility is increased in hyposplenism (e.g. sickle cell disease and nephrotic syndrome)
- vaccination is now included in the standard immunisation schedule.

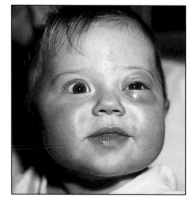

Figure 14.11 Periorbital cellulitis. It should be treated promptly with intravenous antibiotics to prevent spread into the orbit.

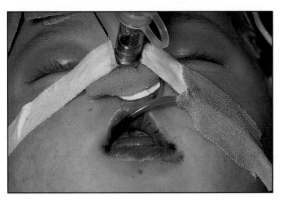

Figure 14.13 A child with toxic shock syndrome receiving intensive care, including artificial ventilation via a nasotracheal tube. The lips are red and the eyelids are oedematous from capillary leak. (Courtesy of Professor Mike Levin.)

Uncommon manifestations of common infections

Toxic shock syndrome

Toxin-producing staphylococci and streptococci can produce this syndrome. The toxin, released from infection at any site, including small abrasions, acts as a superantigen. It causes a systemic illness with high fever, a diffuse macular rash, hypotension and shock. There may be redness of the mucous membranes (Fig. 14.13), vomiting or diarrhoea, severe myalgia, altered consciousness, thrombocytopenia, non-purulent conjunctivitis, coagulopathy, and abnormal hepatic and renal function. About 1–2 weeks after the onset of the illness, there is desquamation of the palms, soles, fingers and toes. Intensive care support is required to manage the shock. Areas of infection should be surgically debrided. Intravenous immunoglobulin may be given to neutralise circulating toxin.

Necrotising fasciitis/necrotising cellulitis

This is a severe subcutaneous infection often involving tissue planes from the skin down to fascia and muscle. The skin surface involved may enlarge rapidly, leaving poorly perfused necrotic areas of tissue, usually at the centre. There is severe pain and systemic illness which may require intensive care. The invading organism may be staphylococcus or group A streptococcus, with or without another synergistic anaerobic organism. Intravenous antibiotic therapy alone is not sufficient to treat this condition. Without surgical intervention and debridement of necrotic tissue, the infection will continue to spread. Clinical suspicion of necrotising fasciitis warrants urgent surgical consultation and intervention.

Kawasaki's disease (acute febrile mucocutaneous syndrome)

Although uncommon, Kawasaki's disease is an important diagnosis to make, as aneurysms of the coronary arteries are an important complication. Prompt treatment reduces their incidence.

Kawasaki's disease mainly affects children of 6 months to 4 years old, with a peak at the end of the first year. The disease is much more common in children of Japanese and, to a lesser extent, Afro-Caribbean ethnicity than it is in Caucasians. Young infants tend to be more severely affected than older children. The cause is unknown, but the many clinical and immunological similarities with the staphylococcal and streptococcal toxic shock syndromes have led to the suggestion that it is also caused by a bacterial toxin acting as a superantigen. The diagnosis is made on clinical findings (Fig. 14.14). The disease is a vasculitis affecting the small and medium-sized vessels. It affects the coronary arteries in about one-third of affected children within the first 6 weeks of the illness. This can lead to aneurysms which are best visualised on echocardiography (see Case history 14.1). Subsequent narrowing of the vessels from scar formation can result in myocardial ischaemia and sudden death. Mortality is 1–2%.

Prompt treatment with intravenous immunoglobulin given within the first 10 days has been shown to lower the risk of coronary artery aneurysms. Aspirin is used to reduce the risk of thrombosis. It is given at a high anti-inflammatory dose until the fever subsides and continued at a low anti-platelet dose when there is an abnormality of the coronary arteries. When the platelet count is very high, anti-platelet aggregation agents may also be used to reduce the risk of coronary thrombosis. Children suspected of having the disease but who do not have all the clinical features should still be considered for treatment.

Prolonged fever – is it Kawasaki's disease?

Summary

Kawasaki's disease:
- mainly affects infants and young children
- the diagnosis is made on clinical features of fever >5 days and four other features of conjunctival injection, red mucous membranes, cervical lymphadenopathy, rash, red and oedematous palms and soles or peeling of fingers and toes
- complications – coronary artery aneurysms and sudden death
- treatment – intravenous immunoglobulin and aspirin.

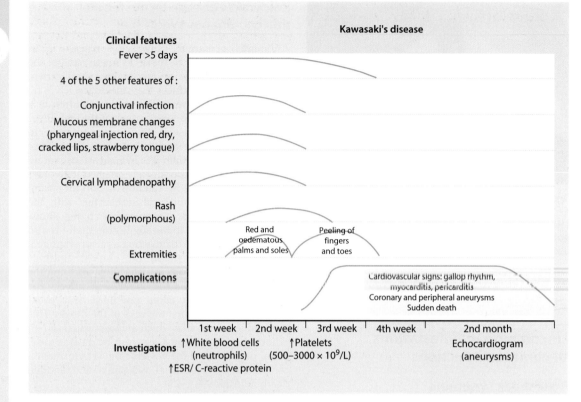

Kawasaki's disease

| Clinical features | | | | | |

Figure 14.14 Clinical features and investigations in Kawasaki's disease.

Case History
14.1 Kawasaki's disease

This 3-year-old boy developed a high fever of 3 days' duration. Examination showed a miserable child with mild conjunctivitis, a rash and cervical lymphadenopathy. A viral infection was diagnosed and his mother was reassured. When he presented to hospital 4 days later, he was noted to have cracked red lips (Fig. 14.15a). He was admitted and a full septic screen, including a lumbar puncture, was performed and antibiotics started. Despite this, 5 days later he was still febrile and irritable and the antibiotics were changed after a repeat blood count, blood and urine culture. He remained febrile and irritable. Four days later the neutrophil count was 15 × 10^9/L, platelet count 800 × 10^9/L and ESR (erythrocyte sedimentation rate) 125. Sixteen days into the illness, there was peeling of the skin of the fingers and toes (Fig. 14.15b) and Kawasaki's disease was suspected. An echocardiogram showed aneurysms of the coronary arteries. He was treated with intravenous immunoglobulins and oral aspirin, following which his clinical condition improved and he became afebrile. Delayed diagnosis meant that the potential benefit from immunoglobulin therapy and aspirin in preventing coronary artery aneurysms was missed.

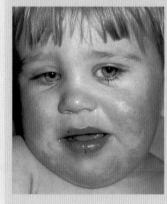

Figure 14.15a Red, cracked lips and conjunctival inflammation.

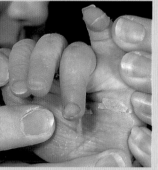

Figure 14.15b Peeling of the fingers, which developed on the 15th day of the illness.

Rare but important infections

Septicaemia

This is considered in Chapter 6 on paediatric emergencies.

Meningitis

Meningitis occurs when there is inflammation of the meninges covering the brain. This can be confirmed by finding inflammatory cells in the cerebrospinal fluid (CSF). Viral infections are the most common cause of meningitis, and most are self-resolving. Bacterial meningitis may have severe consequences. Other causes of non-infectious meningitis include malignancy and autoimmune diseases.

Bacterial meningitis

Over 80% of patients with bacterial meningitis in the UK are younger than 16 years old. Bacterial meningitis remains a serious infection in children, with a 5–10% mortality. Over 10% of survivors are left with long-term neurological impairment.

Pathophysiology

Bacterial infection of the meninges usually follows bacteraemia. It is now thought that much of the damage caused by meningeal infection results from the host response to infection and not from the organism itself. The release of inflammatory mediators and activated leucocytes, together with endothelial damage, leads to cerebral oedema, raised intracranial pressure and decreased cerebral blood flow.

Organisms

The organisms which commonly cause bacterial meningitis vary according to the child's age (Table 14.2).

Presentation

The clinical features are listed in Figure 14.16. The early signs and symptoms of meningitis are non-specific, which makes early diagnosis difficult. Infants and young children may present with any combination of fever, poor feeding, vomiting, irritability, lethargy, drowsiness, seizures or reduced

Table 14.2 Organisms causing bacterial meningitis according to age

Neonatal–3 months	Group B streptococcus
	E. coli and other coliforms
	Listeria monocytogenes
1 month–6 years	Neisseria meningitidis
	Streptococcus pneumoniae
	Haemophilus influenzae
>6 years	Neisseria meningitidis
	Streptococcus pneumoniae

consciousness. A bulging fontanelle, neck stiffness and the infant lying with an arched back (opisthotonos) are late signs. Children old enough to talk are likely to describe the classical meningitis symptoms of headache, neck stiffness and photophobia. Neck stiffness may also be seen in some children with tonsillitis and cervical lymphadenopathy. As children with meningitis may also be septicaemic, signs of shock, such as tachycardia, prolonged capillary refill time, oliguria and hypotension, should be sought. Purpura in a febrile child of any age should be assumed to be due to meningococcal sepsis, even if the child does not appear unduly ill at the time; meningitis may or may not be present.

Investigations

The essential investigations are listed in Figure 14.16. A lumbar puncture is performed to obtain CSF to confirm the diagnosis, identify the organism responsible, and its antibiotic sensitivity. If any of the contraindications listed in Figure 14.16 are present, a lumbar puncture should not be performed, as under these circumstances the procedure carries a risk of coning of the cerebellum through the foramen magnum. If necessary, a lumbar puncture can be performed once the child's condition has stabilised. Although by this stage the organism will rarely be grown, the cytological and biochemical abnormalities of bacterial meningitis will still be present for several days after starting treatment. Even without a lumbar puncture, bacteriological diagnosis can be achieved in at least 50% of cases from the blood by culture, rapid antigen screen or PCR. A throat swab should also be taken. Scrapings from a purpuric skin lesion may also be cultured. A serological diagnosis can be made on convalescent serum 4–6 weeks after the presenting illness.

Management

It is imperative that there is no delay in the administration of antibiotics and supportive therapy in a child with meningitis. The choice of antibiotics will depend on the likely pathogen. A third-generation cephalosporin, e.g. cefotaxime or ceftriaxone, is the preferred choice to cover the most common bacterial causes. Although still rare in the UK, pneumococcal resistance to penicillin and cephalosporins is increasing rapidly in certain parts of the world. Whilst waiting for the sensitivity of pneumococcal cultures, rifampicin or vancomycin may be added. Ampicillin with chloramphenicol is an alternative in certain countries where third-generation cephalosporins are not available, but resistance to these drugs means that they cannot be relied upon when used as single agents. Below 3 months of age, ceftriaxone (or cefotaxime if there is neonatal jaundice) should be combined with ampicillin, which is added to cover *Listeria monocytogenes* infection. The length of the course of antibiotics given depends on the causative organism and the clinical progress of the patient. Beyond the neonatal period, dexamethasone administered

239

Assessment & investigation of meningitis/encephalitis

History	Examination	Investigations
Fever	Fever	Full blood count and differential count
Headache	Purpuric rash (meningococcal disease)	Blood glucose and blood gas (for acidosis)
Photophobia	Neck stiffness (not always present in infants)	Coagulation screen, C-reactive protein
Lethargy		Urea and electrolytes, liver function tests
Poor feeding/vomiting	Positive Brudzinski's/Kernig's signs	Culture of blood, throat swab, urine, stool for bacteria and viruses
Irritability	Signs of shock	Rapid antigen test for meningitis organisms (can be done on blood, CSF, or urine)
Hypotonia	Focal neurological signs	Lumbar puncture for CSF unless contraindicated (see below for tests on CSF)
Drowsiness	Altered conscious level	Serum for comparison of convalescent titres
Loss of consciousness	Papilloedema (rare)	PCR of blood and CSF for possible organisms
Seizures		If TB suspected: chest X-ray, Mantoux test, gastric washings or sputum, early morning urines
		Consider CT/MRI brain scan and EEG

Signs associated with neck stiffness

Brudzinski's sign – flexion of the neck with the child supine causes flexion of the knees and hips

Kernig's sign – with the child lying supine and with the hips and knees flexed, there is back pain on extension of the knee

Contraindications to lumbar puncture:

- Cardiorespiratory instability
- Focal neurological signs
- Signs of raised intracranial pressure, e.g. coma, high BP, low heart rate or papilloedema
- Coagulopathy
- Thrombocytopenia
- Local infection at the site of LP
- If it causes undue delay in starting antibiotics

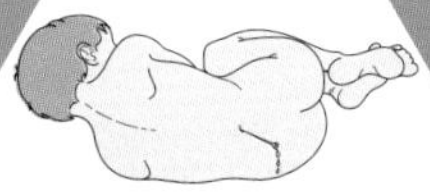

Best time for LP?
Diagnostically useful but potentially dangerous

Typical changes in the CSF in meningitis or encephalitis, beyond the neonatal period

	Aetiology	Appearance	White blood cells	Protein	Glucose
Normal	—	Clear	0–5/mm³	0.15–0.4 g/L	≥50% of blood
Meningitis	Bacterial	Turbid	Polymorphs:↑↑	↑↑	↓↓
	Viral	Clear	Lymphocytes:↑ (initially may be polymorphs)	Normal/↑	Normal/↓
	Tuberculosis	Turbid/clear/viscous	Lymphocytes:↑	↑↑↑	↓↓↓
Encephalitis	Viral/unknown	Clear	Normal/↑ lymphocytes	Normal/↑	Normal/↓

Figure 14.16 Assessment and investigation of meningitis and encephalitis.

with the antibiotics reduces the risk of long-term complications such as deafness. Any child who develops bacterial meningitis with an organism against which they have been immunised should be investigated for underlying immunodeficiency.

Cerebral complications

These include:

- *Hearing loss*. Inflammatory damage to the cochlear hair cells may lead to deafness. All children who have had meningitis should have an audiological assessment promptly, as children who become deaf may benefit from hearing amplification or a cochlear implant.
- *Local vasculitis*. This may lead to cranial nerve palsies or other focal lesions.
- *Local cerebral infarction*. This may result in focal or multifocal seizures which may subsequently lead to epilepsy.
- *Subdural effusion*. Particularly associated with

Meningococcal septicaemia

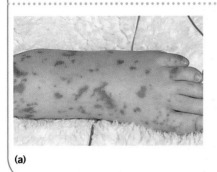

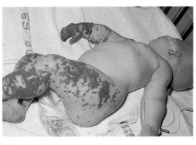

Figure 14.17 Rash of meningococcal infection. **(a)** Characteristic purpuric skin lesions, irregular in size and outline and with a necrotic centre. **(b)** The lesions may be extensive, when it is called 'purpura fulminans'.

(a)   (b)

Haemophilus influenzae and pneumococcal meningitis. This is confirmed by CT scan. Most resolve spontaneously.

- *Hydrocephalus*. May result from impaired resorption of CSF. A ventricular shunt may be required.
- *Cerebral abscess*. The child's clinical condition deteriorates with the emergence of signs of a space-occupying lesion. The temperature will continue to fluctuate. It is confirmed on CT scan. Drainage of the abscess is required.

Prophylaxis

Prophylactic treatment with rifampicin is given to all household contacts for meningococcal meningitis and for young children in the household for *Haemophilus influenzae* infection. It is not required for the patient if he has received a third-generation cephalosporin as this will eradicate nasopharyngeal carriage. Household contacts of patients who have had group C meningococcal meningitis should be vaccinated with the meningococcal group C vaccine.

Specific causes

Meningococcal infection

In the UK, *Neisseria meningitidis* (meningococcus) is the most common cause of meningitis. The incidence increased in the late 1990s but since then has fallen markedly following the introduction of the conjugate vaccine against group C disease in 1999. In countries where it remains endemic, outbreaks may occur. Meningococcal infection is a disease that strikes fear into both parents and doctors as it can kill previously healthy children within hours. While meningitis is the main clinical form of infection with this organism, meningococcal septicaemia carries a worse prognosis (Case history 14.2). Of the three main causes of bacterial meningitis, meningococcal has the lowest risk of long-term neurological sequelae, with most survivors recovering fully. The septicaemia is accompanied by a purpuric rash which may start anywhere on the body and then spread. The rash may or may not be present with meningococcal meningitis. Characteristic lesions are non-blanching on palpation, irregular in size and outline and have a necrotic centre (Fig. 14.17a, b). Any febrile child who develops a purpuric rash should be treated immediately, at home or in the general practitioner's surgery, with systemic antibiotics such as penicillin before urgent admission to hospital. Although there are now polysaccharide conjugate vaccines against groups A and C

Case History
14.2 Meningococcal septicaemia

This 7-month-old boy presented with a 12-hour history of lethargy and a spreading purpuric rash. In hospital, he required immediate resuscitation and transfer to a paediatric intensive care unit for multi-organ failure (Fig. 14.18a). The gross oedema is from leak of capillary fluid into the tissues. He required colloid and inotropic support and peritoneal dialysis for renal failure. He made a full recovery (Fig. 14.18b).

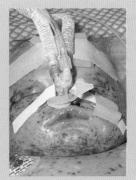

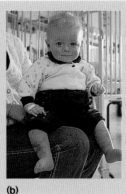

Figure 14.18 (a) A boy with meningococcal septicaemia receiving intensive care. **(b)** After full recovery. (Courtesy of Dr. Parviz Habibi)

(a)   (b)

meningococcus, there is still no effective vaccine for group B meningococcus, which accounts for the majority of isolates in the UK.

> 🌼 **Meningococcal septicaemia can kill children in hours. Optimal outcome requires immediate recognition, prompt resuscitation and antibiotics.**

Haemophilus meningitis

Before the introduction of Hib vaccine, *H. influenzae* type b was the second most common cause of meningitis in the UK and the most common in the USA. Immunisation has been highly effective and this is now a rare cause of meningitis.

Pneumococcal meningitis

While this organism was responsible for only 10% of meningitis before Hib vaccine was introduced, its prominence has now increased. Routine immunisation with the new protein-polysaccharide conjugate vaccine should reduce the high mortality (10%) and morbidity associated with this disease, as more than 30% of survivors develop neurological impairment.

Partially treated bacterial meningitis

Children are frequently given oral antibiotics for a non-specific febrile illness. If they have early meningitis, this partial treatment with antibiotics may cause diagnostic problems. CSF examination shows a raised number of white cells, but cultures are usually negative. Rapid antigen screen or PCR is sometimes helpful in these circumstances. Where the diagnosis is suspected clinically, a full course of antibiotics should be given.

Tuberculous meningitis

Tuberculous meningitis is rare in the UK. The onset of the illness is often insidious, over 2–3 weeks. Meningism may be minimal. There may be a history of TB contact. Most, but not all, affected children have a positive Mantoux test and abnormal chest X-ray. The acid-fast bacilli may be identified on Ziehl–Nielsen or auramine staining of the CSF or in early morning urine samples or gastric aspirates. As there are few organisms, they are easily missed. PCR may aid diagnosis. The mycobacteria may take 2–3 months to culture, but ascertainment of the sensitivities of the organism is important as multidrug resistance is increasing. Treatment should be started empirically when the CSF shows the features suggestive of TB meningitis. The disease is associated with a high mortality and morbidity, especially when treatment is only started after reduced consciousness or when focal neurological signs are present. Four anti-tuberculous drugs will be required for 2 months (e.g. rifampicin, pyrazinamide, isoniazid and ethambutol), decreasing if the organism is fully sensitive to two drugs (isoniazid and rifampicin) to complete a total of at least one year of treatment. Dexamethasone should be given for the first month at least, to decrease the risk of long-term sequelae.

Viral meningitis

Overall, two-thirds of CNS infections are viral. Causes include enteroviruses, Epstein–Barr virus, adenoviruses and mumps. Mumps meningitis is now rare in the UK due to MMR vaccine. The illness is usually much less severe than bacterial meningitis and a full recovery can be anticipated. Diagnosis of viral meningitis can be confirmed by culture or PCR of CSF; culture of stool, urine, nasopharyngeal aspirate, throat swabs; and serology.

Uncommon pathogens and other causes

Where the clinical course is atypical or there is failure to respond to antibiotic and supportive therapy, unusual organisms, e.g. *Mycoplasma* or *Borrelia burgdorferi* (Lyme disease), or fungal infections need to be considered. Uncommon pathogens are particularly likely in children who are immunocompromised. Rarely, recurrent bacterial meningitis may occur in the immuno-deficient or in children with congenital abnormalities of the ears or meninges which facilitate bacterial access. Aseptic meningitis may be seen in malignancy or autoimmune disorders.

> 🌼 **Any febrile child with a purpuric rash should be given intramuscular benzylpenicillin immediately and transferred urgently to hospital.**

Neonatal meningitis

See Chapter 10.

🔘 Summary

Meningitis:

- predominantly affects infants and children
- incidence has been reduced by meningococcal C and Hib immunisation; should be further reduced by pneumococcal immunisation
- clinical features: non-specific in children under 18 months – fever, poor feeding, vomiting, irritability, lethargy, drowsiness, seizures or reduced consciousness; late signs – bulging fontanelle, neck stiffness and arched back (opisthotonos)
- septicaemia can kill in hours; good outcome requires prompt resuscitation and antibiotics
- any febrile child with a purpuric rash should be given intramuscular benzylpenicillin immediately and transferred urgently to hospital.

Encephalitis/Encephalopathy

Whereas in meningitis there is inflammation of the meninges, in encephalitis there is inflammation of the brain substance, although the meninges are often also affected. Encephalitis may be caused by:

- direct invasion of the cerebrum by a neurotoxic virus
- delayed brain swelling following a disordered neuroimmunological response to an antigen, usually a virus (post-infectious encephalopathy), e.g. following chickenpox
- slow virus infection, such as HIV infection or subacute sclerosing panencephalitis (SSPE) following measles.

In encephalopathy from a non-infectious cause, e.g. a metabolic abnormality, the clinical features may be similar to an infectious encephalitis.

The clinical features and investigation of encephalitis are described in Figure 14.16. Most children present with fever, altered consciousness and often seizures. Initially, it is not possible to clinically differentiate encephalitis from meningitis, and treatment for both should be started. The underlying causative organism is only detected in up to 50%. In the UK, the most frequent causes of encephalitis are enteroviruses, respiratory viruses and herpesviruses (e.g. varicella and HHV6). Worldwide, microorganisms causing encephalitis include *Mycoplasma*, *Borrelia burgdorferi* (Lyme disease), *Bartonella henselae* (cat scratch disease), rickettsial infections (e.g. Rocky mountain spotted fever) and the arbovirusues.

Herpes simplex virus (HSV) is a very rare cause of childhood encephalitis but it may have devastating long-term consequences. All children with encephalitis should therefore be treated initially with aciclovir to cover this possibility. Most affected children do not have outward signs of herpes infection, such as cold sores, gingivostomatitis or skin lesions. The PCR of the CSF may be positive for HSV. As HSV encephalitis is a destructive infection, the EEG and CT/MRI scan may show focal changes, particularly within the temporal lobes (Fig. 14.19). These tests may initially give non-specific results and require to be repeated after a few days if the child is not improving. Later confirmation of the diagnosis may be made from HSV antibody production in the CSF. Proven cases of HSV encephalitis or cases where there is a high index of suspicion should be treated with intravenous aciclovir for 3 weeks, as relapses have occurred after shorter courses of treatment. Untreated, the mortality rate from HSV encephalitis is over 70% and survivors usually have severe neurological sequelae.

 Encephalitis may present insidiously and includes behavioural change.

Summary

Encephalitis:
- onset can be insidious and includes behavioural change
- consider if HSV (herpes simplex virus) could be the cause
- treat potential HSV with parenteral aciclovir until diagnosis is excluded.

Tuberculosis

The decline in the incidence and mortality from tuberculosis (TB) in developed countries was hailed as an example of how public health measures and antimicrobial therapy can dramatically modify a disease. However, TB is again becoming a public health problem, partly through its increasing incidence in patients with HIV infection, and with the emergence of multiresistant strains.

With the decline in TB from infected dairy cattle, the spread is usually by the respiratory route. Close proximity, infectious load and underlying immunodeficiency enhance the risk of transmission. Children are usually infected by adults within the same household. Child-to-child transmission is rare.

Clinical features

These are outlined in Figure 14.20.

Diagnosis

Diagnosing TB in children is even more difficult than in adults. The clinical features of the disease, which include prolonged fever, malaise, anorexia, weight loss and focal signs of infection, may be the only clues and empirical treatment may be necessary. Children usually swallow sputum, so gastric washings on three consecutive mornings are required to visualise or culture acid-fast bacilli originating from the lung. To obtain these, a

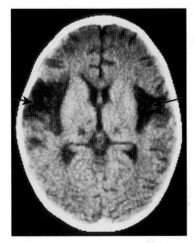

Figure 14.19
Herpes simplex encephalitis. The CT scan shows gross atrophy from loss of neural tissue in the temporoparietal regions (*arrows*).

Clinical features of TB

Primary infection

Asymptomatic

Nearly half of infants and 90% of older children will show minimal signs and symptoms of infection. A local inflammatory reaction limits the progression of infection. However, the disease is latent and may therefore develop into active disease at a later time. A Mantoux test may become positive and is sufficient evidence to initiate treatment.

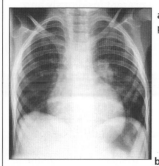

a) Chest X-ray of pulmonary TB.

b) Example of a positive Mantoux test (24 mm induration)
Positive Mantoux test (2 units):
  > 10 mm induration (no BCG given)
  > 15 mm induration (BCG given)
Implies active infection.

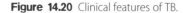

Symptomatic

In this case the local host response fails to contain the inhaled tubercle bacilli, allowing spread via the lymphatic system to regional lymph nodes.
The lung lesion plus the lymph node constitutes the 'Ghon (or primary) complex'.
When the host's cellular immune system responds to the infection (3–6 weeks), bacterial replication diminishes but systemic symptoms develop:
• fever
• anorexia and weight loss
• cough
• chest X-ray changes.
The primary complex usually heals and may calcify
The inflammatory reaction may lead to local enlargement of peribronchial lymph nodes which may cause bronchial obstruction, with collapse and consolidation of the affected lung. Pleural effusions may also be present. Further progression may be halted by the host's immunological response, or there may be local dissemination to other regions of the lung.

Although primary infection most commonly occurs in the lung, it may also involve other organs including gut, skin and superficial lymph nodes. The latter may occasionally caseate forming a 'cold abscess'. Multiple sites may be colonised by metastatic lesions released during the primary infection.

Dormancy and dissemination

Both asymptomatic and symptomatic infections may become dormant but subsequently reactivate and spread by lymphohaematological routes.

Reactivation

Post-primary TB

This may present as local disease or may be widely disseminated, miliary TB to sites such as bones, joints, kidneys, pericardium and CNS. In infants and young children, seeding of the CNS is particularly likely, causing tuberculous meningitis. This was always fatal before antimicrobial therapy was available, and is still associated with significant morbidity and mortality if treatment is not initiated early in the disease.

Figure 14.20 Clinical features of TB.

nasogastric tube is passed and secretions are rinsed out of the stomach with saline on three consecutive mornings before food. Urine, lymph node, CSF and radiological examinations should also be performed where appropriate. Although it is difficult to culture TB from children, the presence of multidrug-resistant strains makes it important to try to grow the organism so that antibiotic sensitivity can be assessed. If TB is suspected, a Mantoux test is performed – 2 units of purified protein derivative of tuberculin (2TU ssi, 0.1 m intradermal and read after 48–72 hours). Induration of greater than 10 mm is positive where no BCG has been given, 15 mm where no BCG has been given. Heaf tests are no longer used for screening for TB.

Treatment

Triple or Quadruple therapy (rifampicin, isoniazid, pyrazinamide, ethambutol) is the recommended initial combination. This is decreased to the two drugs rifampicin and isoniazid after 2 months and by this time antibiotic sensitivities are often known. After puberty, pyridoxine should be given weekly to prevent the peripheral neuropathy associated with isoniazid therapy, a complication which does not occur in young children. Asymptomatic children who are Mantoux-positive and therefore latently infected should also be treated (e.g. with rifampicin and isoniazid for 3 months) as this will decrease the risk of reactivation of infection later in life.

Prevention and contact tracing

BCG immunisation has been shown to be helpful in preventing or modifying TB in the UK. However, its usefulness worldwide in preventing the disease is controversial. In the UK, BCG is recommended at birth for high-risk groups (communities with a relatively high prevalence of TB; i.e. Asian or African origin or TB in a family member in the previous 5 years or if the local area has a high prevalence rate). The UK programme of routine BCG for all tuberculin-negative children between 10 and 14 years has been discontinued. BCG should not be given to HIV-positive or other immuno-suppressed children due to the potential risk of dissemination.

As most children are infected from a household contact, it is essential to screen other family members for the disease. Children who are exposed to smear-positive individuals (where organisms are visualised on sputum) should be assessed for evidence of asymptomatic infection. Mantoux-negative children over 5 years should receive BCG immunisation and some clinicians suggest that those who are Mantoux-negative and less than 5 years old should receive chemoprophylaxis (e.g. rifampicin and isoniazid for 3 months). If at the end of this time they remain Mantoux-negative they should also receive BCG immunisation. Again, the aim of treatment is to decrease the risk of reactivation of TB infection later in life.

Summary

TB:
- affects millions of children worldwide, low but increasing incidence in many developed countries
- clinical features follow a sequence – primary infection, then dormancy, which may be followed by reactivation to post-primary TB
- diagnosis often difficult, so decision to treat is usually based on contact history, Mantoux test, chest X-ray and clinical features
- adherence to drug therapy can be problematic but is essential for successful treatment
- contact tracing is important
- is more likely to disseminate in the immunosuppressed.

Atypical mycobacteria

There are numerous mycobacteria found in the environment. Immunocompetent individuals rarely suffer from diseases caused by these organisms. They occasionally cause persistent lymphadeno-pathy in children, which is usually treated surgically. These organisms, however, may cause disseminated infection in immunocompromised individuals. *Mycobacterium avium intracellulare* (MAI) infections are particularly common in patients with advanced HIV disease. These organisms do not respond well to treatment and require a cocktail of anti-tuberculous drugs.

TB affects millions of children worldwide; incidence is low but increasing in many developed countries

HIV infection

Worldwide, over 2 million children have HIV infection (Fig. 14.21). The major route of HIV transmission to children is vertically from mother to child, usually intrapartum, but also intrauterine or via breast-feeding. The virus is also rarely transmitted to children by infected blood products and contaminated needles. In the UK, late in 2005, 1300 children were recorded as being infected with HIV. Each year over 1000 infants are born to HIV-positive mothers in the UK, but less than 20 are now infected as women can be offered inter-ventions to prevent vertical transmission.

Diagnosis

In children over 18 months old, HIV infection is diagnosed by detecting antibodies to the virus. As infants born to infected mothers will have circulating maternal HIV antibodies, the test is unreliable before this age and their status will be indeterminate. The most sensitive test for HIV in infants is by detection of the viral genome by PCR (HIV DNA PCR). Two negative HIV DNA PCRs

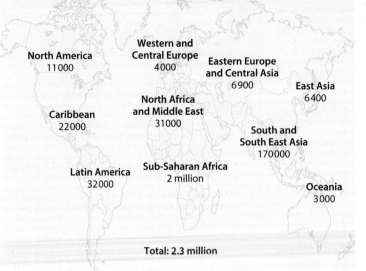

Figure 14.21 Children (<15 years) estimated to be living with HIV as of end of 2004 (UNAIDS, WHO, 2005).

North America
11 000

Western and
Central Europe
4000

Eastern Europe
and Central Asia
6900

East Asia
6400

Caribbean
22 000

North Africa
and Middle East
31 000

South and
South East Asia
170 000

Latin America
32 000

Sub-Saharan Africa
2 million

Oceania
3000

Total: 2.3 million

within the first three months of life, at least 2 weeks after completion of postnatal anti-retroviral therapy, indicate the infant is not infected, although this is confirmed by the loss of transplacental maternal HIV antibodies from the infant's circuation by 18 months of age. Other less sensitive tests in infants include HIV culture, p24 antigen, elevated immunoglobulins, low CD4 T helper-cell count for age and clinical features of infection.

Reduction of vertical transmission

Mothers who are most likely to transmit HIV to their infants are those with a high load of HIV virus and more advanced disease. Where mothers breast-feed, 25–40% of infants become infected with HIV and it is known that avoidance of breast feeding reduces the rate of transmission. In developed countries, vertical transmission of HIV is now <2% by using a combination of interventions:

- avoidance of breast-feeding
- use of antenatal, perinatal and postnatal anti-retroviral drugs to suppress viral replication
- avoidance of labour and contact with the birth canal by elective caesarean section delivery.

Unfortunately this effective combination of interventions is not available to the majority of women with HIV throughout the world.

Clinical features

Infected children may remain asymptomatic for months or years before progressing to severe disease and immunodeficiency (or an AIDS diagnosis). Clinical presentation varies with the degree of immunosuppression. Children with mild immunosuppression may have lymphadenopathy or parotitis; if moderate, they may have recurrent bacterial infections, candidiasis, chronic diarrhoea and lymphocytic interstitial pneumonitis (LIP) (Fig. 14.22). This lymphocytic infiltration of the

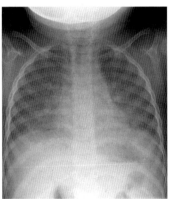

Figure 14.22 Lymphocytic interstitial pneumonitis (LIP) in a child with HIV infection. There is diffuse reticulonodular shadowing with hilar lymphadenopathy.

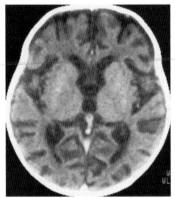

Figure 14.23 A CT scan in a child with HIV encephalopathy showing diffuse increase in CSF spaces from cerebral atrophy and volume loss.

lungs may be caused by a response to the HIV infection itself, or it may be related to EBV infection.

Severe AIDS diagnoses include opportunist infections, e.g. *Pneumocystis jiroveci (carinii)* infection, severe failure to thrive, encephalopathy (Fig. 14.23) and malignancy, which is rare in children. More than one clinical feature is often present. An unusual constellation of symptoms, especially if due to an infectious cause, should alert the clinician to consider HIV infection.

Treatment

Prophylaxis against primary pneumocystis pneumonia (PCP), now reclassified as *Pneumocystis jiroveci* pneumonia (PJP), with co-trimoxazole is prescribed for infants who are HIV-infected, and for older children with low CD4 counts.

Infants of indeterminate status and infected infants should be immunised according to the normal immunisation schedule. Infants born to mothers with HIV are at increased risk of exposure to TB, but only once confirmed uninfected with HIV should these babies be given BCG. As it is a live mycobacterial vaccine, BCG should not be given to immunosuppressed infants (including those with HIV) due to the risk of dissemination.

The two most important criteria which predict long-term morbidity and mortality from HIV infection are the plasma HIV viral load and the CD4 count. A child who has symptomatic HIV disease is likely to have a reduced CD4 count for age and a high viral load. Asymptomatic or mildly symptomatic children require regular monitoring of viral load and CD4 count. Deleterious changes in these parameters may mean that these children will require anti-retroviral therapy. As with HIV-infected adults, combination anti-retroviral therapy is most effective in suppressing viral replication and maintaining health in children. Adherence to anti-retroviral therapy regimens is onerous and required long-term; this can be very difficult for families to cope with. Short- and long-term side-effects of therapy can also be problematic. There are three families of anti-retroviral therapy currently available for children:

- the nucleoside analogue reverse transcriptase inhibitors (NRTIs) (e.g. zidovudine, abacavir, emtricitabine, didanosine, lamivudine, stavudine)
- the non-nucleoside reverse transcriptase inhibitors (NNRTIs) (e.g. nevirapine, efavirenz)
- the protease inhibitors (PIs) (e.g. ritonavir boosted lopinivir (combined as Kaletra), nelfinavir).

Current regimens for children starting anti-retroviral therapy include two NRTIs with either an NNRTI or a PI. In view of rapid new drug developments, the advice of a specialist should be sought before prescribing for children. More effective anti-retroviral therapy means that most children are now surviving into their teenage years, which brings new challenges in the management of this chronic disease.

Social, psychological and family support

Providing coordinated medical, psychological and social support for all family members is an important part of managing children and families with HIV. A coordinated service for parents and children helps to streamline therapy for the family and reduce the number of hospital visits. The multidisciplinary team can help the family cope with complicated issues, including adherence to treatment, when and what to tell children, confidentiality, schooling and planning for the future.

> Antenatal anti-retroviral drugs, elective caesarean section and avoidance of breast-feeding can reduce vertical transmission to <2%.

Summary

HIV:

- affects >2 million children worldwide but is rare in children in the UK
- antenatal anti-retroviral drugs, elective caesarean section and avoidance of breast-feeding can reduce vertical transmission to <2%
- treatment includes combination anti-retroviral therapy
- raises complex psychosocial issues for the family and caregivers, including when and what to tell the child and siblings and confidentiality.

Lyme disease

This disease, caused by the spirochaete *Borrelia burgdorferi*, was first recognised in 1975 in a cluster of children with arthritis in Lyme, Connecticut. Some cases have been reported in the UK. *Borrelia burgdorferi* is transmitted by the hard tick, which has a range of hosts but favours deer and moose. Infections occur most commonly in the summer months in susceptible persons in rural settings.

Clinical features

Following an incubation period of 4–20 days, an erythematous macule at the site of the tick bite enlarges to cause the classical skin lesion known as erythema migrans, a painless red expanding lesion with a bright red outer spreading edge. During early disease, the skin lesion is often accompanied by fever, headache, malaise, myalgia, arthralgia and lymphadenopathy. Usually these features fluctuate over several weeks and then resolve. Dissemination of infection in the early stages is rare and may lead to cranial nerve palsies, meningitis, arthritis or carditis.

The late stage of Lyme disease occurs after weeks to months with neurological, cardiac and joint manifestations. Neurological disease includes meningoencephalitis and cranial (particularly facial nerve) and peripheral neuropathies. Cardiac disease includes myocarditis and heart block. Joint disease occurs in about 50% and varies from brief migratory arthralgia to acute asymmetric mono- and oligoarthritis of the large joints. Recurrent attacks of arthritis are common. In 10%, chronic erosive joint disease occurs months to years after the initial attack.

Diagnosis

This is based on clinical and epidemiological features and serology. Serology may be negative in early disease, so repeat titres after 2–4 weeks are advised. Isolation of the organism is difficult.

Treatment

The drug of choice for early uncomplicated cases over 12 years of age is doxycycline, and for younger children, amoxicillin. Intravenous treatment with ceftriaxone is required for carditis or neurological disease.

Tropical infections

When approaching an unwell child returning from the tropics, tropical infections must be considered, although it is important to remember that these children are still susceptible to the usual range of infections found in temperate climes. The most common or most serious imported infections are outlined in Figure 14.24.

> **A febrile child returning from the tropics – commonest causes are non-tropical infections, but consider malaria typhoid fever and other tropical infections.**

Immunisation

Immunisation is one of the most effective and economic public health measures to improve the health of both children and adults. The most notable success has been the worldwide eradication of smallpox achieved in 1979, but the prevalence of many other diseases has been dramatically reduced by immunisation programmes (Fig. 14.25). The World Health Organization (WHO) aimed to eradicate poliomyelitis from the world by the year 2000, and there are now only occasional outbreaks in Africa and Asia.

Differences exist in the composition and scheduling of immunisation programmes in different countries, and schedules change as new vaccines become available (Table 14.3). The UK schedule from 2006 is shown in Figure 14.26. Features are:

- In the newborn – BCG is given to infants at high risk of infection, but has otherwise been withdrawn from the routine vaccination schedule.
- At 2, 3 and 4 months of age – the '5 in 1' vaccination is given, against diphtheria, tetanus, pertussis, *H. influenzae* type b and polio.
  The oral, live polio vaccine has been replaced by killed-vaccine given by injection, owing to the risk of polio in unvaccinated children and to immunocompromised people from gastrointestinal excretions of vaccine recipients.
- At 2, 4 and 13 months the pneumococcal conjugate vaccine has been added to the immunisation programme.
- At 3, 4 and 12 months the conjugate vaccine against group C meningococcus (MenC) is given by separate injection.
- At 12 months a booster Hib vaccine is given (combined with the MenC).
- At about 13 months – measles, mumps, rubella (MMR) is given.
- Older children – booster doses as in the immunisation schedule.

Rationale behind immunisation programme

Diphtheria infection causes local disease with membrane formation affecting the nose, pharynx or larynx or systemic disease with myocarditis and neurological manifestations. Immunisation has eradicated the disease in the UK (Fig. 14.25a).

The effect of immunisation on the number of notifications of **pertussis (whooping cough), poliomyelitis and measles** is shown in Figures 14.25b, c and e.

Table 14.3   Immunisations available for children

Routine immunisations in the UK	Diphtheria (T), tetanus (T), pertussis (I)
	Poliomyelitis (I)
	Conjugated *Haemophilus influenzae* b (S)
	Conjugated meningococcal C (S)
	Conjugated pneumococcal (S)
	Measles (L), mumps (L), rubella (L)
Additional routine immunisations in the USA	Hepatitis B (S)
	Varicella (L)
Immunisations available for children at risk	BCG for TB (L)
	Hepatitis A (S) and B (I)
	Influenza (S)
Immunisations available for children travelling abroad	Typhoid – oral (L), parenteral (I)
	Cholera (I)
	Yellow fever (L)
	Rabies (I)
	Japanese encephalitis (I), tick-borne encephalitis (I)

L: live attenuated; I: inactivated; T: toxoid; S: subunit.

An approach to the febrile child returning from the tropics

History
All places visited and duration of stay. Immunisation, malaria prophylaxis. History of food, drink (infected water), accommodation (exposure to vectors), contacts, swimming (infected rivers and lakes).

Examination
Particular reference to: fever, jaundice, anaemia, enlarged liver or spleen

Non-tropical causes of fever
Consider non-tropical causes of fever in childhood – urinary tract infection, upper and lower respiratory tract infections, gastroenteritis, septicaemia, meningitis, osteomyelitis, hepatitis, viral infections including the childhood exanthems.

Tropical infections

Malaria

40% of the world's population live in an area where the female *Anopheles* mosquito transmits malaria. Causes over 1 million child deaths in Africa each year, predominantly from *Plasmodium falciparum* malaria. The clinical features include fever (often not cyclical), diarrhoea, vomiting, flu-like symptoms, jaundice, anaemia and thrombocytopenia. Whilst typically the onset is 7–10 days after inoculation, infections can present many months later. Children are particularly susceptible to severe anaemia and the gravest form of the disease, cerebral malaria. The infection is diagnosed by examination of a thick film. The species (*falciparum, vivax, ovale or malariae*) is confirmed on a thin film. Repeated blood films may be necessary.

Quinine is required in most cases seen in the UK.Plasmodium falciparum because of the emergence of chloroquine-resistant strains worldwide.Travellers to endemic areas should always seek up-to-dateinformation onmalaria prevention. Prophylaxis reduces but does not eliminatethe risk of infection. Prevention of mosquito bites with repellants and bed nets is also important.

Typhoid

A child with worsening fever, headaches, cough, abdominal pain, anorexia, malaise and myalgia may be suffering from infection with *Salmonella typhi* or *paratyphi*. Gastrointestinal symptoms (diarrhoea or constipation) may not appear until the second week. Splenomegaly, bradycardia and rose-coloured spots on the trunk may be present. The serious complications of this disease include gastrointestinal perforation, myocarditis, hepatitis and nephritis. The recent increase in multi-resistant strains, particularly from the Indian subcontinent, means that treatment with cotrimoxazole, chloramphenicol or ampicillin may be inadequate. A third-generation cephalosporin or ciprofloxacin is usually effective.

Dengue fever

This viral infection is widespread in the tropics, and it is transmitted by mosquitoes. The primary infection is characterised by a fine erythematous rash, myalgia, arthralgia and high fever. After resolution of the fever, a secondary rash with desquamation may occur. Dengue haemorrhagic fever, also known as dengue shock syndrome, occurs when a previously infected child has a subsequent infection with a serologically different strain of the virus. Unfortunately, the partially effective host immune response serves to augment the severity of the infection. The child presents with severe capillary leak syndrome leading to hypotension as well as haemorrhagic manifestations. With fluid resuscitation, most children will recover fully. A patient with this condition is not infectious as direct person-to-person spread does not occur.

Gastroenteritis and dysentery

Gastroenteritis frequently accompanies foreign travel. 'Traveller's diarrhoea' is commonly caused by a change in gut flora, viruses including rotavirus and by *E. coli*. It rarely needs more than attention to rehydration. Fever accompanied by loose stools with blood or mucus suggests dysentery caused by *Shigella, Salmonella, Campylobacter* or *Entamoeba histolytica*. Blood cultures and stool cultures should be taken and appropriate antibiotics started, if indicated

Viral haemorrhagic fevers

Causes include the Lassa, Marburg, Ebola and Crimean–Congo viruses. These infections are imported, although Hantavirus has recently been isolated from within the UK. These are highly contagious, often lethal, infections. If suspected, strict isolation procedures should be initiated for any symptomatic patient who has returned from an endemic area within the 21-day incubation period of these infections. Specialist advice should be sought.

Figure 14.24 An approach to the febrile child returning from the tropics.

Haemophilus influenzae **type b** causes invasive disease in young children including otitis media, pneumonia, epiglottitis, septic arthritis and meningitis. The number of reports of infection dropped dramatically after the introduction of Hib vaccination (Fig. 14.25d), but a gradual rise from 1988 occurred because protection was not maintained throughout childhood. This was managed with a

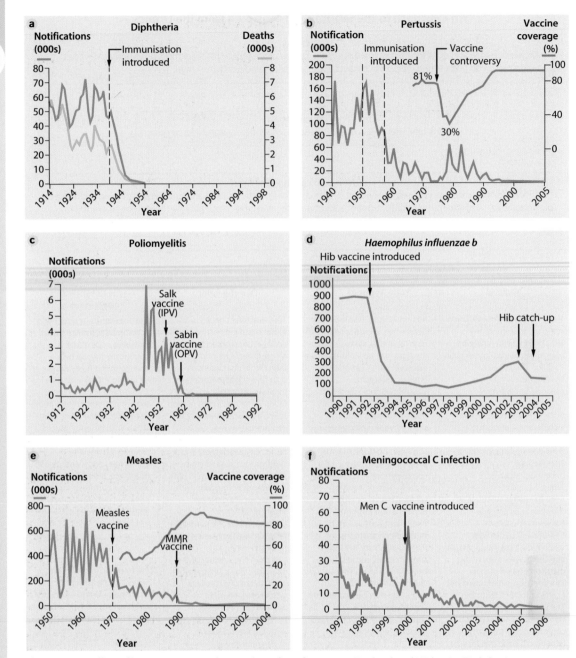

Figure 14.25 Effect of immunisation on the number of notifications in England and Wales. **(a)** Diphtheria. **(b)** Pertussis. **(c)** Poliomyelitis. **(d)** *Haemophilus influenzae* type b. **(e)** Measles. **(f)** Meningococcal disease. (Courtesy of Dr Mary Ramsey and Mrs Anjna Mistry, Health Protection Agency Communicable Disease Surveillance Unit.)

Hib catch-up programme, and to prevent a further resurgence a Hib booster dose has been introduced at 12 months of age.

Meningococcal C was an uncommon but serious pathogen causing septicaemia and meningitis. The marked fall in the number of reports in all age groups is shown in Figure 14.25f. The number of vaccinations in the first year of life has been reduced from three to two as this has been shown to provide the same level of protection. A booster is given at 12 months to extend protection through early childhood.

Pneumococcal vaccination was introduced into the immunisation programme in 2006. About 530 children under 2 years of age develop invasive pneumococcal disease in England and Wales each year. About a third develop pneumococcal meningitis, which has a high mortality, and more than 30% of survivors are left with permanent disabilities. The vaccine protects against seven common strains which are responsible for about 80% of invasive disease. Its introduction into the USA has resulted in a marked decline of invasive pneumococcal infection, not only in young

Immunisation schedule in the UK (2006)

	Birth	1 month	2 months	3 months	4 months	12 months	13 months	3½– 5 years	13–18 years
BCG	BCG if at risk								
Hep B	Hep B if at risk	Hep B if at risk	Hep B if at risk			Hep B if at risk			
1 in 5 Diptheria, tetanus, pertussis, polio, Hib (DTaP/IPV/Hib)			1 in 5	1 in 5	1 in 5				
Pneumococcal conjugate vaccine			Pneumo vaccine		Pneumo vaccine		Pneumo vaccine		
Men C				Men C	Men C				
Hib/Men C						Hib/Men C			
MMR							MMR	MMR	
Diptheria, tetanus, pertussis, polio, (DTaP/IPV)								DTaP/IPV	
Diptheria tetanus, polio (Td/IPV)									Td/IPV

Figure 14.26 Immunisation schedule in the UK. (See www.immunisation.org.uk.)

immunised children but also in older children from a more widespread population effect.

Although the number of notifications of **TB** is rising, it remains uncommon and mainly confined to high risk populations. BCG immunisation in the neonatal period is therefore targeted to those at increased risk. Routine immunisation of all skin test negative schoolchildren has been discontinued as its efficacy was unproven.

In the USA and many other countries, vaccination against **hepatitis B** and **varicella** are part of the immunisation programme.

In many developing countries immunisation uptake is low for logistical and economic reasons, resulting in the preventable death of millions of young children every year. US and WHO recommended schedules are available at www.cdc.gov and www.who.org, respectively.

Complications and contraindications

Following vaccination, there may be swelling and discomfort at the injection site and a mild fever and malaise. Some vaccines, such as measles and rubella, may be followed by a mild form of the disease. More serious reactions, including anaphylaxis, may occur but are very rare. Local guidelines about vaccination and its contraindications should be followed. Vaccination should be postponed if the child has an acute illness; however, a minor infection without fever or systemic upset is not a contraindication. If there is a personal or family history of febrile convulsions, advice on fever prevention should be given. Live vaccines should not be given to children with impaired immune responsiveness (except in children with HIV infection in whom MMR vaccine can be given).

Following pertussis vaccination, seizures and encephalopathy are rare complications, but publicity in the UK in the 1970s surrounding this risk resulted in a marked fall in vaccine uptake and was followed by several whooping cough epidemics (see Fig. 14.25b). It is now recognised that in many instances the complications were falsely attributed to the vaccine and that the neurological complications from the whooping cough itself are more frequent than from the vaccine. The only contraindication to pertussis vaccination is if the child has experienced a severe local or general reaction to a preceding dose. If there is an evolving neurological problem, immunisation should be deferred until the condition is stable.

The recent controversy regarding a possible association between MMR vaccination and autism and inflammatory bowel disease has been discredited, but adversely affected uptake of the vaccine and public confidence in the immunisation programme (see Fig. 14.25e). The MMR vaccine is only contraindicated in children with proven non-HIV-related immunodeficiency and those who are allergic to neomycin or kanamycin, which may be present in small quantities in the vaccine. Children with a history of anaphylaxis to egg (the virus is grown in fibroblast cultures generated from chick embryos) should be immunised with MMR under medical supervision. The website www.mmrthefacts.nhs.uk gives health professionals and parents detailed information on the MMR vaccine.

Infection

Further reading

American Academy of Pediatrics 2006 Report of the committee on infectious diseases. 'Red Book', 27th edn. AAP, Illinois. *Useful manual on paediatric infection and immunisation in the USA*

Feigin R D, Cherry J D 2004 Textbook of pediatric infectious diseases, 5th edn. Saunders, Philadelphia. *Large comprehensive textbook*

Internet sites for updates on immunisation and current information on infectious diseases

Meningitis Research Foundation www.meningitis.org.uk (useful teaching material on meningitis
American Academy of Pediatrics: www.aap.org
Centers for Disease Control, Atlanta, USA: www.CDC.gov
CHIVA: Childrens' HIV Association of UK and Ireland: www.bhiva.org/chiva (guidelines to reduce HIV vertical transmission)
Health Protection Agency (previously Public Health Laboratory Service), UK: www.hpa.org.uk
MMR The facts: www.mmrthefacts.nhs.uk (information about the MMR vaccine)
NHS Immunisation Information: www.immunisation.nhs.uk (up-to-date information on the immunisation programme in the UK)
UNAIDS: www.unaids.org (worldwide information on HIV)
World Health Organization: www.who.org

15

Allergy and immunity

An abnormal immune system may result in:

- allergic disorders
- primary immune deficiencies
- secondary immune deficiencies
  - to infection, drugs, protein loss, metabolic disorders and lack of splenic function
- autoimmune disorders
  - organ specific, e.g. diabetes mellitus, Graves' disease, myasthenia gravis
  - systemic, e.g. juvenile idiopathic arthritis (JIA), systemic lupus erythematosus (SLE).
- malignancy
  - following high dose immunosuppressive therapy.

Paediatric allergy

This comprises asthma, allergic rhinitis, conjunctivitis, eczema, urticaria and hypersensitivity to food, drugs and insect bites or stings. These diseases are important as they:

- are common, up to 40% of children developing allergic rhinitis, eczema and asthma and up to 8% developing food allergy
- are increasing in prevalence throughout the developed world
- account for ≥ 6% of primary care consultations and 7% of acute hospital attendances in the UK
- cause significant morbidity and can be fatal, with about 20 children dying each year from asthma and 2 from anaphylaxis, in the UK.

An explanation of some of the terms used in allergy are listed in Box 15.1.

Mechanisms of allergic disease

Many genes have been linked to the development of allergic disease. Polymorphisms in these genes lead to a genetic susceptibility to allergy.

In early life, infants are exposed to a wide variety of non-specific environmental antigens which prime the immune system. In allergy, this priming is abnormal and in a genetically susceptible individual leads to the individual becoming atopic. If the individual is then exposed to a specific antigen (e.g. food) this may lead to the develop-

Box 15.1 Allergy definitions

- **Hypersensitivity** – objectively reproducible symptoms or signs following a defined stimulus (e.g. food, drug, venom) at a dose tolerated by normal persons.
- **Allergy** – a hypersensitivity reaction initiated by specific immunological mechanisms. This can be IgE mediated (e.g. peanut allergy) or non-IgE mediated (e.g. coeliac disease).
- **Atopy** – a personal and/or familial tendency, usually in childhood or adolescence, to become sensitised and produce IgE antibodies in response to ordinary exposures to allergens, usually proteins. Results in asthma, allergic rhinitis, conjunctivitis or eczema.
- **Anaphylaxis** – a severe, life-threatening, generalised or systemic hypersensitivity reaction.

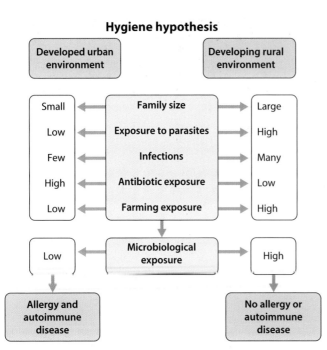

Figure 15.1 Hygiene hypothesis.

ment of allergic sensitisation. Subsequent exposure to the allergen results in an allergic reaction, which may occur in two phases:

- immediate, within minutes from histamine release from mast cells
- delayed response, after 4–6 hours, from tissue damage at the site of exposure from inflammatory cells, particularly eosinophils.

The hygiene hypothesis

The hygiene hypothesis is a proposed explanation for the increase in allergy which accompanies improved living conditions and hygiene. The hypothesis is that allergy results from a reduction in microbiological and other environmental exposures in infancy (Fig. 15.1). Circumstantial epidemiological evidence supports this theory, but it remains unproven.

However, although those living in a developing rural environment are at very low risk of allergy and autoimmune disease, they do have the great disadvantage of a higher incidence of infectious diseases.

Age of presentation

Many children with allergic disease have a family history of allergy. Infants with a strong family history are at high risk of developing allergy.

Allergic children develop individual allergic disorders at different ages:

- eczema and food allergy in infancy
- asthma and allergic rhinitis in childhood.

In addition, the presence of eczema or food allergy in infancy is predictive of asthma and allergic rhinitis in later childhood.

This progression is referred to as the 'allergic march'.

Prevention of allergic diseases

Attempts have been made to prevent the onset of allergic disease and to interrupt the allergic march. These include: environmental manipulation (avoidance of allergens in pregnancy, during lactation or in infancy), probiotics (orally administered microorganisms which alter intestinal microflora), prebiotics (immunologically active oligosaccharides) and nutritional supplements (e.g. antioxidants, fish oils, trace elements). However, none have been shown to reduce, long term, the prevalence of allergic diseases.

Examination of an allergic child

In addition to the signs of individual allergic diseases, examination may reveal:

- Morgan–Dennie folds (Fig. 15.2a), extra folds under the eyes
- an allergic salute (Fig. 15.2b), from rubbing an itchy nose
- enlarged cervical lymph nodes
- pale and swollen nasal turbinates
- mouth breathing.

Management

The individual diseases are managed by general practitioners, general paediatricians or organ-specific specialists, e.g. eczema by dermatologists, asthma by respiratory paediatricians. However, allergic diseases coexist and it is therefore helpful to consider allergy as a systemic disease. The role of paediatric allergists is to identify triggers to avoid

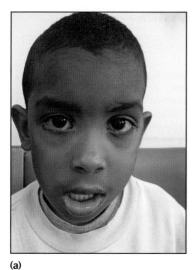
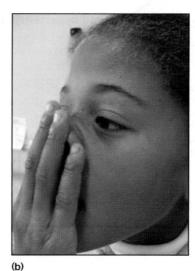

Figure 15.2 Allergic facies.
(a) There are Morgan–Dennie folds (extra folds under the eyes), rhinitis and lip smacking eczema. **(b)** An allergic salute, from rubbing an itchy nose. (Courtesy Dr George Du Toit.)

(a)

(b)

and to manage children with systemic or severe disease.

Management of specific conditions are described below. In addition, specific immunotherapy, though uncommon in the UK, is widely used in many other countries especially the USA and Europe for allergic rhinitis, insect sting hypersensitivity and increasingly for asthma. Standardised solutions of the allergen are injected subcutaneously, starting with a low dose and increasing to a maintenance dose, with the aim of developing immune tolerance. The maintenance injections are then continued every 4–6 weeks for 3–5 years, with the protective effects lasting many years after the end of the treatment. Newer modalities such as sublingual immunotherapy are also being introduced.

🎯 Summary

Paediatric allergy:
- includes asthma, allergic rhinitis, conjunctivitis, eczema, urticaria and hypersensitivity to food, drugs and insect bites or stings
- occurs when a genetically susceptible person reacts abnormally to an environmental antigen; subsequent exposure to a specific antigen may lead to allergic sensitisation
- there is an 'allergic march' of disorders
- different allergic diseases often coexist – if a child has one, look for others.

Food allergy and food hypersensitivity

A food allergy occurs when a pathological immune response is mounted against a specific food protein. Food allergy may be IgE mediated or non-IgE mediated. If a non-immunological reaction to a specific food occurs this is called non-allergic food hypersensitivity. An example of each in relation to cow's milk is shown in Figure 15.3.

Presentation of food allergy varies with the agent and the child's age:

- in infants the most common causes are milk, egg and peanut
- in older children peanut, tree nut and fish.

Regional differences reflect national diets (e.g. birds nest soup allergy is common in S.E. Asia). Fruit allergy, although common, is usually mild, causing an itchy mouth but no systemic symptoms. This is called 'oral allergy syndrome' and is usually associated with spring hay fever due to cross-reaction with tree pollens. Kiwi fruit, however, can cause anaphylaxis.

Food hypersensitivity is not related to food aversion, where the person refuses the food for psychological or behavioural reasons.

Diagnosis

The diagnosis of IgE-mediated food allergy is based on a suggestive history of allergic symptoms, usually occurring within minutes of ingestion, each time the food is eaten. If this history is not present, the child does not have food allergy.

Although many tests to identify allergies are promoted to the general public, most have no scientific basis. The clinically helpful screening tests for allergy are skin prick tests (Fig. 15.4) and measurement of specific IgE antibodies in blood.

With both tests, the greater the response the more likely the child is to be allergic. In cases of doubt, the gold standard investigation is the double-blind placebo-controlled food challenge. This involves the child being given increasing amounts of the food or placebo, starting with a tiny quantity of food until a full portion is reached. The test should be performed in hospital with monitoring for signs of an allergic reaction.

Example of food allergy and hypersensitivity to milk

Condition	Clinical manifestation

IgE-mediated food allergy
- Immediate cow's milk allergy

This 6-month old breastfed infant developed an allergic reaction, **a** , with widespread urticaria immediately after the first formula feed. Skin prick tests were strongly positive to cow's milk. Widespread urticaria and lip swelling during milk challenges are shown in **b** and **c**

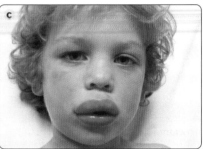

a Clinical features of an acute allergic reaction:
Mild reaction
- Urticaria and itchy skin
- Facial swelling

Severe reaction
- Wheeze
- Stridor
- Itchy throat
- Abdominal pain, vomiting, diarrhoea
- Shock, collapse

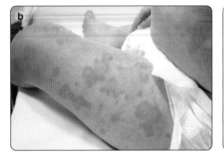

Non IgE-mediated food allergy
- Cow's milk protein intolerance

A 4-month-old infant, formula fed since birth, always a poor feeder, has loose stools and is failing to thrive. Skin tests are all negative. Elimination of cow's milk results in resolution of symptoms which return on trial reintroduction.

Non-allergic food hypersensitivity
- Temporary lactose intolerance

Previously well 12-month-old infant develops diarrhoea and vomiting. The vomiting settles but watery stools continue for several weeks.
Stool sample - no pathogens but positive for reducing substances.
Diagnosis - temporary lactose intolerance.

Figure 15.3 Examples of food allergy and hypersensitivity to milk. **(a)** Clinical features of an acute allergic reaction. **(b and c)** Widespread urticaria and lip swelling during milk challenge. (Courtesy Dr Pete Smith.)

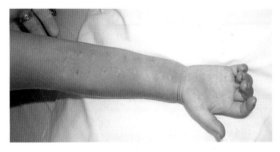

Figure 15.4 Skin prick testing. A drop of the allergen is placed on the skin, the site is marked and pricked with a needle, and any weals measured. Multiple positive results are present. (Courtesy Dr Pete Smith.)

⊚ Summary

Food allergy:
- most common causes in infants are milk, egg and peanut; in older children it is peanuts
- peanut allergy affects 1 in 70 children
- diagnosis of IgE-mediated food allergy is based on a suggestive history and, if necessary, skin prick tests, specific IgE antibodies in blood and double-blind placebo-controlled food challenge.
- with previous severe reaction or asthma – carry an epinephrine (adrenaline) auto-injector.

Management

The management of a food allergic child involves avoidance of the food but, especially for milk and nuts, this is very difficult as they may be present in small quantities in many foods and food labels are often unclear. The advice of a paediatric dietician is essential.

In addition, the child and family must be able to manage an allergic attack. Written self-management plans and adequate training are essential. Drug management for mild reactions (no cardiorespiratory symptoms) is with antihistamines. If the child had a severe reaction or has asthma, treatment is with epinephrine (adrenaline) given intramuscularly by auto-injector (e.g. Epipen), which the child or parent should carry with them at all times.

Eczema

Eczema is classed as an allergic disease as many children will have a family history of allergy, up to 50% develop other allergic diseases and it is associated with allergic sensitisation (i.e. raised IgE levels). However, the role of allergen avoidance is controversial. Infants and young children with eczema may have food allergy (in particular cow's milk allergy) and exposure to the offending food can cause worsening of disease or immediate allergic symptoms. If the eczema is severe and a food allergy is suspected on the basis of history, and the allergy skin and blood tests are positive, it should be confirmed or refuted by a food elimination diet. It is important to ensure that the child maintains an adequate diet and dietician support is essential. A food challenge to the causative food can subsequently be performed.

Allergic rhinitis

Allergic rhinitis (hay fever) is an underestimated cause of childhood morbidity. It affects up to 20% of children and can severely disrupt their lives. In addition to its classic presentation of coryza and conjunctivitis, it can also present as 'cough-variant rhinitis' due to post-nasal drip and may be detrimental to concentration. It is associated with eczema, asthma, sinusitis and adenoidal hypertrophy. Treatment of allergic rhinitis has been shown to improve coexistent asthma.

Seasonal allergic rhinitis is predominantly due to sensitisation and exposure to airborne pollens and spores (tree pollens in the spring, grass pollens in the summer, and mould spores in the autumn). Perennial allergic rhinitis is usually due to sensitisation and exposure to house dust mite or ongoing exposure to an allergen such as a pet to which the child is sensitised. Treatment options are listed in Box 15.2.

Box 15.2 Range of treatment for allergic rhinitis

- Antihistamines (used singly or in combination)
- Steroid nasal sprays
- Cromoglicate eye drops
- Leukotriene inhibitors
- Oral steroids
- Specific immunotherapy

Asthma

Allergy is an important component of asthma. There may be sensitisation to aeroallergens (house dust mite; tree, grass and weed pollens; moulds; animal danders) and foods. In sensitised children, targeted avoidance measures (such as using dust mite mattress covers to minimise exposure to house dust mite) can lead to improvement in symptoms and reduction in need for medication. Management is described in Chapter 16 on respiratory disorders.

Urticaria

Acute urticaria usually results from exposure to an allergen or a viral infection, which triggers an urticarial skin reaction. It may also involve deeper tissues to produce swelling of the lips and soft tissues around the eyes (angioedema), and even anaphylaxis, the management of which is described in Chapter 6, Figure 6.15.

Chronic urticaria (persisting >6 weeks) is usually non-allergic in origin. It results from a local increase in the permeability of capillaries and venules. These changes are dependent on activation of skin mast cells which contain a range of mediators including histamine. A cause may be identified, such as cow's milk allergy in infants, but most are idiopathic (Box 15.3).

Box 15.3 Causes of urticaria

- Idiopathic (common)
- Infection
- IgE-mediated
  - Specific food – cow's milk, nuts (especially peanuts), fish
  - Blood products
  - Drugs – penicillins, cephalosporins
- Pharmacological
  - Foods containing histamine-releasing substances, e.g. strawberries, egg white, cheese
  - Aspirin and other non-steroidal anti-inflammatory agents
- Physical agents
  - Heat, cold, pressure

Drug allergy

Drug allergies do occur in children, especially to antibiotics, but only a minority who are labelled drug allergic are truly allergic. This is usually because viral illnesses, for which children are often prescribed antibiotics, themselves cause skin rashes. A detailed history is required of the nature and timing of the rash in relation to taking the antibiotics.

As allergy skin and blood tests are unreliable in predicting drug allergy, a drug challenge is the only way to confirm or refute the diagnosis.

Insect bite or sting hypersensitivity

This arises mainly from bee and wasp stings, also from fire ants in the USA, Asia and Australia. The severity of the allergic reaction may be:

* mild – local swelling
* moderate – generalised urticaria
* severe – systemic symptoms with wheeze or shock.

Children with a previous mild or moderate reaction are unlikely to develop a severe reaction in the future and the families can be reassured. Those who had a severe reaction should carry an epinephrine (adrenaline) auto-injector and be desensitised using specific immunotherapy.

Summary

Insect bite or sting hypersensitivity:
* is mainly to bee and wasp stings
* following a severe reaction, an epinephrine (adrenaline) auto-injector should be carried
* immunotherapy is highly effective in children who have had a severe reaction.

Immunodeficiency disorders

Immunodeficiencies may be primary or secondary. In primary disorders there is an intrinsic defect in the immune system. Secondary immune deficiency is more common and may occur with malignant disease, immunosuppressive therapy, HIV infection, malnutrition, splenectomy, nephrotic syndrome and many bacterial and viral infections.

Clinical features

Many of the primary immunodeficiencies (Fig. 15.5) are inherited as X-linked or autosomal recessive disorders. There may be a family history of parental consanguinity and unexplained death, particularly in boys. Children with an immunodeficiency will usually have a history of infections which are recurrent, persistent or unusual (Table 15.1). There may also be evidence of a protein-losing enteropathy and failure to thrive.

Investigation of immunological competence

This is directed towards the most likely cause (Table 15.2). Investigations can quantify the essential components of the immune system and also provide a functional assessment of immunocompetence.

Treatment

The recent discovery of the genetic basis of many of the primary immunodeficiencies is likely to have a profound impact on future management. It is hoped that, in the future, gene therapy, in which a normally functioning gene is transfected into defective progenitor cells, may become a feasible treatment for many conditions. Until such corrective therapy becomes available, management will continue to comprise:

Table 15.1 Specific defects in the components of the immune system lead to particular types of infection (only the most common/important are listed)

Immune defect	Infectious susceptibility	
Antibody/humoral (B lymphocytes)	Bacteria	*Pneumococcus, Staphylococcus, Streptococcus, Haemophilus influenzae, Moraxella catarrhalis*
	Viruses	Enteroviruses
Cellular immunity (T lymphocytes)	Bacteria	*Mycobacterium, Listeria*
	Viruses	CMV, VZV, HSV, EBV, measles, respiratory viruses
	Fungi	*Candida, Aspergillus, Pneumocystis jiroveci* (previously *carinii*)
Combined cellular and humoral (T and B lymphocytes)	Bacteria	All of above
	Viruses	
	Fungi	
Neutrophils	Bacteria	Gram-positive, Gram-negative
	Fungi	*Aspergillus, Candida*
Opsonisation (complement, mannose binding lectin)	Bacteria	*Neisseria meningitidis, Staphylococcus*
	Fungi	*Candida*

Immunodeficiency disorders

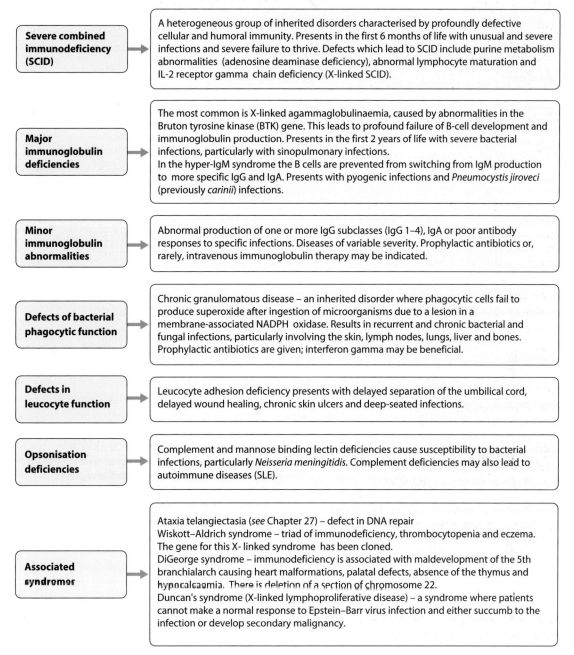

Severe combined immunodeficiency (SCID)	A heterogeneous group of inherited disorders characterised by profoundly defective cellular and humoral immunity. Presents in the first 6 months of life with unusual and severe infections and severe failure to thrive. Defects which lead to SCID include purine metabolism abnormalities (adenosine deaminase deficiency), abnormal lymphocyte maturation and IL-2 receptor gamma chain deficiency (X-linked SCID).
Major immunoglobulin deficiencies	The most common is X-linked agammaglobulinaemia, caused by abnormalities in the Bruton tyrosine kinase (BTK) gene. This leads to profound failure of B-cell development and immunoglobulin production. Presents in the first 2 years of life with severe bacterial infections, particularly with sinopulmonary infections. In the hyper-IgM syndrome the B cells are prevented from switching from IgM production to more specific IgG and IgA. Presents with pyogenic infections and *Pneumocystis jiroveci* (previously *carinii*) infections.
Minor immunoglobulin abnormalities	Abnormal production of one or more IgG subclasses (IgG 1–4), IgA or poor antibody responses to specific infections. Diseases of variable severity. Prophylactic antibiotics or, rarely, intravenous immunoglobulin therapy may be indicated.
Defects of bacterial phagocytic function	Chronic granulomatous disease – an inherited disorder where phagocytic cells fail to produce superoxide after ingestion of microorganisms due to a lesion in a membrane-associated NADPH oxidase. Results in recurrent and chronic bacterial and fungal infections, particularly involving the skin, lymph nodes, lungs, liver and bones. Prophylactic antibiotics are given; interferon gamma may be beneficial.
Defects in leucocyte function	Leucocyte adhesion deficiency presents with delayed separation of the umbilical cord, delayed wound healing, chronic skin ulcers and deep-seated infections.
Opsonisation deficiencies	Complement and mannose binding lectin deficiencies cause susceptibility to bacterial infections, particularly *Neisseria meningitidis*. Complement deficiencies may also lead to autoimmune diseases (SLE).
Associated syndromes	Ataxia telangiectasia (*see* Chapter 27) – defect in DNA repair Wiskott–Aldrich syndrome – triad of immunodeficiency, thrombocytopenia and eczema. The gene for this X-linked syndrome has been cloned. DiGeorge syndrome – immunodeficiency is associated with maldevelopment of the 5th branchial arch causing heart malformations, palatal defects, absence of the thymus and hypocalcaemia. There is deletion of a section of chromosome 22. Duncan's syndrome (X-linked lymphoproliferative disease) – a syndrome where patients cannot make a normal response to Epstein–Barr virus infection and either succumb to the infection or develop secondary malignancy.

Figure 15.5 Immunodeficiency disorders.

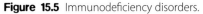

- antibiotic prophylaxis to prevent infection, e.g. co-trimoxazole to prevent *Pneumocystis jaroveci* (previously *carinii*) pneumonia
- appropriate antibiotics to treat infection
- immunoglobulin replacement therapy for defects in antibody function or production
- bone marrow transplantation for severe immunodeficiency.

Table 15.2 Some of the more commonly used tests of immune function in children

Test	Function
Full blood count	Number of white blood cells, and differential count of neutrophils, lymphocytes, platelets
Blood film	Morphology of cells
Lymphocytes	
Lymphocyte subsets	Determines the number of T and B cells, monocytes and natural killer cells
Immunoglobulins	Level of IgG, IgM, IgA and IgE and IgG subclasses. If total IgG is low, IgG subclasses may be measured
Specific immunoglobulin	Tests the ability to mount an appropriate antibody response to known antigens, e.g. vaccine responses
T-cell proliferation in response to mitogens and antigens, e.g. phytohaemagglutin and *Candida*	Functional test of cell-mediated immunity
Tests of purine and pyrimidine metabolism	Abnormal in some forms of severe combined immunodeficiency
Chromosomal fragility test	Test for ataxia telangiectasia
Neutrophils	
Nitroblue tetrazolium test (NBT)	Abnormal response in chronic granulomatous disease
Surface adhesion molecules (CD18, CD11b)	Test for leucocyte adhesion deficiency
Tests of chemotaxis	Test of leucocyte motility
Complement	
Individual complement components	Reduced in complement deficiency states and other diseases
Total haemolytic complement	Functional test for complement
Mannose binding lectin (MBL) level	MBL deficiency
Identification of genetic polymorphisms	Specific abnormal genes have been identified for a number of conditions (e.g. Wiskott–Aldrich syndrome, Bruton's agammaglobulinaemia, DiGeorge's syndrome, severe combined immunodeficiency, MBL deficiency, Duncan's syndrome)

Further reading

www.allergyuk.org
www.anaphylaxis.org.uk

Respiratory disorders

Respiratory disorders are important as:

- they account for 50% of consultations with general practitioners for acute illness in young children and a third of consultations in older children
- respiratory illness leads to 20–35% of acute paediatric admissions to hospital, some of which are life-threatening
- asthma is the most common chronic illness of childhood in the UK
- cystic fibrosis is the most common inherited life-limiting disorder in Caucasians.

Respiratory infections

These are the most frequent infections of childhood. The preschool child has, on average, six to eight respiratory infections a year. Most are mild self-limiting illnesses of the upper respiratory tract (ear, nose, throat) but some, such as bronchiolitis or pneumonia, are potentially life-threatening.

Pathogens

Viruses cause 80–90% of childhood respiratory infections. The most important are the respiratory syncytial virus (RSV), rhinoviruses, parainfluenza, influenza, metapneumovirus and adenoviruses. An individual virus can cause several different patterns of illness; e.g. RSV can cause bronchiolitis, croup, pneumonia or a common cold.

The important bacterial pathogens of the respiratory tract are *Streptococcus pneumoniae* (pneumococcus) and other streptococci, *Haemophilus influenzae*, *Bordetella pertussis* which causes whooping cough, and *Mycoplasma pneumoniae*. Dual infections, with two viral pathogens or with a viral and bacterial pathogen, may occur. *Mycobacterium tuberculosis* remains an important pathogen. Some pathogens cause predictable epidemics, such as RSV bronchiolitis every winter, whereas others, e.g. pneumococcus, show little seasonal variation.

Host and environmental factors

An increased risk of symptomatic respiratory infection is associated with:

- poor socioeconomic status (such as overcrowded, damp housing and poor nutrition)
- large family size
- parental, especially maternal smoking
- gender, boys more than girls
- prematurity – especially those who required artificial ventilation or prolonged oxygen therapy
- cystic fibrosis
- congenital abnormalities of the heart or lungs
- rarely, immune deficiency – either congenital (e.g. hypogammaglobulinaemia) or acquired (e.g. as a result of therapy for malignant disease or from HIV infection).

The child's age influences the prevalence and severity of infections (Fig. 16.1). It is in infancy that serious respiratory illness requiring hospital admission is most common and the risk of death is greatest. There is an increased frequency of infections when the child or older siblings start nursery or school. Repeated upper respiratory tract infection is common and rarely indicates underlying disease.

Classification of respiratory infections

Respiratory infections are classified according to the level of the respiratory tree most involved:

- upper respiratory tract infection
- laryngeal/tracheal infection
- bronchitis
- bronchiolitis
- pneumonia.

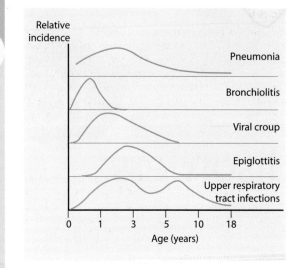

Figure 16.1 Age distribution of acute respiratory infections in children.

Upper respiratory tract infection (URTI)

Approximately 80% of all respiratory infections involve only the nose, throat, ears or sinuses. The term URTI embraces a number of different conditions.

- common cold (coryza)
- sore throat (pharyngitis, including tonsillitis)
- acute otitis media
- sinusitis (relatively uncommon).

The commonest presentation is a child with a combination of a nasal discharge and blockage, fever, painful throat and earache. Cough may be troublesome. URTIs may cause:

- difficulty in feeding in infants as their noses are blocked and this obstructs breathing
- febrile convulsions
- acute exacerbations of asthma.

In infants, hospital admission may be required to exclude a more serious infection, if feeding is inadequate, or for parental reassurance.

The common cold (coryza)

This is the commonest infection of childhood. Classical features include a clear or mucopurulent nasal discharge and nasal blockage. The commonest pathogens are viruses – rhinoviruses (of which there are over 100 different serotypes), coronaviruses and RSV. Health education to advise parents that colds are self-limiting and have no specific curative treatment may reduce anxiety and save unnecessary visits to doctors. Fever and pain are best treated with paracetamol or ibuprofen. Antibiotics are of no benefit as the common cold is viral in origin and secondary bacterial infection is very uncommon.

Sore throat (pharyngitis)

Sore throats are usually due to viral infection with respiratory viruses (mostly adenoviruses, enteroviruses and rhinoviruses). In the older child, group A β-haemolytic *Streptococcus* is a very common pathogen. The pharynx and soft palate are inflamed and local lymph nodes are enlarged and tender.

Tonsillitis

This is a form of pharyngitis where there is intense inflammation of the tonsils, often with a purulent exudate. Group A β-haemolytic streptococci and the Epstein–Barr virus (in infectious mononucleosis) are common pathogens.

Although viruses are the commonest cause of pharyngitis or tonsillitis, especially in preschool children, it is not possible to distinguish clinically between viral and bacterial causes. Marked constitutional disturbance, such as headache, apathy and abdominal pain, tonsillar exudate and cervical lymphadenopathy, is more common with bacterial infection.

Antibiotics (often penicillin, or erythromycin if there is penicillin allergy) are often prescribed for severe pharyngitis and tonsillitis even though only a third are caused by bacteria. They may hasten recovery from streptococcal infection, but 10 days of treatment is required to eradicate the organism to prevent rheumatic fever, and this is now exceedingly rare in the UK. Amoxicillin is best avoided as it may cause a widespread maculopapular rash if the tonsillitis is due to infectious mononucleosis.

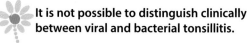

It is not possible to distinguish clinically between viral and bacterial tonsillitis.

Acute infection of the middle ear (acute otitis media)

Most children will have at least one episode of acute otitis media (OM). This is most common at 6–12 months of age. Up to 20% will have three or more episodes (recurrent OM). Infants and young children are prone to OM because their Eustachian tubes are short, horizontal and function poorly. There is pain in the ear and fever. The child is irritable and may pull at the affected ear. Every child with a fever must have the tympanic membranes examined (Fig. 16.2a–d). In acute otitis media, the tympanic membrane is seen to be bright red and bulging with loss of the normal light reflection. Occasionally there is acute perforation of the eardrum with pus visible in the external canal. Pathogens include viruses, especially RSV and rhinovirus, and pneumococcus, non-typeable *H. influenzae* and *Moraxella catarrhalis*. Serious complications such as mastoiditis and meningitis are now uncommon. Pain should be treated with paracetamol or ibuprofen. Around 80% of cases of acute otitis media resolve spontaneously. Antibiotics shorten the duration of pain but have not been shown to reduce the risk of hearing loss (see section on evidence-based medicine in Ch. 5). It is

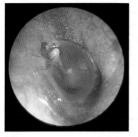
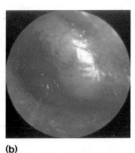

(a)   (b)

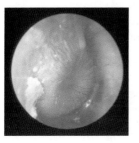
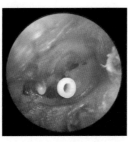

(c)   (d)

Figure 16.2 Appearance of the eardrum. **(a)** Normal. **(b)** Acute otitis media. **(c)** Otitis media with effusion. **(d)** Grommet. ((a) and (d) courtesy of Mr N Shah & Mr N Tolley, (b) and (c) from Stafford N D, Youngs R *Colour Guide ENT*, Churchill Livingstone Edinburgh, 1999, with permission.)

often useful to give the parents a prescription, but ask them to use it only if the child remains unwell after 2–3 days. Amoxicillin is widely used. Neither decongestants nor antihistamines are beneficial.

Recurrent ear infections can lead to otitis media with effusion (OME or glue ear or serous otitis media). Children are asymptomatic apart from possible decreased hearing. The eardrum is seen to be dull and retracted, often with a fluid level visible. Otitis media with effusion is very common, peak incidence is 1 year of age, and usually resolves spontaneously. Although antibiotics improve the appearance of the tympanic membrane in the short term, they give no long-term benefit. Otitis media with effusion is the most common cause of conductive hearing loss in children and can interfere with normal speech development and result in learning difficulties in school. In such children insertion of ventilation tubes (grommets) can be beneficial, and adenoidectomy considered.

ⓘ Summary

Acute otitis media (OM):
- can only be diagnosed by examining the tympanic membrane
- antibiotics shorten the duration of pain but do not reduce hearing loss
- if recurrent, many result in otitis media with effusion, which may cause speech and learning difficulties from hearing loss.

Sinusitis

Infection of the paranasal sinuses may occur with viral URTIs. Occasionally there is secondary bacterial infection, with pain, swelling and tenderness over the cheek from infection of the maxillary sinus. As the frontal sinuses do not develop until late childhood, frontal sinusitis is uncommon in the first decade of life. Antibiotics and analgesia are used for acute sinusitis.

Tonsillectomy and adenoidectomy

Children with recurrent URTIs are often referred for removal of their tonsils and adenoids, one of the commonest operations performed in children. Many children have large tonsils but this in itself is not an indication for tonsillectomy as they shrink spontaneously in late childhood.

The indications for tonsillectomy are controversial but include:

- recurrent tonsillitis (as opposed to recurrent URTIs) – tonsillectomy reduces the number of episodes of tonsillitis by a third, e.g. from three to two per year
- a peritonsillar abscess (quinsy)
- obstructive sleep apnoea.

Like the tonsils, adenoids increase in size until about the age of 8 years and then gradually regress. In young children the adenoids grow proportionately faster than the airway, so that their effect of narrowing the airway lumen is greatest between 2 and 8 years of age. They may narrow the posterior nasal space sufficiently to justify adenoidectomy. Indications for the removal of both the tonsils and adenoids are controversial but include:

- otitis media with effusion with hearing loss, when it gives a small additional benefit to the insertion of grommets (ventilation tubes).
- obstructive sleep apnoea (an absolute indication).

Sleep-disordered breathing

Up to 10% of children will snore, but less than 1% will have sleep-disordered breathing. Obstructive sleep apnoea (OSA) in childhood is usually due to upper airway obstruction secondary to adeno-tonsillar hypertrophy. There may be a history of loud snoring, apnoea for 30–45 seconds with struggling for breath, and disturbed sleep. Whilst affected children may be obese, others may have growth failure and they may have daytime hyperactivity rather than sleepiness. Overnight sleep studies show intermittent hypoxia and hypercarbia. Adeno-tonsillectomy is usually curative (Fig. 16.3a,b).

It is now recognised that children with a range of disorders may be prone to sleep-disordered breathing, particularly those with craniofacial disorders (e.g. Pierre Robin), neuromuscular disorders (e.g. muscular dystrophy) or hypotonia (e.g. Down's syndrome). There may be a mixture of obstructive and central hypoventilation. Many improve with overnight ventilation at home via a nasal mask.

Respiratory infections

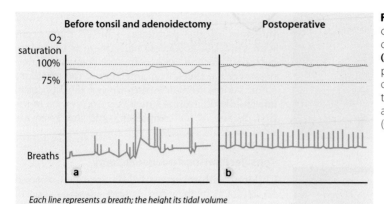

Before tonsil and adenoidectomy   **Postoperative**

Each line represents a breath; the height its tidal volume

Figure 16.3 Extract from cardiorespiratory monitoring in a child with obstructive sleep apnoea. **(a)** Irregular breathing with periodic pauses associated with oxygen desaturation. **(b)** Post adenotonsillectomy, the breathing is regular and the desaturation has resolved. (Courtesy of Dr Parviz Habibi.)

> ### Summary
>
> **Sleep disordered breathing:**
> * from adeno-tonsillar hypertrophy – surgical removal is almost always curative
> * from craniofacial disorders or neuromuscular weakness or hypotonia – improved by overnight nasal mask ventilation.

Laryngeal and tracheal infections

The mucosal inflammation and swelling produced by laryngeal and tracheal infections can rapidly cause life-threatening obstruction of the airway in young children. Several conditions can cause acute upper airways obstruction (Box 16.1). They are characterised by:

* stridor, a rasping sound heard predominantly on inspiration
* hoarseness due to inflammation of the vocal cords

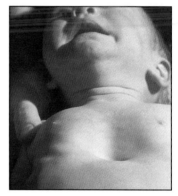

Figure 16.4 The degree of subcostal, intercostal and sternal recession is a more useful indicator of severity of upper airways obstruction than the respiratory rate (© Boehringer Ingelheim International GmbH).

* a barking cough like a sea lion
* a variable degree of dyspnoea.

The severity of upper airways obstruction is best assessed clinically by the degree of chest retraction (none, only on crying, at rest or biphasic) and degree of stridor (none, only on crying, at rest or biphasic) (Fig. 16.4).

Severe obstruction leads to increasing respiratory rate, heart rate and agitation. Central cyanosis or drowsiness indicates severe hypoxaemia and the need for urgent intervention – the measurement of oxygen saturation by pulse oximetry is the most reliable objective measure of hypoxaemia.

Box 16.1 Differential diagnosis of acute upper airways obstruction

Croup
* Viral laryngotracheitis (very common)
* Acute-on-chronic stridor, e.g. from a floppy larynx (laryngomalacia)
* Bacterial tracheitis (rare)

Rare causes
* Epiglottitis
* Inhalation of smoke and hot air in fires
* Trauma to the throat
* Retropharyngeal abscess
* Laryngeal foreign body
* Allergic laryngeal oedema (angioedema)
* Tetany due to poor vitamin D intake
* Infectious mononucleosis
* Measles
* Diphtheria

> **Basic management of acute upper airways obstruction:**
> * **Don't examine the throat!**
> * **Reduce anxiety by staff being calm, confident and well organised.**
> * **Observe carefully for signs of hypoxia or deterioration.**
> * **If in doubt, administer nebulised epinephrine (adrenaline).**
> * **If respiratory failure develops from increasing airways obstruction, exhaustion or secretions blocking the airway, urgent tracheal intubation is required.**

Total obstruction of the upper airway may be precipitated by examination of the throat using a spatula. One must avoid looking at the throat of a child with upper airways obstruction unless full resuscitation equipment and personnel are at hand.

Croup

Viral croup accounts for over 95% of laryngo-tracheal infections. Parainfluenza viruses are the commonest cause, but other viruses, such as metapneumovirus, RSV and influenza, can produce a similar clinical picture. There is mucosal inflammation and increased secretions affecting the larynx, trachea and bronchi, but it is the oedema of the subglottic area that is potentially dangerous in young children because it may result in critical narrowing of the trachea. Croup occurs from 6 months to 6 years of age but the peak incidence is in the second year of life. Croup is commonest in the autumn. The typical features are of a barking cough, harsh stridor and hoarseness usually preceded by fever and coryza. The symptoms often start, and are worse, at night.

The child with mild viral croup can usually be managed at home. When the upper airway obstruction is mild, the stridor and chest recession disappear when the child is at rest. The parents need to observe the child closely for the signs of increasing severity. The decision to manage the child at home or in hospital is influenced by the severity of the illness, time of day, ease of access to hospital, the child's age (with a low threshold for admission for those <12 months old) and parental understanding and confidence about the disorder.

Inhalation of warm moist air is widely used but is of unproven benefit. Oral dexamethasone, oral prednisolone and nebulised steroids (budesonide) reduce the severity and duration of croup and the need for hospitalisation. Nebulised epinephrine (adrenaline) provides transient improvement in severe upper airways obstruction, and children with the clinical features of severe croup, or an oxygen saturation of less than 93% in air, should be given nebulised epinephrine (adrenaline) with oxygen by face mask and closely monitored. Few children with croup require tracheal intubation since the introduction of steroid therapy.

Bacterial tracheitis (pseudomembranous croup)

This rare but dangerous condition is usually caused by infection with *Staphylococcus aureus* or *H. influenzae*. The clinical picture is similar to severe viral croup except that the child has a high fever, appears toxic and has rapidly progressive airways obstruction with copious thick airway secretions. Treatment is intravenous antibiotics and intubation and ventilation if required.

Acute epiglottitis

Acute epiglottitis is a life-threatening emergency due to respiratory obstruction. It is caused by *H. influenzae* type b. In the UK and many other

Table 16.1 Clinical features of croup (viral laryngotracheitis) and epiglottitis

	Croup	Epiglottitis
Onset	Over days	Over hours
Preceding coryza	Yes	No
Cough	Severe, barking	Absent or slight
Able to drink	Yes	No
Drooling saliva	No	Yes
Appearance	Unwell	Toxic, very ill
Fever	<38.5° C	>38.5° C
Stridor	Harsh, rasping	Soft, whispering
Voice, cry	Hoarse	Muffled, reluctant to speak

countries, the introduction of universal Hib immunisation in infancy has led to a decrease of over 99% in the incidence of epiglottitis and other invasive *H. influenzae* type b infections.

There is intense swelling of the epiglottis and surrounding tissues associated with septicaemia. Epiglottitis is most common in children aged 1–6 years but affects all age groups. It is important to distinguish between epiglottitis and croup (Table 16.1) as they require quite different treatment.

The onset of epiglottitis is often very acute (see Case history 16.1), with:

- high fever in an ill, toxic-looking child
- an intensely painful throat that prevents the child from speaking or swallowing; saliva drools down the chin
- soft inspiratory stridor and rapidly increasing respiratory difficulty over hours
- the child sits immobile, upright, with an open mouth to optimise the airway.

In contrast to viral croup, cough is minimal or absent. Attempts to lie the child down or examine the throat with a spatula or perform a lateral neck X-ray must not be undertaken as they can precipitate total airway obstruction and death.

If the diagnosis of epiglottitis is suspected, urgent hospital admission and treatment are required. A senior anaesthetist, paediatrician and ENT surgeon should be summoned and treatment initiated without delay. The child should be transferred directly to the intensive care unit or an anaesthetic room, and must be accompanied by senior medical staff in case respiratory obstruction occurs. The child should be intubated under controlled conditions with a general anaesthetic. Rarely, this is impossible and urgent tracheostomy is life-saving. Only after the airway is secured should blood be taken for culture and intravenous antibiotics such as cefuroxime started. The tracheal tube can usually be removed after 24 hours and antibiotics given for 3–5 days. With appropriate treatment, most children recover completely within 2–3 days. As with other serious *H. influenzae*

Case History
16.1 Acute epiglottis

This 5-year-old girl developed a severe sore throat, drooling of saliva, a high fever and increasing difficulty breathing over 8 hours (Fig. 16.5A) Epiglottitis was diagnosed and her airway was guaranteed with a nasotracheal tube. Antibiotics were started immediately (Fig. 16.5b, c). She made a full recovery.

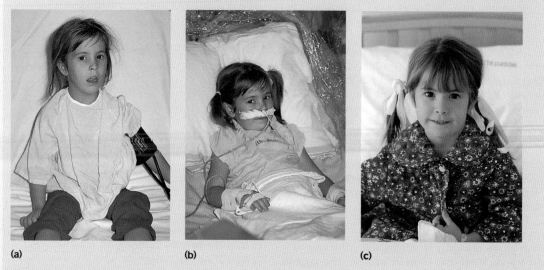

(a)　　　　　　　　　(b)　　　　　　　　　(c)

Figure 16.5 Acute epiglottitis. **(a)** At presentation. **(b)** At 16 hours, with nasotracheal and nasogastric tubes and an indwelling cannula for intravenous antibiotics. **(c)** At 36 hours, following removal of the nasotracheal and nasogastric tubes.

infections, prophylaxis with rifampicin is offered to close household contacts.

Minutes count in acute epiglottitis.

Bronchitis

There is controversy about the term bronchitis in childhood. Whilst some inflammation of the bronchi producing a mixture of wheeze and coarse crackles is often a feature of respiratory infections, bronchitis in children is very different from the chronic bronchitis of adults. In acute bronchitis in children, cough and fever are the main symptoms. The cough may persist for about 2 weeks, or longer with pertussis or *Mycoplasma* infections. There is no evidence that antibiotics, cough suppressants or expectorants speed recovery.

Whooping cough (pertussis)

This is a highly infectious form of bronchitis, caused by *Bordetella pertussis*. It is endemic, with epidemics every 3–4 years. After a week of coryza (catarrhal phase), the child develops a characteristic paroxysmal or spasmodic cough followed by a characteristic inspiratory whoop (paroxysmal phase). The spasms of cough are often worse at night and may culminate in vomiting. During a paroxysm, the child goes red or blue in the face, and mucus flows from the nose and mouth. The whoop may be absent in infants, but apnoea is a feature at this age. Epistaxes and subconjunctival haemorrhages can occur after vigorous coughing. The paroxysmal phase lasts 3–6 weeks. The symptoms gradually decrease (convalescent phase) but may persist for many months. Complications of pertussis, such as pneumonia, convulsions and bronchiectasis, are uncommon, but there is still a significant mortality, particularly in infants who develop apnoea. Infants and young children suffering severe spasms of cough or cyanotic attacks should be admitted to hospital.

The organism can be identified early in the disease from culture of a per-nasal swab. Characteristically, there is a marked lymphocytosis ($>15 \times 10^9$/L). Although erythromycin eradicates the organism, it decreases symptoms only if started during the catarrhal phase. Siblings, parents and school contacts may develop a similar cough, and close contacts should receive erythromycin prophylaxis, and unvaccinated infant contacts should be vaccinated. Immunisation reduces the risk of developing pertussis and the severity of disease in those affected, but does not guarantee protection. The level of protection declines steadily during childhood.

Summary

The child with stridor

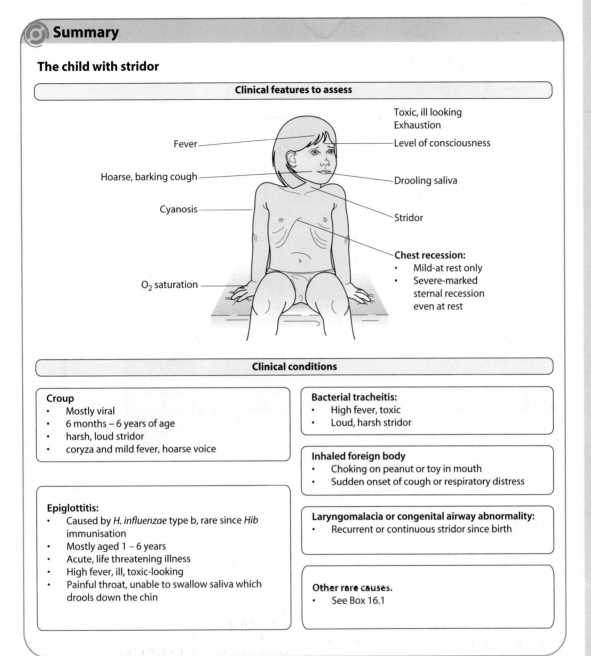

Clinical features to assess

Fever

Hoarse, barking cough

Cyanosis

O₂ saturation

Toxic, ill looking
Exhaustion

Level of consciousness

Drooling saliva

Stridor

Chest recession:
- Mild-at rest only
- Severe-marked sternal recession even at rest

Clinical conditions

Croup
- Mostly viral
- 6 months – 6 years of age
- harsh, loud stridor
- coryza and mild fever, hoarse voice

Epiglottitis:
- Caused by *H. influenzae* type b, rare since *Hib* immunisation
- Mostly aged 1 – 6 years
- Acute, life threatening illness
- High fever, ill, toxic-looking
- Painful throat, unable to swallow saliva which drools down the chin

Bacterial tracheitis:
- High fever, toxic
- Loud, harsh stridor

Inhaled foreign body
- Choking on peanut or toy in mouth
- Sudden onset of cough or respiratory distress

Laryngomalacia or congenital airway abnormality:
- Recurrent or continuous stridor since birth

Other rare causes.
- See Box 16.1

Summary

Pertussis:
- caused by *Bordetella pertussis*
- paroxysmal cough followed by inspiratory whoop and vomiting; in infants, apnoea rather than whoop, which is potentially dangerous
- diagnosis – culture of organism on per-nasal swab, marked lymphocytosis on blood film.

Bronchiolitis

Bronchiolitis is the commonest serious respiratory infection of infancy: 2–3% of all infants are admitted to hospital with the disease each year during annual winter epidemics; 90% are aged 1–9 months (bronchiolitis is rare after 1 year of age). Respiratory syncytial virus (RSV) is the pathogen in 80% of cases. Human metapneumovirus is a recently identified virus causing respiratory symptoms in children, and with the other respiratory viruses accounts for the remainder.

Clinical features

Coryzal symptoms precede a dry cough and increasing breathlessness. Wheezing is often, but not always, present. Feeding difficulty associated with increasing dyspnoea is often the reason for admission to hospital. Recurrent apnoea is a serious complication, especially in young infants. Infants born prematurely who develop bronchopulmonary

Bronchiolitis

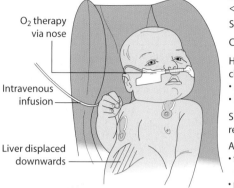

O₂ therapy via nose

Intravenous infusion

Liver displaced downwards

Apnoea in infants
<4 months

Sharp, dry cough

Cyanosis or pallor

Hyperinflation of the chest:
• sternum prominent
• liver displaced downwards

Subcostal and intercostal recession

Auscultation:
• fine end-inspiratory crackles
• prolonged expiration

Figure 16.6 Clinical features of severe bronchiolitis in an infant.

dysplasia and infants with congenital heart disease are most at risk from this disease. The characteristic findings on examination (Fig. 16.6) are:

- sharp, dry cough
- tachypnoea
- subcostal and intercostal recession
- hyperinflation of the chest
  - sternum prominent
  - liver displaced downwards
- fine end-inspiratory crackles
- high-pitched wheezes – expiratory > inspiratory
- tachycardia
- cyanosis or pallor.

Investigations

RSV can be identified rapidly on nasopharyngeal secretions demonstrating binding of a fluorescent antibody. A chest X-ray shows hyperinflation of the lungs due to small airways obstruction, air trapping (Fig. 16.7) and often focal atelectasis. Blood gas analysis, which is required in only the most severe cases, shows lowered arterial oxygen and raised CO_2 tension.

Management

This is supportive. Humidified oxygen is delivered via nasal cannulae or into a headbox; the concentration required is determined by pulse oximetry. The infant is monitored for apnoea. Mist, antibiotics and steroids are not helpful. Nebulised broncho-dilators, such as salbutamol or ipratropium, though often used, have not been shown to reduce the severity or duration of the illness. Fluids may need to be given by nasogastric tube or intravenously. Mechanical ventilation is required in about 2% of infants admitted to hospital. RSV is highly infectious, and infection control measures, particularly good hand hygiene, are needed to prevent cross-infection to other infants in hospital.

Prognosis

Most infants recover from the acute infection within 2 weeks. However, as many as half will have recurrent episodes of cough and wheeze (see section on asthma, below). Rarely, usually follow-

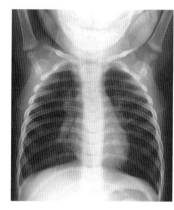

Figure 16.7 In acute bronchiolitis, the chest X-ray shows hyperinflation of the lungs with flattening of the diaphragm, horizontal ribs and increased hilar bronchial markings. Note: chest X-ray is rarely helpful in bronchiolitis.

ing adenovirus infection, the illness may result in permanent damage to the airways (bronchiolitis obliterans).

Prevention

A monoclonal antibody to RSV (palivizumab, given monthly by intramuscular injection) reduces the number of hospital admissions in high-risk preterm infants. Its use is limited by cost and the need for several injections.

Pneumonia

The incidence of pneumonia is highest in infancy, remains relatively high in childhood, is low in adults and increases again in old age. Pneumonia is caused by a variety of viruses and bacteria, although in half of cases no causative pathogen is identified. Viruses are the most common cause in younger children, while bacteria are commoner in older children. In clinical practice it is difficult to distinguish between viral and bacterial pneumonia, although viral pneumonia tends to peak during autumn and winter, while bacterial pneumonia exhibits less seasonal fluctuation.

The pathogens causing pneumonia vary according to the child's age:

- Newborn – organisms from the mother's genital tract, particularly group B *Streptococcus*, but also Gram-negative enterococci.

- Infants and young children – respiratory viruses, particularly RSV, are most common, but bacterial infections include *Streptococcus pneumoniae* or *Haemophilus influenzae*. *Bordetella pertussis* and *Chlamydia trachomatis* can also cause pneumonia at this age. An infrequent but serious cause is *Staph. aureus*.
- Children over 5 years – *Mycoplasma pneumoniae*, *Streptococcus pneumoniae* and *Chlamydia pneumoniae* are the main causes. *Mycobacterium tuberculosis* should be considered at all ages.

Clinical features

Fever and difficulty in breathing are the commonest presenting symptoms, usually preceded by an upper respiratory tract infection. Other symptoms include cough, lethargy, poor feeding and an 'unwell' child. Localised chest, abdominal, or neck pain is a feature of pleural irritation and suggests bacterial infection.

Examination reveals tachypnoea, nasal flaring and chest indrawing. Chest hyperinflation and wheeze are more suggestive of viral or mycoplasma infection. There may be end-inspiratory respiratory coarse crackles over the affected area, but the classic signs of consolidation with dullness on percussion, decreased breath sounds and bronchial breathing over the affected area are usually absent. Oxygen saturation readings may be decreased.

A chest X-ray may confirm the diagnosis, but with the exception of a classic lobar pneumonia characteristic of *Streptococcus pneumoniae* (Fig. 16.8), a chest X-ray cannot differentiate between bacterial and viral pneumonia. In younger children a nasopharyngeal aspirate is useful to identify viral causes, but blood tests, including full blood count and acute-phase reactants, are generally unhelpful in differentiating between a viral and bacterial cause. A chest X-ray showing cavities containing fluid and air is characteristic of staphylococcal pneumonia. A small proportion of pneumonias are associated with a parapneumonic effusion, where there may be blunting of the costophrenic angle on the chest X-ray. Some of these effusions develop into empyema and fibrin strands may form leading to septations, which make drainage difficult (Fig. 16.9). Ultrasound of the chest will distinguish between parapneumonic effusion and empyema.

Management

Evidence-based guidelines for the management of pneumonia in childhood have been published (British Thoracic Society).

Most cases can be managed at home, but indications for admission include oxygen saturations <93%, severe tachypnoea and difficulty breathing, grunting, apnoea, not feeding or family unable to provide appropriate care. General supportive care should include analgesia for pain, and oxygen for hypoxia. Fluids should be given if necessary, ensuring that an excessive volume is not given because of potential inappropriate ADH secretion. Physiotherapy has no role.

The choice of antibiotic is determined by the child's age, severity of illness and appearance on chest X-ray. Newborns require broad-spectrum intravenous antibiotics. Most older infants can be managed with oral amoxicillin, with broader-spectrum antibiotics such as co-amoxiclav being reserved for those who are complicated or unresponsive. For children >5 years of age either amoxicillin or an oral macrolide such as erythromycin is the treatment of choice.

Parapneumonic effusions usually resolve with appropriate antibiotics, but the small proportion that develop an empyema require drainage of the fluid, either by placement of a pigtail catheter and installation of intrapleural urokinase to break down any intrapleural septations, or by surgery.

Prognosis

Follow-up is not generally required for children with simple consolidation on chest X-ray and who recover clinically. Those with evidence of collapse or empyema should have a repeat chest X-ray after 4–6 weeks. Virtually all children with pneumonia, even those with empyema, make a full recovery. Long-term follow-up in adults shows measurable, but clinically insignificant, decreases in lung function.

Consider pneumonia in children with neck stiffness or acute abdominal pain.

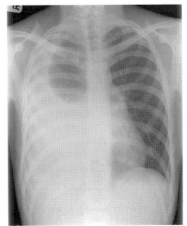

Figure 16.9 Right-sided empyema.

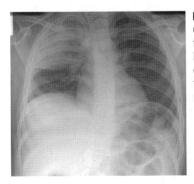

Figure 16.8 Consolidation of the right upper lobe. Lobar consolidation is a feature of pneumococcal pneumonia.

⊙ Summary

The infant with tachypnoea or wheeze

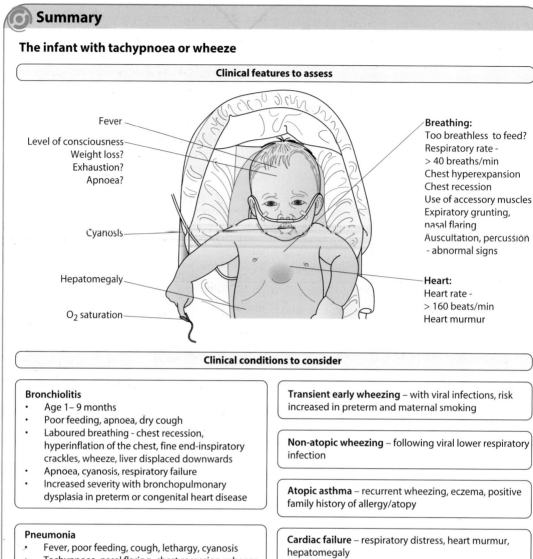

Clinical features to assess

Fever

Level of consciousness
Weight loss?
Exhaustion?
Apnoea?

Cyanosis

Hepatomegaly

O₂ saturation

Breathing:
Too breathless to feed?
Respiratory rate -
> 40 breaths/min
Chest hyperexpansion
Chest recession
Use of accessory muscles
Expiratory grunting,
nasal flaring
Auscultation, percussion
- abnormal signs

Heart:
Heart rate -
> 160 beats/min
Heart murmur

Clinical conditions to consider

Bronchiolitis
- Age 1– 9 months
- Poor feeding, apnoea, dry cough
- Laboured breathing - chest recession, hyperinflation of the chest, fine end-inspiratory crackles, wheeze, liver displaced downwards
- Apnoea, cyanosis, respiratory failure
- Increased severity with bronchopulmonary dysplasia in preterm or congenital heart disease

Pneumonia
- Fever, poor feeding, cough, lethargy, cyanosis
- Tachypnoea, nasal flaring, chest recession, wheeze and end-inspiratory coarse crackles over the affected area
- O₂ saturation may be decreased
- Chest X-ray – consolidation, parapneumonic effusion or empyema

Transient early wheezing – with viral infections, risk increased in preterm and maternal smoking

Non-atopic wheezing – following viral lower respiratory infection

Atopic asthma – recurrent wheezing, eczema, positive family history of allergy/atopy

Cardiac failure – respiratory distress, heart murmur, hepatomegaly

Inhaled foreign body – choking on peanut or toy, etc.
Aspiration of feeds – especially with neuromuscular disorder
Other causes – see Box 16.2

Asthma

Asthma and wheeze

Asthma is the most common chronic respiratory disorder in childhood, affecting 15–20% of children. Worldwide there appears to have been a significant increase in the incidence of asthma over the last 30 years, although this has plateaued. The highest rates are in the developed world. In most children, the symptoms of asthma are readily controlled, but it is an important cause of school absenteeism, restricted activity and anxiety for the child and family. There are still about 20 deaths from asthma in children each year in the UK.

Asthma is a heterogeneous condition of different clinical phenotypes, with wheezing being the major clinical expression. Three wheezing phenotypes have been identified in children with asthma:

- transient early wheezing
- non-atopic wheezing in the preschool child
- IgE-mediated wheezing (atopic asthma).

Transient early wheezing

Wheezing is very common in infancy, with approximately half of all children wheezing at some stage. The majority of infant wheezers have transient early virus associated wheezing (also known as wheezy bronchitis).

Transient early wheezing is thought to result from small airways being more likely to obstruct due to inflammation secondary to viral infections. Transient early wheezers have decreased lung function from birth, reflecting small airway calibre. Main risk factors are the mother smoking during and/or after pregnancy and prematurity. A family history of asthma or allergy is not a risk factor. Transient early wheezing is commoner in males than in females. It usually resolves by 5 years of age, presumably from the increase in airway calibre.

Non-atopic wheezing

In contrast, non-atopic wheezers have normal lung function early in life, but a lower respiratory illness due to a viral infection (usually RSV) leads to increased wheezing during the first ten years of life. This phenotype seems to cause less severe persistent wheezing, and symptoms improve during adolescence.

IgE-mediated wheezing (atopic asthma)

Atopic wheezing is the usual perception of asthma. Lung function is normal at birth, but recurrent wheeze develops with allergic sensitisation, with increased blood IgE and positive skin prick tests to common allergens. Atopic wheezers have persistence of symptoms and have decreased lung function later in childhood. Risk factors for the development of atopic wheeze (asthma) are family history of asthma or allergy and a history of

eczema, while exposure to tobacco smoke or prematurity are not risk factors.

Other causes of recurrent wheeze are listed in Box 16.2.

Pathophysiology

An outline of the pathophysiology of asthma is shown in Figure 16.10. Asthma results in chronic inflammation of the airways involving eosinophils, lymphocytes, mast cells and neutrophils. The inflammation causes widespread but variable airflow obstruction, with bronchoconstriction, mucosal oedema and excessive mucus production. The airflow obstruction is often reversible, either spontaneously or with treatment, and is associated with an increase in airway responsiveness to a variety of stimuli such as exercise, cold air or allergen exposure.

Figure 16.10 Pathophysiology of asthma.

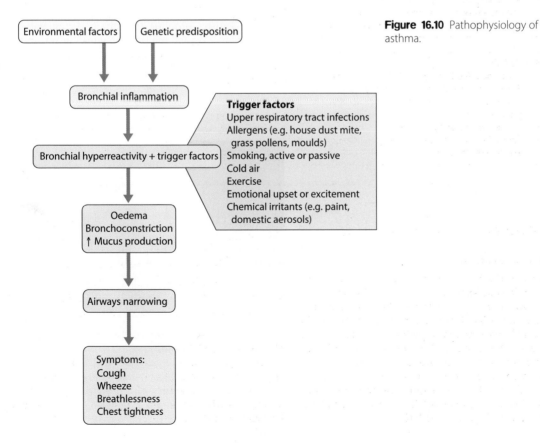

Atopy and allergy

Atopy is an inherited predisposition to sensitisation to allergens, and is present in up to 40% of children, most of whom are asymptomatic. Atopic children are at increased risk of allergic disease (see Box 16.3 and Ch. 15) The presence of one allergic condition within a child increases the risk of another; for example, half of children with allergic asthma will have eczema at some stage during their lives.

Diagnosis

The diagnosis of asthma in children should be suspected in any child with wheezing on more than one occasion, ideally heard on auscultation by a health professional, and distinguished from transmitted upper respiratory noises (BTS/SIGN Guideline on Asthma Management). Wheezing is a whistling noise heard from the chest, and parents' perception of wheezing often varies from health professionals. In practice, the diagnosis is usually made on a history of recurrent wheeze, with exacerbations usually precipitated by viral respiratory infections.

The pattern of asthma should be assessed by asking:

- How frequent are the symptoms?
- How much school has been missed due to asthma?
- Are sport and general activities affected by the asthma?
- How often is sleep disturbed by asthma?
- How severe are the interval symptoms between exacerbations?

Examination of the chest is usually normal between attacks. In long-standing asthma there may be hyperinflation of the chest, generalised polyphonic expiratory wheeze and a prolonged expiratory phase. Onset of the disease in infancy may result in Harrison's sulci (Fig. 16.11). Evidence of eczema should be sought, as should examination of the nasal mucosa for allergic rhinitis. Growth is normal unless the asthma is extremely severe. The presence of a wet cough or sputum production, finger clubbing, or poor growth suggests a more severe condition such as cystic fibrosis or bronchiectasis.

Investigations

Usually the diagnosis is clear from the history and no investigations are needed. Skin prick testing for common allergens is often considered both as an aid to the diagnosis of atopy and to identify allergens which may be acting as triggers. A chest X-ray is usually normal but may help to rule out other conditions. If there is uncertainty, recording peak expiratory flow rate (PEFR) may be useful (Fig. 16.12 and Appendix). Most children over 5 years of age can use a peak flow meter. Asthma results in increased variability in peak flow, both diurnal variability (morning PEFR usually lower than evening PEFR) and day-to-day variability (change in PEFR over the course of a week). There may also be bronchodilator responsiveness, where PEFR will increase by more than 10–15% after inhaling a bronchodilator. Often response to treatment is the most helpful investigation.

Management

The aim of management is to allow the child to lead as normal a life as possible by controlling symptoms and preventing exacerbations, optimising pulmonary function, while minimising treatment and side-effects. An evidence-based and regularly updated British Guideline on Asthma Management gives guidance on asthma treatment in children and adults.

Medications used to treat children with asthma are shown in Table 16.2.

● ●

Box 16.3 Allergic disorders

- Asthma
- Eczema
- Allergic rhinitis
- Allergic conjunctivitis
- Urticaria and angioedema
- Food and drug allergies

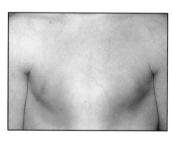

Figure 16.11 The depressions at the base of the thorax associated with the muscular insertion of the diaphragm are called Harrison's sulcus, and are often associated with respiratory symptoms in infancy.

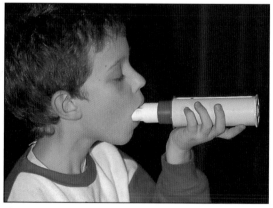

Figure 16.12 Measurement of the peak expiratory flow rate (PEFR) provides a simple objective measurement of the severity of airflow obstruction in asthma. Regular measurements recorded in a diary provide information about disease control. Normal values of PEFR are related to height (see Appendix).

Table 16.2 Drugs in asthma

Type of drug	Drug
Bronchodilators	
β₂-agonists (relievers)	Salbutamol
	Terbutaline
Anticholinergic bronchodilator	Ipratropium bromide
Preventative/prophylactic treatment	
Inhaled steroids	Budesonide
	Beclometasone
	Fluticasone
	Mometasone
Long-acting β₂-bronchodilators	Salmeterol
	Formoterol
Methylxanthines	Theophylline
Leukotriene inhibitors	Montelukast
Oral steroids	Prednisolone

All are given by inhalation, except prednisolone, leukotriene modulators and theophylline preparations.

Bronchodilator therapy

Inhaled β₂-agonists are the most commonly used and most effective bronchodilators. *Short-acting β₂-agonists* (often called *relievers*) such as salbutamol or terbutaline have a rapid onset of action, are effective for 2–4 hours, and have few side-effects. They are used as required for increased symptoms, and in high doses for acute asthma attacks.

In contrast, *long-acting β₂-agonists (LABAs)* such as salmeterol or formoterol are effective for 12 hours and are used in conjunction with regular inhaled corticosteroids. They are not used in acute asthma, and should not be used without an inhaled corticosteroid. Long-acting β₂-agonists are useful in exercise-induced asthma.

Ipratropium bromide, an anticholinergic bronchodilator, is sometimes given to young infants when other bronchodilators are found to be ineffective, or in the treatment of severe acute asthma.

Inhaled steroids

Prophylactic drugs are effective only if taken regularly. *Inhaled steroids* (often called *preventers*) are the most effective inhaled prophylactic therapy. They decrease airway inflammation, resulting in decreased symptoms, asthma exacerbations and bronchial hyperactivity. They are increasingly used in conjunction with an inhaled long-acting β₂-agonist. They have no clinically significant side-effects when given in conventional licensed doses. They can produce systemic side-effects, including impaired growth, adrenal suppression and altered bone metabolism, when high doses are used.

Other agents

Oral leukotriene receptor antagonists such as montelukast are helpful as add-on therapy when inhaled steroids with a LABA fail to control symptoms.

Summary

Assessment of the child with chronic asthma

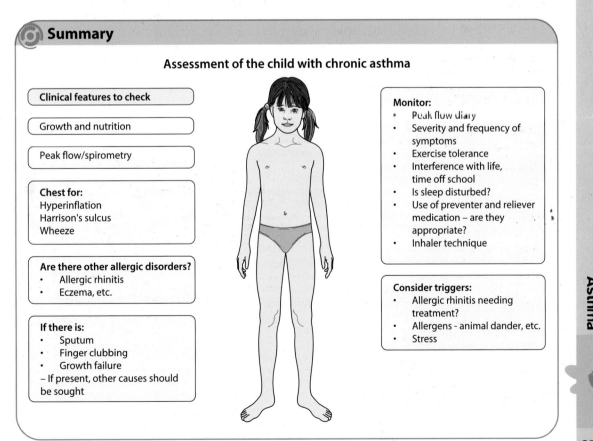

Clinical features to check

Growth and nutrition

Peak flow/spirometry

Chest for:
Hyperinflation
Harrison's sulcus
Wheeze

Are there other allergic disorders?
- Allergic rhinitis
- Eczema, etc.

If there is:
- Sputum
- Finger clubbing
- Growth failure
– If present, other causes should be sought

Monitor:
- Peak flow diary
- Severity and frequency of symptoms
- Exercise tolerance
- Interference with life, time off school
- Is sleep disturbed?
- Use of preventer and reliever medication – are they appropriate?
- Inhaler technique

Consider triggers:
- Allergic rhinitis needing treatment?
- Allergens - animal dander, etc.
- Stress

Slow-release oral theophylline is an alternative, However it has a high incidence of side-effects (vomiting, insomnia, headaches, poor concentration) and blood levels need to be monitored, so it is now rarely used in children.

Oral prednisolone, usually given on alternate days to minimise the adverse effect on height, is required only in severe persistent asthma where other treatment has failed.

Antibiotics are of no value in the absence of a bacterial infection and neither cough medicines nor decongestants are helpful. Antihistamines, e.g. loratadine and nasal steroids, are useful in the treatment of allergic rhinitis.

The British asthma guideline uses a stepwise approach, starting treatment with the step most appropriate to the severity of the asthma. Treatment increases from step 1 (mild intermittent asthma) to step 5 (chronic severe asthma), stepping down when control is good (Fig. 16.13).

Allergen avoidance and other non-pharmacological measures

Although many children's asthma is precipitated or worsened by specific allergens, complete avoidance of the allergen is difficult and therefore the value of identifying such triggers by history or allergy testing is controversial. There is currently no conclusive evidence that allergen avoidance measures (such as removal of furry animals or using dust mite impermeable mattress covers) are beneficial, although they may be considered in selected cases.

There is little evidence that any complementary or alternative therapy is effective. Parents should be advised about the harmful effects of cigarette smoking in the house Although exercise improves general fitness, there is no evidence that physical training improves asthma itself. Psychological intervention may be useful in chronic severe asthma.

Exercise-induced asthma

Some children's asthma is brought on only by vigorous exercise. With appropriate treatment asthma should not restrict exercise, and there are many elite athletes with asthma. For most, a short-acting β_2-agonist bronchodilator taken immediately before exercise is sufficient, but if there are more marked symptoms a LABA taken in conjunction with an inhaled steroid will give greater protection.

A stepwise approach to the treatment of chronic asthma

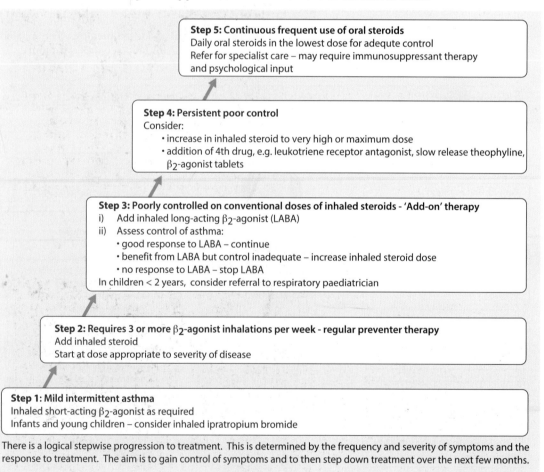

Step 5: Continuous frequent use of oral steroids
Daily oral steroids in the lowest dose for adequte control
Refer for specialist care – may require immunosuppressant therapy and psychological input

Step 4: Persistent poor control
Consider:
• increase in inhaled steroid to very high or maximum dose
• addition of 4th drug, e.g. leukotriene receptor antagonist, slow release theophyline, β_2-agonist tablets

Step 3: Poorly controlled on conventional doses of inhaled steroids - 'Add-on' therapy
i) Add inhaled long-acting β_2-agonist (LABA)
ii) Assess control of asthma:
• good response to LABA – continue
• benefit from LABA but control inadequate – increase inhaled steroid dose
• no response to LABA – stop LABA
In children < 2 years, consider referral to respiratory paediatrician

Step 2: Requires 3 or more β_2-agonist inhalations per week - regular preventer therapy
Add inhaled steroid
Start at dose appropriate to severity of disease

Step 1: Mild intermittent asthma
Inhaled short-acting β_2-agonist as required
Infants and young children – consider inhaled ipratropium bromide

There is a logical stepwise progression to treatment. This is determined by the frequency and severity of symptoms and the response to treatment. The aim is to gain control of symptoms and to then step down treatment over the next few months.

Figure 16.13 A stepwise approach to the treatment of asthma. (Adapted from British guideline on the management of asthma, 2003.)

Acute asthma

With each acute attack, the duration of symptoms, the treatment already given and the course of previous attacks should be noted. Clinical features are:

- Wheeze and tachypnoea (respiratory rate >50 breaths/min in children 2–5 years, >30 breaths/min in children 5 or over) – but poor guide to severity.
- Increasing tachycardia (>130 beats/min in children aged 2–5 years, >120 beats/min in children 5 or over) – better guide to severity.
- The use of accessory muscles and chest recession – also better guide to severity.
- The presence of marked pulsus paradoxus (the difference between systolic pressure on inspiration and expiration) indicates moderate to severe in children but is difficult to measure accurately and is therefore unreliable.

- If breathlessness interferes with talking, the attack is severe.
- Cyanosis, fatigue and drowsiness are late signs, indicating life-threatening asthma; this may be accompanied by a silent chest on auscultation as little air is being exchanged.

However, the severity of an acute asthma may be underestimated by clinical examination alone. Therefore:

- Arterial oxygen saturation should be measured with a pulse oximeter in all children presenting to hospital with acute asthma. Oxygen saturations <92% in air imply severe or life-threatening asthma.
- Measurement of the peak expiratory flow rate should be routine in school-age children.

The features of a severe and life-threatening acute attack are shown in Figure 16.17.

Choosing the correct inhaler

Inhaled drugs may be administered via a variety of devices, chosen according to the child's age and preference:
- metered dose inhaler
- breath-actuated metered dose inhaler, e.g. Autohaler or Easi-Breathe
- dry powder devices, e.g. terbutaline sulphate (Bricanyl Turbohaler) and salbutamol (Ventolin Accuhaler).

The pressurised metered-dose inhaler (MDI) requires the greatest coordination and should never be used alone in children. Using an MDI through a spacer device such as the Nebuhaler or aerochamber significantly increases the proportion of the drug reaching the airways, reduces impaction of drug on the throat and requires less coordination. In young children, a soft face mask can be attached to the spacer (Fig. 16.15). Ideally inhaled steroids should

always be given by MDI and spacer, and spacers should be used in young children and for delivering beta agonists during acute asthma attacks. Spacers are very effective at delivering bronchodilators and inhaled steroids to the preschool child.

Breath-actuated devices and dry-powder inhalers require less coordination than MDIs and can be used for delivering beta agonists in school-age children (Fig. 16.14).

Nebulised treatment is now only given for severe life-threatening asthma, or rarely for children who need inhaled therapy but are unable to use any of these devices or require high doses (Fig. 16.16).

Many children fail to gain the benefit of their treatment because they cannot use the inhaler they have been given. The correct way to use an inhaler must be demonstrated and the child's ability to use it checked.

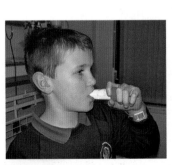

Figure 16.14 4–10 years old: dry-powder inhaler as shown or metered dose inhaler with spacer.

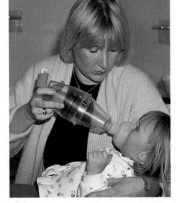

Figure 16.15 Less than 4 years old: metered dose inhaler with spacer. Use a mask if <2 years old.

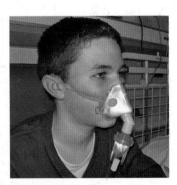

Figure 16.16 Nebulisers deliver high-dose therapy and are used in severe acute attacks.

Criteria for hospital admission

Children require hospital admission if, after high-dose inhaled bronchodilator therapy, they:

- have not responded adequately clinically – persisting breathlessness, tachypnoea
- are exhausted
- still have a marked reduction in their predicted (or usual) peak flow rate
- have a reduced oxygen saturation (<92% in air).

A chest X-ray is indicated only if there is severe dyspnoea or unusual features (e.g. asymmetry of chest signs suggesting pneumothorax, lobar collapse) or signs of severe infection. In children, arterial blood gases are only indicated in life-threatening or refractory cases.

Treatment

Acute breathlessness is frightening for both the child and the parents. Calm and skilful management is the key to their reassurance. High-dose inhaled bronchodilators, steroids and oxygen form the foundation of therapy of severe acute asthma.

Management is summarised in Figure 16.17. As soon as the diagnosis has been made, the child should be given a β_2-bronchodilator. For severe

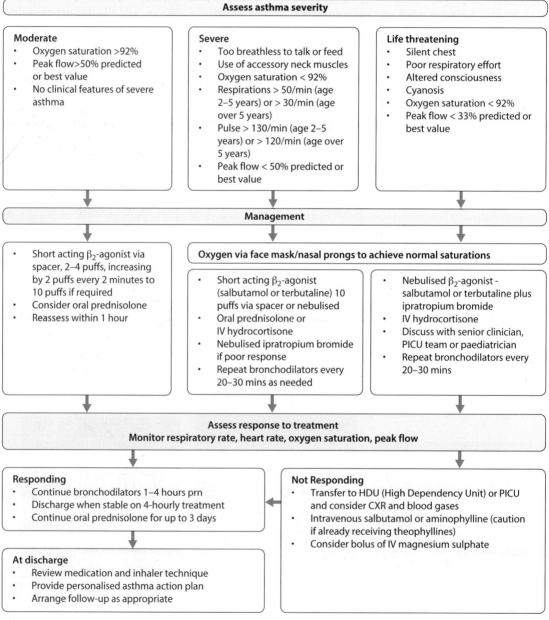

Assessment and management of acute asthma

Assess asthma severity

Moderate
- Oxygen saturation >92%
- Peak flow>50% predicted or best value
- No clinical features of severe asthma

Severe
- Too breathless to talk or feed
- Use of accessory neck muscles
- Oxygen saturation < 92%
- Respirations > 50/min (age 2–5 years) or > 30/min (age over 5 years)
- Pulse > 130/min (age 2–5 years) or > 120/min (age over 5 years)
- Peak flow < 50% predicted or best value

Life threatening
- Silent chest
- Poor respiratory effort
- Altered consciousness
- Cyanosis
- Oxygen saturation < 92%
- Peak flow < 33% predicted or best value

Management

- Short acting β_2-agonist via spacer, 2–4 puffs, increasing by 2 puffs every 2 minutes to 10 puffs if required
- Consider oral prednisolone
- Reassess within 1 hour

Oxygen via face mask/nasal prongs to achieve normal saturations

- Short acting β_2-agonist (salbutamol or terbutaline) 10 puffs via spacer or nebulised
- Oral prednisolone or IV hydrocortisone
- Nebulised ipratropium bromide if poor response
- Repeat bronchodilators every 20–30 mins as needed

- Nebulised β_2-agonist - salbutamol or terbutaline plus ipratropium bromide
- IV hydrocortisone
- Discuss with senior clinician, PICU team or paediatrician
- Repeat bronchodilators every 20–30 mins

Assess response to treatment
Monitor respiratory rate, heart rate, oxygen saturation, peak flow

Responding
- Continue bronchodilators 1–4 hours prn
- Discharge when stable on 4-hourly treatment
- Continue oral prednisolone for up to 3 days

Not Responding
- Transfer to HDU (High Dependency Unit) or PICU and consider CXR and blood gases
- Intravenous salbutamol or aminophylline (caution if already receiving theophyllines)
- Consider bolus of IV magnesium sulphate

At discharge
- Review medication and inhaler technique
- Provide personalised asthma action plan
- Arrange follow-up as appropriate

Figure 16.17 Assessment and management of acute asthma. Adapted from British guideline on asthma management, 2003.

exacerbations, high-dose therapy should be given and repeated every 20–30 minutes For moderate to severe asthma, 10 puffs of β₂-bronchodilator should be given via metered-dose inhaler (MDI) and large volume spacer. For severe to life-threatening asthma, a β₂-bronchodilator may need to be given via nebuliser. The addition of nebulised ipratropium to the initial therapy in severe asthma is beneficial. Oxygen is given when there is any evidence of arterial oxygen desaturation. A short course (2–5 days) of oral prednisolone expedites the recovery from moderate or severe acute asthma.

Intravenous therapy has a role in the minority of children who fail to respond adequately to inhaled bronchodilator, either aminophylline or intravenous salbutamol. For intravenous amino-phylline, a loading dose is given over 20 minutes, followed by continuous infusion. Seizures, severe vomiting and fatal cardiac arrhythmias may follow a rapid infusion. If the child is already on oral theophylline, the loading dose should be omitted. With both aminophylline and salbutamol, the ECG should be monitored and blood electrolytes checked. There is increasing evidence that intra-venous magnesium is helpful in life-threatening asthma. Antibiotics are only given if there are clinical features of bacterial infection. Occasionally, these measures are insufficient and artificial ventilation is required.

After an acute exacerbation, the child's mainte-nance treatment and inhaler technique should be reviewed and altered if inadequate. The child should be given a written individualised asthma action plan. Follow-up arrangements should be made to monitor progress by the general practi-tioner or, for the more problematic patients, by a paediatrician.

Patient education

In order for families to make rational decisions, they need to know:

- when drugs should be used (regularly or 'as required')
- how to use the drug (inhaler technique)
- what each drug does (relief vs. prevention)
- how often and how much can be used (frequency and dosage)
- what to do if asthma worsens (management of acute attacks).

The child and parents need to know that increasing cough, wheeze and breathlessness and difficulty in walking, talking and sleeping, or decreasing relief from bronchodilators all indicate poorly controlled asthma. Some asthmatics find it difficult to perceive gradual deterioration – measurement of peak flow rate at home allows

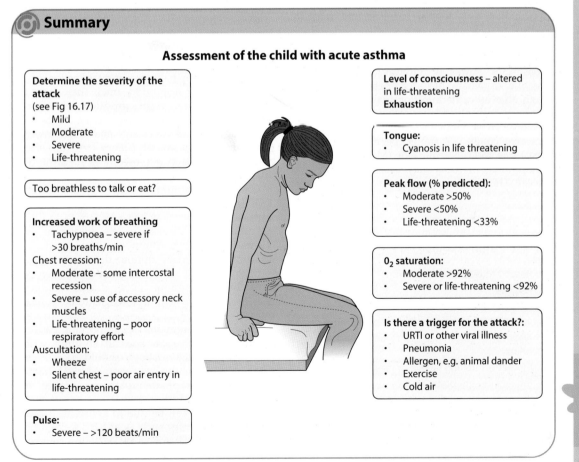

Summary

Assessment of the child with acute asthma

Determine the severity of the attack
(see Fig 16.17)
- Mild
- Moderate
- Severe
- Life-threatening

Too breathless to talk or eat?

Increased work of breathing
- Tachypnoea – severe if >30 breaths/min

Chest recession:
- Moderate – some intercostal recession
- Severe – use of accessory neck muscles
- Life-threatening – poor respiratory effort

Auscultation:
- Wheeze
- Silent chest – poor air entry in life-threatening

Pulse:
- Severe – >120 beats/min

Level of consciousness – altered in life-threatening
Exhaustion

Tongue:
- Cyanosis in life threatening

Peak flow (% predicted):
- Moderate >50%
- Severe <50%
- Life-threatening <33%

O₂ saturation:
- Moderate >92%
- Severe or life-threatening <92%

Is there a trigger for the attack?:
- URTI or other viral illness
- Pneumonia
- Allergen, e.g. animal dander
- Exercise
- Cold air

earlier recognition. Parents need to know when to start steroids at home and what dose to give. Written personalised asthma action plans improve control of asthma, particularly in those with more severe disease or who have had a recent exacerbation. They should be written specifically for each individual patient. Based on symptoms and/or peak flow, treatment is increased with increased severity of attack. Patients with troublesome asthma are usually given a supply of oral steroids to keep at home, with instructions in the asthma action plan on when to start them.

Recurrent cough

Cough is the most common symptom of respiratory disease and indicates irritation of nerve receptors in the pharynx, larynx, trachea or large bronchi. While recurrent cough may simply indicate that the child is having recurrent respiratory infections, other causes need to be considered (Box 16.4).

Asthma is the commonest cause of recurrent cough in childhood. Although there is usually associated wheeze and breathlessness triggered by characteristic factors, in the preschool child a troublesome night-time cough may sometimes be the only symptom, and often responds to treatment. Many children have a persistent nasal discharge due to allergic rhinitis; their nocturnal cough may be due to their postnasal drip or may be caused by coexisting asthma. A trial of therapy with a bronchodilator or topical nasal steroid may be required to make the diagnosis.

Certain infections, such as pertussis, RSV and *Mycoplasma* infection, can cause a cough that persists for weeks or months, long after the infective organism has disappeared. Persistent cough after an acute infection may indicate cystic fibrosis or unresolved lobar collapse, which will be seen on a chest X-ray. In any child with a severe, persistent cough, TB should be excluded with a chest X-ray and tuberculin skin (Mantoux) test.

Aspiration of feeds may cause coughing and wheeze. This may be caused by gastro-oesophageal

reflux in infants or as a result of swallowing disorders, e.g. in children with cerebral palsy.

Some older children and adolescents develop a barking, unproductive, habit cough following an infection or an asthma attack. The cough characteristically disappears during sleep. Reassurance and explanation after a thorough examination are usually effective.

The importance of parental smoking on children is generally underestimated. If both parents smoke, young children are twice as likely to have recurrent cough and wheeze than in non-smoking households. In the older child, active smoking is common – 10% of 11–15-year-olds and 30% of 16–19-year-olds smoke regularly.

Chronic lung infection

Children with recurrent pneumonia or who produce purulent sputum may have bronchiectasis, which is permanent dilatation of the bronchi.

It is helpful to determine if recurrent pneumonia affects different lobes of the lung (generalised), or only one lobe (focal). Generalised causes include cystic fibrosis, primary ciliary dyskinesia, immunodeficiency or chronic aspiration. Bronchiectasis following severe pneumonia, particularly tuberculosis, pertussis or measles, has now become uncommon. Although a plain chest X-ray may show gross bronchiectasis, it is best seen on a CT scan of the chest (Fig. 16.18a and b).

Cystic fibrosis is considered below. In primary ciliary dyskinesia, the microcilia of the respiratory epithelium, which are an important defence against infection, are abnormal in structure or function. Affected children have recurrent infection of the upper and lower respiratory tract. They characteristically have recurrent productive cough, a purulent nasal discharge and chronic ear infections; 50% also have dextrocardia and situs inversus (Kartagener's syndrome). Ciliary structure can be assessed by electron microscopy of nasal mucosal brushings.

Children with immunodeficiency may develop severe, unusual or recurrent chest infections. The immune deficiency may be secondary to an illness, e.g. malignant disease or its treatment with chemotherapy. Less commonly it is due to HIV infection or a primary immune deficiency.

Many neurologically impaired children will have chronic aspiration, either due to oropharyngeal incoordination or due to gastro-oesophageal reflux.

Tuberculosis remains an important cause of chronic lung infection and all children with a persistent productive cough should have a chest X-ray and tuberculin skin test. Marked hilar or paratracheal lymphadenopathy is highly suggestive of tuberculosis.

Focal disease can be due to generalised causes but also local causes such as inhaled foreign body (e.g. peanut; see Case history 16.2), or a congenital abnormality of the lungs, such as congenital cysts

---

Box 16.4 Causes of recurrent or persistent cough

- Recurrent respiratory infections
- Asthma
- Allergic rhinitis
- Infection (e.g. pertussis, RSV, *Mycoplasma*)
- Recurrent aspiration (± gastro-oesophageal reflux)
- Cigarette smoking (active or passive)
- Inhaled foreign body
- Suppurative lung diseases (e.g. cystic fibrosis or ciliary dyskinesia)
- Tuberculosis
- Habit cough

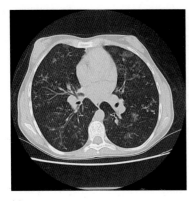 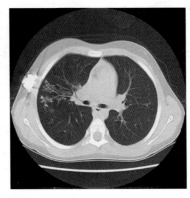

Figure 16.18 Bronchiectasis on CT scan of the chest. **(a)** Generalised and **(b)** focal, in the right upper lobe.

(a)

(b)

Case History
16.2 Foreign body inhalation

A previously well 3-year-old boy presented with a 5-day history of severe cough and wheeze. His symptoms developed after choking on some peanuts. A chest X-ray revealed a hyperlucent right lung (Fig. 16.19). Bronchoscopy was performed and revealed a peanut wedged in the right main bronchus.

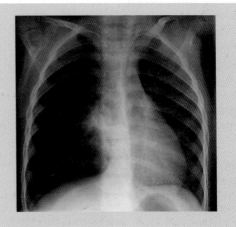

Figure 16.19 Hyperlucency of the right lung and mediastinal shift to the left. (Courtesy of Dr Abbas Khakoo.)

or a sequestrated lobe. Bronchoscopy is usually required for focal disease.

Cystic fibrosis

Cystic fibrosis (CF) is the commonest life-limiting inherited condition in Caucasians. Average life expectancy has increased from a few years to the mid-thirties, with a projected life expectancy for current newborns into the forties. CF is an autosomal recessive disease. In Caucasians the carrier rate is 1 in 25, with 1 in 2500 affected births. The disease is much less common in other ethnic groups. A gene located on chromosome 7 codes for the protein called cystic fibrosis transmembrane regulator (CFTR), which is defective in CF. CFTR is a cyclic AMP-dependent chloride channel blocker. Over 1000 different gene mutations have been discovered in CF, but the ΔF508 mutation is found in 75% of cases in the UK. The gene mutation affects the severity of disease, and life expectancy. Identification of the gene mutation involved within a family allows prenatal diagnosis and carrier detection in the wider family.

In CF, the abnormal ion transport across the epithelial cells of the exocrine glands of the respiratory tract and pancreas results in increased viscosity of secretions. Abnormal function of the sweat glands results in excessive concentrations of sodium and chloride in the sweat (60–125 mmol/L in cystic fibrosis, 10–30 mmol/L in normal children). This forms the basis of the essential diagnostic procedure, the sweat test, in which sweating is stimulated by pilocarpine iontophoresis. The sweat is collected into a special capillary tube or absorbed onto a weighed piece of filter paper. Diagnostic errors are common if there is an inadequate volume of sweat collected, so the test must be performed by experienced staff. Thick and viscid mucus is not the only basis of the pathogenesis of CF. Abnormality of the CFTR also affects inflammatory processes and defence against infection.

Clinical features

In the UK, screening of newborn is performed. Clinically, most children with CF will present with malabsorption and failure to thrive from birth, accompanied by recurrent or persistent chest

Box 16.5 Clinical features of cystic fibrosis

Newborn
Diagnosed through newborn screening.

Infancy
- Meconium ileus in newborn period
- Prolonged neonatal jaundice
- Failure to thrive
- Recurrent chest infections
- Malabsorption, steatorrhoea

Young child
- Bronchiectasis
- Rectal prolapse
- Nasal polyp
- Sinusitis

Older child and adolescent
- Allergic bronchopulmonary aspergillosis (ABPA)
- Diabetes mellitus (often not insulin-dependent)
- Cirrhosis and portal hypertension
- Distal intestinal obstruction (DIOS, meconium ileus equivalent)
- Pneumothorax or recurrent haemoptysis
- Sterility in males
- Increasing psychological problems

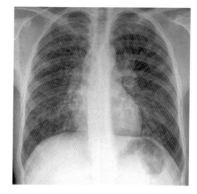

Figure 16.20 A chest X-ray in cystic fibrosis showing hyperinflation, marked peribronchial shadowing, bronchial wall thickening and ring shadows.

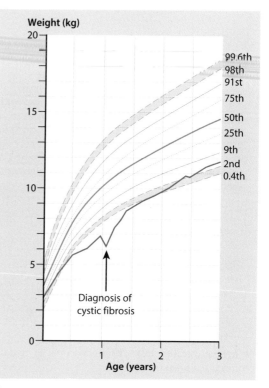

Figure 16.21 Growth chart of a child with cough and recurrent wheeze. Only when the diagnosis of cystic fibrosis was made and appropriate treatment started did he gain weight. (Adapted from growth chart © Child Growth Foundation.)

infections (Box 16.5). In the lungs, viscid mucus in the smaller airways predisposes to chronic infection, initially with *Staph. aureus* and *H. influenzae* and subsequently with *Pseudomonas aeruginosa*. This leads to damage of the bronchial wall, bronchiectasis and abscess formation (Fig. 16.20). The child has a persistent, loose cough productive of purulent sputum. On examination there is hyperinflation of the chest due to air trapping, coarse inspiratory crepitations and/or expiratory wheeze. With established disease, there is finger clubbing. Ultimately 95% of patients with CF will die of respiratory failure.

Over 90% of children with CF have pancreatic exocrine insufficiency (lipase, amylase and proteases) resulting in maldigestion and malabsorption. This leads to failure to thrive (Fig. 16.21), passing frequent large, pale, very offensive and greasy stools (steatorrhoea). Pancreatic insufficiency can be diagnosed by demonstrating low elastase in faeces.

About 10–20% of CF infants present in the neonatal period with meconium ileus, in which inspissated meconium causes intestinal obstruction with vomiting, abdominal distension and failure to pass meconium in the first few days of life. Initial treatment is with Gastrografin enemas, but most cases require surgery.

Management

The effective management of CF requires a multidisciplinary team approach, including paediatricians, physiotherapists, dieticians, specialist nurses, the primary care team, teachers and, most importantly, the child and parents. All patients with CF should be reviewed at least annually in a specialist centre. The condition cannot be cured. The aims of therapy are to prevent progression of the lung disease and to maintain adequate nutrition and growth.

Respiratory management

Recurrent and persistent bacterial chest infection is the major problem. In younger children respiratory status is monitored on symptoms; older children should have their lung function measured regularly by spirometry. The forced expiratory volume in 1

Summary

Assessment of the adolescent with cystic fibrosis

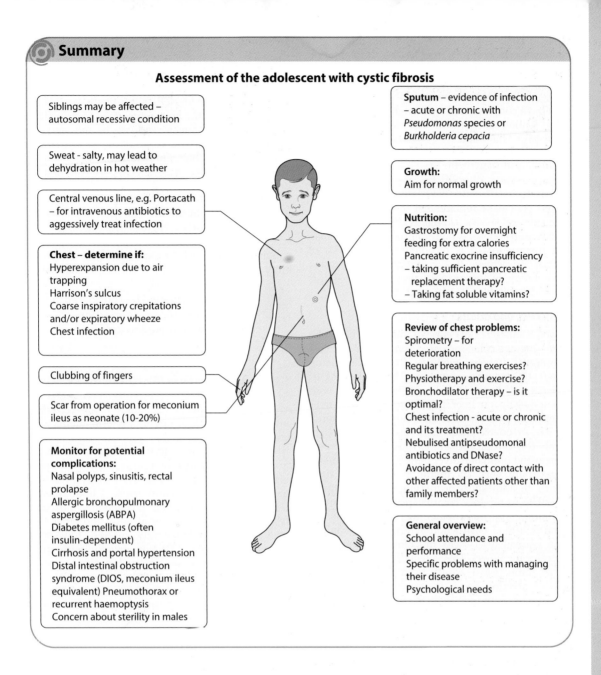

Siblings may be affected – autosomal recessive condition

Sweat - salty, may lead to dehydration in hot weather

Central venous line, e.g. Portacath – for intravenous antibiotics to aggessively treat infection

Chest – determine if:
Hyperexpansion due to air trapping
Harrison's sulcus
Coarse inspiratory crepitations and/or expiratory wheeze
Chest infection

Clubbing of fingers

Scar from operation for meconium ileus as neonate (10-20%)

Monitor for potential complications:
Nasal polyps, sinusitis, rectal prolapse
Allergic bronchopulmonary aspergillosis (ABPA)
Diabetes mellitus (often insulin-dependent)
Cirrhosis and portal hypertension
Distal intestinal obstruction syndrome (DIOS, meconium ileus equivalent) Pneumothorax or recurrent haemoptysis
Concern about sterility in males

Sputum – evidence of infection – acute or chronic with *Pseudomonas* species or *Burkholderia cepacia*

Growth:
Aim for normal growth

Nutrition:
Gastrostomy for overnight feeding for extra calories
Pancreatic exocrine insufficiency
– taking sufficient pancreatic replacement therapy?
– Taking fat soluble vitamins?

Review of chest problems:
Spirometry – for deterioration
Regular breathing exercises?
Physiotherapy and exercise?
Bronchodilator therapy – is it optimal?
Chest infection - acute or chronic and its treatment?
Nebulised antipseudomonal antibiotics and DNase?
Avoidance of direct contact with other affected patients other than family members?

General overview:
School attendance and performance
Specific problems with managing their disease
Psychological needs

second (FEV_1), expressed as a percentage predicted for age, sex and height, is an indicator of clinical severity and declines with disease progression.

With regular treatment, most infants and children with CF should have no respiratory symptoms, and often have no abnormal sign. From diagnosis, children should have physiotherapy at least twice a day, aiming to clear the airways of secretions. In younger children parents are taught to perform airway clearance at home using chest percussion and postural drainage. Older patients perform controlled deep breathing exercises and use a variety of physiotherapy devices for airway clearance. Physical exercise is beneficial in CF, and is encouraged. Many CF specialists recommend continuous prophylactic oral antibiotics (usually flucloxacillin), with additional rescue oral antibiotics for any increase in respiratory symptoms or

decline in lung function. Persisting symptoms or signs require prompt and vigorous intravenous therapy to limit lung damage, usually administered for 14 days via a peripheral venous long line. Increasingly, parents are taught to administer courses of intravenous antibiotics at home, so decreasing disruption of normal activities such as school. Chronic *Pseudomonas* infection is associated with a more rapid decline in lung function, and this is slowed by the use of daily nebulised antipseudomonal antibiotics. Nebulised DNase may be helpful to decrease the viscosity of sputum and so increase its clearance. The macrolide antibiotic azithromycin given regularly decreases respiratory exacerbations, probably due to an immunomodulatory effect rather than to antibiotic actions. Regular, nebulised hypertonic saline may decrease the number of respiratory exacerbations. More severe CF requires more regular intravenous antibiotic therapy. If venous access becomes troublesome, implantation of a central venous catheter with a subcutaneous port (e.g. Portacath) simplifies venous access, although they require monthly flushing and they may have complications. Although lung transplant is an option in terminal disease, this is rarely required in childhood.

Nutritional management

Dietary status should be assessed regularly. Pancreatic insufficiency is treated with oral enteric-coated pancreatic replacement therapy taken with all meals and snacks. Dosage is adjusted according to clinical response. A high-calorie diet is essential, and dietary intake is recommended at 150% of normal. To achieve this, overnight feeding via a gastrostomy is increasingly used. Most patients require fat-soluble vitamin supplements.

Teenagers and adults

Most CF sufferers now survive into adult life. With increasing age come increased complications, most commonly diabetes mellitus due to decreasing pancreatic endocrine function. Up to a third of patients will have evidence of liver disease with hepatomegaly on liver palpation, abnormal liver function on blood tests or an abnormal ultrasound; regular ursodeoxycholic acid may be beneficial. Rarely this can progress to cirrhosis, portal hypertension and ultimately liver failure. Liver transplant is generally very successful in CF-related liver failure. In addition to increasing chest infections, other late respiratory complications include pneumothorax and life-threatening haemoptysis. In distal intestinal obstruction syndrome (meconium ileus equivalent), viscid mucofaeculent material obstructs the bowel. This is usually cleared by oral Gastrografin. Most adults have chronic *Pseudomonas* infection, and in most the strain of *Pseudomonas* is unique to them. There is increasing concern over transmission of virulent strains of *Pseudomonas* and *Burkholderia cepacia* between patients, causing rapid decline in lung function. Consequently, patients are often segregated and advised not to socialise with other CF sufferers.

Females have normal fertility, and unless they have severe lung disease, tolerate pregnancy well. Males are virtually always infertile due to absence of the vas deferens, although they can father children through intracytoplasmic sperm injection (ICSI). The psychological repercussions on the affected child and family of a chronic and ultimately fatal illness which requires regular physiotherapy and drugs, frequent hospital admissions and absences from school are considerable. The CF team should provide psychological and emotional support. Adolescents have particular needs which must receive special consideration. Older adolescents with CF should transfer to specialist adult CF care.

Gene therapy is currently being assessed but is unlikely to be of practical value in the immediate future.

Screening

Newborn screening for CF leads to better lung function in childhood, decreases malnutrition and improves neurodevelopment. Screening of all newborn infants for CF is routinely performed throughout the UK. Immunoreactive trypsin (IRT) is raised in CF patients and can be measured in routine heelprick blood taken for biochemical screening of all babies (Guthrie test). Those samples with a raised IRT are then screened for common CF gene mutations, and infants with two mutations have a sweat test to confirm the diagnosis. Identifying cases in the neonatal period allows the early introduction of regular treatment. It also enables early genetic counselling for the parents about the 1 in 4 risk of recurrence and the possibility of prenatal diagnosis in future pregnancies.

> **Cystic fibrosis should be considered in any child with recurrent infections, loose stools or failure to thrive.**

Long-term respiratory support

An increasing number of children are receiving long-term respiratory support. Preterm infants with severe bronchopulmonary dysplasia (chronic lung disease) may require additional oxygen for many months, and may also require respiratory support with CPAP (continuous positive airway pressure) via nasal prongs or nasal mask. Children with a muscle weakness from Duchenne's muscular dystrophy, spinal muscular atrophy and other rare conditions are increasingly offered long-term ventilatory support. This is usually with non-invasive ventilation and bilevel positive airway pressure (BiPAP) (Fig. 16.22), but may be full ventilation via a tracheostomy (Fig. 16.23). In Duchenne's muscular dystrophy and some other conditions causing muscle weakness, non-invasive ventilation at night may provide additional quality years of life. This service can often be provided at home, with considerable specialist community support. With progressive neurological disorders, difficult ethical decisions need to be made about admission for intensive care and initiation of long-term full ventilation.

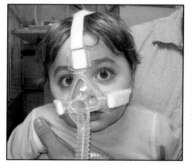

Figure 16.22
Long-term non-invasive respiratory support given overnight to a child with muscle weakness.

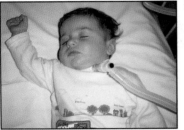

Figure 16.23
Long-term ventilation via a tracheostomy.

Further reading

British Thoracic Society Guidelines on community acquired pneumonia in childhood. Thorax (www.sign.ac.uk)

British Thoracic Society/Scottish Intercollegiate Guideline Network 2005 The British guideline on asthma management

Butler C C, Williams R G 2003 The etiology, pathophysiology, and management of otitis media with effusion. Current Infectious Disease Reports 5:205–212

Silverman M 2001 Childhood asthma and other wheezing disorders. Chapman Hall, London

Taussig L M, Landau L I 1997 Pediatric respiratory medicine. Mosby, St Louis. *Definitive textbook*

17

Cardiac disorders

Recent developments in paediatric cardiac disease are:

- lesions are increasingly identified on antenatal ultrasound screening
- most lesions are diagnosed by echocardiography, the mainstay of diagnostic imaging
- MRI allows three-dimensional reconstruction of complex cardiac disorders, assessment of haemodynamics and flow patterns and assists interventional cardiology, reducing the need for cardiac catheterisation
- most complex defects can be corrected completely at the initial operation, e.g. transposition of the great arteries
- an increasing number of defects (60%) are treated non-invasively, e.g. persistent ductus arteriosus
- new therapies are available to treat pulmonary hypertension and delay transplantation
- the overall infant cardiac surgical mortality has been reduced from approximately 20% in 1970 to 4% in 2007.

Epidemiology

Heart disease in children is mostly congenital. It is the most common single group of structural malformations in infants:

- 8 per 1000 live-born infants have significant cardiac malformations
- some abnormality of the cardiovascular system, e.g. a bicuspid aortic valve, is present in 1–2% of live births
- about 1 in 10 stillborn infants have a cardiac anomaly.

The nine most common anomalies account for 80% of all lesions (Box 17.1), but:

- about 10–15% have complex lesions with more than one cardiac abnormality
- about 10–15% also have a non-cardiac abnormality.

Congenital heart disease is the most common group of structural malformations in children.

Little is known about the aetiology of congenital heart disease. A small proportion are related to external teratogens and about 8% are associated

---

Box 17.1 The most common congenital heart lesions

Acyanotic
Left-to-right shunts
Ventricular septal defect 30%
Persistent ductus arteriosus 12%
Atrial septal defect 7%

Outflow obstruction
Pulmonary stenosis 7%
Aortic stenosis   5%
Coarctation of the aorta 5%

Cyanotic
Tetralogy of Fallot 5%
Transposition of the great arteries 5%
Atrioventricular septal defect (complete) 2%

with major chromosomal abnormalities (Table 17.1), but recently more subtle chromosomal abnormalities have been identified; for example abnormalities of chromosome 22 have been detected in many patients with aortic arch abnormalities. The less obvious, polygenic abnormalities probably explain why a previous child with congenital heart disease doubles the risk for subsequent children and the risk is higher still if either parent has congenital heart disease.

> When structural abnormalities of other systems are present, consider echocardiography for associated cardiac disorders.

Circulatory changes at birth

In the fetus, the left atrial pressure is low, as relatively little blood returns from the lungs. The pressure in the right atrium is higher than in the left, as it receives all the systemic venous return including blood from the placenta. The flap valve of the foramen ovale is held open, blood flows across the atrial septum into the left atrium and then into the left ventricle, which in turn pumps it to the upper body (Fig. 17.1).

With the first breaths, resistance to pulmonary blood flow falls and the volume of blood flowing through the lungs increases sixfold. This results in a rise in the left atrial pressure. Meanwhile, the volume of blood returning to the right atrium falls

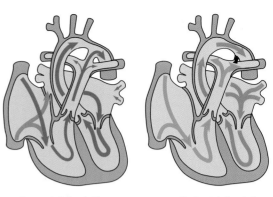

Antenatal circulation   Postnatal circulation

Figure 17.1 Changes in the circulation from the fetus to the newborn. When congenital heart lesions rely on blood flow through the duct (a duct-dependent circulation), there will be dramatic deterioration in the clinical condition when the duct closes.

as the placenta is excluded from the circulation. The change in the pressure difference causes the flap valve of the foramen ovale to be closed. The ductus arteriosus, which connects the pulmonary artery to the aorta in fetal life, will normally close within the first few hours or days. Some babies with congenital heart lesions rely on blood flow through the duct (duct-dependent circulation). Their clinical condition will deteriorate dramatically when the duct closes, which is usually at 1–2 days of age but occasionally later.

Table 17.1 Causes of congenital heart disease

	Cardiac abnormalities	Frequency
Maternal disorders		
Rubella infection	Peripheral pulmonary stenosis, PDA	30–35%
Systemic lupus erythematosus (SLE)	Complete heart block (anti-Ro and anti-La antibody)	35%
Diabetes mellitus	Incidence increased overall	2%
Maternal drugs		
Warfarin therapy	Pulmonary valve stenosis, PDA	5%
Fetal alcohol syndrome	ASD, VSD, tetralogy of Fallot	25%
Chromosomal abnormality		
Down's syndrome (trisomy 21)	Atrioventricular septal defect, VSD	30%
Edwards' syndrome (trisomy 18), Patau's syndrome (trisomy 13)	Complex	60–80%
Turner's syndrome (45XO)	Aortic valve stenosis, coarctation of the aorta	15%
Chromosome 22q11.2 deletion	Aortic arch anomalies, tetralogy of Fallot	
Williams' syndrome (chromosome 7 microdeletion)	Supravalvular aortic stenosis, peripheral pulmonary artery stenosis	

ASD, atrial septal defect; PDA, persistent ductus arteriosus; VSD, ventricular septal defect.

Presentation

Congenital heart disease presents with:

- antenatal cardiac ultrasound diagnosis
- detection of a heart murmur
- cyanosis
- heart failure
- shock.

Antenatal diagnosis

Checking the anatomy of the fetal heart has become a routine part of the fetal anomaly scan performed in the UK between 18 and 20 weeks' gestation. Over 70% of infants requiring surgery in the first six months of life are diagnosed antenatally. If an abnormality is detected, detailed fetal echocardiography is performed by a paediatric cardiologist, who also checks any fetus at increased risk, e.g. where Down's syndrome is suspected, where the parents have had a previous child with heart disease or where the mother has congenital heart disease. Early diagnosis allows the parents to be counselled. Depending on the diagnosis, some choose termination of pregnancy; the majority continue with the pregnancy and can have their child's management planned antenatally. Mothers of infants with duct-dependent lesions likely to need treatment within the first 2 days of life may be offered delivery close to the cardiac centre.

Heart murmurs

The most common presentation of congenital heart disease is with a heart murmur. However, the vast majority of children with murmurs have a normal heart. They have an 'innocent murmur', from turbulent flow in the outflow tracts or great vessels on either side of the heart, which can be heard at some time in almost 30% of children. It is obviously important to be able to distinguish an innocent murmur from a pathological one

There are two types of innocent murmur:

- Ejection murmur – generated in the ventricle, outflow tracts or great vessels on either side of the heart by turbulent blood flow. It is not associated with any structural abnormality.
- Venous hum – from turbulent blood flow in the head and neck veins. It is a continuous low-pitched rumble heard beneath either clavicle. It may increase on inspiration and will be louder after exercise. It may be mistaken for a persistent ductus arteriosus, but can be distinguished by its disappearance on lying flat or with compression of the jugular veins on the same side.

Hallmarks of an innocent ejection murmur are:

- soft blowing systolic murmur (usually from the right side pulmonary outflow in the second left interspace) or short 'buzzing' murmur (usually from the left side of the heart – aortic blood flow – in the fourth left interspace)
- localised to left sternal edge

- no diastolic component
- normal heart sounds with no added sounds
- no parasternal thrill
- no radiation
- asymptomatic patient.

During a febrile illness or anaemia, innocent murmurs are often heard because of increased cardiac output.

Differentiating between innocent and pathological murmurs can be difficult. If a murmur is thought to be significant, or if there is uncertainty about whether it is innocent, the child should be seen by an experienced paediatrician to decide about referral to a paediatric cardiologist for echocardiography. A chest X-ray and ECG may help with the diagnosis beyond the neonatal period.

Many newborn infants with potential shunts have neither symptoms nor a murmur at birth, as the pulmonary vascular resistance is still high. Therefore conditions such as a ventricular septal defect or ductus arteriosus may only become apparent at several weeks of age when the pulmonary vascular resistance falls.

> **The features of an innocent murmur can be remembered as the five S's:**
> **InnoSent murmur = Soft, Systolic, aSymptomatic, left Sternal edge.**

Cyanosis

Peripheral cyanosis (blueness of the hands and feet) may occur when a child is cold or unwell from any cause. This should be distinguished from central cyanosis, seen on the tongue as a slate blue colour, which is associated with a fall in arterial blood oxygen tension. Central cyanosis can only be recognised clinically if the concentration of reduced haemoglobin in the blood exceeds 5 g/dl, so it is less pronounced if the child is anaemic. Clinically, it may be evident only intermittently and difficult to identify with certainty; if any doubt is expressed by a parent or health care professional, check with a pulse oximeter that the infant's oxygen saturation is normal. Persistent cyanosis in an otherwise well infant is nearly always a sign of structural heart disease.

Cyanosis in a newborn infant with respiratory distress (respiratory rate >60 breaths/min) may be due to:

- cardiac disorders – cyanotic congenital heart disease
- respiratory disorders, e.g. surfactant deficiency, meconium aspiration, pulmonary hypoplasia, etc.
- persistent pulmonary hypertension of the newborn (PPHN) – failure of the pulmonary vascular resistance to fall after birth
- infection – septicaemia, group B streptococcus and other organisms
- inborn error of metabolism – metabolic acidosis and shock
- polycythaemia.

In the neonatal period, cardiac cyanosis may be caused by

- *Reduced pulmonary blood flow* – infants may have a duct-dependent pulmonary circulation that relies on blood flowing from left to right across the ductus arteriosus (e.g. see Fig. 17.2). They become severely cyanosed when the duct closes shortly after birth.
- *Abnormal mixing of systemic venous and pulmonary venous blood* – most infants present with cyanosis in the first day or two of life. In transposition of the great arteries, the systemic and pulmonary circulations are in parallel but there must be some mixing of blood between the two circulations.

The diagnosis of cyanotic congenital heart disease can be confirmed by the hyperoxia (nitrogen washout) test if detailed echocardiography is not readily available. The infant is placed in 100% oxygen for 10 minutes. If the right radial arterial PaO_2 remains low (<15 kPa, 113 mmHg) after this time, a diagnosis of 'cyanotic' congenital heart disease can be made if lung disease and persistent pulmonary hypertension of the newborn (persistent fetal circulation) have been excluded. If the PaO_2 is >20 kPa it is not cyanotic heart disease. Blood gas analysis must be performed as oxygen saturations are not reliable enough in this range of values.

Immediate management is to stabilise the airway, breathing and circulation, with artificial ventilation if necessary. Most infants with cyanotic heart disease presenting in the first few days of life are duct dependent; i.e. there is reduced mixing between the pink oxygenated blood returning from the lungs and the blue deoxygenated blood from the body. Maintenance of ductal patency is the key to early survival of these children. This is achieved with intravenous prostaglandin (PGE), whilst observing for potential side-effects – apnoea, jitteriness and seizures, flushing, vasodilatation and hypotension.

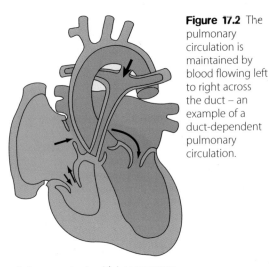

Figure 17.2 The pulmonary circulation is maintained by blood flowing left to right across the duct – an example of a duct-dependent pulmonary circulation.

Pulmonary atresia with intact septum

Box 17.2 Causes of heart failure

1. Neonates – obstructed (duct-dependent) systemic circulation
Hypoplastic left heart syndrome
Critical aortic valve stenosis
Severe coarctation of the aorta
Interruption of the aortic arch

2. Infants
Ventricular septal defect
Atrioventricular septal defect
Large persistent ductus arteriosus

Heart failure

Heart failure is difficult to define but in children is best summarised as a clinical syndrome.

Symptoms
- Breathlessness (particularly on feeding or exertion)
- Sweating
- Poor feeding
- Recurrent chest infections.

Signs
- Poor weight gain or 'failure to thrive'
- Tachypnoea
- Tachycardia
- Heart murmur, gallop rhythm
- Enlarged heart
- Hepatomegaly
- Cool peripheries.

Heart failure in the neonatal period (Box 17.2) usually results from left heart obstruction, e.g. coarctation of the aorta. If the obstructive lesion is very severe then arterial perfusion may be predominantly by right-to-left flow of blood via the arterial duct, so-called duct-dependent systemic circulation (e.g. see Fig. 17.3). Closure of the duct under these circumstances rapidly leads to severe acidosis, collapse and death unless ductal patency is restored (Case history 17.1).

Beyond the neonatal period, progressive heart failure is most likely due to a left-to-right shunt (Case history 17.2). During the first few weeks of life, as the pulmonary vascular resistance falls, there is a progressive increase in pulmonary blood flow. Symptoms of heart failure will increase up to the age of about 3 months, but may subsequently improve as the pulmonary vascular resistance rises in response to the left-to-right shunt. If left untreated, some of these children may develop Eisenmenger's syndrome, which is irreversibly raised pulmonary vascular resistance resulting from chronically raised pulmonary arterial pressure and flow. If this develops, the only surgical option is a heart–lung transplant.

Case History
17.1 Shock

A 2-day-old baby had been discharged home the day after delivery following a normal routine examination. He suddenly collapsed and was rushed to hospital. He was pale, with grey lips. The right brachial pulse could just be felt, the femoral pulses were impalpable and his liver was significantly enlarged. Blood gases showed a severe metabolic acidosis. The differential diagnosis was:

- congenital heart disease
- septicaemia
- inherited disorder of metabolism.

He was ventilated and treated with volume support. Blood cultures were taken and antibiotics started for possible sepsis. Blood and urine samples were taken for an amino acid screen and urine for organic acids. As the femoral pulses remained impalpable, a prostaglandin infusion was started. Within 2 hours he was pink and well perfused and the acidosis was resolving. Severe coarctation of the aorta (Fig. 17.3) was diagnosed on echocardiography. He had developed shock from left heart outflow tract obstruction once the arterial duct had closed.

> Maintaining ductal patency is the key to early survival in neonates with a duct-dependent circulation.

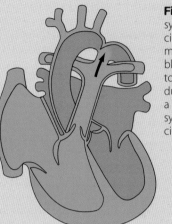

Figure 17.3 The systemic circulation is maintained by blood flowing right to left across the ductus arteriosus – a duct-dependent systemic circulation.

Duct-dependent coarctation

Case History
17.2 Heart failure

A 5-week-old female infant was referred to hospital because of wheezing, poor feeding and poor weight gain during the previous 2 weeks. Before this, she had been well. Her routine neonatal examination had been normal. She was tachypnoeic (50–60 breaths/min) and there was some sternal and intercostal recession. The pulses were normal. There was a thrill, a loud pansystolic murmur at the lower left sternal edge and a slightly accentuated pulmonary component to the second heart sound. There were scattered wheezes. The liver was enlarged, palpable at 2 fingerbreadths below the costal margin. The ECG was unremarkable. The chest X-ray showed cardiomegaly and increased pulmonary vascular markings. An echocardiogram showed a moderate-sized ventricular septal defect (VSD) (Fig. 17.4). Treatment was with diuretics and captopril. The VSD closed spontaneously at 11 months.

This infant developed heart failure from a moderately large VSD presenting at several weeks of age when the pulmonary resistance fell, causing increased left-to-right shunting of blood.

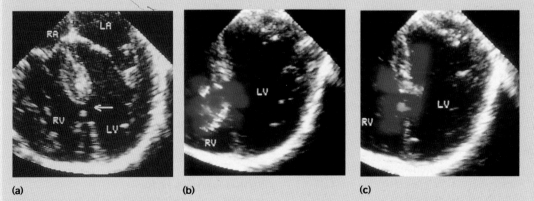

(a)   (b)   (c)

Figure 17.4 (a) Echocardiogram showing a medium-sized muscular ventricular septal defect (arrow). **(b)** The colour Doppler shows a left-to-right shunt (blue) during systole. **(c)** There is also a small right-to-left shunt (red) during diastole (RA, right atrium; LA, left atrium; RV, right ventricle; LV, left ventricle).

Summary

Congenital heart disease presents with:
- antenatal ultrasound screening – increasing proportion detected
- detection of a heart murmur – need to differentiate innocent from pathological murmur
- cyanosis – if duct dependent, prostaglandin to maintain ductal patency is vital for initial survival
- heart failure – usually from left-to-right shunt when pulmonary vascular resistance falls, in neonate from left heart obstruction
- shock – when duct closes in severe left heart obstruction.

Diagnosis

If congenital heart disease is suspected, a chest X-ray and ECG (Box 17.3) should be performed. Although rarely diagnostic, they may be helpful in establishing that there is an abnormality of the cardiovascular system and as a baseline for assessing future changes. Echocardiography, combined with Doppler ultrasound, enables almost all causes of congenital heart disease to be diagnosed. Even when a paediatric cardiologist is not available locally, a specialist echocardiography opinion may be available via telemedicine, or else transfer to the cardiac centre will be necessary. A specialist opinion is required if the child is haemo-dynamically unstable, if there is heart failure, if there is cyanosis, when the oxygen saturations are less than 94% due to heart disease and when there are reduced volume pulses. Cardiac catheterisation is seldom required to make the diagnosis and is now reserved for haemodynamic measurements and intervention.

Box 17.3 ECGs in children

Important features
- Arrhythmias
- Superior QRS axis (negative deflection in AVF) (Fig. 17.5e)
- Right ventricular hypertrophy (upright T wave in V1, over 1 month of age) (Fig. 17.6d)
- Left ventricular strain (inverted T wave in V_6) (Fig. 17.9d)

Pitfalls
- P wave morphology is rarely helpful in children
- Partial right bundle branch block – most are normal children, although it is common in ASD
- Left ventricular hypertrophy is difficult to define (ASD, atrial septal defect)

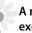

A normal chest X-ray and ECG does not exclude congenital heart disease.

Nomenclature

The European (as opposed to American) system for naming congenital heart disease is referred to as sequential segmental arrangement. The advantage is that it is not necessary to remember the pattern of an eponymous syndrome, e.g. tetralogy of Fallot. The disadvantage is that it is long winded. The idea is that each component is described in turn, naming the way the atria, then the ventricles and then the great arteries are connected. Hence a normal heart will be described as situs solitus (i.e. the atria are in the correct orientation), concordant atrioventricular connection and concordant ventriculo-arterial connection. Therefore a heart of any complexity can be described in a logical step-by-step process. This system is not used in this chapter as it is too complex.

Acyanotic congenital heart disease

1. Left-to-right shunts

Atrial septal defect

There are two main types of atrial septal defect (ASD):
- secundum ASD (80% of ASDs) (Fig. 17.5a)
- partial atrioventricular septal defect (primum ASD, pAVSD) (Fig. 17.5b).

Both present with similar symptoms and signs, but their anatomy is quite different. The secundum ASD is a defect in the centre of the atrial septum involving the foramen ovale. Partial AVSD is a defect of the atrioventricular septum and is characterised by:
- an inter-atrial communication between the bottom end of the atrial septum and the atrioventricular valves (primum ASD)
- abnormal atrioventricular valves, with a left atrioventricular valve which has three leaflets and tends to leak (regurgitant valve).

Clinical features

Symptoms
- None (commonly)
- Recurrent chest infections/wheeze
- Heart failure
- Arrhythmias (fourth decade onwards).

Physical signs (Fig. 17.5d)
- A fixed and widely split second heart sound (often difficult to hear) – due to the right ventricular stroke volume being equal in both inspiration and expiration

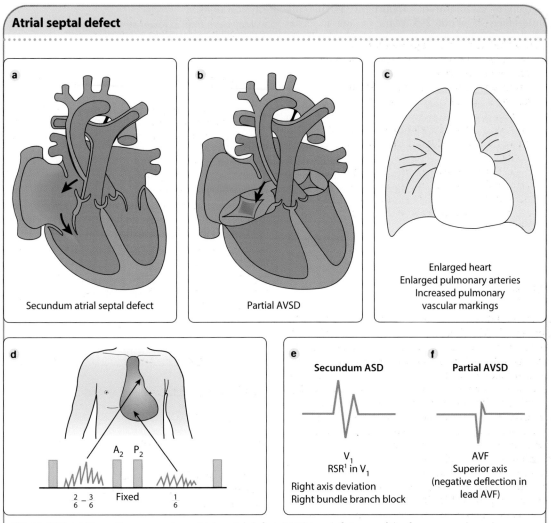

Figure 17.5 (a) The ostium secundum atrial septal defect (ASD) is a deficiency of the foramen ovale and surrounding atrial septum. **(b)** The partial AVSD is a deficiency of the atrioventricular septum. **(c)** Chest X-ray. **(d)** Murmur, **(e, f)** ECG.

- An ejection systolic murmur best heard at the upper left sternal edge – due to increased flow across the right ventricular outflow tract because of the left-to-right shunt
- With a partial AVSD, an apical pansystolic murmur from atrioventricular valve regurgitation.

Investigations

Chest X-ray (Fig. 17.5c)

May show cardiomegaly, enlarged pulmonary arteries and increased pulmonary vascular markings, all non-specific features.

ECG (Fig. 17.5e)

This may provide a strong diagnostic clue:

- Secundum ASD – partial right bundle branch block is common (but may occur in normal children),

right axis deviation due to right ventricular enlargement.
- Partial AVSD – left axis deviation, a so-called 'superior' QRS axis. This occurs because there is a defect of the middle part of the heart where the atrioventricular node is. The displaced node then conducts to the ventricles superiorly giving the abnormal axis.

Cross-sectional echocardiography

This will delineate the anatomy in most cases and is the mainstay of diagnostic investigations.

Management

Children with significant atrial septal defect will require treatment. For secundum ASDs this is by cardiac catheterisation with insertion of an occlusion device, but for partial AVSD surgical correction is required. Treatment is usually undertaken at about 3–5 years of age in order to prevent right heart failure and arrhythmias in later life.

Ventricular septal defects

Ventricular septal defects (VSDs) are common, accounting for 30% of all cases of congenital heart disease. There is a defect anywhere in the ventricular septum, usually perimembranous (adjacent to the tricuspid valve) or muscular (completely surrounded by muscle). They can most conveniently be considered according to the size of the lesion.

Small VSDs

These are smaller than the aortic valve in diameter, perhaps up to 3 mm.

Clinical features

Symptoms
- Asymptomatic.

Physical signs
- May have thrill at lower sternal edge
- Loud pansystolic murmur at lower left sternal edge
- Quiet pulmonary second sound (P2).

Investigations

Chest X-ray
- Normal

ECG
- Normal

Echocardiography
- Demonstrates the precise anatomy of the defect. It is possible to assess its haemodynamic effects using Doppler echocardiography.

Management

Most of these lesions will close spontaneously. This is ascertained by the disappearance of the murmur with a normal ECG on follow-up by a paediatrician or paediatric cardiologist and by a normal echo-

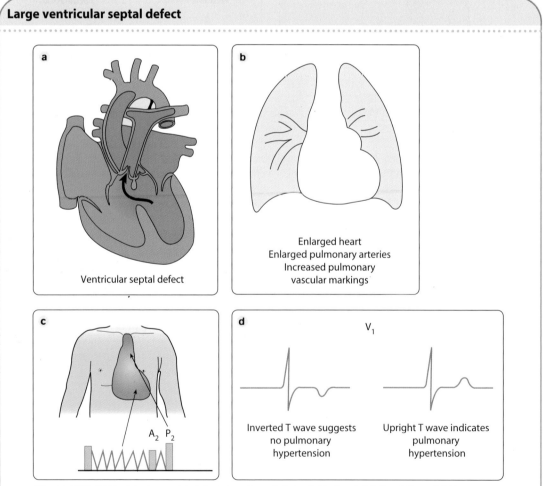

Large ventricular septal defect

Ventricular septal defect

Enlarged heart
Enlarged pulmonary arteries
Increased pulmonary
vascular markings

A₂ P₂

V₁

Inverted T wave suggests
no pulmonary
hypertension

Upright T wave indicates
pulmonary
hypertension

Figure 17.6 (a) Ventricular septal defect showing a left-to-right shunt. **(b)** Chest X-ray. **(c)** Murmur. **(d)** ECG.

cardiogram. Whilst the VSD is present, prevention of bacterial endocarditis is attempted by maintaining good dental hygiene and by antibiotic prophylaxis before dental extraction or any operation where there will be bleeding.

Large VSDs

These defects are the same size or bigger than the aortic valve.

Clinical features

Symptoms
- Heart failure with breathlessness and failure to thrive after 1 week old
- Recurrent chest infections.

Physical signs (Fig. 17.6c)
- Active precordium
- Soft pansystolic murmur or no murmur
- Apical mid-diastolic murmur (from increased flow across the mitral valve after the blood has circulated through the lungs)
- Loud pulmonary second sound (P2) – from raised pulmonary arterial diastolic pressure
- Tachypnoea, tachycardia and enlarged liver from heart failure.

Investigations

Chest X-ray (Fig. 17.6b)
- Cardiomegaly
- Enlarged pulmonary arteries
- Increased pulmonary vascular markings
- Pulmonary oedema.

ECG (Fig. 17.6d)
- Biventricular hypertrophy by 2 months of age and signs of pulmonary hypertension.

Echocardiography
- Demonstrates the anatomy of the defect, haemodynamic effects and severity of pulmonary hypertension.

Management

Drug therapy for heart failure is with diuretics often combined with captopril. Additional calorie input is required. There is always some degree of pulmonary hypertension in children with large left-to-right shunt. This damages the lungs as increased pulmonary blood flow and pulmonary hypertension will ultimately lead to irreversible damage of the pulmonary capillary vascular bed. This pulmonary vascular disease usually becomes established in the second year of life, but Eisenmenger's syndrome (Fig. 17.7), with cyanosis due to intracardiac shunting from right to left, rarely evolves until the second decade. Surgery is usually performed at 3–6 months of age in order to:

- manage heart failure and failure to thrive
- prevent permanent lung damage from pulmonary hypertension and high blood flow.

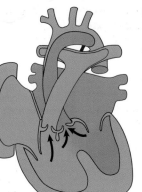

Figure 17.7 Eisenmenger's syndrome with right-to-left shunting from pulmonary vascular disease following increased pulmonary blood flow and pulmonary hypertension.

Eisenmenger's syndrome

Persistent ductus arteriosus

The ductus arteriosus connects the pulmonary artery to the descending aorta. In term infants it normally closes shortly after birth. In persistent ductus arteriosus it has failed to close by a month post term due to a defect in the constrictor mechanism of the duct. The flow of blood across a persistent ductus arteriosus (PDA) is from the aorta to the pulmonary artery (i.e. left to right), following the fall in pulmonary vascular resistance after birth. In the preterm infant, the presence of a persistent ductus arteriosus is not from congenital heart disease but due to prematurity. It is described in Chapter 9.

Clinical features

Most children present with a continuous murmur beneath the left clavicle (Fig. 17.8a). The murmur continues into diastole because the pressure in the pulmonary artery is lower than that in the aorta throughout the cardiac cycle. The pulse pressure is increased, causing a collapsing or bounding pulse. Symptoms are rare, but when the duct is large there will be increased pulmonary blood flow with heart failure and even pulmonary hypertension.

Investigations

The chest X-ray and ECG are usually normal, but if the PDA is large and symptomatic the features on chest X-ray (Fig. 17.8b) and ECG (Fig. 17.8c) are indistinguishable from those seen in a patient with a large VSD. However, the duct should be readily identified with cross-sectional echocardiography assisted by Doppler ultrasound.

Management

In infants with an asymptomatic PDA, closure is recommended to abolish the lifelong risk of bacterial endocarditis. Closure is with a coil or occlusion device introduced via a cardiac catheter at about 1 year of age (Fig. 17.8d–g).

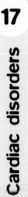

Persistent ductus arteriosus

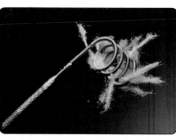

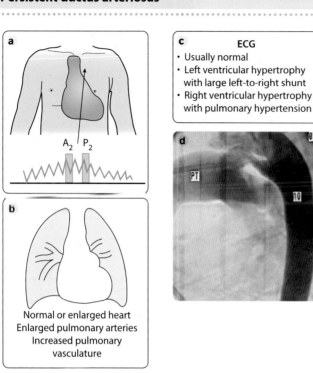

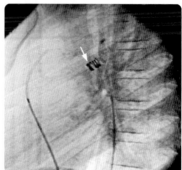

a

A₂ P₂

b

Normal or enlarged heart
Enlarged pulmonary arteries
Increased pulmonary
vasculature

c   ECG
- Usually normal
- Left ventricular hypertrophy
  with large left-to-right shunt
- Right ventricular hypertrophy
  with pulmonary hypertension

d

Figure 17.8 Persistent ductus arteriosus. **(a)** Murmur. **(b)** Chest X-ray. **(c)** ECG. **(d)** A persistent ductus arteriosus visualised on angiography. **(e)** A coil used to close ducts. It is passed through a catheter via the femoral artery. **(f)** Angiogram to show coil in the duct. (PT, pulmonary trunk; AO, aorta).

2. Outflow obstruction in the well child

Aortic stenosis

The aortic valve leaflets are partly fused together, giving a restrictive exit from the left ventricle (Fig. 17.9a). There may be one to three aortic leaflets. Aortic stenosis may not be an isolated lesion. It is often associated with mitral valve stenosis and coarctation of the aorta, and their presence should always be excluded.

Clinical features

Most present with an asymptomatic murmur. Those with severe stenosis may present with reduced exercise tolerance, chest pain on exertion or syncope.

In the neonatal period, there may be severe heart failure or a duct-dependent systemic circulation leading to shock.

Physical signs (Fig. 17.9b)
- Small volume, slow rising pulses
- Carotid thrill (always)
- Ejection systolic murmur maximal at the upper right sternal edge radiating to the neck
- Delayed and soft aortic second sound
- Apical ejection click.

Investigations

Chest X-ray (Fig. 17.9c)
Normal or prominent left ventricle with post-stenotic dilatation of the ascending aorta.

ECG (Fig. 17.9d)
There may be left ventricular hypertrophy.

Management

In children, regular clinical and echocardiographic assessment is required in order to assess when to intervene. Children with symptoms on exercise or who have a high resting pressure gradient (more than 64 mmHg) across the aortic valve will undergo balloon valvotomy. Balloon dilatation in older children is generally safe and uncomplicated, but in neonates this is much more difficult and dangerous.

Summary

Left-to-right shunts

Lesion	Symptoms	Signs	Management
ASD – secundum	None	Ejection systolic murmur at ULSE	Catheter device closure at 3–5 years
AVSD – partial	None, heart failure	Fixed split S2	Surgery at 3 years
VSD – small (80–90%)	None	Pansystolic murmur at LLSE	None
VSD – large (10–20%)	Heart failure	Active precordium, loud P2, soft murmur, tachypnoea, hepatomegaly	Diuretics, captopril, calories Surgery at 3–6 months old
PDA – term	None	Continuous murmur at ULSE ± bounding pulses	Coil or device closure at cardiac catheter
PDA – preterm	None, heart failure	Systolic murmur at ULSE ± bounding pulses	Fluid restriction, indomethacin or ibuprofen, or surgical ligation

ASD, atrial septal defect; AVSD, atrioventricular septal defect; VSD, ventricular septal defect; PDA, persistent or patent ductus arteriosus; ULSE, upper left sternal edge; LLSE, lower left sternal edge.

Aortic stenosis

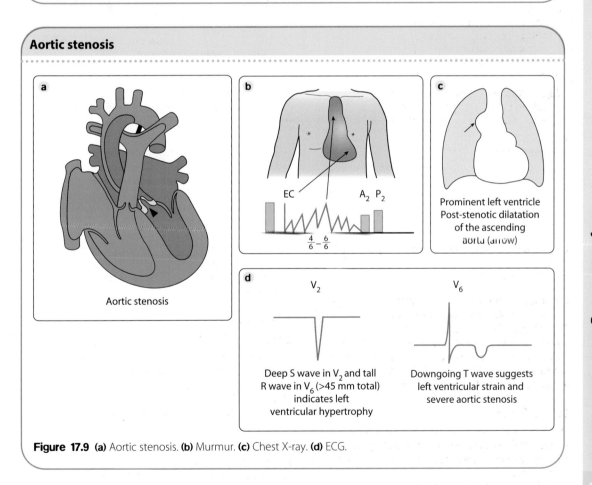

Figure 17.9 **(a)** Aortic stenosis. **(b)** Murmur. **(c)** Chest X-ray. **(d)** ECG.

Most neonates and children with significant aortic valve stenosis requiring treatment in the first few years of life will eventually require aortic valve replacement. Early treatment is therefore palliative and directed towards delaying this for as long as possible.

Pulmonary stenosis

The pulmonary valve leaflets are partly fused together, giving a restrictive exit from the right ventricle.

Pulmonary stenosis

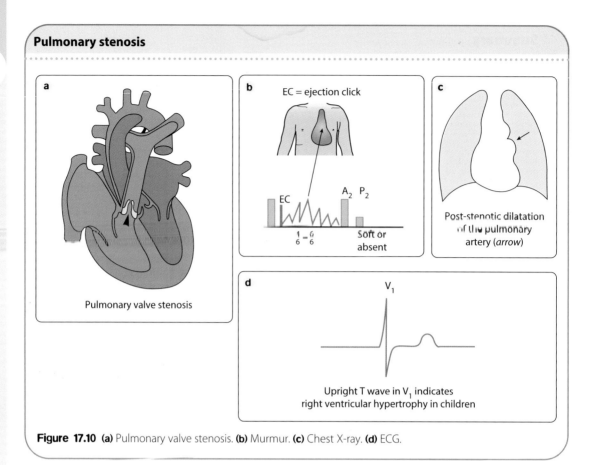

Figure 17.10 **(a)** Pulmonary valve stenosis. **(b)** Murmur. **(c)** Chest X-ray. **(d)** ECG.

Clinical features

Most are asymptomatic (Fig. 17.10a). It is diagnosed clinically. A small number of neonates with critical pulmonary stenosis have a duct-dependent pulmonary circulation and present in the first few days of life.

Physical signs (Fig. 17.10b)

- An ejection systolic murmur best heard at the upper left sternal edge; thrill may be present.
- An ejection click best heard at the upper left sternal edge.
- Soft or absent P2.
- When severe lesion – prolonged right ventricular impulse, with delayed pulmonary valve closure on auscultation.

Investigations

Chest X-ray (Fig. 17.10c)

Normal or post-stenotic dilatation of the pulmonary artery.

ECG (Fig. 17.10d)

Shows evidence of right ventricular hypertrophy.

Management

Although most children are asymptomatic, progressive right ventricular hypertrophy and reduced exercise tolerance eventually occur. When the pressure gradient across the pulmonary valve becomes markedly increased (greater than about 64 mmHg), intervention will be required. Transcatheter balloon dilatation is the treatment of choice in most children.

Adult type coarctation of the aorta

This uncommon lesion (Fig. 17.11a) is not duct dependent. It gradually becomes more severe over many years.

Clinical features

- Asymptomatic.
- Always systemic hypertension in the right arm.
- Ejection systolic murmur at upper sternal edge.
- Collaterals at the back.
- Radio-femoral delay. This is due to blood bypassing the obstruction via collateral vessels in the chest wall and hence the pulse in the legs is delayed.

Investigations

Chest X-ray (Fig. 17.11c)

- 'Rib-notching' due to the development of large collateral intercostal arteries running under the ribs posteriorly to bypass the obstruction.
- '3' sign, with visible notch in the descending aorta at site of the coarctation.

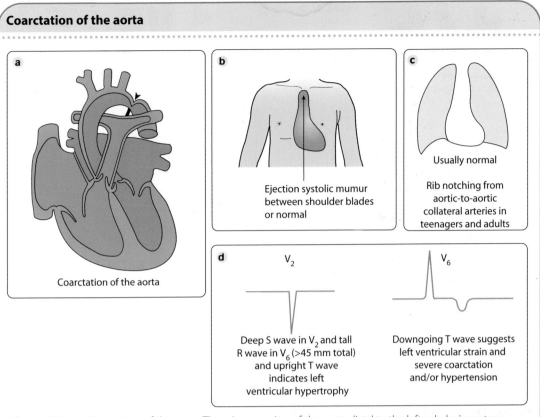

Coarctation of the aorta

a

Coarctation of the aorta

b

Ejection systolic mumur
between shoulder blades
or normal

c

Usually normal

Rib notching from
aortic-to-aortic
collateral arteries in
teenagers and adults

d

V_2

V_6

Deep S wave in V_2 and tall
R wave in V_6 (>45 mm total)
and upright T wave
indicates left
ventricular hypertrophy

Downgoing T wave suggests
left ventricular strain and
severe coarctation
and/or hypertension

Figure 17.11 (a) Coarctation of the aorta. There is narrowing of the aorta distal to the left subclavian artery adjacent to the insertion of the arterial duct. **(b)** Murmur. **(c)** Chest X-ray. **(d)** ECG.

Summary

Outflow obstruction in the well child

Lesion	Signs	Management
Aortic stenosis	Murmur, upper right sternal edge Carotid thrill	Balloon dilatation
Pulmonary stenosis	Murmur, upper left sternal edge No carotid thrill	Balloon dilatation
Coarctation (adult type)	Systemic hypertension Radio-femoral delay	Stent insertion or surgery

ECG

- Left ventricular hypertrophy (Fig. 17.11d).

Management

When the condition becomes severe, as assessed by echocardiography, a stent may be inserted at cardiac catheter. Sometimes surgical repair is required.

3. Outflow obstruction in the sick infant

Interruption of the aortic arch

This is a severe form of coarctation with no connection between the aorta proximal and distal to the arterial duct. A VSD is usually present. Presentation is almost invariably in the neonatal period with features of a duct-dependent systemic circulation (Fig. 17.12). Complete correction with closure of the VSD and repair of the aortic arch is usually performed within the first few days of life. The risk of death is higher than that for simple coarctation of the aorta, being in the order of 10–20%. There is an association with other conditions (DiGeorge syndrome – absence of thymus, palatal defects, immunodeficiency and hypocalcaemia and 22q11.2 gene deletion).

Palpation for absent femoral pulses to detect coarctation of the aorta must be performed during the cardiovascular examination of any child.

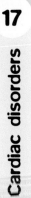

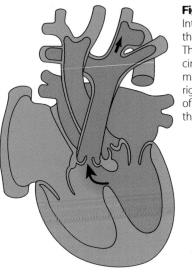

Figure 17.12
Interruption of the aortic arch. The lower body circulation is maintained by right-to-left flow of blood across the duct.

Interrupted aortic arch

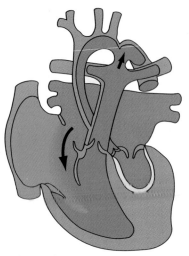

Figure 17.13
Hypoplastic left heart syndrome. The entire left side of the heart is underdeveloped.

Hypoplastic left heart

Hypoplastic left heart syndrome

In this condition there is underdevelopment of the entire left side of the heart (Fig. 17.13). The mitral valve is small or atretic, the left ventricle is diminutive and there is usually aortic valve atresia. The ascending aorta is very small, and there is almost invariably coarctation of the aorta.

Clinical features

These children may be detected antenatally at ultrasound screening. This allows for effective counselling and prevents the child from becoming sick after birth. If they do present after birth, they are the sickest of all neonates presenting with a duct-dependent systemic circulation. There is no flow through the left side of the heart, so ductal constriction leads to profound acidosis and rapid cardiovascular collapse. There is weakness or absence of all peripheral pulses, in contrast to weak femoral pulses in coarctation of the aorta. The infant will fail the hyperoxia (nitrogen washout) test by remaining desaturated in oxygen, as there is common mixing of pulmonary venous and systemic venous blood at atrial level. As in all suspected duct-dependent lesions, prostaglandin

must be commenced and the diagnosis established urgently by echocardiography.

Management

The management of this condition consists of a difficult neonatal operation called the Norwood procedure. This is followed by a further operation (Glenn or hemi-Fontan) at about 6 months and again (Fontan) at about 3 years.

Cyanotic congenital heart disease

In congenital heart disease there are two causes of cyanosis:
- decreased pulmonary blood flow with a right-to-left shunt, e.g. tetralogy of Fallot
- abnormal mixing of systemic and pulmonary venous return, e.g. transposition of the great arteries and tricuspid atresia.

Tetralogy of Fallot

This is the most common cause of cyanotic congenital heart disease (Fig. 17.14a).

⊙ Summary

Left heart outflow obstruction in the sick infant – duct-dependent lesions

Lesion	Clinical features	Management
Coarctation of the aorta and interruption of the aortic arch	Heart murmur, heart failure Circulatory collapse Weak or absent femoral pulses Blood pressure arms > legs	Maintain airway, breathing, circulation Immediately start prostaglandin infusion
Hypoplastic left heart syndrome	Circulatory collapse All peripheral pulses weak or absent	Maintain airway, breathing, circulation Immediately start prostaglandin infusion Surgery (complex)

Tetralogy of Fallot

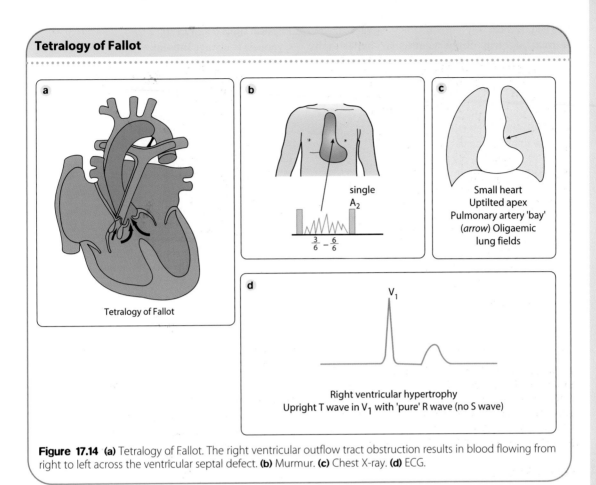

a

Tetralogy of Fallot

b

single
A₂

$\frac{3}{6} - \frac{6}{6}$

c

Small heart
Uptilted apex
Pulmonary artery 'bay'
(*arrow*) Oligaemic
lung fields

d

V₁

Right ventricular hypertrophy
Upright T wave in V₁ with 'pure' R wave (no S wave)

Figure 17.14 (a) Tetralogy of Fallot. The right ventricular outflow tract obstruction results in blood flowing from right to left across the ventricular septal defect. **(b)** Murmur. **(c)** Chest X-ray. **(d)** ECG.

Clinical features

In tetralogy of Fallot, as implied by the name, there are four cardinal anatomical features:

- a large VSD
- overriding of the aorta with respect to the ventricular septum
- subpulmonary stenosis causing right ventricular outflow tract obstruction
- right ventricular hypertrophy as a result.

Symptoms

Most are diagnosed:

- antenatally or
- following the identification of a murmur in the first month or two of life. Cyanosis at this stage may not be obvious, although a few present with severe cyanosis in the first few days of life.

The classical description of severe cyanosis, hypercyanotic spells and squatting on exercise developing in late infancy is now rare. However, it is important to recognise hypercyanotic spells, as they may lead to myocardial infarction, cerebrovascular accidents and even death if left untreated. They are characterised by a rapid increase in cyanosis, usually associated with irritability or inconsolable crying because of severe hypoxia, and breathlessness and pallor because of tissue acidosis.

Signs

Clubbing of the fingers and toes may develop in older children.

A loud harsh ejection systolic murmur at the left sternal edge from day 1 of life, usually with a single second heart sound (A2) (Fig. 17.14b). With increasing right ventricular outflow tract obstruction, which is predominantly muscular and below the pulmonary valve, the murmur will shorten and cyanosis will increase. During a hypercyanotic spell, the murmur will be very short or inaudible.

Investigations

Chest X-ray (Fig. 17.14c)

Usually normal.

If the child is older, X-ray will show a relatively small heart, possibly with an uptilted apex (boot shaped) due to right ventricular hypertrophy. There may be a right-sided aortic arch, but characteristically there is a pulmonary artery 'bay', a concavity on the left heart border where the convex-shaped main pulmonary artery and right ventricular outflow tract are normally profiled. There may also be decreased pulmonary vascular markings reflecting reduced pulmonary blood flow.

ECG (Fig. 17.14d)

Normal at birth. Right ventricular hypertrophy when older.

Echocardiography

This will demonstrate the cardinal features, but cardiac catheterisation may be required to show the detailed anatomy of the pulmonary arteries, which may be small or stenosed.

Management

Initial management is medical, with corrective surgery at around 6 months of age. It involves closing the VSD and relieving right ventricular outflow tract obstruction with an artificial patch, which sometimes extends across the pulmonary valve. Most are free from significant symptoms in childhood.

Infants who are very cyanosed in the neonatal period require a shunt to increase pulmonary blood flow. This is usually done by surgical placement of an artificial tube between the subclavian artery and the pulmonary artery (a modified Blalock–Taussig shunt) or sometimes by balloon dilatation of the right ventricular outflow tract.

Hypercyanotic spells are usually self-limiting and followed by a period of sleep. If prolonged (beyond about 15 minutes), they require prompt treatment with:

- sedation and pain relief (morphine is excellent)
- intravenous propranolol (or an alpha adrenoceptor agonist), which probably works both as a peripheral vasoconstrictor and by relieving the subpulmonary muscular obstruction that is the cause of reduced pulmonary blood flow
- intravenous volume administration
- bicarbonate to correct acidosis
- muscle paralysis and artificial ventilation in order to reduce metabolic oxygen demand.

Transposition of the great arteries

The aorta is connected to the right ventricle, and the pulmonary artery is connected to the left ventricle. The blue blood is therefore returned to the body and the pink blood is returned to the lungs (Fig. 17.15a). There are two parallel circulations – unless there is mixing of blood between them this condition is incompatible with life. Fortunately, there are a number of naturally occurring associated anomalies, e.g. VSD, ASD and PDA, as well as therapeutic interventions which can achieve this.

Clinical features

Symptoms

Cyanosis is the predominant symptom. It may be profound and life-threatening; a PaO_2 of 1–3 kPa is not unusual. Presentation is usually on day 1–2 of life when ductal closure leads to a marked reduction in mixing of the desaturated and saturated blood. Cyanosis will be less severe and presentation delayed if there is more mixing of blood from associated anomalies, e.g. a VSD.

Physical signs (Fig. 17.15b)

Cyanosis is always present.

Finger clubbing is present in the rare child presenting after the first year of life. The remainder of the cardiovascular examination will vary depending on the associated abnormalities. The second heart sound is often single.

Usually no murmur, but may be a systolic murmur from increased flow or stenosis within the left ventricular (pulmonary) outflow tract.

Investigations

Chest X-ray (Fig. 17.15c)

This may reveal the classic findings of a narrow upper mediastinum with an 'egg on side' appearance of the cardiac shadow (due to the anteroposterior relationship of the great vessels and hypertrophied right ventricle, respectively). Increased pulmonary vascular markings are common due to increased pulmonary blood flow.

ECG (Fig. 17.15d)

This is rarely helpful in establishing the diagnosis, as it is usually normal.

Echocardiography

This is essential to demonstrate the abnormal arterial connections and associated abnormalities.

Management

In the sick cyanosed neonate, the key is to improve mixing of saturated and desaturated blood. Maintaining the patency of the ductus arteriosus with a prostaglandin infusion is mandatory. A balloon atrial septostomy is a life-saving procedure which may be performed in children with any form of transposition of the great arteries (Fig. 17.15e,f). A catheter, with an expandable balloon at its tip, is passed through the umbilical or femoral vein and then on through the right atrium and foramen ovale. The balloon is inflated within the left atrium and then pulled through the atrial septum. This tears the atrial septum, renders the flap valve of the foramen ovale incompetent, and so allows mixing of the systemic and pulmonary venous blood within the atrium.

All patients with transposition of the great arteries will require surgery, which is usually the arterial switch procedure. In this operation, performed in the first few days of life, the pulmonary artery and aorta are transected above the arterial valves and switched over. In addition, the coronary arteries have to be transferred across to the new aorta. Thus the left ventricle acts as the systemic ventricle, pumping fully oxygenated blood into the aorta, and the right ventricle assumes its more normal role of pumping blood to the lungs.

Atrioventricular septal defect (complete)

This is most commonly seen in children with Down's syndrome (Fig. 17.16). A complete atrio-

Transposition of the great arteries

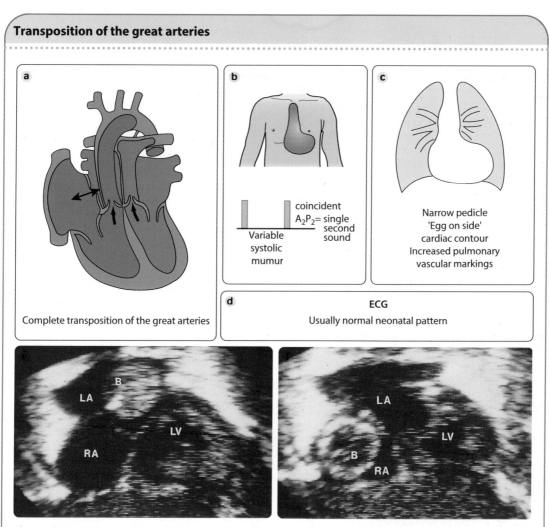

a

Complete transposition of the great arteries

b

Variable systolic mumur

coincident A₂P₂= single second sound

c

Narrow pedicle
'Egg on side'
cardiac contour
Increased pulmonary
vascular markings

d

ECG
Usually normal neonatal pattern

Figure 17.15 **(a)** Transposition of the great arteries. There must be mixing of blood between the two circulations for this to be compatible with life. **(b)** Murmur. **(c)** Chest X-ray. **(d)** ECG. **(e, f)** Echocardiogram showing balloon atrial septostomy in transposition of the great arteries. A balloon (about 2 ml) is pulled through the atrial septum from the left atrium (e) across the atrial septum to the right atrium (f) in order to increase the size of the foramen in the atrial septum (B, balloon; LA, left atrium; RA, right atrium; LV, left ventricle).

ventricular septal defect (cAVSD) has a defect in the middle of the heart with a single five-leaflet valve between the atria and ventricles which stretches across the entire atrioventricular junction and tends to leak. As there is a large defect there is pulmonary hypertension.

Features of a complete atrioventricular septal defect are:

- presentation on antenatal ultrasound screening
- cyanosis at birth or heart failure at 2–3 weeks of life
- none, with no murmur heard, the lesion being detected on routine echocardiography screening in a newborn baby with Down's syndrome. There is always a superior axis on the ECG.

Management is to treat heart failure medically (as for large VSD) and surgical repair at 3–6 months of age.

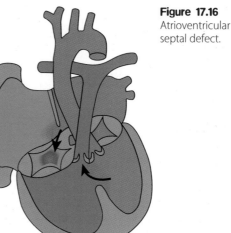

Figure 17.16
Atrioventricular septal defect.

Atrioventricular septal defect

301

Tricuspid atresia

In tricuspid atresia (Fig. 17.17) only the left ventricle is effective, the right being small and non-functional.

Clinical features

There is 'common mixing' of systemic and pulmonary venous return in the left atrium. Presentation is with cyanosis in the newborn period if duct-dependent, or the child may be well at birth and become cyanosed or breathless.

Management

Early palliation is performed to maintain a secure supply of blood to the lungs at low pressure, by:

- a Blalock–Taussig shunt (between the subclavian and pulmonary artery) in children who are severely cyanosed

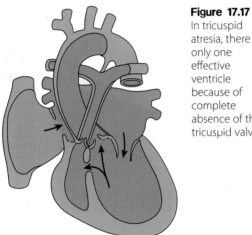

Tricuspid atresia

Figure 17.17
In tricuspid atresia, there is only one effective ventricle because of complete absence of the tricuspid valve.

- pulmonary artery banding to reduce pulmonary blood flow if breathless.

Completely corrective surgery is not possible as there is only one effective functioning ventricle. Palliation is performed (Glenn or hemi-Fontan operation connecting the superior vena cava to the pulmonary artery after 6 months of age and a Fontan operation to also connect the inferior vena cava to the pulmonary artery at 3–5 years).

Thus the left ventricle drives blood around the body and systemic venous pressure supplies blood to the lungs. The Fontan operation results in a less than ideal functional outcome, but has the advantages of relieving cyanosis and removing the long-term volume load on the single functional ventricle.

Care following cardiac surgery

Most children recover rapidly following cardiac surgery and are back at nursery or school within a month. Almost all will require antibiotic prophylaxis against bacterial endocarditis. Exercise tolerance will be variable and most children can be allowed to find their own limits. Restricted exercise is advised only for children with severe residual aortic stenosis and for ventricular dysfunction.

Most of the children are followed up in specialist cardiac clinics. Most lead normal, unrestricted lives, but any change in symptoms, e.g. decreasing exercise tolerance or palpitations, requires further investigation. An increasing number of adolescents and young adults require revision of surgery performed in early life. The most common reason for this is replacement of artificial valves and relief of post-surgical suture line stenosis, for example re-coarctation or pulmonary artery stenosis.

⊙ Summary

Cyanotic congenital heart disease

Lesion	Clinical features	Management
Tetralogy of Fallot	Loud murmur at the upper left sternal edge, with a single second heart sound Clubbing of fingers and toes (older) Hypercyanotic spells (rare)	Surgery at 6–9 months
Transposition of the great arteries	Neonatal cyanosis No murmur	Prostaglandin infusion, some need balloon atrial septostomy at diagnosis Arterial switch operation in neonatal period
Atrioventricular septal defect (complete)	Down's syndrome (often) Cyanosis at birth Murmur, heart failure at 2–3 weeks of life	Treat heart failure medically Surgical repair
Tricuspid atresia	Cyanosis	Shunt (Blalock–Taussig) or pulmonary artery banding Surgery (Fontan operation)

Cardiac arrhythmias

Sinus arrhythmia is normal in children and is detectable as a cyclical change in heart rate with respiration. There is acceleration during inspiration and slowing on expiration (the heart rate changing by up to 30 beats/min).

Supraventricular tachycardia

This is the most common childhood arrhythmia. The heart rate is rapid, between 250 and 300 beats/min. It can cause poor cardiac output and pulmonary oedema. It typically presents with symptoms of heart failure in the neonate or young infant. It is a cause of hydrops fetalis and intrauterine death. The term re-entry tachycardia is used because a circuit of conduction is set up, with premature activation of the atrium via an accessory pathway. There is rarely a structural heart problem, but an echocardiogram should be performed.

Investigation

The ECG will generally show a narrow complex tachycardia of 250–300 beats/min (Fig. 17.18). It may be possible to discern a P wave after the QRS complex due to retrograde activation of the atrium via the accessory pathway. If heart failure is severe, there may be changes suggestive of myocardial ischaemia, with T wave inversion in the lateral precordial leads. When in sinus rhythm, a short P–R interval may be discernible. In the Wolff–Parkinson–White (WPW) syndrome, the early antegrade activation of the ventricle via the pathway results in a short P–R interval and a delta wave.

Management

In the severely ill child, prompt restoration of sinus rhythm is the key to improvement. This is achieved by:

- Circulatory and respiratory support – tissue acidosis is corrected, positive pressure ventilation if required.
- Vagal stimulating manoeuvres, e.g. carotid sinus massage or cold ice pack to face, successful in about 80%.
- Intravenous adenosine – the treatment of choice. This is safe and effective, inducing atrioventricular block after rapid bolus injection. It terminates the tachycardia by breaking the re-entry circuit that is set up between the atrioventricular node and accessory pathway. It is given incrementally in increasing doses.
- Electrical cardioversion with a synchronised DC shock (0.5–2 J/kg body weight) if adenosine fails.

Once sinus rhythm is restored, maintenance therapy will be required, e.g. with flecainide or sotalol. Digoxin can be used on its own when there is no overt pre-excitation wave (delta wave) on the resting ECG, but propranolol can be added in the presence of pre-excitation. Even though the resting ECG may remain abnormal, 90% of children will have no further attacks after infancy. Treatment is therefore stopped at 1 year of age. Those who relapse thereafter are usually treated with percutaneous radiofrequency ablation or cryoablation of the accessory pathway.

Congenital complete heart block

This is a rare condition (Fig. 17.19) which is usually related to the presence of anti-Ro or anti-La antibodies in maternal serum. These mothers will have either manifest or latent connective tissue disorders. Subsequent pregnancies are often affected. This antibody appears to prevent normal development of the electrical conduction system in the developing heart, with atrophy and fibrosis of the atrioventricular node. It may cause fetal hydrops, death in utero and heart failure in the neonatal period. However, most remain symptom-free for many years, but a few become symptomatic with presyncope or syncope. All children with symptoms require insertion of an endocardial pacemaker.

Other arrhythmias

Long QT syndrome may be associated with sudden loss of consciousness during exercise, stress or emotion, usually in late childhood. It may be mistakenly diagnosed as epilepsy. If unrecognised, sudden death from ventricular tachycardia may occur. Inheritance is autosomal dominant; there are several phenotypes. Prolongation of the QT interval on ECG has been associated with the drug cisapride, which was used to treat gastro-oesophageal reflux, and with use of the antibiotic erythromycin.

Atrial fibrillation, atrial flutter, ectopic atrial tachycardia, ventricular tachycardia and ventri-

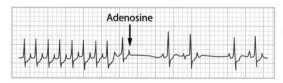

Figure 17.18 Rhythm strip showing supraventricular re-entry tachycardia, in which there is a narrow complex tachycardia (<120 ms or three small squares) of 250–300 beats/min, and response to treatment with adenosine.

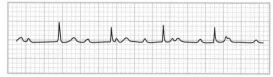

Figure 17.19 ECG of congenital complete heart block. The P waves and QRS complexes are dissociated.

cular fibrillation occur in children, but all are rare. They are most often seen in children who have undergone surgery for complex congenital heart disease.

Rheumatic fever

This is now rare in the UK, but remains the most important cause of heart disease in children worldwide. Improvements in sanitation, social factors, the more liberal use of antibiotics and changes in streptococcal virulence have led to its virtual disappearance in developed countries. In susceptible individuals, there is an abnormal immune response to a preceding infection with group A β-haemolytic streptococcus. The disease mainly affects children aged 5–15 years.

Clinical features

After a latent interval of 2–6 weeks following a pharyngeal infection, polyarthritis, mild fever and malaise develop. The clinical features and diagnostic criteria are shown in Figure 17.20.

Chronic rheumatic heart disease

The most common form of long-term damage from scarring and fibrosis of the valve tissue of the heart is mitral stenosis. If there have been repeated attacks of rheumatic fever with carditis, this may occur as early as the second decade of life, but usually symptoms do not develop until later adult life. Although the mitral valve is the most frequently affected, aortic, tricuspid and, rarely, pulmonary valve disease may occur.

Management

The acute episode is usually treated with bed rest and anti-inflammatory agents. While there is evidence of active myocarditis (echocardiographic changes with a raised ESR), bed rest and limitation of exercise are essential. Aspirin is very effective at suppressing the inflammatory response of the joints

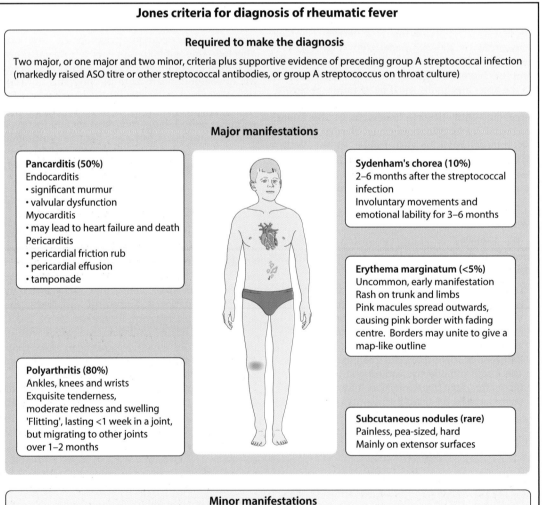

Jones criteria for diagnosis of rheumatic fever

Required to make the diagnosis

Two major, or one major and two minor, criteria plus supportive evidence of preceding group A streptococcal infection (markedly raised ASO titre or other streptococcal antibodies, or group A streptococcus on throat culture)

Major manifestations

Pancarditis (50%)
Endocarditis
• significant murmur
• valvular dysfunction
Myocarditis
• may lead to heart failure and death
Pericarditis
• pericardial friction rub
• pericardial effusion
• tamponade

Polyarthritis (80%)
Ankles, knees and wrists
Exquisite tenderness, moderate redness and swelling
'Flitting', lasting <1 week in a joint, but migrating to other joints over 1–2 months

Sydenham's chorea (10%)
2–6 months after the streptococcal infection
Involuntary movements and emotional lability for 3–6 months

Erythema marginatum (<5%)
Uncommon, early manifestation
Rash on trunk and limbs
Pink macules spread outwards, causing pink border with fading centre. Borders may unite to give a map-like outline

Subcutaneous nodules (rare)
Painless, pea-sized, hard
Mainly on extensor surfaces

Minor manifestations

Fever	Raised acute-phase reactants: ESR, C-reactive protein, leucocytosis
Polyarthralgia	Prolonged P–R interval on ECG
History of rheumatic fever	

Figure 17.20 Jones criteria for diagnosis of rheumatic fever.

and heart. It needs to be given in high dosage and serum levels monitored. If the fever and inflammation do not resolve rapidly, corticosteroids will be required. Symptomatic heart failure is treated with diuretics and ACE inhibitors, and significant pericardial effusions will require pericardiocentesis. Anti-streptococcal antibiotics may be given if there is any evidence of persisting infection.

Following resolution of the acute episode, recurrence should be prevented. Monthly injections of benzathine penicillin is the most effective prophylaxis. Alternatively, the penicillin can be given orally every day, but compliance may be a problem. Oral erythromycin can be substituted in those sensitive to penicillin. The length of treatment is controversial. Most recommend treatment to the age of 18 or 21 years, but, more recently, lifelong prophylaxis has been advocated. The severity of eventual rheumatic valvular disease relates to the number of childhood episodes of rheumatic fever.

Infective endocarditis

All children of any age with congenital heart disease (except secundum ASD), including neonates, are at risk of infective endocarditis. The risk is highest when there is a turbulent jet of blood, as with a VSD, coarctation of the aorta and persistent ductus arteriosus or if prosthetic material has been inserted at surgery. It may be difficult to diagnose, but should be suspected in any child or adult with a sustained fever, malaise, raised ESR, unexplained anaemia or haematuria. The presence of the classical peripheral stigmata of infective endocarditis should not be relied upon.

Clinical signs

- Fever
- Anaemia and pallor
- Splinter haemorrhages in nailbed
- Clubbing (late)
- Necrotic skin lesions (Fig. 17.21)
- Changing cardiac signs
- Splenomegaly

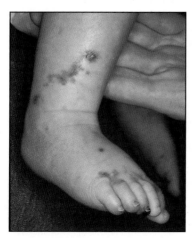

Figure 17.21
Widespread infected emboli and infarcts in a child with bacterial endocarditis. The tip of the third toe is gangrenous.

- Neurological signs from cerebral infarction
- Retinal infarcts
- Arthritis/arthralgia
- Haematuria (microscopic).

Diagnosis

Multiple blood cultures should be taken before antibiotics are started. Detailed cross-sectional echocardiography may confirm the diagnosis by identification of vegetations but can never exclude it. The vegetations consist of fibrin and platelets and contain infecting organisms. Acute-phase reactants are raised and can be useful to monitor response to treatment.

The most common causative organism is α-haemolytic streptococcus (*Streptococcus viridans*). Bacterial endocarditis is usually treated with high-dose penicillin in combination with an aminoglycoside, giving 6 weeks of intravenous therapy and checking that the serum level of the antibiotic will kill the organism. If there is infected prosthetic material, e.g. prosthetic valves, VSD patches or shunts, there is less chance of complete eradication and surgical removal may be required.

Prophylaxis

The most important factor in prophylaxis against endocarditis is good dental hygiene, and this should be strongly encouraged in all children with congenital heart disease. Antibiotic prophylaxis will be required for:

- dental treatment, however trivial
- surgery which is likely to be associated with bacteraemia (e.g. appendicectomy, ENT surgery).

> Antibiotic prophylaxis against bacterial endocarditis must be given to all children with congenital heart disease (except secundum ASD) before dental extraction or any potentially septic operation.

Myocarditis/cardiomyopathy

Dilated cardiomyopathy (a large, poorly contracting heart) may be inherited, secondary to metabolic disease or may result from a direct viral infection of the myocardium. It should be suspected in any child with an enlarged heart and heart failure who has previously been well. The diagnosis is readily made on echocardiography. Treatment is symptomatic with diuretics and ACE inhibitors or carvedilol, a beta-adrenoceptor blocking agent. The role of steroids and immunoglobulin infusion is controversial. Myocarditis usually improves spontaneously, but some children ultimately require heart transplantation. Other cardiomyopathies (hypertrophic/restrictive) are rare in childhood and are usually related to a systemic disease (e.g. Hurler's, Pompe's or Noonan's syndromes).

Kawasaki's disease

This mainly affects children of 6 months to 4 years. Clinical features are described in Chapter 14. It is uncommon but can cause significant cardiac disease. An echocardiogram is performed at diagnosis which may show a pericardial effusion, myocardial disease (poor contractility), endocardial disease (valve regurgitation) or coronary disease with aneurysm formation, which can be giant (more than 8 mm in diameter). If the coronary arteries are abnormal, angiography (Fig. 17.22) or MRI will be required.

Pulmonary hypertension

This is of increasing importance in paediatric cardiology as there is now effective medication for most causes. It can be caused by a number of different diseases (Box 17.4). From the cardiac perspective, most children with pulmonary hypertension (high pulmonary artery pressure, mean >25 mmHg), have a large post-tricuspid shunt with high pulmonary blood flow and low resistance, e.g. VSD, AVSD or PDA. The pressure falls to normal if the defect is corrected by surgery within 3 months of age. If these children are left untreated, however, the high flow and pressure causes irreversible damage to the pulmonary vascular bed (pulmonary vascular disease) which is not correctable other than by heart/lung transplantation.

Many medical therapies are now available, which may act on the pulmonary vasculature on the cyclic GMP pathway (e.g. inhaled nitric oxide, intravenous magnesium sulphate and oral phosphodiesterase inhibitors including sildenafil) or on the cyclic AMP pathway (intravenous prostacyclin or inhaled iloprost. In addition, endothelin antagonists are valuable therapy, e.g. oral bosentan. Anticoagulation is often given with heparin, aspirin or warfarin. These medications allow lung transplantation to be delayed for many years.

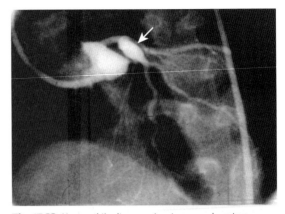

Fig 17.22 Kawasaki's disease. Angiogram showing coronary artery aneurysm.

Box 17.4 Causes of pulmonary hypertension

- Pulmonary arterial hypertension
  Idiopathic: sporadic or familial
  Post-tricuspid shunts (e.g. VSD, AVSD, PDA)
  Collagen vascular disease
  HIV infection
  Persistent pulmonary hypertension of the newborn
- Pulmonary venous hypertension
  Left-sided heart disease
  Pulmonary vein stenosis or compression
- Pulmonary hypertension with respiratory disease
  Chronic obstructive or premature lung disease
  Interstitial lung disease
  Obstructive sleep apnoea or upper airway obstruction
- Pulmonary thromboembolic disease
- Pulmonary inflammatory or capillary disease

Further reading

Anderson R, Baker E, McCartney F, Rigby M, Shinebourne E, Tynan M 2001 Paediatric cardiology, 2nd edn. Churchill Livingstone, Edinburgh

Archer N, Burch M 1998 Paediatric cardiology. Chapman and Hall, London

Kidney and urinary tract disorders

The spectrum of renal disease in children differs from that in adults:

- many structural abnormalities of the kidneys and urinary tract are identified on antenatal ultrasound screening
- urinary tract infection, vesicoureteric reflux and urinary obstruction have the potential to damage the growing kidney
- nephrotic syndrome is usually steroid-sensitive and only rarely leads to chronic renal failure
- chronic renal disorders and the drugs used to treat them may affect growth and development.

Assessment of the kidneys and urinary tract

The glomerular filtration rate (GFR) is low in the newborn infant. It is especially low if premature; the GFR at 28 weeks' gestation is only 10% of the term infant, or 30% if corrected for body surface area. In term infants, the corrected GFR doubles in the first two weeks after birth, increasing fourfold from birth to 1–2 years of age when the adult rate of 120 ml/min per 1.73 m^2 is achieved. The assessment of renal function in children is listed in Box 18.1 and the radiological investigations of the kidneys and urinary tract in Box 18.2.

Antenatal diagnosis of urinary tract anomalies

Before antenatal ultrasound scanning became routine, few congenital malformations of the kidneys and urinary tract were diagnosed until they caused symptoms in infancy, childhood or,

occasionally, adult life. Now the majority are identified in utero and can be managed prospectively. Abnormalities are identified in 1 in 200–400 births. They are potentially important because they may:

- be associated with abnormal renal development or function
- predispose to postnatal infection
- involve urinary obstruction which requires surgical treatment.

Box 18.1 Assessment of renal function in children

Plasma creatinine concentration
Rises progressively throughout childhood according to height and muscle bulk. Plasma creatinine may not rise above normal for age until renal function has fallen to less than half normal.

Glomerular filtration rate (GFR)
A rough estimate of GFR can be obtained using the formula:

$$\frac{\text{height (cm)} \times 40}{\text{plasma creatinine (micromol/L)}}$$

More accurate measurement of GFR is by measuring the clearance from the plasma of a substance that is freely filtered at the glomerulus and is not secreted or reabsorbed by the tubules (e.g. inulin, EDTA). The need for repeated blood tests limits its use in children.

Creatinine clearance
Rarely measured in children because of the difficulties in collecting a complete, timed urine sample.

Box 18.2 Radiological investigation of the kidneys and urinary tract

Ultrasound

Provides a non-invasive anatomical assessment of the whole urinary tract. It is the standard imaging procedure of the kidneys and urinary tract, but it does not give information about function and its accuracy is operator-dependent.

Functional scanning

Radioisotopes give a lower radiation dose than conventional X-rays and allow comparison of individual kidney function. Good images are difficult to obtained in the first month of life.

Static nuclear medicine scanning

This uses an isotope-labelled substance (e.g. DMSA) that is incorporated into the functioning renal tissue. It is particularly good for the detection of renal scars.

Dynamic nuclear medicine scanning

This uses an isotope-labelled substance, usually MAG 3, that is excreted by proximal tubular secretion, and gives information on blood flow, renal function and drainage. It is particularly useful for detecting urinary obstruction. It can also be used to detect vesicoureteric reflux in the older child who can cooperate by stopping and starting micturition on command (indirect radionuclide cystography, IRC).

Micturating cystourethrography (MCUG)

Filling the bladder with contrast via a urethral catheter outlines the bladder and is used to identify vesicoureteric reflux. Urethral obstruction is demonstrated on views during voiding without the catheter. As infection may be introduced on catheterisation, prophylactic antibiotics are given. Other disadvantages are that catheterisation is unpleasant and the radiation dose is high, particularly to the gonads. Using radioisotope scanning lowers the radiation dose but will not identify urethral obstruction.

Intravenous urography (IVU)

This is rarely indicated in children unless detailed anatomy of the calyces or ureter is required.

The antenatal detection and early treatment of urinary tract anomalies provide an opportunity to minimise or prevent progressive renal damage. A disadvantage is that minor abnormalities are also detected, most commonly mild unilateral pelvic dilatation, which do not require intervention but may lead to over-investigation, unnecessary treatment and unwarranted parental anxiety.

Anomalies detectable on antenatal ultrasound screening

Absence of both kidneys (renal agenesis) – as amniotic fluid is mainly derived from fetal urine, there is severe oligohydramnios resulting in Potter's syndrome (Fig. 18.1a and b).

Multicystic dysplastic kidney (MCDK) results from the failure of union of the ureteric bud (which forms the ureter, pelvis, calyces and collecting ducts) with the nephrogenic mesenchyme. It is a non-functioning structure with large fluid-filled cysts with no renal tissue and no connection with the bladder (Fig. 18.2). Half will have involuted by 2 years of age, and nephrectomy is indicated only if it remains very large or hypertension develops, but this is rare. Since MCDKs produce no urine, Potter's syndrome will result if the lesion is bilateral. Other causes of large cystic kidneys are *autosomal recessive polycystic kidney disease (ARPKD)* (Fig. 18.3) and *autosomal dominant polycystic kidney disease (ADPKD)* (Fig. 18.4) and tuberous sclerosis. In contrast to a multicystic kidney, in these disorders some or normal renal function is maintained but both kidneys are always affected.

Abnormal caudal migration may result in a *pelvic kidney* or a *horseshoe kidney* (Fig. 18.5). The abnormal position may predispose to infection or obstruction to urinary drainage.

Premature division of the ureteric bud gives rise to a *duplex system*, which can vary from simply a bifid renal pelvis to complete division with two ureters. These ureters frequently have an abnormal drainage so that the ureter from the lower pole moiety often refluxes, whereas the upper pole ureter may drain ectopically into the urethra or vagina or may prolapse into the bladder (ureterocele) and obstruct urine flow (Fig. 18.6).

Failure of fusion of the infraumbilical midline structures results in exposed bladder mucosa (*bladder extrophy*). Absence or severe deficiency of the anterior abdominal wall muscles is frequently associated with a large bladder and dilated ureters (megacystis-megaureters) and cryptorchidism, the *absent musculature syndrome* (Fig. 18.7).

Obstruction to urine flow may occur at the pelvi-ureteric or vesicoureteric junction, at the *bladder neck* (e.g. due to disruption of the nerve supply, *neuropathic bladder*) or at the *posterior urethra* in a boy due to mucosal folds or a membrane, known as a *posterior urethral valve*. The consequences of obstruction to urine flow are shown in Figure 18.8. At worst, this results in a *dysplastic kidney* which is small, poorly functioning and may contain cysts and aberrant embryonic tissue such as cartilage. In the most severe cases Potter's syndrome is present. Renal dysplasia can also occur in association with severe intrauterine vesicoureteric reflux, in isolation or in certain rare, inherited syndromes affecting multiple systems.

Some anomalies of the urinary tract

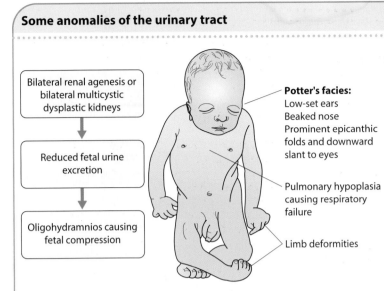

Bilateral renal agenesis or bilateral multicystic dysplastic kidneys

↓

Reduced fetal urine excretion

↓

Oligohydramnios causing fetal compression

Potter's facies:
Low-set ears
Beaked nose
Prominent epicanthic folds and downward slant to eyes

Pulmonary hypoplasia causing respiratory failure

Limb deformities

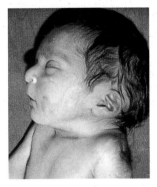

Figure 18.1b Facies in Potter's syndrome.

Figure 18.1a Potter's syndrome. Intrauterine compression of the fetus from oligohydramnios caused by lack of fetal urine causes a characteristic facies, lung hypoplasia and postural deformities including severe talipes. The infant may be stillborn or die soon after birth from respiratory failure.

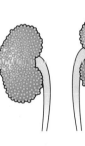

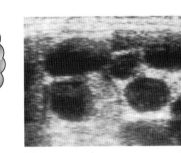

(a)　　　(b)

Figure 18.2 (a) Multicystic renal dysplasia. The kidney is replaced by cysts of variable size, with atresia of the ureter. **(b)** Renal ultrasound showing discrete cysts of variable size.

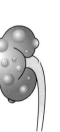

Figure 18.3 (left) Autosomal recessive polycystic kidney disease (ARPKD). There is diffuse bilateral enlargement of both kidneys.
Figure 18.4 (right) Autosomal dominant polycystic kidney disease (ADPKD). There are separate cysts of varying size between normal renal parenchyma. The kidneys are enlarged.

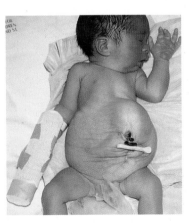

Figure 18.7 Absent musculature syndrome. The name arises from the wrinkled appearance of the abdomen. It is associated with a large bladder, dilated ureters and cryptorchidism. (Courtesy of Dr Jane Deal.)

Figure 18.5 (left) Horseshoe kidney.
Figure 18.6 (right) Duplex kidney showing ureterocele of upper moiety and reflux into lower pole moiety.

Urinary tract obstruction

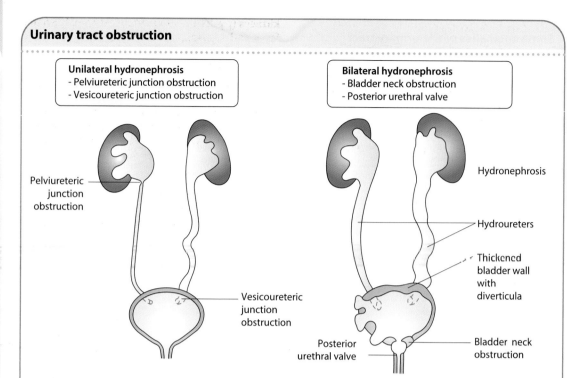

Unilateral hydronephrosis
- Pelviureteric junction obstruction
- Vesicoureteric junction obstruction

Bilateral hydronephrosis
- Bladder neck obstruction
- Posterior urethral valve

Pelviureteric junction obstruction

Vesicoureteric junction obstruction

Hydronephrosis

Hydroureters

Thickened bladder wall with diverticula

Posterior urethral valve

Bladder neck obstruction

Figure 18.8a Obstruction to urine flow results in dilatation of the urinary tract proximal to the site of obstruction. Obstruction may be at the pelviureteric or vesicoureteric junction (left), the bladder neck or urethra (right).

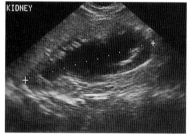

Figure 18.8b An ultrasound showing a dilated renal pelvis from pelviureteric junction obstruction.

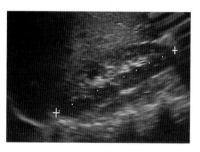

Figure 18.8c A normal ultrasound of the kidney is shown for comparison.

Figure 18.8d Graph from dynamic nuclear medicine scan (MAG 3) showing delayed excretion from a pelviureteric junction obstruction.

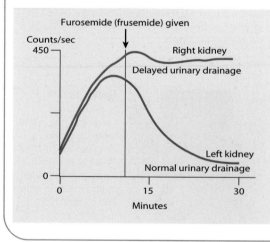

Furosemide (frusemide) given

Counts/sec
450

Right kidney

Delayed urinary drainage

Left kidney

Normal urinary drainage

0

0   15   30

Minutes

Antenatal treatment

The male fetus with a posterior urethral valve may develop severe urinary outflow obstruction resulting in progressive bilateral hydronephrosis, poor renal growth and declining liquor volume with the potential to induce pulmonary hypoplasia. Intrauterine bladder drainage procedures to prevent severe renal damage have been attempted but results have been disappointing. Early delivery is rarely indicated.

Postnatal management

An example of a protocol for infants with ante-natally diagnosed anomalies is shown in Figure 18.9. Prophylactic antibiotics should be started at birth to try to prevent urinary tract infection. As the newborn kidney has a low GFR, urine flow is low and mild outflow obstruction may not be evident in the first few days of life. The scan should therefore be repeated several weeks later. Bilateral hydro-nephrosis in a male infant warrants urgent further investigation to exclude a posterior urethral valve, which always requires surgery (see Case history 18.1).

Urinary tract infection

Three per cent of girls and 1% of boys have a symptomatic urinary tract infection (UTI) before the age of 11 years, and 50% of them have a recurrence within a year. UTI may involve the kidneys (pyelonephritis), when it is associated with fever and systemic involvement, or may be due to cystitis, when fever is absent or low grade. UTI in childhood is important because:

- up to half have a structural abnormality of their urinary tract
- pyelonephritis may damage the growing kidney by forming a scar, predisposing to hypertension and to chronic renal failure if the scarring is bilateral.

Clinical features

Presentation of UTI varies with age (Box 18.3). In the newborn, symptoms are non-specific and include vomiting and jaundice; septicaemia may

Box 18.3 Presentation of UTI in infancy and childhood

Infancy	Childhood
Fever	Dysuria and frequency
Lethargy or irritability	Fever with or without
Vomiting, diarrhoea	rigors
Poor feeding/failure to thrive	Lethargy and anorexia
Prolonged neonatal jaundice	Vomiting, diarrhoea
	Abdominal or loin pain
	Febrile convulsion
Septicaemia	(not to be confused with
Febrile convulsion	rigors)
(>6 months)	Recurrence of enuresis

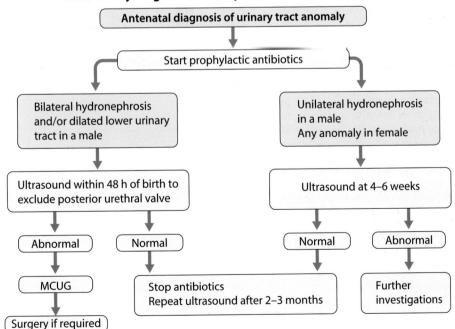

Antenatally diagnosed urinary tract anomalies–a protocol

Figure 18.9 An example of a protocol for the management of infants with antenatally diagnosed urinary tract anomalies (MCUG, micturating cystourethrogram).

Case History
18.1 Posterior urethral valve

Bilateral hydronephrosis was noted on antenatal ultrasound at 20 weeks' gestation in a male fetus. There was poor renal growth, progressive hydronephrosis and decreasing volume of amniotic fluid (Fig. 18.10a) on repeated scans. After birth, prophylactic antibiotics were started. An urgent ultrasound showed bilateral hydronephrosis with small dysplastic kidneys. The bladder and ureters were grossly distended. The plasma creatinine was raised. A micturating cystourethrogram (MCUG) (Fig. 18.10b) showed vesicoureteric reflux, a dilated posterior urethra and a posterior urethral valve which

was treated endoscopically. Renal function initially improved but then progressed to chronic renal failure. He had a renal transplant at 10 years of age.

> Bilateral hydronephrosis in a male infant requires urgent investigation to exclude a posterior urethral valve.

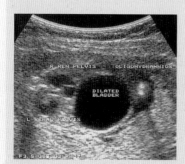

Figure 18.10a Antenatal ultrasound scan in an infant with urinary outflow obstruction from a posterior urethral valve. (Courtesy of Mr Karl Murphy.)

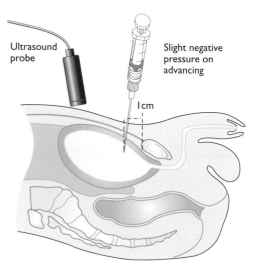

Gross vesicoureteric reflux

Distended bladder with trabeculated wall

Dilated posterior urethra

Posterior urethral valve

Figure 18.10b Micturating cystourethrogram (MCUG) in the same patient.

develop rapidly. The classical symptoms of dysuria, frequency and loin pain become more common with increasing age. It is rare for renal involvement to occur without fever, and dysuria alone is usually due to cystitis, or vulvitis in girls or balanitis in uncircumcised boys. Symptoms suggestive of a UTI may also occur following sexual abuse.

Collection of samples

The commonest error in the management of UTI in children, and especially in infants, is failure to establish the diagnosis properly in the first place. If the diagnosis of a UTI is not made, the opportunity to prevent renal damage may be missed, or, if incorrectly diagnosed, may lead to unnecessary invasive investigations.

For the child in nappies, urine can be collected by:

- absorbent pads in the nappy
- a 'clean-catch' sample into a waiting clean pot when the nappy is removed; this is easier in boys
- an adhesive plastic bag applied to the perineum after careful washing, although there may be contamination from the skin
- suprapubic aspiration (SPA) using ultrasound guidance, the method of choice in the severely ill infant under 1 year old requiring urgent diagnosis and treatment (Fig. 18.11); catheter samples are used as an alternative in some centres.

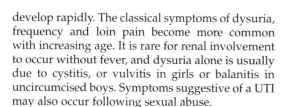

Ultrasound probe

Slight negative pressure on advancing

1cm

Figure 18.11 Suprapubic aspiration should be undertaken using ultrasound guidance. In an infant, the bladder extends into the abdomen. Negative pressure is applied to the syringe while advancing the needle until urine appears. This should avoid puncture of the rectum.

In the older child, urine can be obtained by collecting a midstream sample. Careful cleaning and collection are necessary, as contamination with both white cells and bacteria can occur from under the foreskin in boys, and from reflux of urine into the vagina during voiding in girls.

Ideally, the urine sample should be microscoped to identify organisms and cultured straight away. If this is not possible, it should be refrigerated to prevent the overgrowth of contaminating bacteria. Alternatively, delay in culture can be circumvented by the use of boric acid or dipslides. Urinary white cells are not a reliable feature of a UTI, as they may lyse during storage and may be present in febrile children without a UTI and in children with balanitis or vulvovaginitis. Positive testing of the urine with sticks for nitrite and white cell esterase is also suggestive of infection but there may be both false-negative and false-positive results, so sticks should only be used as a screening test.

A bacterial culture of $>10^5$ colony-forming units of a single organism per millilitre in a properly collected specimen gives a 90% probability of infection. If the same result is found in a second sample, the probability rises to 95%. A growth of mixed organisms usually represents contamination, but if there is doubt, another sample should be collected. Any bacterial growth of a single organism per millilitre in a suprapubic aspirate or catheter sample is considered diagnostic of infection.

Bacterial and host factors that predispose to infection

Infecting organism

UTI is usually the result of bowel flora entering the urinary tract via the urethra, except in the newborn when it is more likely to be haematogenous. The commonest organism is *E. coli*, followed by *Proteus* and *Pseudomonas*. The virulence of *E. coli* varies with its cell wall antigens and possession of endotoxin and cell wall appendages called P-fimbriae. *Proteus* infection is more commonly diagnosed in boys than in girls, possibly because of its presence under the prepuce. *Proteus* infection predisposes to the formation of phosphate stones by splitting urea to ammonia and thus alkalinising the urine. *Pseudomonas* infection may indicate the presence of some structural abnormality in the urinary tract affecting drainage.

Incomplete bladder emptying

Contributing factors in some children are:
- infrequent voiding, resulting in bladder enlargement
- vulvitis
- hurried micturition
- obstruction by a loaded rectum from constipation
- neuropathic bladder
- vesicoureteric reflux.

Vesicoureteric reflux

Vesicoureteric reflux (VUR) is a developmental anomaly of the vesicoureteric junctions. The ureters are displaced laterally and enter directly into the bladder rather than at an angle, with a shortened or absent intramural course. Severe cases may be associated with renal dysplasia. It is familial, with a 30–50% chance of occurring in first-degree relatives. It may also occur with bladder pathology, e.g. a neuropathic bladder or urethral obstruction, or temporarily after a UTI. Its severity varies from reflux into the lower end of an undilated ureter during micturition to the severest form with reflux during bladder filling and voiding, with a distended ureter, renal pelvis and clubbed calyces (Fig. 18.12). Mild reflux is unlikely to be of significance, but the more severe degrees of VUR may be associated with *intrarenal reflux* (IRR), the backflow of urine from the renal pelvis into the papillary collecting ducts; IRR is associated with a particularly high risk of renal scarring if UTIs occur. The incidence of renal defects increases with increasing severity of reflux; however, many children with renal defects do not have reflux. With growth, reflux resolves in 10% each year.

Reflux with associated ureteric dilatation is important, as:

- urine returning to the bladder from the ureters after voiding results in incomplete bladder emptying, which encourages infection
- the kidneys may become infected (pyelonephritis), particularly if there is intrarenal reflux
- bladder voiding pressure is transmitted to the renal papillae; this may contribute to renal damage if voiding pressures are high.

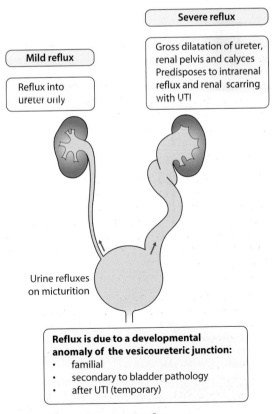

Mild reflux

Reflux into ureter only

Severe reflux

Gross dilatation of ureter, renal pelvis and calyces Predisposes to intrarenal reflux and renal scarring with UTI

Urine refluxes on micturition

Reflux is due to a developmental anomaly of the vesicoureteric junction:
- familial
- secondary to bladder pathology
- after UTI (temporary)

Figure 18.12 Vesicoureteric reflux.

Infection may destroy renal tissue, leaving a scar, resulting in a shrunken, poorly functioning segment of kidney (reflux nephropathy). If scarring is bilateral and severe, chronic renal failure may develop. The risk for hypertension in childhood or early adult life is variously estimated to be up to 10%.

Management

Prompt treatment reduces the risk of renal scarring. Most children can be treated with oral antibiotics (e.g. co-amoxiclav for 5 days, or for 10 days if the child was systemically unwell), adjusting the choice of antibiotic according to sensitivity on urine culture. All infants, and all children who are severely ill, require intravenous antibiotic therapy (e.g. cefotaxime or amoxicillin and an amino-glycoside such as gentamicin, monitoring its serum levels) until the temperature has settled, when oral treatment is substituted. (See Case history 18.2.)

Medical measures for the prevention of UTI

The aim is to ensure washout of organisms that ascend into the bladder from the perineum; and to reduce the presence of aggressive organisms in the stool, perineum and under the foreskin:

- high fluid intake to produce a high urine output
- regular voiding
- ensuring complete bladder emptying by encouraging the child to try a second time to empty his bladder after a minute or two, commonly known as double micturition; this empties any urine residue or refluxed urine returning to the bladder
- prevention or treatment of constipation
- good perineal hygiene
- *Lactobacillus acidophilus*, a probiotic to encourage colonisation of the gut by this organism and reduce the number of pathogenic organisms that might potentially cause invasive disease
- antibiotic prophylaxis, although this is controversial. It is often used in those under 2 years of age and those with severe reflux. Trimethoprim (2 mg/kg at night) is used most often, but nitrofurantoin or nalidixic acid may be given. Broad-spectrum, poorly absorbed antibiotics such as amoxicillin should be avoided.

First urinary tract infection – a protocol for initial management and investigation

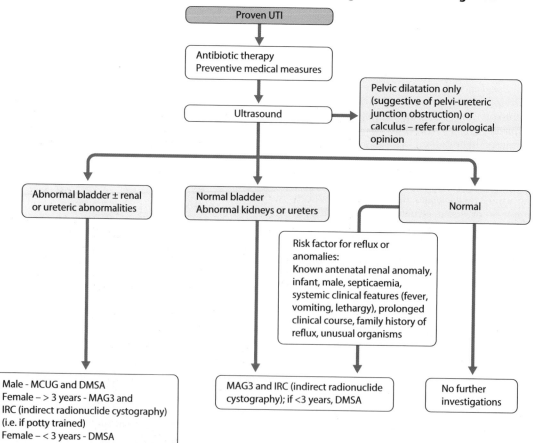

Figure 18.13 An example of a protocol for the initial management and investigation of a first urinary tract infection.

Investigation

The extent to which a child with a UTI should be investigated is controversial. This is not only because of the invasive nature and radiation burden of the tests, but also because of the lack of an evidence base to show that outcome is improved (unless urinary obstruction is demonstrated). Mild reflux usually resolves spontaneously, and operative intervention to stop reflux has not been shown to decrease renal damage. Furthermore, there is no evidence that antibiotic prophylaxis is any better than prompt treatment. There has, therefore, been a move away from the traditional view that uses age to determine which children to investigate, to protocols that identify children for investigation who are at the most risk of renal damage. Such children would be considered to be those who:

- have a known antenatal renal anomaly
- are infants
- are boys
- have had more than one UTI
- have had septicaemia
- have had a prolonged clinical course or fever >48 hours
- have a family history of reflux
- have unusual organisms (i.e. not *E. coli*).

An initial ultrasound will identify:

- serious structural abnormalities and urinary obstruction
- renal defects.

Subsequent investigations will depend on the results of the ultrasound. The need for any investigations in a child with only bladder symptoms is controversial. If urethral obstruction is suspected (abnormal bladder in a boy), MCUG should be performed promptly. Functional scans should be deferred for 3 to 6 months after a UTI, unless the ultrasound is suggestive of obstruction, to avoid missing a newly developed scar and because of false-positive results due to transient inflammation. Medical measures for the prevention of UTI should be initiated.

A suggested schema for investigation of the first proven UTI is shown in Figure 18.13, but varies between centres.

Follow-up of children with recurrent UTIs, renal scarring or reflux

In these children:
- Urine culture should be checked with a non-specific illness in case it is caused by a UTI (urine should not be cultured routinely).

Case History
18.2 Urinary tract infection

Jack, a 2-month-old infant, stopped feeding and had a high, intermittent fever. He was referred to hospital, where he had an infection screen. Urine examination showed >100 white blood cells, $>10^5$ *E. coli*/ml. He was treated with intravenous antibiotics. An ultrasound showed a small right kidney with a dilated renal pelvis and a dilated ureter. He was started on prophylactic antibiotics. A DMSA scan (Fig. 18.14) performed 3 months later confirmed bilateral renal scarring, with the right kidney contributing only 17%

of renal function. The MCUG (Fig. 18.15) showed bilateral vesicoureteric reflux. At 3 years of age, the reflux had resolved and antibiotic prophylaxis was stopped. His blood pressure and renal growth and function continue to be monitored.

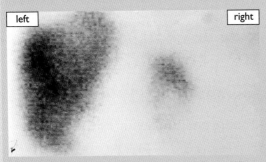

Figure 18.14 DMSA scan showing a small scarred right kidney and scars at the upper and lower poles of the left kidney.

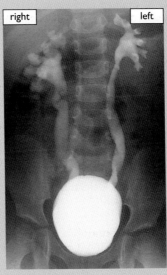

Figure 18.15 Micturating cystourethrogram showing bilateral vesicoureteric reflux with ureteric dilatation and dilated, clubbed calyces on the right.

⊙ Summary

A child with a first urinary tract infection

Why important?
Up to half have a structural abnormality of their urinary tract
Pyelonephritis may damage the growing kidney by forming a renal scar, which may result in hypertension and chronic renal failure

Diagnosis secure?
- Suggestive clinical features?
- Urine sample properly collected and processed?
- Culture of single organism >10^5/ml if clean catch or mid-stream urine or else any organisms on suprapubic aspirate or catheter sample?

Predisposing factors?
Incomplete bladder emptying
Constipation
Vesicoureteric reflux

Why investigate?
To identify serious structural abnormalities, urinary obstruction, renal scars, vesicoureteric reflux.

What investigation?
- Ultrasound of kidneys and urinary tract
- MAG3 and IRC (Indirect radionuclide scan) In this child as systemic features

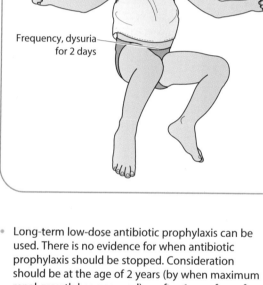

Fever, feeling unwell

Frequency, dysuria for 2 days

Management
Treat infection with antibiotics
Advice about medical preventive measures:
- High fluid intake
- Regular voiding, double micturition
- Prevent or treat constipation
- Good perineal hygiene
- *Lactobacillus acidophilus*
Advise to check urine culture if develops clinical features suggestive of non-specific illness

If renal scarring or reflux on investigation, or develops recurrent UTIs:
- Long term low-dose antibiotic prophylaxis
- Monitor blood pressure, renal growth and function

- Long-term low-dose antibiotic prophylaxis can be used. There is no evidence for when antibiotic prophylaxis should be stopped. Consideration should be at the age of 2 years (by when maximum renal growth has occurred) or after 1 year free of UTIs.
- Circumcision in boys may be considered as there is evidence that it reduces the incidence of urinary tract infection.
- Anti-reflux surgery may be indicated if there is progression of scarring with ongoing reflux, but it has not been shown to improve outcome.
- Blood pressure should be checked annually if renal defects are present.
- Regular assessment of renal growth and function is necessary if there are bilateral defects because of the risk of chronic renal failure.

If there are further symptomatic UTIs in younger children, investigations are required to determine whether there are new scars or continuing reflux. New scars are rare in previously unscarred kidneys after 4 years of age, even in the presence of continuing VUR, and reinvestigation is rarely indicated after this age.

Asymptomatic bacteriuria

Occasionally bacteriuria may be discovered during investigation of another problem in an asymptomatic child. Although treatment with antibiotics will eradicate the bacteriuria, recurrence is common. Asymptomatic bacteriuria does not need treatment as it does not cause renal damage.

Enuresis

Primary nocturnal enuresis

This is considered on page 394.

Daytime enuresis

This is a lack of bladder control during the day in a child old enough to be continent (over the age of 3–5 years). Nocturnal enuresis is also usually present. It may be caused by:

- lack of attention to bladder sensation, a manifestation of a developmental or psychogenic problem which may be secondary to stress or part of a general behavioural problem, although it may occur in otherwise normal children who are too preoccupied with what they are doing to respond to the sensation of a full bladder
- detrusor instability (uncoordinated bladder contractions)
- bladder neck weakness
- a neuropathic bladder
- a urinary tract infection (although rarely in the absence of other symptoms)
- constipation
- an ectopic ureter.

Examination may reveal evidence of a neuropathic bladder, i.e. the bladder may be distended, there may be abnormal perineal sensation and anal tone or abnormal leg reflexes and gait. Sensory loss in the distribution of the S2, 3 and 4 dermatomes should be sought. A spinal lesion may be present. Girls who are dry at night but wet on getting up are likely to have pooling of urine from an ectopic ureter opening into the vagina.

A urine sample is examined for microscopy, culture and sensitivity. Other investigations are performed if indicated. An ultrasound may show bladder pathology, with incomplete bladder emptying or thickening of the bladder wall. Urodynamic studies may be required. An X-ray of the spine may reveal a vertebral anomaly. An MRI scan may be required to confirm or exclude a non-bony spinal defect such as tethering of the cord.

Affected children in whom a neurological cause has been excluded may benefit from star charts, bladder training and pelvic floor exercises. Constipation should be treated. A small portable alarm with a pad in the pants, which is activated by urine, can be used when there is lack of attention to bladder sensation. Anticholinergic or adrenergic drugs, such as oxybutynin to damp down bladder contractions or ephedrine to increase tone at the bladder neck, may be helpful if other measures fail.

Secondary (onset) enuresis

The loss of previously achieved urinary continence may be due to:

- emotional upset, the commonest cause
- UTI
- polyuria from an osmotic diuresis in diabetes mellitus or a renal concentrating disorder, e.g. sickle cell disease or chronic renal failure.

Investigation should include:

- testing a urine sample for infection, glycosuria and proteinuria
- assessment of urinary concentrating ability by measuring the osmolality of an early morning urine sample. Rarely, a formal water deprivation

Summary

Enuresis
Daytime enuresis:

- consider causes – developmental or psychogenic, bladder instability or neuropathy, urinary tract infection, constipation, ectopic ureter.

Secondary (onset) enuresis:

- consider – emotional upset, UTI, polyuria from an osmotic diuresis in diabetes mellitus or a renal concentrating disorder.

test may be needed to exclude a urinary concentrating defect.
- ultrasound of the renal tract.

Proteinuria

Transient proteinuria may occur during febrile illnesses or after exercise and does not require investigation. Persistent proteinuria can be quantified by a 24-hour urine, a timed collection (protein excretion should not exceed 4 mg/h per m^2) or, more usefully in younger children, by measuring the urine protein/creatinine ratio in an early morning sample (protein should not exceed 20 mg/mmol of creatinine).

A common cause is orthostatic (postural) proteinuria, where proteinuria is only found when the child is upright, i.e. during the day. It can be diagnosed by measuring the urine protein/creatinine ratio in a series of early morning urine specimens. The prognosis is excellent and further investigations are not necessary. Other causes of proteinuria are listed in Box 18.4.

Nephrotic syndrome

In nephrotic syndrome, heavy proteinuria results in a low plasma albumin and oedema. The cause of the condition is unknown, but a few cases are secondary to systemic diseases such as Henoch–Schönlein purpura (HSP) and other vasculitides, e.g. systemic lupus erythematosus (SLE), infections (e.g. malaria) or allergens (e.g. bee sting).

Box 18.4 Causes of proteinuria

Orthostatic proteinuria
Glomerular abnormalities
   Minimal change disease
   Glomerulonephritis
   Abnormal glomerular basement membrane (familial nephritides)
Increased glomerular perfusion pressure
Reduced renal mass
Hypertension
Tubular proteinuria

Nephrotic syndrome

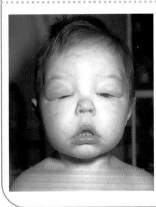

Figure 18.16 Facial oedema in nephrotic syndrome.

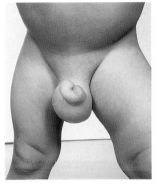

Figure 18.17 Gross oedema of the scrotum and legs as well as abdominal distension from ascites.

Clinical signs of the nephrotic syndrome are:

- periorbital oedema (particularly on waking), the earliest sign (Fig. 18.16)
- scrotal or vulval, leg and ankle oedema (Fig. 18.17)
- ascites
- breathlessness due to pleural effusions and abdominal distension.

The initial investigations are listed in Box 18.5.

Box 18.5 Investigations performed at presentation of nephrotic syndrome

Urine protein – on test strips ('Dipstick')
Full blood count and ESR
Urea, electrolytes, creatinine, albumin
Complement levels – C3, C4
Antistreptolysin O titre and throat swab
Urine microscopy and culture
Urinary sodium concentration
Hepatitis B antigen

Steroid-sensitive nephrotic syndrome

In 85–90% of children with nephrotic syndrome, the proteinuria resolves with corticosteroid therapy (steroid-sensitive nephrotic syndrome). These children do not progress to renal failure. It is commoner in boys than in girls, in Asian children than in Caucasians and there is a weak association with atopy. It is often precipitated by respiratory infections. Features suggesting steroid-sensitive nephrotic syndrome are:

- age between 1 and 10 years
- no macroscopic haematuria
- normal blood pressure
- normal complement levels
- normal renal function.

Management

The most widely used protocol is to initially give oral corticosteroids (60 mg/m² per day of prednisolone, unless there are atypical features. After 4 weeks the dose is reduced to 40 mg/m² on alternate days for 4 weeks and then stopped. The median time for the urine to become free of protein is 11 days. However, there is now good evidence that extending the initial course of steroids to about 6 months, by gradually tapering the alternate day part of the course, leads to a marked reduction in the proportion of children who develop a frequently relapsing or steroid dependent course, and this scheme is increasingly replacing the standard protocol. Children who do not respond to 4–8 weeks of corticosteroid therapy or have atypical features may have a more sinister diagnosis and require a renal biopsy. Renal histology in steroid-sensitive nephrotic syndrome is usually normal on light microscopy but fusion of the specialised epithelial cells that invest the glomerular capillaries (podocytes) is seen on electron microscopy. For this reason it is called minimal change disease.

The child with nephrotic syndrome is susceptible to several serious complications at presentation or relapse:

- *Hypovolaemia*. During the initial phase of oedema formation the intravascular compartment may become volume depleted. The child who becomes hypovolaemic characteristically complains of abdominal pain and may feel faint. There is peripheral vasoconstriction and urinary sodium retention. A low urinary sodium (<20 mmol/L) and a high packed cell volume are indications of hypovolaemia, which requires urgent treatment with intravenous albumin as the child is at risk of vascular thrombosis and shock. Increasing peripheral oedema, assessed clinically and by daily weight, may cause discomfort and respiratory compromise. If severe, this may need treatment with intravenous albumin. Care must be taken with the use of colloid, as it may precipitate pulmonary oedema and hypertension from fluid overload, and also with diuretics, which may cause or worsen hypovolaemia.

- *Thrombosis.* A hypercoagulable state, due to urinary losses of antithrombin, thrombocytosis which may be exacerbated by steroid therapy, increased synthesis of clotting factors and increased blood viscosity from the raised haematocrit, predisposes to thrombosis. This is usually arterial and may affect the brain, limbs and splanchnic circulation with potentially catastrophic results.
- *Infection.* Children in relapse are at risk of infection with capsulated bacteria, especially *Pneumococcus*. Peritonitis may occur.
- *Hypercholesterolaemia.* This correlates inversely with the serum albumin, but the cause of the hyperlipidaemia is not fully understood.

Prognosis

This is summarised in Figure 18.18. Relapses are identified by parents on urine testing. The side-effects of corticosteroid therapy may be reduced by an alternate-day regimen. If relapses are frequent or if a high maintenance dose is required, involvement of a paediatric nephrologist is advisable as other drug therapy may be considered. Levamisole, an immunomodulator, may maintain remission. An 8-week course of alkylating agents (for example cyclophosphamide or chlorambucil) maintains remission in 25–30% of steroid-dependent children for 2 years. Ciclosporin A maintains remission in about 75% of patients while it is being taken, but relapse almost always occurs when it is stopped. The drug mycophenolate mofetil shows promise.

Steroid-resistant nephrotic syndrome (Table 18.1)

These children should be referred to a paediatric nephrologist. Management of the oedema is by diuretic therapy, salt restriction, ACE inhibitors and sometimes NSAIDs (non-steroidal anti-inflammatory drugs), which may reduce proteinuria.

Congenital nephrotic syndrome

Congenital nephrotic syndrome presents in the first 3 months of life. It is rare. The commonest kind is recessively inherited and the gene frequency is particularly high in Finns. It is associated with a high mortality, usually due to complications of hypoalbuminaemia rather than renal failure. The albuminuria is so severe that bilateral nephrectomy may be necessary for its control, inevitably

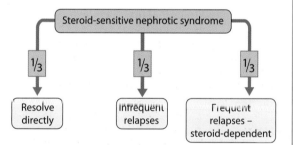

Figure 18.18 Clinical course in steroid-responsive nephrotic syndrome.

⊙ Summary

Nephrotic syndrome:
- clinical signs – oedema (periorbital, scrotal or vulval, leg and ankle oedema, ascites), pleural effusions
- diagnosis – heavy proteinuria and low plasma albumin.

Steroid-sensitive nephrotic syndrome:
- characteristic features – 1 to 10 years old, no macroscopic haematuria, and blood pressure, complement levels and renal function are normal
- management – oral corticosteroids, renal biopsy if unresponsive or atypical features
- complications – hypovolaemia, thrombosis, infection (pneumococcal), hypercholesterolaemia
- prognosis – may resolve or else there may be infrequent or frequent relapse.

Table 18.1 Steroid-resistant nephrotic syndrome

Cause	Specific features	Prognosis
Focal segmental glomerulosclerosis	Most common Familial or idiopathic	30% progress to end-stage renal failure in 5 years; 20% respond to cyclophosphamide, vincristine or ciclosporin. Recurrence post transplant is common
Mesangiocapillary glomerulonephritis (membranoproliferative glomerulonephritis)	More common in older children Haematuria and low complement level present	Decline in renal function over many years
Membranous nephropathy	Associated with hepatitis B May precede SLE	Most remit spontaneously within 5 years

Proteinuria

precipitating the need for dialysis, which is then continued until the child is large and fit enough for renal transplantation.

🌼 **An oedematous child – test for proteinuria to diagnose nephrotic syndrome**

Haematuria

Urine which is red in colour or tests positive for haemoglobin on urine sticks should be examined under the microscope to confirm haematuria (>10 red blood cells per high power field). Glomerular haematuria is suggested by brown urine, the presence of deformed red cells (which occurs as they pass through the basement membrane) and casts, and is often accompanied by proteinuria. Lower urinary tract haematuria is usually red, occurs at the beginning or end of the urinary stream, is not accompanied by proteinuria and is unusual in children.

Urinary tract infection is the most common cause of haematuria (Box 18.6), although seldom as the only symptom. The history and examination may suggest the diagnosis, e.g. a family history of stone formation or nephritis or a history of trauma. A plan of investigation is outlined in Box 18.7.

A renal biopsy may be indicated if:

- there is recurrent macroscopic haematuria
- a familial nephritis is suspected
- renal function is abnormal

- the complement levels are persistently abnormal
- there is proteinuria.

Acute nephritis

Acute nephritis in childhood usually follows a streptococcal sore throat or skin infection. Streptococcal nephritis is a common condition in the developing world, but has become uncommon in the UK. Other less common causes of acute nephritis are listed in Box 18.8. In acute nephritis, increased glomerular cellularity restricts glomerular blood flow and therefore filtration is decreased. This leads to:

- decreased urine output and volume overload
- hypertension, which may cause seizures
- oedema, characteristically around the eyes
- haematuria and proteinuria.

Management is by attention to both water and electrolyte balance and the use of diuretics when

- -

Box 18.8 Causes of acute nephritis

- Post-infectious (including streptococcus)
- Vasculitis (Henoch–Schönlein purpura or, rarely, SLE, Wegener's granulomatosis, microscopic polyarteritis, polyarteritis nodosa)
- IgA nephropathy and mesangiocapillary glomerulonephritis
- Anti-glomerular basement membrane disease (Goodpasture's syndrome) – very rare

---

Haematuria

- -

Box 18.6 Causes of haematuria

Non-glomerular
- Infection (bacterial, viral, TB, schistosomiasis)
- Trauma to genitalia, urinary tract or kidneys
- Stones
- Tumours
- Sickle cell disease
- Bleeding disorders
- Renal vein thrombosis
- Hypercalciuria

Glomerular
- Acute glomerulonephritis (usually with proteinuria)
- Chronic glomerulonephritis (usually with proteinuria)
- IgA nephropathy
- Familial nephritis
- Thin basement membrane disease

Box 18.7 Investigation of haematuria

All patients
- Urine microscopy (with phase contrast) and culture
- Protein and calcium excretion
- Kidney and urinary tract ultrasound
- Plasma urea, electrolytes, creatinine, calcium, phosphate, albumin
- Full blood count, platelets, clotting screen, sickle cell screen

If suggestive of glomerular haematuria
- ESR, complement levels and anti-DNA binding
- Throat swab and antistreptolysin O titre
- Hepatitis B antigen
- Renal biopsy if indicated
- Test mother's urine for blood (if Alport's syndrome suspected)
- Hearing test (if Alport's syndrome suspected)

necessary. Rarely, there may be a rapid deterioration in renal function (rapidly progressive glomerulonephritis). This may occur with any cause of acute nephritis, but is uncommon when the cause is post-streptococcal. If left untreated, irreversible renal failure may occur over weeks or months, so renal biopsy and treatment with immunosuppression and plasma exchange should be undertaken promptly.

Post-streptococcal nephritis

This is diagnosed by evidence of a recent streptococcal infection (culture of the organism, raised ASO titre) and low complement C3 levels that return to normal after 3–4 weeks. Long-term prognosis is good.

Henoch–Schönlein purpura

Henoch–Schönlein purpura is the combination of:

- characteristic skin rash
- arthralgia
- periarticular oedema
- abdominal pain
- glomerulonephritis.

It usually occurs between the ages of 3 and 10 years, is twice as common in boys, peaks during the winter months and is often preceded by an upper respiratory infection. Despite much research, the cause is unknown. It is postulated that genetic predisposition and antigen exposure increase circulating IgA levels and disrupt IgG synthesis. The IgA and IgG interact to produce complexes that activate complement and are deposited in affected organs, precipitating an inflammatory response with vasculitis.

Clinical findings (Fig. 18.19)

At presentation, affected children often have a fever. The *rash* is the most obvious feature. It is symmetrically distributed over the buttocks, the extensor surfaces of the arms and legs, and the ankles. The trunk is spared unless lesions are induced by trauma. The rash may initially be urticarial, rapidly becoming maculopapular and purpuric, is characteristically palpable and may recur over several weeks. The rash is the first clinical feature in about 50% and is the cornerstone of the diagnosis, which is clinical.

Joint pain occurs in two-thirds of patients, particularly of the knees and ankles. There is *periarticular oedema*. Long-term damage to the joints does not occur, and symptoms usually resolve before the rash goes.

Colicky abdominal pain occurs in many children and, if severe, can be treated with corticosteroids. Gastrointestinal petechiae can cause haematemesis and melaena. Intussusception can occur and can be particularly difficult to diagnose under these circumstances. Ileus, protein-losing enteropathy, orchitis and occasionally central nervous system involvement are rare complications.

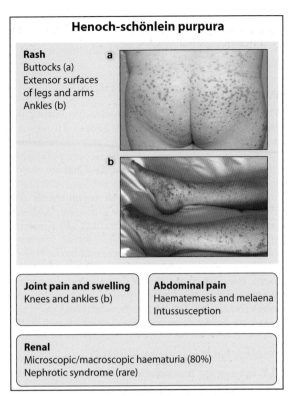

Henoch-schönlein purpura

Rash
Buttocks (a)
Extensor surfaces of legs and arms
Ankles (b)

Joint pain and swelling
Knees and ankles (b)

Abdominal pain
Haematemesis and melaena
Intussusception

Renal
Microscopic/macroscopic haematuria (80%)
Nephrotic syndrome (rare)

Figure 18.19 Main clinical manifestations of Henoch–Schönlein purpura. **(a)** Rash on buttocks. (Courtesy of Dr Michael Markiewicz) **(b)** Rash around the extensor surfaces of the legs and slight joint swelling. (Courtesy of Professor Tauny Southwood.)

Renal involvement is common, but is rarely the first symptom. Over 80% have microscopic or macroscopic haematuria or mild proteinuria. These children usually make a complete recovery. If proteinuria is more severe, nephrotic syndrome may result. Risk factors for progressive renal disease are heavy proteinuria, oedema, hypertension and deteriorating renal function, when a renal biopsy will determine if treatment is necessary. All children with renal involvement are followed for a year to detect those with persisting urinary abnormalities (5–10%) who require long term follow-up. This is necessary as hypertension and declining renal function may develop after an interval of several years.

IgA nephropathy

This may present with episodes of macroscopic haematuria, commonly in association with upper respiratory tract infections. Histological findings and management are as for Henoch–Schönlein purpura, which may be a variant of the same pathological process but not restricted to the kidney. The prognosis in children is better than that in adults.

Familial nephritis

The commonest familial nephritis is Alport's syndrome. This is usually an X-linked recessive disorder that progresses to end-stage renal failure by early adult life in males and is associated with nerve deafness and ocular defects. The mother may have haematuria.

Vasculitis

The commonest vasculitis to involve the kidney is Henoch–Schönlein purpura (see above). However, renal involvement may occur in rarer vasculitides such as polyarteritis nodosa, microscopic polyarteritis and Wegener's granulomatosis. Characteristic symptoms are fever, malaise, weight loss, skin rash and arthropathy with prominent involvement of the respiratory tract in Wegener's disease. ANCA (antineutrophil cytoplasm antibodies) are present and diagnostic in these diseases. Renal arteriography, to demonstrate the presence of aneurysms, will diagnose polyarteritis nodosa. Renal involvement may be severe and rapidly progressive. Treatment is with steroids, plasma exchange and intravenous cyclophosphamide, which may need to be continued for many months.

Systemic lupus erythematosus (SLE)

SLE is a disease that presents mainly in adolescent girls and young women. It is much commoner in Asians and Afro-Caribbeans than Caucasians. It is characterised by the presence of multiple autoantibodies, including antibodies to double-stranded DNA. The C3 component of complement may be low, particularly during active phases of the disease. Haematuria and proteinuria are indications for renal biopsy, as immunosuppression is always necessary and its intensity will depend on the severity of renal involvement.

> ### Summary
>
> **Acute nephritis:**
> - cause – usually follows a streptococcal infection, but also vasculitis (including Henoch–Schönlein purpura), IgA nephropathy and familial nephritis
> - clinical features – oedema (around the eyes), hypertension, decreased urine output, haematuria and proteinuria
> - management – fluid and electrolyte balance, diuretics, monitor for rapid deterioration in renal function.

Renal masses

An abdominal mass identified on palpating the abdomen should be investigated promptly by ultrasound scan. The causes of palpable kidneys are shown in Box 18.9. Bilaterally enlarged kidneys in early life are most frequently due to autosomal recessive polycystic kidney disease, which is associated with hypertension, hepatic fibrosis and progression to chronic renal failure. This form of polycystic kidney disease must be distinguished

> **Box 18.9** Causes of palpable kidneys
>
> **Unilateral**
> - Multicystic kidney
> - Compensatory hypertrophy
> - Obstructed hydronephrosis
> - Renal tumour (Wilms' tumour)
> - Renal vein thrombosis
>
> **Bilateral**
> - Autosomal recessive (infantile) polycystic kidneys
> - Autosomal dominant (adult) polycystic kidneys
> - Tuberous sclerosis
> - Renal vein thrombosis

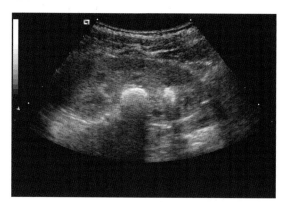

Figure 18.20 Renal ultrasound showing a staghorn calculus.

from the autosomal dominant adult-type polycystic kidney disease, which has a more benign prognosis.

Renal calculi

Renal stones are uncommon in childhood (Fig. 18.20). When they occur, predisposing causes must be sought:

- urinary tract infection
- structural anomalies of the urinary tract
- metabolic abnormalities.

The commonest are phosphate stones associated with infection, especially with *Proteus*. Calcium-containing stones occur in idiopathic hypercalciuria, the most common metabolic abnormality, and with increased urinary urate and oxalate excretion. Deposition of calcium in the parenchyma (nephrocalcinosis) may occur with hypercalciuria, hyperoxaluria and distal renal tubular acidosis. Nephrocalcinosis may be a complication of furosemide therapy in the neonate. Cystine and xanthine stones are rare.

Presentation may be with haematuria, loin or abdominal pain, UTI or passage of a stone.

Stones that are not passed spontaneously should be removed, by either lithotripsy or surgery, and any predisposing structural anomaly repaired. A high fluid intake is recommended in all affected children. If the cause is a metabolic abnormality, specific therapy may be possible.

Renal tubular disorders

Abnormalities of renal tubular function may occur at any point along the length of the nephron and affect any of the substances handled by it.

Generalised proximal tubular dysfunction (Fanconi syndrome)

The cardinal features are excessive urinary loss of amino acids, glucose, phosphate, bicarbonate, sodium, calcium, potassium and urate. The causes are listed in Box 18.10. Fanconi syndrome should be considered in a child presenting with:

Box 18.10 Causes of Fanconi syndrome

Idiopathic

Secondary to inborn errors of metabolism
- Cystinosis (an autosomal recessive disorder causing intracellular accumulation of cystine)
- Glycogen storage disorders
- Lowe's syndrome (oculocerebrorenal dystrophy)
- Galactosaemia
- Fructose intolerance
- Tyrosinaemia
- Wilson's disease

Acquired
- Heavy metals
- Drugs and toxins
- Vitamin D deficiency

- polydipsia and polyuria
- salt depletion and dehydration
- hyperchloraemic metabolic acidosis
- rickets and osteoporosis
- failure to thrive/poor growth.

Specific transport defects

(See Fig. 18.21.)

Acute renal failure

Acute renal failure is a sudden, potentially reversible, reduction in renal function. Oliguria (<0.5 ml/kg per hour) is usually present. It can be classified as (Box 18.11):

- prerenal – the commonest cause in children
- renal – there is salt and water retention; blood, protein and casts are often present in the urine; and there may be symptoms specific to an accompanying disease (e.g. Henoch–Schönlein purpura)
- postrenal – from urinary obstruction.

Acute-on-chronic renal failure is suggested by the child having growth failure, anaemia and disordered bone mineralisation (renal osteodystrophy).

Management

Children with acute renal failure should have their circulation and fluid balance meticulously monitored. Investigation by ultrasound scan will identify obstruction of the urinary tract, the small kidneys of chronic renal failure, or large, bright kidneys with loss of cortical medullary differentiation typical of an acute process.

Prerenal failure

This is suggested by hypovolaemia. The urinary sodium concentration is very low as the body tries

Box 18.11 Causes of acute renal failure

Prerenal	Renal	Postrenal
Hypovolaemia:	*Vascular:*	*Obstruction:*
Gastroenteritis	Haemolytic uraemic syndrome (HUS)	Congenital
Burns	Vasculitis	Acquired
Sepsis	Embolus	
Haemorrhage	Renal vein thrombosis	
Nephrotic syndrome	*Tubular:*	
Circulatory failure	Acute tubular necrosis (ATN)	
	Ischaemic	
	Toxic	
	Obstructive	
	Glomerular:	
	Glomerulonephritis	
	Interstitial:	
	Interstitial nephritis	
	Pyelonephritis	
	Acute-on-chronic renal failure	

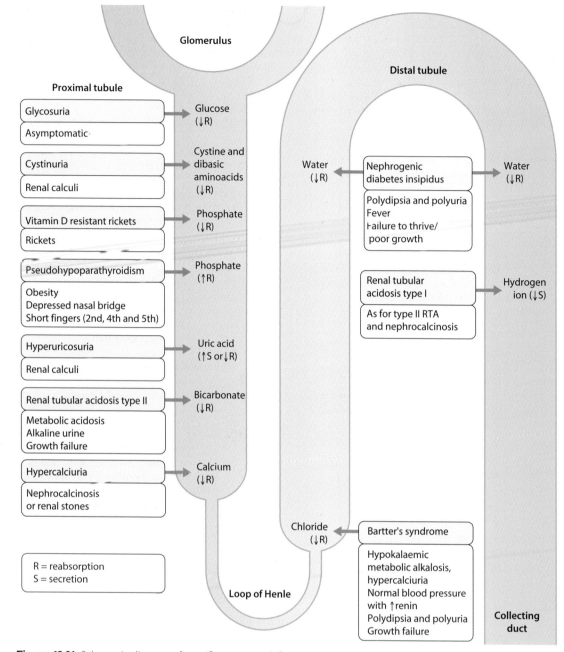

Figure 18.21 Schematic diagram of specific transport defects in some renal tubular disorders.

to retain fluid. The hypovolaemia needs to be urgently corrected with fluid replacement and circulatory support if acute tubular necrosis is to be avoided.

Renal failure

If there is circulatory overload, restriction of fluid intake and challenge with a diuretic may increase urine output sufficiently to allow gradual correction of sodium and water balance. A high-calorie, low-protein feed will decrease catabolism, uraemia and hyperkalaemia. Emergency management of metabolic acidosis, hyperkalaemia and hyperphosphataemia is shown in Box 18.12. If the cause

of renal failure is not obvious, a renal biopsy should be performed to identify rapidly progressive glomerulonephritis, as this needs immediate treatment with immunosuppression. The two commonest renal causes of acute renal failure in children in the UK are the haemolytic uraemic syndrome and acute tubular necrosis, the latter usually in the setting of multisystem failure in the intensive care unit or following cardiac surgery.

Postrenal failure

This requires assessment of the site of obstruction and relief by nephrostomy or bladder catheterisation. Surgery can be performed once fluid volume and electrolyte abnormalities have been corrected.

Dialysis in acute renal failure is indicated when there is:

- failure of conservative management
- hyperkalaemia
- severe hypo- or hypernatraemia
- pulmonary oedema or hypertension
- severe acidosis
- multisystem failure.

Peritoneal dialysis is the most common choice for children with acute renal failure due to primary renal disease as it is easier to perform than haemodialysis. If plasma exchange is part of the treatment, haemodialysis is used. If there is cardiac decompensation or hyper-catabolism, continuous arteriovenous or venovenous haemofiltration or dialysis provides gentle, continuous dialysis and fluid removal. One of these techniques should be instituted electively in multisystem failure since peritoneal dialysis is inadequate to remove the products of catabolism in this setting.

Acute renal failure in childhood generally carries a good prognosis for renal recovery unless complicating a life-threatening condition, e.g. severe infection, following cardiac surgery or multisystem failure.

Summary

Acute renal failure:
- prerenal – commonest cause in children, from hypovolaemia and circulatory failure
- renal – most often haemolytic uraemic syndrome or multisystem failure
- postrenal – from urinary obstruction
- management – treat underlying cause, metabolic abnormalities, dialysis if necessary.

Haemolytic uraemic syndrome

Haemolytic uraemic syndrome (HUS) is a triad of acute renal failure, microangiopathic haemolytic anaemia and thrombocytopenia. The patho-physiology of the disorder is not well understood; it is thought to be due to activation of neutrophils which damage vascular endothelium. Typical

HUS is secondary to gastrointestinal infection with verocytotoxin-producing *E. coli* O157:H7 or, less often, *Shigella*. It follows a prodrome of bloody diarrhoea. Although the platelet count is reduced, the clotting is normal (unlike in disseminated intravascular coagulation, DIC). Other organs such as the brain, pancreas and heart may also be involved.

With early supportive therapy, including dialysis, the typical diarrhoea-associated HUS usually has a good prognosis, although follow-up is necessary as there may be persistent proteinuria and the development of hypertension and declining renal function in subsequent years. In contrast, atypical HUS has no diarrhoeal prodrome, may be familial and frequently relapses. It has a high risk of hypertension and chronic renal failure and has a high mortality. Children with intracerebral involvement or with atypical HUS may be treated with prostacyclin or plasma exchange, but their efficacy is unproven.

> Haemolytic uraemic syndrome (HUS) – the triad of:
> - acute renal failure
> - haemolytic anaemia
> - thrombocytopenia.

Hypertension

Symptomatic hypertension in children is usually secondary and of renal origin. Most often, this is due to renal parenchymal disease. Coarctation of the aorta is another important cause in children. Other causes are rare (Box 18.13).

Presentation includes vomiting, headaches, facial palsy, hypertensive retinopathy, convulsions or proteinuria. Failure to thrive and cardiac failure are the most common features in infants. Phaeochromocytoma may cause paroxysmal palpitations and sweating.

Some causes are correctable, e.g. nephrectomy for unilateral scarring, angioplasty for renal artery stenosis, surgical repair of coarctation of the aorta, resection of a phaeochromocytoma, but in most cases medical treatment is necessary with antihypertensive drugs.

Early detection of hypertension is important. Any child with a renal abnormality should have their blood pressure checked annually throughout life. Children with a family history of essential hypertension should be encouraged to restrict their salt intake, avoid obesity and have their blood pressure checked regularly.

Chronic renal failure

Chronic renal failure is much less common in children than in adults, with an incidence of only 10 per million of the child population each year. Congenital and familial causes are more common in childhood than are acquired diseases (Table 18.2).

Clinical features

Chronic renal failure presents with:

- anorexia and lethargy
- polydipsia and polyuria
- failure to thrive/growth failure
- bony deformities from renal osteodystrophy (renal rickets)
- hypertension
- acute-on-chronic renal failure (precipitated by infection or dehydration)
- incidental finding of proteinuria
- unexplained normochromic, normocytic anaemia.

Many children with chronic renal failure have had their renal disease detected before birth by antenatal ultrasound or have previously identified renal disease. Symptoms rarely develop before renal function falls to less than one third of normal.

Management

The aims of management are to prevent the symptoms and metabolic abnormalities of chronic renal failure, to allow normal growth and development and to preserve residual renal function. The management of these children should be conducted in a specialist paediatric nephrology centre.

Table 18.2 Causes of chronic renal failure

Structural malformations	40%
Glomerulonephritis	25%
Hereditary nephropathies	20%
Systemic diseases	10%
Miscellaneous/unknown	5%

Diet

Anorexia and vomiting are common. Improving nutrition using calorie supplements and nasogastric or gastrostomy feeding is often necessary to optimise growth. Protein intake should be sufficient to maintain growth and a normal albumin, whilst preventing the accumulation of toxic metabolic by-products.

Prevention of renal osteodystrophy

Phosphate retention and hypocalcaemia due to decreased activation of vitamin D result in secondary hyperparathyroidism, osteitis fibrosa and osteomalacia. Phosphate restriction by decreasing the dietary intake of milk products, calcium carbonate as a phosphate binder, and activated vitamin D supplements help to prevent renal osteodystrophy.

Control of salt and water balance and acidosis

Many children with chronic renal failure caused by congenital structural malformations and renal dysplasia have an obligatory loss of salt and water. They need salt supplements and free access to water. Treatment with bicarbonate supplements is necessary to prevent acidosis.

Anaemia

Reduced production of erythropoietin and circulation of metabolites that are toxic to the bone marrow result in anaemia. This responds well to the administration of recombinant human erythropoietin.

Hormonal abnormalities

Many hormonal abnormalities occur in chronic renal failure. Most importantly, there is growth hormone resistance with high growth hormone levels but poor growth. Recombinant human growth hormone has been shown to be effective in improving growth for up to 5 years of treatment, but whether it improves final height remains unknown. Many children with chronic renal failure have delayed puberty and a subnormal pubertal growth spurt.

Dialysis and transplantation

It is now possible for all children, no matter how small, to enter renal replacement therapy programmes when end-stage renal failure is reached. The optimum management is by renal transplantation. Technically this is difficult in very small children, but infants weighing less than 10 kg have been successfully transplanted. Kidneys obtained from parents or other living donors have a higher success rate than cadaveric donor kidneys, which are matched as far as possible to the recipient's HLA type. Patient survival is high and first-year graft survival is around 80%, although technical difficulties reduce this rate in very young recipients and with small donor kidneys. Graft losses

⊚ Summary

Chronic renal failure:

- causes – congenital (structural malformations and hereditary nephropathies) most common
- presentation – abnormal antenatal ultrasound, anorexia and lethargy, polydipsia and polyuria, failure to thrive/growth failure, renal rickets, hypertension, proteinuria, anaemia
- management – diet and nasogastric or gastrostomy feeding, phosphate restriction and activated vitamin D to prevent renal osteodystrophy, salt supplements and free access to water to control salt and water balance, bicarbonate supplements to prevent acidosis, erythropoietin to prevent anaemia, growth hormone (rarely) and dialysis and transplantation.

from both acute and chronic rejection or recurrent disease mean that the 5-year graft survival is reduced to 70% and some children need re-transplantation. Current immunosuppression is mainly with combinations of prednisolone, azathioprine and ciclosporin A, although tacrolimus, mycophenolate mofetil and other newer agents are increasingly used.

Ideally a child is transplanted before dialysis is required, but if this is not possible, a period of dialysis may be necessary. Peritoneal dialysis, either by cycling overnight using a machine (continuous cycling peritoneal dialysis) or by manual exchanges over 24 hours (continuous ambulatory peritoneal dialysis), is preferable to haemodialysis as it can be done by the parents at home and is therefore less disruptive to family life and the child's schooling.

Further reading

Avner E D, Harmon W E, Niaudet P 2004 Pediatric nephrology. Lippincott Williams & Wilkins, Philadelphia. *A comprehensive textbook*

Rees L, Brogan P, Webb N 2006 Handbook of paediatric nephrology. Oxford University Press, Oxford

Webb N, Postlethwaite R J 2003 Clinical paediatric nephrology. Oxford University Press, Oxford. *Short textbook*

19

Genitalia

Most abnormalities of the genitalia in male infants are due to abnormal embryogenesis.

Inguinoscrotal disorders

Embryology

The testis is formed from the urogenital ridge on the posterior abdominal wall close to the developing kidney. Gonadal induction to form a testis is regulated by genes on the Y chromosome. During gestation, the testis migrates down towards the inguinal canal, guided by mesenchymal tissue known as the gubernaculum, probably under the influence of anti-Mullerian hormone (Fig. 19.1a).

Inguinoscrotal descent of the testis requires the release of testosterone from the fetal testis. A tongue of peritoneum, the processus vaginalis, precedes the migrating testis through the inguinal canal. This

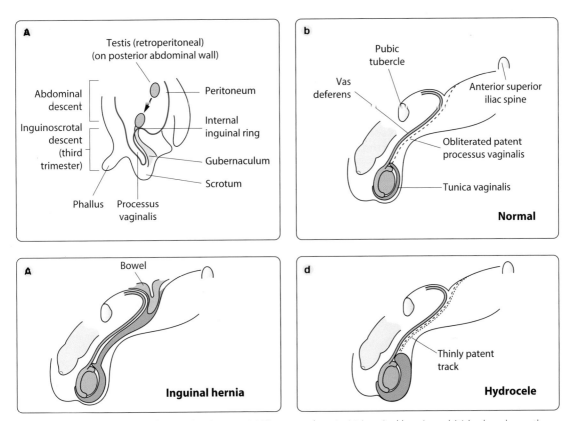

Figure 19.1 **(a)** Embryology of testicular descent. **(b)** The normal testis. **(c)** Inguinal hernia and **(d)** hydrocele are the result of incomplete obliteration of the processus vaginalis.

peritoneal extension normally becomes obliterated after birth, but failure of this process may lead to the development of an inguinal hernia or hydrocele (Fig. 19.1b–d).

Inguinal hernia

Inguinal hernias in children are almost always indirect and due to a patent processus vaginalis. They are much more frequent in boys and are particularly common in premature infants. Hernias are more common on the right side. At least 1 in 50 boys will develop an inguinal hernia.

Inguinal hernias usually present as an intermittent swelling in the groin or scrotum on crying or straining. Unless the hernia is observed as an inguinal swelling (Figs 19.2 and 19.3), diagnosis relies on the history and the identification of thickening of the spermatic cord (or round ligament in girls). The groin swelling may become visible on raising the intra-abdominal pressure by gently pressing on the abdomen or asking the child to cough.

An inguinal hernia in an infant may present as an irreducible lump in the groin or scrotum. The lump is firm and tender. The infant may be unwell with irritability and vomiting. Most 'irreducible' hernias can be successfully reduced following opioid analgesia and sustained gentle compression. Surgery is delayed for 24–48 hours to allow resolution of oedema. If reduction is impossible, emergency surgery is required because of the risk of strangulation of bowel and damage to the testis.

Surgery

The operation is carried out via an inguinal skin crease incision and involves ligation and division of the hernial sac (processus vaginalis). Except in small infants, this can usually be undertaken as a day-case procedure, provided there is appropriate anaesthetic and surgical support.

> **Inguinal hernias in infants should be repaired promptly to avoid the risk of strangulation.**

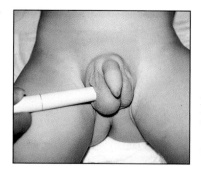

Figure 19.4
Right-sided hydrocele. This scrotal swelling often has a bluish discoloration and will transilluminate in a darkened room.

Hydrocele

A patent processus vaginalis, which is sufficiently narrow to prevent the formation of an inguinal hernia, may still allow peritoneal fluid to track down around the testis to form a hydrocele (Fig. 19.4). Hydroceles are asymptomatic scrotal swellings, often bilateral, and sometimes with a bluish discoloration. They may be tense or lax but are non-tender and transilluminate. The majority resolve spontaneously as the processus continues to obliterate, but surgery is required in children older than 18 months. A hydrocele of the cord forms a non-tender mobile swelling in the spermatic cord.

Undescended testis

An undescended testis has been arrested along its normal pathway of descent (Fig. 19.5). At birth, about 4% of full-term male infants will have a unilateral or bilateral undescended testis (cryptorchidism). It is more common in preterm infants because testicular descent through the inguinal canal occurs in the third trimester. Testicular descent may continue during early infancy and by 3 months of age the overall rate of cryptorchidism in boys is 1.5%, with little change thereafter. Contrary to previous teaching it is now recognised that occasionally a testis which is fully descended at birth can *ascend* to an inguinal position during childhood, accounting for some late-presenting 'undescended' testes. This phenomenon may be due to a relative shortening of cord structures during growth of the child.

Inguinal hernia in infants

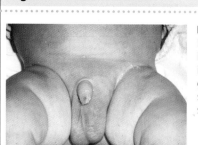

Figure 19.2
Left inguinal hernia in an infant. The left groin is only slightly swollen.

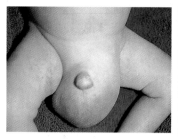

Figure 19.3
Bilateral inguinal hernias in a preterm infant. Inguinal hernia is primarily a groin swelling; only when it is large does it extend into the scrotum.

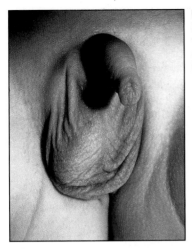

Figure 19.5 A left undescended testis with an empty hemiscrotum.

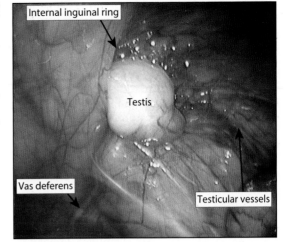

Internal inguinal ring

Testis

Vas deferens

Testicular vessels

Figure 19.6 Laparoscopic appearance of an intra-abdominal testis.

Examination

This should be carried out in a warm room, with warm hands and a relaxed child. The testes can then be brought down into a palpable position by gently massaging the contents of the inguinal canal towards the scrotum.

Classification

Retractile

The testis can be manipulated into the bottom of the scrotum without tension, but subsequently retracts into the inguinal region, pulled up by the cremasteric muscle. The testis has usually been found in the scrotum at a neonatal check. With age, the testis resides permanently in the scrotum. Follow-up is advisable as, rarely, the testis subsequently ascends into the inguinal canal.

Palpable

The testis can be palpated in the groin but cannot be manipulated into the scrotum. Occasionally, a testis is ectopic, when it lies outside its normal line of descent and may then be found in the perineum or femoral triangle.

Impalpable

No testis can be felt on detailed examination. The testis may be in the inguinal canal, intra-abdominal or absent.

Investigations

Useful investigations include:

- ultrasound – this has a limited role in identifying testes in the inguinal canal in obese boys but cannot reliably distinguish between an intra-abdominal or absent testis
- hormonal – for bilateral impalpable testes, the presence of testicular tissue can be confirmed by recording a rise in serum testosterone in response to intramuscular injections of human chorionic gonadotropin (HCG); these boys may require specialist endocrine review

- laparoscopy – the investigation of choice for the impalpable testis to determine if it is intra-abdominal or absent (Fig. 19.6).

Management

Surgical placement of the testis in the scrotum (*orchidopexy*) is undertaken for several reasons:

- *Fertility* – to optimise spermatogenesis, the testis needs to be in the scrotum below body temperature. The timing of orchidopexy is controversial, but evidence suggests that early orchidopexy during the second year of life may optimise reproductive potential. Fertility after orchidopexy for a unilateral undescended testis is close to normal. In contrast, fertility is reduced to around 50% after bilateral orchidopexy for palpable undescended testes, and men with a history of bilaterally impalpable testes are usually sterile.
- *Malignancy* – undescended testes have histological abnormalities and an increased risk of malignancy. The risk is greater for bilateral undescended testes and the greatest risk is for testes which are intra-abdominal. Although the evidence is somewhat contradictory, some studies have suggested that early orchidopexy for a unilateral undescended testis reduces the risk to nearly the same as a normal testis.
- *Cosmetic and psychological* – if a testis is absent, a prosthesis can be used but this is best delayed until a larger adult-sized prosthesis can be inserted.

Surgery

Most boys with an undescended testis undergo an orchidopexy via an inguinal incision. The testis is mobilised, preserving the vas deferens and testicular vessels, the associated patent processus vaginalis is ligated and divided, and the testis is placed in the scrotal pouch. The operation is usually performed as a day-case procedure. Orchidectomy is often advised for a unilateral intra-abdominal testis which cannot be corrected by simple orchidopexy, because of the future risk of malignancy. Microvascular orchidopexy or staged orchidopexy are two of the options available to preserve the testis in the rare cases of bilateral intra-abdominal testes, when the testicular vessels are too short to allow a single-stage procedure. Although intra-abdominal testes have profoundly defective spermatogenesis, they are capable of producing male hormones.

Varicocele

Varicosities of the testicular veins may develop in boys around puberty. They are usually on the left side and there is an association with subfertility. Treatment is indicated for symptoms (dragging, aching), impaired testicular growth and, in later life, for infertility. Obliteration of the testicular veins can be achieved by conventional surgery, laparoscopic techniques or radiological embolisation. The role of such interventions in asymptomatic boys is uncertain.

The acute scrotum

Torsion of the testis

Testicular torsion is most common in adolescents but may occur at any age, including the perinatal period (Fig. 19.7). The pain is not always centred on the scrotum but may be in the groin or lower abdomen. Atypical presentation is not unusual and the testes must always be examined whenever a boy or young man presents with inguinal or lower abdominal pain of sudden onset (see Case history 19.1). There may be a history of previous self-limiting episodes. Torsion of the testis must be relieved within 6–12 hours of the onset of symptoms for there to be a good chance of testicular viability. Surgical exploration is mandatory unless torsion can be excluded. If torsion is confirmed, fixation of the contralateral testis is essential because there may be an anatomical predisposition to torsion, for example the bell clapper testis, where the testis is not anchored properly. An undescended testis is at increased risk of torsion. Expert Doppler ultrasound looking at flow in the testicular blood vessels may allow torsion of the testis to be differentiated from epididymitis.

Torsion of testicular appendage

A hydatid of Morgagni is an embryological remnant found on the upper pole of the testis. Torsion of this appendage characteristically affects boys just prior to puberty. This may be because of rapid enlargement of the hydatid in response to gonadotrophins. The pain may increase over 1 or 2 days and occasionally the torted hydatid can be seen or felt (the blue dot sign). Surgical exploration and excision of the appendage leads to rapid resolution of the problem.

Other causes

Viral or bacterial epididymo-orchitis or epididymitis may cause an acute scrotum in infants and toddlers, and scrotal exploration is often necessary to confirm the diagnosis. If an associated urinary tract infection is present, antibiotic treatment and full investigation of the urinary tract will be required. Other conditions which may cause scrotal symptoms and signs are idiopathic scrotal oedema (usually painless, bilateral scrotal swelling and redness in a preschool child) or an incarcerated inguinal hernia.

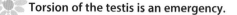

Torsion of the testis is an emergency.

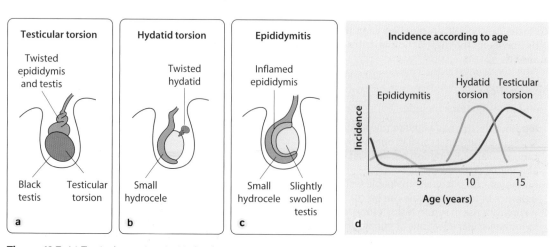

Figure 19.7 **(a)** Testicular torsion. **(b)** Hydatid torsion. **(c)** Epididymitis. **(d)** Incidence in relation to age.

Case History
19.1 Torsion of the testis

A 13-year-old boy presents to the Accident and Emergency Department with a 2-hour history of right lower abdominal pain of sudden onset. He has vomited once. Temperature 37.4° C. He indicates that his pain is in the right lower quadrant. Urine dipstick testing was normal. Appendicitis is suspected. However, examination of the abdomen does not reveal any guarding or other signs of peritoneal irritation in the right iliac fossa. When his testes are examined, the right testis is found to be slightly swollen and lying higher in the scrotum than the left testis (Fig. 19.8). Although he has not complained of testicular pain the testis is tender on palpation. Urgent surgical exploration confirms testicular torsion (Fig. 19.9). After detorsion, the testis appears

viable and is conserved. It is fixed with sutures to minimise the risk of further torsion. The left testis is also fixed as the anatomical variant which predisposes to torsion occurs bilaterally.

This case highlights:

- the clinical features of testicular torsion are variable and can be potentially misleading, with pain predominantly referred to the abdomen or inguinal region and minimal pain felt in the testis itself
- abdominal examination is never complete without inspection and gentle palpation of both testes
- with torsion, the testis is always tender.

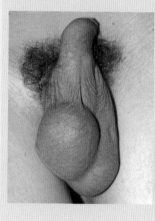

Figure 19.8 Enlarged, raised right testis, which was tender on palpation.

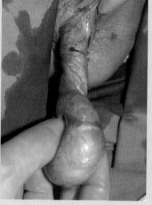

Figure 19.9 Torsion of the testis at surgery.

Abnormalities of the penis

Hypospadias

In the male fetus, urethral tubularisation occurs in a proximal to distal direction under the influence of fetal testosterone. Failure to complete this process leaves the urethral opening proximal to the normal meatus on the glans and this is termed hypospadias (Fig. 19.10). This is a common congenital anomaly, affecting about 1 in every 200 boys. Recent studies suggest that the incidence is increasing.

Hypospadias consists of:

- a ventral urethral meatus – in most cases the urethra opens on or adjacent to the glans penis, but in severe cases the opening may be on the penile shaft or in the perineum (Fig. 19.11)
- a hooded dorsal foreskin – the foreskin has failed to fuse ventrally
- chordee – a ventral curvature of the shaft of the penis, most apparent on erection. This is only marked in the more severe forms of hypospadias (Fig. 19.12).

Glanular hypospadias may be a solely cosmetic concern but more proximal varieties may cause functional problems including an inability to micturate in a normal direction and erectile deformity. With more severe varieties of hypospadias, additional genitourinary anomalies should be excluded and sometimes it is necessary to consider ambiguous genitalia and intersex disorders.

Surgery

Correction is often undertaken before 2 years of age, often as a single-stage operation. The aims of surgery are to produce:

- a terminal urethral meatus so that the boy can micturate in a normal standing position like his peers
- a straight erection
- a penis that looks normal.

> **Infants with hypospadias must not be circumcised, as the foreskin is often needed for later reconstructive surgery.**

Abnormalities of the penis

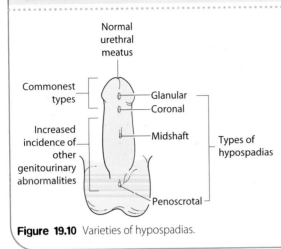

Figure legend labels:
Normal urethral meatus

Commonest types — Glanular, Coronal

Increased incidence of other genitourinary abnormalities

Midshaft — Types of hypospadias

Penoscrotal

Figure 19.10 Varieties of hypospadias.

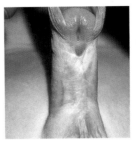

Figure 19.11 Penile shaft hypospadias with dorsal hooded foreskin.

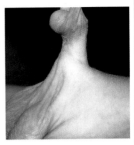

Figure 19.12 In lateral view, the ventral curvature of the penis (chordee) can be seen.

Circumcision

At birth, the foreskin is adherent to the surface of the glans penis. These adhesions separate spontaneously with time, allowing the foreskin to become more mobile and eventually retractile. At 1 year of age, approximately 50% of boys have a *non-retractile foreskin*, but by 4 years this has declined to 10%, and by 16 years to only 1%. A non-retractile foreskin often leads to ballooning on micturition, which is physiological. Gentle retraction of the foreskin at bathtimes helps to maintain hygiene, but forcible retraction of a healthy non-retractile foreskin should be avoided.

Two conditions that require reassurance are preputial adhesions (when the foreskin remains partially adherent to the glans) and the presence of white 'pearls' under the foreskin due to trapped epithelial squames. Both conditions are usually asymptomatic and resolve spontaneously.

Circumcision is one of the earliest recorded operations and remains an important tradition in the Jewish and Muslim religions. Although routine neonatal circumcision is still common in some Western countries such as the USA, the arguments generally used to justify on medical grounds have been discredited and no national or international medical association currently advocates routine neonatal circumcision. Neonatal circumcision is not without risk of significant morbidity. Nevertheless, the issue is still hotly debated (see 'Further reading').

There are only a few medical indications for circumcision:

- *Phimosis* (Fig. 19.13). This term is often wrongly used to describe a normal, non-retractile foreskin. Genuine phimosis is seen as a whitish scarring of the foreskin and is rare before the age of 5 years. The condition is due to a localised skin disease known as balanitis xerotica obliterans (BXO), which involves the glans penis as well and can cause urethral meatal stenosis.

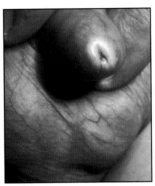

Figure 19.13 True phimosis.

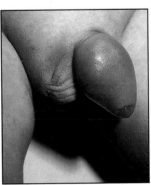

Figure 19.14 Balanoposthitis.

- *Recurrent balanoposthitis* (Fig. 19.14). A single attack of redness and inflammation of the foreskin, sometimes with a purulent discharge, is common and usually responds rapidly to warm baths and a broad-spectrum antibiotic. Recurrent attacks of balanoposthitis (inflammation of the glans and foreskin) are uncommon and circumcision is occasionally indicated.
- *Recurrent urinary tract infections*. Although urinary infection is more common in uncircumcised boys the overall incidence is low and routine circumcision is not justified as a preventative measure. However, circumcision may be helpful in reducing the risk of urinary tract bacterial

colonisation in boys with upper urinary tract anomalies complicated by recurrent urinary infection. It may also be appropriate in boys with spina bifida who need to perform clean intermittent urethral catheterisation.

Surgery

Circumcision for medical indications is performed under a general anaesthetic as a day case. During the procedure, a long-acting local anaesthetic block can be given to reduce postoperative pain. Circumcision is not a trivial operation. Healing can take up to 10 days, with discomfort for several days. Bleeding and infection are well-recognised complications, but more serious hazards, such as damage to the glans, may occur if the procedure is not carried out by appropriately trained personnel. The procedure also carries the risk of psychological trauma.

Preputioplasty can be offered as an effective alternative to circumcision in selected cases. After retraction of the foreskin the tight preputial ring is incised longitudinally and then sutured transversely. Unlike circumcision, preputioplasty conserves the foreskin and results in less postoperative discomfort and fewer complications. However, regular retraction of the foreskin is required in the first few weeks after surgery and for this reason preputioplasty is better suited to older boys who are willing to do this.

Topical corticosteroids

Application of a topical steroid ointment to the prepuce has been shown to facilitate retraction of a non-retractile prepuce, with success rates of up to 80%. Different treatment regimens have been described but typically the ointment is applied twice daily for 2 to 3 months. The mode of action is unclear.

Paraphimosis

The foreskin becomes trapped in the retracted position proximal to a swollen glans. The foreskin can usually be reduced, but adequate analgesia (often a general anaesthetic) is needed to achieve this. The problem is not usually recurrent and circumcision is rarely required.

Summary

Genital conditions in male infants and children

Inguinal hernia:
- Presentation – intermittent swelling in the groin or scrotum on crying or as an irreducible lump
- Repair promptly to avoid the risk of strangulation
- If irreducible – sustained gentle compression with analgesia to reduce, followed by delayed surgery

Hypospadias:
- Consists of – ventral urethral meatus, a hooded dorsal foreskin, chordee
- When severe, exclude other genitourinary anomalies
- Affected infants must not be circumcised, as the foreskin is often needed for later reconstructive surgery

An undescended testis:
- Is present in about 4% of full-term male infants but only 1.3% at 3 months of age
- May be **retractile**, if it can be brought to bottom of scrotum without tension but subsequently retracts – is usually normal
- Is **palpable** if felt in the groin but cannot be manipulated into the scrotum
- Is **impalpable** if no testis can be felt – may be in the inguinal canal, intra-abdominal or absent
- Orchidopexy – performed to optimise fertility, avoid malignant change, and for cosmetic and psychological reasons

Torsion of the testis:
- Must always be considered in a boy with an acutely painful scrotum
- Must be treated within hours for the testis to be viable

Circumcision:
- Is not recommended routinely, but is a tradition for Jews and Muslims and still common in the USA
- The only medical indications are – phimosis, recurrent balanoposthitis and possibly some boys with recurrent urinary tract infections
- Complications include pain, bleeding, infection and damage to the glans

Genital disorders in girls

Inguinal hernias

These are much less common than in boys. Sometimes the ovary becomes incarcerated in the hernial sac and can be difficult to reduce. Rarely, androgen insensitivity syndrome (testicular feminisation) can present as a hernia in a phenotypic female who actually has a male genotype.

Labial adhesions

If the labia minora are adherent in the midline, this may give the appearance of absence of the vagina, except there is a characteristic translucent midline raphe partially or totally occluding the vaginal opening. Asymptomatic adhesions can be left alone and will often lyse spontaneously. If there is perineal soreness or urinary irritation, treatment with an oestrogen cream often dissolves the adhesions. The cream should be applied sparingly and for a brief course to limit absorption. Active separation of the adhesions under anaesthesia is sometimes required.

Vulvovaginitis/vaginal discharge

Vulvovaginitis and vaginal discharge are common in young girls. They may result from infection (bacterial or fungal), specific irritants, poor hygiene or sexual abuse, although none of these factors is present in most cases. Vulvovaginitis may rarely be associated with threadworm infestation. Parents should be advised about hygiene, the avoidance of bubble bath and scented soaps and the use of loose-fitting cotton underwear. Swabs should be taken to identify any pathogens, which can then be specifically treated. Salt baths may be helpful. Oestrogen cream applied sparingly to the vulva may relieve the problem in resistant cases by increasing vaginal resistance to infection. If there are any concerns about sexual abuse, the child must be seen by a paediatrician (see Ch. 7). Rarely, if the vaginal discharge is persistent or purulent, examination under anaesthesia may be needed to exclude a vaginal foreign body or unusual infections.

Ambiguous genitalia is considered in Chapter 11.

Further reading

Circumcision. *British Journal of Urology International* 1999, Volume 83, Supplement 1

Hutson J M, Beasley S W, Woodward A A 1999 Jones' clinical paediatric surgery: diagnosis and management, 5th edn. Blackwell Science, Oxford

Thomas D F M, Rickwood A M K, Duffy P G (eds) 2002 Essentials of paediatric urology. Martin Dunitz, London

Liver disorders

In children:

- prolonged (persistent) neonatal jaundice is the most common presentation of liver disease in the neonatal period
- the earlier in life biliary atresia is diagnosed and treated surgically, the better the prognosis
- transmission of hepatitis B surface antigen-positive mothers is prevented by immunising their babies at birth
- chronic liver disease (Fig. 20.1), cirrhosis and portal hypertension are uncommon and should be treated in tertiary or national centres
- liver transplantation is an effective therapy for acute or chronic liver failure with greater than 80% 5-year survival.

Hepatic dysfunction

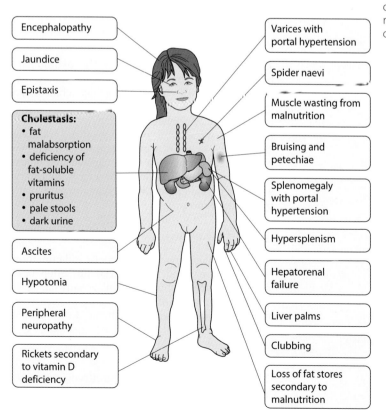

Encephalopathy

Jaundice

Epistaxis

Cholestasis:
- fat malabsorption
- deficiency of fat-soluble vitamins
- pruritus
- pale stools
- dark urine

Ascites

Hypotonia

Peripheral neuropathy

Rickets secondary to vitamin D deficiency

Varices with portal hypertension

Spider naevi

Muscle wasting from malnutrition

Bruising and petechiae

Splenomegaly with portal hypertension

Hypersplenism

Hepatorenal failure

Liver palms

Clubbing

Loss of fat stores secondary to malnutrition

Figure 20.1 Clinical features of liver disease. In addition, these children may have growth failure and developmental delay.

Neonatal liver disease

Most newborn infants become clinically jaundiced. About 5–10% are still jaundiced at more than 3 weeks of age, when it is called 'prolonged (or persistent) neonatal jaundice'. This is usually an unconjugated hyperbilirubinaemia, which resolves shortly afterwards (Box 20.1). Prolonged neonatal jaundice caused by liver disease is a conjugated hyperbilirubinaemia and is usually accompanied by:

- pale stools
- dark urine
- bleeding tendency
- failure to thrive.

The urgency to diagnose liver disease as early in the neonatal period as possible is because early diagnosis and management improve the prognosis.

> Prolonged (persistent) neonatal jaundice – check if it is due to liver disease i.e. conjugated hyperbilirubinaemia.

Bile duct obstruction

Biliary atresia (see Case history 20.1)

Box 20.1 Causes of prolonged (persistent) neonatal jaundice

Unconjugated
Breast milk jaundice
Infection (particularly urinary tract)
Haemolytic anaemia, e.g. G6PD deficiency
Hypothyroidism
High gastrointestinal obstruction
Crigler–Najjar syndrome

Conjugated (>20% of total bilirubin)

Bile duct obstruction
Biliary atresia
Choledochal cyst

Neonatal hepatitis
Congenital infection
Inborn errors of metabolism
   α_1–Antitrypsin deficiency
   Galactosaemia
   Tyrosinaemia (type 1)
Cystic fibrosis
Total Parenteral Nutrition (PN) cholestasis

Intrahepatic biliary hypoplasia
Alagille's syndrome

This occurs in 1 in 14 000 live births. It is a progressive disease in which there is destruction or absence of the extrahepatic biliary tree and intrahepatic biliary ducts. This leads to chronic liver failure and death unless surgical intervention is performed. Babies with biliary atresia have a normal birthweight but fail to thrive as the disease progresses. They are jaundiced and from the second day their stools are pale and their urine dark, although both the jaundice and stool colour may fluctuate. Hepatomegaly is present and splenomegaly will develop secondary to portal hypertension.

Standard liver function tests are of little value in the differential diagnosis. A fasting abdominal ultrasound may be normal, or demonstrate a contracted or absent gall bladder. A radioisotope scan with TBIDA (iminodiacetic acid derivatives) shows good uptake by the liver, but no excretion into the bowel. Liver biopsy demonstrates features of extrahepatic biliary obstruction, i.e. fibrosis and proliferation of bile ductules, although there may be features of neonatal hepatitis. The diagnosis is confirmed at laparotomy by operative cholangiography, which fails to outline a normal biliary tree.

Treatment consists of surgical bypass of the fibrotic ducts, hepatoportoenterostomy (Kasai procedure), in which the jejunum is anastomosed to patent ducts in the cut surface of the porta hepatis. If surgery is performed before the age of 60 days, 80% of children achieve bile drainage. The success rate diminishes with increasing age – hence the need for early diagnosis and treatment. Postoperative complications include cholangitis and fat malabsorption. Even when bile drainage is successful, there may be progression to cirrhosis and portal hypertension. If the operation is unsuccessful, liver transplantation has to be considered.

Choledochal cysts

These are cystic dilatations of the extrahepatic biliary system. About 25% present in infancy with cholestasis. In the older age group, choledochal cysts present with abdominal pain, a palpable mass and jaundice or cholangitis. The diagnosis is established by ultrasound or radionuclide scanning. Treatment is by surgical excision of the cyst with the formation of a roux-en-Y anastomosis to the biliary duct. Future complications include cholangitis and a 2% risk of malignancy, which may develop in any part of the biliary tree.

Neonatal hepatitis

In neonatal hepatitis there is hepatic inflammation. Its causes are listed in Box 20.1, but often none is identified. In contrast to biliary atresia, these infants may have intrauterine growth restriction and hepatosplenomegaly at birth. Liver biopsy (Fig. 20.6) may be non-specific.

α_1-antitrypsin deficiency

Deficiency of the protease α_1-antitrypsin is associated with liver disease in infancy and childhood

A term infant was given oral vitamin K shortly after birth. He was breast-fed. He became mildly jaundiced on the third day of life. At 5 weeks of age he presented with poor feeding and vomiting and a history of bruising on his forehead and shoulders. His urine had become dark and stools intermittently pale. He was pale, jaundiced, had several bruises and hepatomegaly. Investigations showed:

- Hb 8.8 g/L
- Platelets 465 × 10^9/L
- Prothrombin time – grossly prolonged
- Bilirubin 178 mmol/L – 80% conjugated.

The investigation of conjugated hyperbilirubinaemia is shown in Figure 20.2. The TBIDA radionuclide scan showed no excretion at 24 hours (Fig. 20.3) and a liver biopsy suggested biliary atresia (Fig. 20.4). A hepatoportoenterostomy was performed at 6 weeks of age (Fig. 20.5).

In persistent neonatal jaundice, early diagnosis of biliary atresia improves the prognosis.

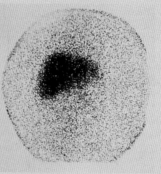

In persistent jaundice, always ask if the stools are pale – suggests bile duct obstruction.

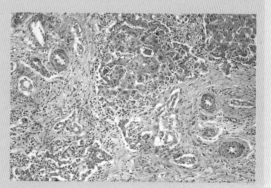

Figure 20.3
Radioisotope scan (TBIDA) of liver showing good hepatic uptake of isotope and no excretion into bowel. This scan suggests extrahepatic biliary obstruction or atresia or severe intrahepatic cholestasis.

Evaluation of neonatal conjugated hyperbilirubinaemia

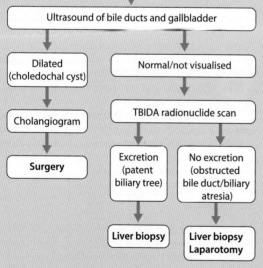

Screen for:
- infection – congenital, hepatitis
- genetic causes – α_1-antitrypsin deficiency, cystic fibrosis, galactosaemia
- metabolic – plasma aminoacids and urinary organic acids

↓

Ultrasound of bile ducts and gallbladder

Dilated (choledochal cyst) → Normal/not visualised

Cholangiogram → TBIDA radionuclide scan

Surgery → Excretion (patent biliary tree) / No excretion (obstructed bile duct/biliary atresia)

Liver biopsy → Liver biopsy Laparotomy

Figure 20.2 Evaluation of neonatal conjugated hyperbilirubinaemia.

Figure 20.4 Liver biopsy of biliary atresia showing bands of fibrous tissue with bile duct proliferation.

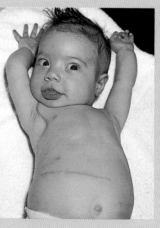

Figure 20.5
Shortly after successful bile drainage by hepatoporto-enterostomy (Kasai procedure) for biliary atresia.

Neonatal liver disease

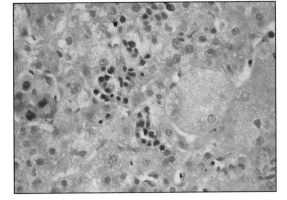

Figure 20.6 Liver biopsy in neonatal hepatitis showing inflammatory infiltrate throughout the liver, and giant cell and rosette formation of liver cells.

and emphysema in adults. It is inherited as an autosomal recessive disorder with an incidence of 1 in 2000–4000 in the UK. There are many phenotypes of the protease inhibitor (Pi) which are coded on chromosome 14. Liver disease is associated with the phenotype PiZZ.

The majority of babies present with prolonged (persistent) neonatal jaundice, but some develop bleeding, including intracranial haemorrhage, from vitamin K deficiency, particularly if they are breast-fed. Hepatomegaly is present. Splenomegaly develops with cirrhosis and portal hypertension. The diagnosis is confirmed by estimating the level of α_1-antitrypsin in the plasma and identifying the phenotype. Approximately 30% of children will recover, but the remainder will develop chronic liver disease, some of whom will develop cirrhosis and portal hypertension and require liver transplantation. Pulmonary disease is not significant in childhood. The disorder can be diagnosed antenatally.

Galactosaemia

This very rare disorder has an incidence of 1 in 40 000. The infants develop poor feeding, vomiting, jaundice and hepatomegaly when fed milk. Chronic liver failure, cataracts and developmental delay are inevitable if galactosaemia is untreated. A rapidly fatal course with shock, haemorrhage and disseminated intravascular coagulation, often due to Gram-negative sepsis, may occur.

The condition can be screened for in prolonged (persistent) jaundice by detecting galactose, a reducing substance, in the urine. The diagnosis is made by measuring the enzyme galactose-1-phosphate-uridyl transferase in red cells. A galactose-free diet prevents progression of liver disease, but ovarian failure and learning difficulties may occur later.

Other causes

Neonatal hepatitis may be caused by tyrosinaemia type 1, cystic fibrosis, lipid and glycogen storage disorders, peroxisomal disorders, or may be associated with parenteral nutrition.

Intrahepatic biliary hypoplasia

Syndromic causes

Alagille's syndrome is an autosomal dominant condition. Infants have characteristic triangular facies, skeletal abnormalities, peripheral pulmonary stenosis, renal tubular disorders, defects in the eye and intrahepatic biliary hypoplasia with severe pruritus and failure to thrive. Prognosis is variable, with 50% of children surviving into adult life without liver transplantation.

Progressive familial intrahepatic cholestasis (PFIC) is a heterogeneous group of cholestatic disorders of bile acid transporter defects. Children present with jaundice, itching, failure to thrive, diarrhoea and a variable progression of liver disease. Prognosis is variable, but some children will require liver transplantation.

Viral hepatitis

The clinical features of viral hepatitis include nausea, vomiting, abdominal pain, lethargy and jaundice; however, 30–50% of children do not develop jaundice. A large tender liver is common and 30% will have splenomegaly. The liver transferases are usually elevated 10-fold. Coagulation is usually normal.

Hepatitis A

Hepatitis A virus (HAV) is an RNA virus which is spread by faecal–oral transmission. The incidence of hepatitis A in childhood has fallen as socio-economic conditions have improved. Many adults are not immune. Vaccination is required for travellers to endemic areas.

The disease may be asymptomatic, but the majority of children have a mild illness and recover both clinically and biochemically within 2–4 weeks. Some may develop prolonged cholestatic hepatitis (which is self-limiting), or fulminant hepatitis. Chronic liver disease does not occur.

The diagnosis can be confirmed by detecting IgM antibody to the virus.

There is no treatment and no evidence that bed rest or change of diet is effective. Close contacts should be given prophylaxis with human normal immunoglobulin (HNIG) or vaccinated within 2 weeks of the onset of the illness.

Hepatitis B

Hepatitis B virus (HBV) is a DNA virus which is an important cause of acute and chronic liver disease worldwide, with high prevalence and carrier rates in the Far East, sub-Saharan Africa and parts of North and South America (Fig. 20.7). HBV is transmitted by:

- perinatal transmission from carrier mothers
- blood transfusions, needlestick injuries or biting insects

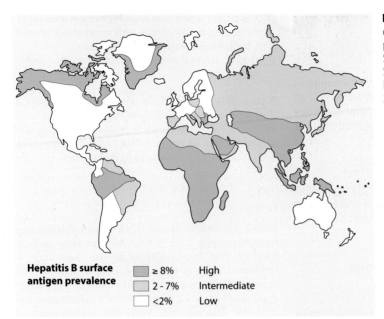

Figure 20.7 Worldwide prevalence of hepatitis B (HBsAg), showing high prevalence in the Far East, sub-Saharan Africa and parts of North and South America (CDC, Centers for Disease Control and Prevention, 2002).

Hepatitis B surface antigen prevalence

≥ 8%	High
2 - 7%	Intermediate
<2%	Low

- renal dialysis
- horizontal spread within families.

Children with HBV may be asymptomatic or have classical features of acute hepatitis. The majority will resolve spontaneously, but 1–2% develop fulminant hepatic failure, while 5–10% become chronic carriers. The diagnosis is made by detecting HBV antigens and antibodies. IgM antibodies to the core antigen (anti-HBc) are positive in acute infection. There is no treatment for acute HBV infection.

Chronic hepatitis B

Infants infected with HBV by vertical transmission from their mothers usually become asymptomatic carriers. Approximately 30–50% of carrier children will develop chronic HBV liver disease, which may progress to cirrhosis in 10%. There is a long-term risk of hepatocellular carcinoma. Treatment for chronic HBV is unsatisfactory. Interferon treatment for chronic hepatitis B is successful in 50% of children infected horizontally and 30% of children infected perinatally. Oral antiviral therapy such as lamivudine is effective in 23% but is limited by the development of resistance. Newer drugs such as adefovir or long-acting (peg) interferon may be more effective.

Prevention

Prevention of HBV infection is important. All pregnant women should have antenatal screening for the hepatitis surface antigen (HBsAg). Babies of all HBsAg-positive mothers should receive a course of hepatitis B vaccination, with hepatitis B immunoglobulin also being given if the mother is also hepatitis B e antigen (HBeAg)-positive. Other members of the family should also be vaccinated. There is evidence that effective neonatal vaccination reduces the incidence of HBV-related cancer.

Summary

Hepatitis B virus (HBV):
- perinatal transmission from carrier mothers should be prevented by maternal screening and giving the infant a course of hepatitis B vaccine with hepatitis B immunoglobulin if indicated
- infection may result in chronic HBV liver disease, which may progress to cirrhosis and hepatocellular carcinoma.

Hepatitis C

Hepatitis C virus (HCV) is an RNA virus which was responsible for 90% of post-transfusion hepatitis until screening of donor blood was introduced in 1991. In the UK, about 1 in 2000 donors have HCV antibodies. The prevalence is high among intravenous drug users. Children previously at risk were those who have received unscreened blood or blood products, in particular those with haemoglobinopathies or haemophilia. Vertical transmission from infected mothers is rare unless there is co-infection with HIV, but is now the commonest cause of HCV transmission in children. It seldom causes an acute infection, but at least 50% develop chronic liver disease, with cirrhosis and hepatocellular carcinoma occurring after a number of years. The combination of interferon or peg-interferon (long-acting) and ribavirin therapy in children is effective in 50% of children.

Hepatitis D virus

Hepatitis D virus (HDV) is a defective RNA virus which depends on hepatitis B virus for replication. It occurs as a co-infection with hepatitis B virus or as a superinfection causing an acute exacerbation of chronic hepatitis B virus infection. Cirrhosis develops in 50–70% of those who develop chronic HDV infection.

Hepatitis E virus

This is an RNA virus which is enterally transmitted, usually by contaminated water. Epidemics occur in some developing countries. When a viral aetiology of hepatitis is suspected but not identified, it is known as non-A to G hepatitis.

Epstein–Barr virus

Children with Epstein–Barr virus (EBV) infection are usually asymptomatic. Forty per cent have hepatitis which may become fulminant. Less than 5% are jaundiced.

Acute liver failure (fulminant hepatitis)

Acute liver failure in children is the development of massive hepatic necrosis with subsequent loss of liver function, with or without hepatic encephalopathy. The disease is uncommon, but has a high mortality. Most of the cases in childhood are attributed to a viral hepatitis non-A to G and metabolic conditions (Table 20.1). The child may present within hours or weeks with jaundice, encephalopathy, coagulopathy, hypoglycaemia and electrolyte disturbance. Early signs of encephalopathy include alternate periods of irritability and confusion with drowsiness. Older children may be aggressive and unusually difficult. Complications include cerebral oedema, haemorrhage from gastritis or coagulopathy, sepsis and pancreatitis.

Diagnosis

Bilirubin may be normal in the early stages, particularly with metabolic disease. Transaminases are greatly elevated (10–100 times normal), alkaline phosphatase is increased, coagulation is very abnormal and plasma ammonia is elevated. It is essential to monitor the acid–base balance, blood glucose and coagulation times. An EEG will show acute hepatic encephalopathy and a CT scan may demonstrate cerebral oedema.

Management

This includes:

- maintaining the blood glucose (>4 mmol/L) with intravenous dextrose

- preventing sepsis with broad-spectrum antibiotics
- preventing haemorrhage with intravenous vitamin K, fresh frozen plasma and H_2-blockers
- treating cerebral oedema by fluid restriction and mannitol diuresis.

A poor prognosis is likely when the liver begins to shrink in size, if there is a rising bilirubin with falling transaminases, an increasing coagulopathy or progression to coma. Without liver transplantation, 70% of children who progress to coma will die.

Reye's syndrome and Reye-like syndrome

Reye's syndrome is an acute non-inflammatory encephalopathy with microvesicular fatty infiltration of the liver. Although the aetiology is unknown, there is a close association with aspirin therapy. Since stopping giving aspirin to children aged less than 12 years, Reye's syndrome has virtually disappeared. With the introduction of tandem mass spectroscopy in the neonatal screening programme, the commonest beta oxidation defect, medium chain acyl-CoA dehydrogenase deficiency (MCAD), is diagnosed early in many regions of the UK. Many of these patients would have presented with acute liver failure and a Reye-like syndrome later in life.

Chronic liver disease

The causes of chronic liver disease are given in Box 20.2. The clinical presentation varies from acute hepatitis to the insidious development of hepato-splenomegaly, cirrhosis and portal hypertension with lethargy and malnutrition. The commonest causes of chronic hepatitis are post-viral hepatitis (B, C or non-A to G) and autoimmune hepatitis, but Wilson's disease should always be excluded. Histology may demonstrate varying degrees of hepatitis, with an inflammatory infiltrate in the portal tracts that spreads into the liver lobules.

Box 20.2 Causes of chronic liver disease in children

Chronic hepatitis
    Post-viral hepatitis B, C, non-A to G
    Autoimmune hepatitis
    Drugs (nitrofurantoin, non-steroidal anti-inflammatory)
    Inflammatory bowel disease
    Primary sclerosing cholangitis (± ulcerative colitis)
Wilson's disease (>3 years)
Alpha-1-antitrypsin deficiency
Cystic fibrosis

Secondary to:
    Neonatal liver disease
    Bile duct lesions

Table 20.1 Causes of acute liver failure in children

Infection	Viral hepatitis A, B, C, non-A to G
Poisons/drugs	Paracetamol, isoniazid, halothane, *Amanita phalloides* (poisonous mushroom)
Metabolic	Wilson's disease, tyrosinaemia
Autoimmune hepatitis	
Reye's syndrome	

Autoimmune hepatitis

The mean age of presentation is 7–10 years. It is more common in girls. It may present as an acute hepatitis, as fulminant hepatic failure or chronic liver disease with autoimmune features such as skin rash, lupus erythematosus, arthritis, haemolytic anaemia or nephritis. Diagnosis is based on hypergammaglobulinaemia (IgG >20 g/L); positive autoantibodies, e.g. smooth muscle antibodies (SMAs), antinuclear antibodies (ANAs) or liver/kidney microsomal antibodies (LKMs); a low serum complement (C4); and typical histology. Ninety per cent of children will respond to prednisolone and azathioprine.

Cystic fibrosis

Abnormal bile acid concentration and biliary disease is seen in cystic fibrosis as the CFTR (cystic fibrosis transmembrane regulator) is found in biliary epithelial cells. Cirrhosis and portal hypertension develop in 20% of children by mid-adolescence. Early liver disease is difficult to detect by biochemistry, ultrasound or radioisotope scanning. Liver histology includes fatty liver, focal biliary fibrosis or focal nodular cirrhosis. Therapy includes standard supportive and nutritional therapy with ursodeoxycholic acid. Liver transplantation should be considered for those with end-stage liver disease, either alone or in combination with a heart–lung transplant.

Wilson's disease

Wilson's disease is an autosomal recessive disorder with an incidence of 1 in 200 000. Many mutations have now been identified (on chromosome 13). The basic genetic defect is a combination of reduced synthesis of caeruloplasmin (the copper-binding protein) and defective excretion of copper in the bile, which leads to an accumulation of copper in the liver, brain, kidney and cornea. Wilson's disease rarely presents in children under the age of 3 years. A hepatic presentation is likely in children less than 12 years. They may present with almost any form of liver disease, including acute hepatitis, fulminant hepatitis, cirrhosis and portal hypertension. Neurological features are common in the second decade and include deterioration in school performance, mood and behaviour change, and extrapyramidal signs such as incoordination, tremor and dysarthria. Renal tubular dysfunction, with vitamin D-resistant rickets, and haemolytic anaemia also occur. Copper accumulation in the cornea (Kayser–Fleischer rings) (Fig. 20.8) are not seen before 7 years of age.

The diagnosis is confirmed by detecting low serum caeruloplasmin, low serum copper, excess urine copper and increased hepatic copper.

Penicillamine is a chelating agent and promotes urinary copper excretion. It reduces hepatic and central nervous system copper but also has a detoxifying effect on the copper deposition. It is the

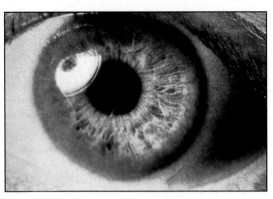

Figure 20.8 Kayser–Fleischer rings from copper in the cornea in a child with Wilson's disease.

drug of choice in combination with zinc to reduce copper absorption. Pyridoxine is given to prevent peripheral neuropathy. Neurological improvement may take up to 12 months of therapy. Thirty per cent of children with Wilson's disease will die from hepatic complications if untreated. Liver transplantation is considered for children with acute liver failure or severe end-stage liver failure.

Congenital hepatic fibrosis

Congenital hepatic fibrosis (CHF) presents in children over 2 years old with hepatosplenomegaly, abdominal distension and portal hypertension. Renal disease may coexist. Congenital hepatic fibrosis differs from cirrhosis in that liver function tests are normal in the early stage. Liver histology shows large bands of hepatic fibrosis containing abnormal bile ductules. The consequent portal hypertension causes bleeding from varices.

Non-alcoholic fatty liver disease

Non-alcoholic fatty liver disease (NAFLD) is diagnosed in up to 60% of overweight children but it can also be found in lean individuals and in certain metabolic syndromes. The term NAFLD includes benign fatty infiltration of the liver as well as more aggressive forms with inflammation and fibrosis that may progress to cirrhosis in childhood. The pathogenesis is not understood but may be linked to insulin resistance. In obese children liver function tests improve with weight loss.

Cirrhosis and portal hypertension

Cirrhosis is the end stage of many forms of liver disease. It is defined pathologically as extensive fibrosis with regenerative nodules. It may be secondary to hepatocellular disease or to chronic bile duct obstruction (biliary cirrhosis). The main pathophysiological effects of cirrhosis are diminished hepatic function and portal hypertension with splenomegaly, varices and ascites (see Fig. 20.1). Hepatocellular carcinoma may develop.

Children with compensated cirrhosis may be asymptomatic if liver function is adequate. They

343

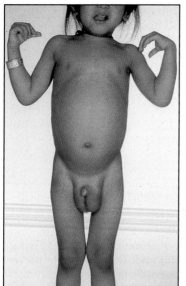

Figure 20.9
Cirrhosis and portal hypertension. This picture shows:
(i) malnutrition with loss of fat and muscle bulk
(ii) distended abdomen from hepatospleno-megaly and ascites
(iii) scrotal swelling from ascites
(iv) no jaundice despite advanced liver disease.

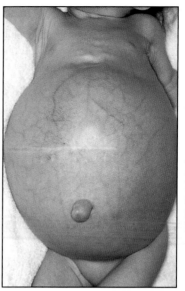

Figure 20.10
This infant has a grossly distended abdomen from ascites. There are dilated abdominal veins secondary to portal hypertension and an umbilical hernia from increased abdominal pressure. There is a surgical scar.

will not be jaundiced and may have normal liver function tests. As the cirrhosis increases, however, the results of deteriorating liver function and portal hypertension become obvious (Fig. 20.9). Physical signs include palmar and plantar erythema and spider naevi, malnutrition and hypotonia. Dilated abdominal veins and splenomegaly suggest portal hypertension, although the liver may be impalpable.

Investigations include:

* screening for the known causes of chronic liver disease (see Box 20.2)
* upper gastrointestinal endoscopy to detect the presence of oesophageal varices and/or erosive gastritis
* abdominal ultrasound – may show a shrunken liver and splenomegaly with gastric and oesophageal varices
* liver biopsy – may be difficult because of increased fibrosis but may indicate the aetiology (e.g. typical changes in congenital hepatic fibrosis, copper storage).

As cirrhosis decompensates, biochemical tests may demonstrate an elevation of aminotransferases and alkaline phosphatase. The plasma albumin is low and the prothrombin time is prolonged.

Oesophageal varices

These are an inevitable consequence of portal hypertension and may develop rapidly in children. They are best diagnosed by upper gastrointestinal endoscopy, as a barium swallow may miss small varices. Acute bleeding is treated conservatively with blood transfusions and H_2-blockers (e.g. ranitidine) or omeprazole. If bleeding persists, octreotide infusion, vasopressin analogues, sclero-therapy or band ligation may be effective. Porta-caval shunts may preclude liver transplantation,

but radiological placement of a stent between the hepatic and portal veins can be used as a temporary measure if transplantation is being considered.

Ascites (Fig. 20.10)

This is a major problem. The cause of ascites is uncertain, but contributory factors are hypo-albuminaemia, sodium retention, renal impairment and fluid redistribution. It is treated by sodium and fluid restriction and diuretics. Additional therapy for refractory ascites includes albumin infusions or paracentesis.

Spontaneous bacterial peritonitis

This should always be considered if there is undiagnosed fever, abdominal pain, tenderness or an unexplained deterioration in hepatic or renal function. A diagnostic paracentesis should be performed and the fluid sent for white cell count and differential and culture. Treatment is with broad-spectrum antibiotics.

Encephalopathy

This is precipitated by gastrointestinal haemor-rhage, sepsis, sedatives, renal failure or electrolyte imbalance. It is difficult to diagnose in children as the level of consciousness may vary throughout the day. Infants present with irritability and sleepiness, while older children present with abnormalities in mood, sleep rhythm, intellectual performance and behaviour. Plasma ammonia may be elevated and an EEG is always abnormal.

Renal failure

This may be secondary to renal tubular acidosis, acute tubular necrosis or functional renal failure.

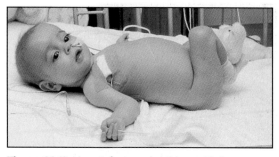

Figure 20.11 Many infants and children with liver disease need intensive nutritional supplementation. This malnourished infant is having both parenteral nutrition via a central line and continuous nasogastric feeding.

Management of children with liver disease

The management of children with liver disease is supportive, with the emphasis on correction of nutritional abnormalities, prevention of complications and intensive family support.

Nutrition

Malnutrition may be due to protein malnutrition, fat malabsorption, anorexia or fat-soluble vitamin deficiency (vitamins A, D, E and K).

Treatment is to provide a high-protein, high-carbohydrate diet with 50% more calories than the recommended dietary allowance. In children with cholestasis, medium-chain triglycerides, which are absorbed by the portal circulation, will provide fat, but 20–40% long-chain triglycerides are required to prevent essential fatty acid deficiency. Many children will require nasogastric tube feeding or parenteral nutrition (Fig. 20.11).

Fat-soluble vitamins

Vitamin K deficiency in liver disease may be due to malabsorption or diminished synthesis. Water-soluble forms of vitamin K are available.

Vitamin A deficiency causes night blindness in adults and retinal changes in infants. It is easily prevented with oral vitamin A.

Vitamin E deficiency causes peripheral neuropathy, haemolysis and ataxia. It is very poorly absorbed in cholestatic conditions and high oral doses are required.

Vitamin D deficiency causes rickets and pathological fractures. It is prevented by using a water-soluble form of vitamin D. Vitamin D-resistant rickets indicates renal tubular acidosis.

Pruritus

Many children with cholestasis have severe pruritus. It is alleviated by phenobarbital to stimulate bile flow, cholestyramine, which is a bile salt resin, ursodeoxycholic acid, an oral bile acid or evening primrose oil (arachidonic acid) applied to the skin.

Encephalopathy

In children, encephalopathy is managed by treating the precipitating factor (sepsis, gastrointestinal haemorrhage), by protein restriction or by using oral lactulose to reduce ammonia reabsorption by lowering colonic pH and increasing colonic transit.

Liver transplantation

Liver transplantation is accepted therapy for acute or chronic end-stage liver failure and has revolutionised the prognosis for these children. Transplantation is also considered for some hepatic malignancy.

The indications for transplantation in chronic liver failure are:

* severe malnutrition unresponsive to intensive nutritional therapy
* recurrent complications (bleeding varices, resistant ascites)
* failure of growth and development
* poor quality of life.

Liver transplant evaluation includes assessment of the vascular anatomy of the liver and exclusion of irreversible disease in other systems. Absolute contraindications include sepsis, untreatable cardiopulmonary disease or cerebrovascular disease.

There is considerable difficulty in obtaining small organs for children. Most children receive part of an adult's liver, which is either reduced to fit the child's abdomen (reduction hepatectomy) or split (shared between an adult and child). Complications post transplantation include:

* primary non-function of the liver (5%)
* hepatic artery thrombosis (10–20%)
* biliary leaks and strictures (20%)
* rejection (30–60%)
* sepsis, the main cause of death.

In large national centres, the overall 1-year survival is approximately 90%, and the overall 5-year survival is more than 80%. Most deaths occur in the first 3 months. Children who survive the initial postoperative period usually do well. Long-term studies indicate normal psychosocial development and quality of life in survivors.

Further reading

Booth I W, Kelly D A 1996 Paediatric gastroenterology and hepatology. Mosby-Wolfe, London

Kelly D A 2004 Diseases of the liver and biliary system in childhood, 2nd edn. Blackwell Science, Oxford

Malignant disease

Cancer in children is not common:

- around 1 child in 500 develops cancer by 15 years of age
- each year there are 120–140 new cases per million children aged under 15 years, about 1500 in the UK.

The types of malignant disease (Fig. 21.1) are very different from those in adults, where carcinomas of the lung, breast, gut and skin predominate. The age at presentation varies with the different types of disease:

- leukaemia affects children at all ages
- neuroblastoma and Wilms' tumour are most frequent in the first 5 years of life

- Hodgkin's disease and bone tumours have their peak incidence in adolescence and early adult life.

The survival rate for many tumours has increased dramatically over the last four decades (Fig. 21.2). However, after accidents, cancer is the most common cause of death in children over 1 year of age. The overall 5-year survival of children with malignant disease is about 75%, most of whom can be considered cured. This improved life expectancy can be attributed mainly to the introduction of multi-agent chemotherapy and specialist multi-disciplinary care. However, for some children, the

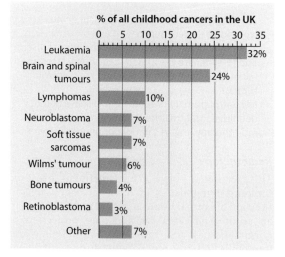

Figure 21.1 Relative frequency of different types of cancer in children.

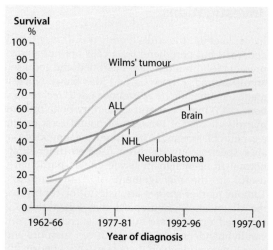

Figure 21.2 Five-year survival rates showing the considerable improvement over the last 30 years. (ALL, acute lymphoblastic leukaemia; NHL, Non-Hodgkin's lymphoma.)

price of survival is long-term medical or psycho-social difficulties.

> 🌼 **In children, leukaemia is the most common malignancy followed by brain tumours.**

Aetiology

In most cases, the precise aetiology of childhood cancer is unclear, but it is likely to involve an interaction between environmental factors (e.g. viral infection) and host genetic susceptibility (e.g. gene mutation). In fact, there are very few established environmental risk factors and although cancer occurs as a result of mutation in cell growth-controlling genes, which may be either inherited or sporadic, in most cases a specific gene mutation is unknown. One example of an inherited cancer is bilateral retinoblastoma, which is associated with a mutation within the RB gene located on chromosome 13. There is a wide range of syndromes associated with an increased risk of cancer in childhood, e.g. Down's syndrome and leukaemia, neurofibromatosis and glioma. In time, the identification of biological characteristics of tumour cells may also help elucidate the basic pathogenetic mechanisms behind their origin.

Clinical presentation

Cancer presents with:

- a localised mass
- the consequences of disseminated disease, e.g. bone marrow infiltration, causing systemic ill-health
- the consequences of pressure from a mass on local structures or tissue, e.g. airway obstruction secondary to enlarged lymph nodes.

Investigations

In leukaemia the full blood count is usually abnormal but peripheral blast cells are not always present. Solid tumours are identified and localised on ultrasound, X-rays, CT and MRI scans. Nuclear medicine imaging (e.g. radiolabelled technetium bone scan) may be useful to identify bone or bone marrow disease or tumours of neural crest origin, e.g. neuroblastomas. More recently, magnetic resonance spectroscopy has been used to differentiate normal from malignant tissue and is particularly useful in the management of brain tumours. Tumour marker studies are helpful for confirming the diagnosis of neuroblastoma, when there is increased urinary catecholamine excretion (VMA, vanillylmandelic acid) and germ cell tumours and liver tumours in which there is usually abnormally high alphafetoprotein (AFP) production. However, all diagnoses must be confirmed histologically, either by bone marrow aspiration for most cases of leukaemia or by biopsy for most solid tumours,

although this may not always be possible for brain tumours. The differentiation between some solid tumours may be difficult by standard microscopy, and further differentiation requires specialised histopathology investigation such as immuno-histochemistry and electron microscopy. Molecular and genetic techniques can identify specific characteristics of certain tumour types and such tests are used in a clinical setting to predict prognosis (e.g. amplification of the 'N-*myc*' oncogene associated with a poor prognosis in neuroblastoma) or to confirm an uncertain histological diagnosis (e.g. translocation of chromosomes 11 and 22 in Ewing's sarcoma).

Management

Once a tumour has been diagnosed, the parents and child need to be seen and the diagnosis explained to them in a realistic, yet positive way. Detailed investigation to define the extent of the disease and, in solid tumours, to assess the presence of metastatic disease, is essential to plan treatment. Considerable progress has been made in improving outcome by evaluating new treatment regimens through national and international collaborative studies.

Most children with cancer in the UK are initially investigated and treated in regional centres, which provide experienced multidisciplinary teams with facilities for the intensive medical and psychosocial support required. Subsequent management is often shared between the specialist centre, referral hospital and local services within the community to provide the optimum care with the least disruption to the family.

Treatment

Treatment may involve chemotherapy, surgery or radiotherapy, alone or in combination.

Chemotherapy

This is used:

- as primary curative treatment, e.g. in acute lymphoblastic leukaemia
- as adjuvant treatment to deal with residual disease and to eliminate presumed micrometastases after initial local treatment with surgery, e.g. in Wilms' tumour
- to control primary or metastatic disease before definitive local treatment with surgery and/or radiotherapy, e.g. in sarcoma or neuroblastoma.

Radiotherapy

This retains a role in the treatment of some tumours, but the risk of damage to growth and function of normal tissue is greater in a child than in an adult. The need for adequate protection of normal tissues and for careful positioning and immobilisation of the patient during treatment raises practical difficulties, particularly in young children.

Surgery

Initial surgery is increasingly restricted to biopsy to establish the diagnosis, and more extensive operations are usually undertaken to remove residual tumour after chemotherapy and/or radiotherapy.

High-dose therapy with bone marrow rescue

The limitation of both chemotherapy and radiotherapy is the risk of irreversible damage to normal tissues, particularly bone marrow. Transplantation of bone marrow stem cells can be used as a strategy to treat patients after administering potentially lethal doses of chemotherapy and/or radiation. The source of the marrow stem cells may be allogeneic (from a compatible donor) or autologous (from the patient's harvested beforehand while the marrow is uninvolved or in remission). Allogeneic transplantation is principally used in the management of high-risk or relapsed leukaemia and autologous stem cell support is used most commonly in the treatment of children with solid tumours whose prognosis is poor using conventional chemotherapy, e.g. advanced neuroblastoma.

Side-effects of chemotherapy

Chemotherapy causes a range of side-effects (Fig. 21.3).

Infection from immunosuppression

Children receiving chemotherapy (or wide-field radiation) are immunocompromised. Neutropenia induced by chemotherapy places children at risk of septicaemia. Children with fever and neutropenia must be admitted to hospital for cultures and broad-spectrum antibiotics. Some important infections associated with therapy for cancer include *Pneumocystis jiroveci (carinii)* pneumonia (especially in children with leukaemia), disseminated fungal infection (e.g. aspergillosis and candidiasis) and coagulase-negative staphylococcal infections of central venous catheters.

Most common viral infections are no worse in children with cancer than in other children, but measles and varicella zoster (chickenpox) may have atypical presentation and be life-threatening. If non-immune, these children are at risk from contact with measles or varicella, although some protection can be afforded by prompt administration of immunoglobulin or zoster immune globulin. Aciclovir is used to treat established varicella infection, but no treatment is available for measles. During chemotherapy and from 6 months to a year subsequently, the use of live vaccines is contraindicated due to depressed immunity. After this period, reimmunisation against the common childhood infections is recommended.

Bone marrow suppression

Anaemia may necessitate blood transfusions. Thrombocytopenia presents the hazard of bleeding, and considerable blood product support may be required, particularly for children with leukaemia, those undergoing intensive therapy requiring bone marrow transplantation and in the more intensive solid tumour protocols.

Gastrointestinal damage, nausea and vomiting, and nutritional compromise

Mouth ulcers are common and painful. When severe, they can prevent the child eating adequately. Many chemotherapy agents are nauseating and induce vomiting which may be only partially prevented by the routine use of antiemetic drugs. These two complications can result in significant nutritional compromise. Chemotherapy-induced gut mucosal damage also causes diarrhoea and may predispose to Gram-negative infection.

Other side-effects

Many individual drugs have very specific side-effects, e.g. cardiotoxicity with doxorubicin, renal failure and deafness with cisplatin, haemorrhagic cystitis with cyclophosphamide, and neuropathy with vincristine. These side-effects are not always predictable and require careful monitoring during, and in some cases, after treatment is complete.

> **Fever with neutropenia requires hospital admission, cultures and intravenous antibiotics.**

Supportive care

Cancer treatment produces frequent, and often severe multisystem side-effects. Supportive care is an important part of management and improvements in this aspect of cancer care have contrib-

Short-term side-effects of chemotherapy

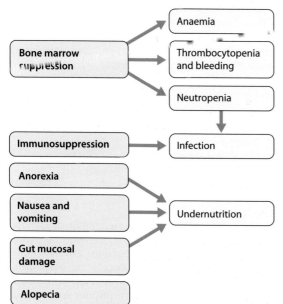

Figure 21.3 Short-term side-effects of chemotherapy.

uted to the increasing survival rates (see Fig. 21.2). Supportive care includes prompt management of potential infections, early nutritional support with regular dietetic input, pharmacological control of nausea and vomiting and considered use of blood products where necessary. The discomfort of multiple venepunctures for blood sampling and intravenous infusions can be avoided with central venous catheters, although these do carry a risk of infection (Fig. 21.4). Some patients may be at risk of infertility as a result of their cancer treatment. Appropriate fertility preservation techniques may involve surgically moving a testis or ovary out of the radiotherapy field, sperm banking (in those boys mature enough to achieve this) and consideration of newer techniques such as cryopreservation of ovarian cortical tissue, although the long-term benefit of this is still uncertain.

Psychosocial support

The diagnosis of a potentially fatal illness has an enormous and long-lasting impact on the whole family. They need the opportunity to discuss the implications and their anxiety, fear, guilt and sadness. Most will benefit from the counselling and practical support provided by health professionals. Help with practical issues, including transport, finances, accommodation and care of siblings, is an early priority. The provision of detailed written material for parents will help them understand their child's disease and treatment. The children themselves and their siblings need an age-appropriate explanation of the disease. Once treatment is established and the disease appears to be under control, families should be encouraged to return to as normal a lifestyle as possible. Early return to school is important and children with cancer should not be allowed to underachieve the expectations previously held for them. It is easy to underestimate the severe stress that persists within families in relation to the uncertainty of the long-term outcome. This often manifests itself as marital problems in parents and behavioural difficulties in both the child and siblings.

Summary

Malignant disease in children:

- is uncommon, but affects 1 in 500 by 15 years of age
- the overall 5-year survival rate is 75%
- presents with a localised mass or its pressure effects or disseminated disease
- treatment may involve chemotherapy, surgery, radiotherapy or high-dose therapy with bone marrow rescue
- fever with neutropenia must be investigated and treated urgently
- measles and varicella zoster infection are potentially life-threatening
- requires a multidisciplinary team to provide supportive care and psychosocial support
- supportive care – includes not only management of side-effects but also pain management and fertility preservation
- psychosocial support – includes not only the patient and parents, but also siblings and other family and community members.

Leukaemia

Acute lymphoblastic leukaemia (ALL) accounts for 80% of leukaemia in children. Most of the remainder are acute myeloid/acute non-lymphocytic (AML/ANLL) leukaemia. Chronic myeloid leukaemia and other myeloproliferative disorders are rare.

Clinical presentation

Clinical symptoms and signs result from infiltration of the bone marrow or other organs with leukaemic blast cells (Fig. 21.5). In most children, leukaemia presents insidiously over several weeks (see Case history 21.1) with some or all of the following signs and symptoms:

- malaise
- infections
- pallor
- abnormal bruising
- hepatosplenomegaly
- lymphadenopathy
- bone pain.

In some children the illness progresses very rapidly.

In most but not all children, the blood count is abnormal, with low haemoglobin and thrombocytopenia and evidence of circulating blast cells. Bone marrow examination is essential to confirm the diagnosis and to identify immunological and cytogenetic characteristics which give useful prognostic information.

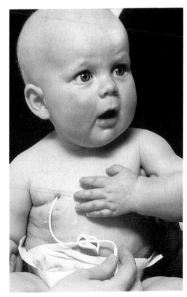

Figure 21.4 The central venous catheter allows pain-free blood tests and injections for this child on chemotherapy, which has caused the alopecia.

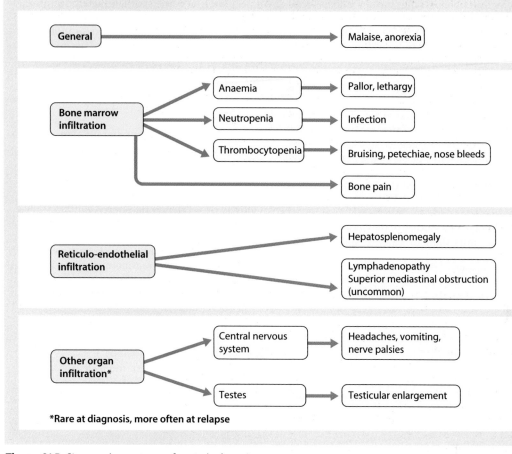

Figure 21.5 Signs and symptoms of acute leukaemia.

Case History
21.1 Acute lymphoblastic leukaemia

A 4-year-old girl was generally unwell, feeling lethargic, looking pale and occasionally febrile over a period of 9 weeks. Two courses of antibiotics for recurrent sore throat failed to result in any benefit. Her parents returned to their general practitioner when she developed a rash. Examination showed pallor, petechiae, modest lymphadenopathy and mild hepatosplenomegaly. The results of full blood count showed:

- Hb 8.3 g/dl
- WBC 15.6×10^9/L
- Platelets 44×10^9/L.

Blast cells were seen on the peripheral blood film. Cerebrospinal fluid (CSF) examination was normal. Bone marrow examination confirmed acute lymphoblastic leukaemia (Fig. 21.6).

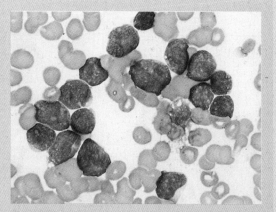

Figure 21.6 Leukaemic blast cells on a bone marrow smear.

Leukaemia

351

Both ALL and AML are classified by morphology. Immunological phenotyping further subclassifies ALL: the common (75%) and T-cell (15%) subtypes are the most common. Prognosis and some aspects of clinical presentation vary according to different subtypes, and treatment is adjusted accordingly.

The prognosis in ALL is related to age, tumour load (measured by the white cell count, WBC), speed of response to initial chemotherapy and the presence or absence of specific cytogenetic/molecular genetic abnormalities in tumour cells. High WBC ($>50 \times 10^9$/L), age <1 year or >10 years, persistence of leukaemic blasts in the bone marrow and the presence of submicroscopic levels of leukaemia (minimal residual disease, MRD) at the end of the first phase (induction) of treatment are all important variables in determining treatment intensity. Cytogenetic studies of the bone marrow at diagnosis are important to identify specific prognostic factors which may require adjustment to the intensity of therapy.

Treatment of acute lymphoblastic leukaemia

A typical treatment schema is shown in Figure 21.7.

Remission induction

Before starting treatment of the disease, anaemia is corrected with blood transfusion, the risk of bleeding minimised by transfusion of platelets and infection is treated. Additional hydration and allopurinol (or urate oxidase when the white cell count is high and the risk is greater) are given to protect renal function against the effects of rapid cell lysis. Remission implies eradication of the leukaemic blasts and restoration of normal marrow function. Four weeks of combination chemotherapy is given and current induction schedules achieve remission rates of 95%.

Intensification

Blocks of intensive chemotherapy are given to consolidate remission. They improve cure rates but at the expense of increased toxicity.

Central nervous system (CNS)

Cytotoxic drugs penetrate poorly into the CNS. As leukaemic cells in this site may survive effective systemic treatment, additional treatment with intrathecal chemotherapy is used to prevent CNS relapse. Previously, treatment included cranial radiation or high-dose methotrexate, but there are concerns that these result in adverse neuropsychological effects and they are now omitted from first-line treatment schedules.

Continuing maintenance therapy

Chemotherapy of modest intensity is continued over a relatively long period of time, up to 3 years from diagnosis. Co-trimoxazole is given routinely to prevent *Pneumocystis jiroveci (carinii)* pneumonia.

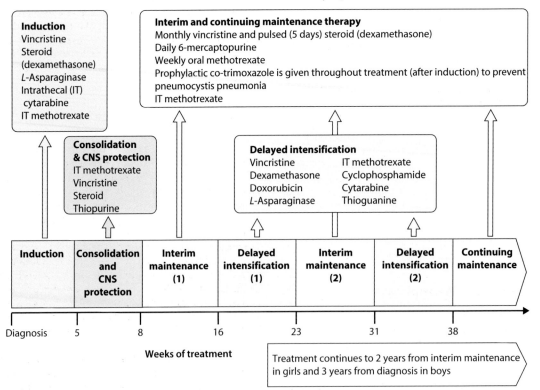

Figure 21.7 Treatment schema for standard-risk acute lymphoblastic leukaemia.

Treatment of relapse

High-dose chemotherapy, usually with total body irradiation (TBI) and bone marrow transplantation, is used as an alternative to conventional chemotherapy after a relapse.

Brain tumours

In contrast to adults, brain tumours in children are almost always primary and 60% are infratentorial (Fig. 21.8). Signs and symptoms are often related to evidence of raised intracranial pressure but focal neurological signs may be detected depending on the site of the tumour. The most common findings are:

- headache (classically worse on lying down)
- vomiting (especially on waking in the mornings)
- papilloedema
- squint secondary to VIth nerve palsy
- nystagmus
- ataxia
- personality or behaviour change.

Tumours are best characterised on MRI scan (Case history 21.2). Lumbar puncture must not be performed without neurosurgical advice if there is suspicion of raised intracranial pressure. Brain tumours may present particular diagnostic difficulties as the histological appearance may not always be representative of subsequent tumour behaviour. Furthermore, in some cases, biopsy is not always safe, for example, when tumours are located in the brainstem. The outcome of treatment is often strongly influenced by the anatomical position of the tumour as this determines the surgical strategy, as well as the histological subtype.

The functional implications of the site of the tumour, the potential hazards of surgery and the importance of radiotherapy in treatment, all combine to place children with brain tumours at particular risk of neurological disability and of growth, endocrine and neuropsychological problems. Survivors may present complex combinations of these problems.

Lymphomas

Lymphoma can be divided into Hodgkin's disease and non-Hodgkin's lymphoma (NHL). NHL is more common in childhood, while Hodgkin's disease is seen more frequently in adolescence.

Non-Hodgkin's lymphoma

Lymphomas are malignancies of the cells of the immune system. A firm distinction between solid and haematological lymphoid malignancy is somewhat artificial as some subtypes of ALL and NHL may represent a continuum of the same disease. In most cases of childhood NHL, the clinical features reflect the pattern of migration of normal lymphoid cells, with lymph nodes being the predominant site of disease.

Presentation will depend on the site of disease. T-cell malignancies may present as ALL or NHL, with both being characterised by a mediastinal mass with varying degrees of bone marrow infiltration. B-cell malignancies present more commonly as NHL, with localised lymph node disease usually in the head and neck or abdomen. Abdominal disease presents with pain, a palpable mass or even intussusception in cases with involvement of the ileum.

Staging must include radiological assessment of all nodal sites (CT or MRI) and examination of the bone marrow and CSF. Treatment is multi-agent chemotherapy, a more intensive course being employed for advanced B-cell disease.

Hodgkin's disease

This is relatively uncommon in prepubertal children. It usually presents as painless lymphadenopathy, most frequently in the neck. Lymph nodes are much larger and firmer than the benign lymphadenopathy commonly seen in children. The clinical history is often long, and systemic symptoms (sweating, pruritus, weight loss and fever – the so-called 'B' symptoms) are uncommon, even in more advanced disease.

After diagnostic biopsy, the disease is staged to determine treatment. Intra-abdominal disease is generally assessed radiologically, and staging laparotomy, with biopsies and splenectomy, is no longer performed. Lymphangiography is a technically difficult examination in small children and is rarely required. Combination chemotherapy, with or without radiotherapy, is the recommended treatment for all stages of the disease. Overall, about 80% of all patients can be cured; even for those with disseminated disease, about 60% can be cured.

Neuroblastoma

Neuroblastoma and related tumours arise from neural crest tissue in the adrenal medulla and sympathetic nervous system. It is an unusual tumour in that spontaneous regression sometimes occurs in very young infants. There is a spectrum of disease from the benign (ganglioneuroma) to the malignant (neuroblastoma).

Neuroblastoma is most common before the age of 5 years. Most children present with an abdominal mass, but the primary tumour can lie anywhere along the sympathetic chain from the neck to the pelvis. Classically, the abdominal primary is of adrenal origin, but at presentation the tumour mass is often large and complex, crossing the midline and enveloping major blood vessels and lymph nodes. Paravertebral tumours may invade through the adjacent intervertebral foramen and cause spinal cord compression. Over the age of 2 years, clinical symptoms are mostly from metastatic disease,

Case History
21.2 Brain tumour

Ben, who was 7 years old, began to complain of occasional headaches but seemed otherwise well. His headaches were at all times of the day, even on waking. Over a few weeks his parents noted that he had lost interest in his schoolwork. He also became less interested in watching TV or in playing with his friends after school. He had some occasional vomits. Two weeks later he developed an unusual neck posture, holding his head to one side. On direct referral to hospital an MRI scan was performed which showed a large posterior fossa tumour (Fig. 21.9). A near complete tumour resection was achieved. Histology confirmed a medulloblastoma.

> 🌼 Headaches with behaviour and personality changes – consider raised intracranial pressure.

Brain tumours

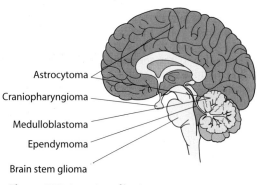

Astrocytoma

Craniopharyngioma

Medulloblastoma

Ependymoma

Brain stem glioma

Figure 21.8 Location of brain tumours.

Ependymoma (8%)
Mostly occurs in the posterior fossa where it behaves like medulloblastoma, but can also arise in the ventricles or spinal cord.

Brain stem glioma (6%)
Peak incidence is in early childhood. It presents with cranial nerve defects, ataxia and pyramidal tract signs, but frequently without raised intracranial pressure. The diagnosis is often based on clinical findings and CT/MRI scan, as biopsy can be hazardous. The prognosis for this group of children is particularly poor (<20% survival) and radiotherapy is usually only palliative. Chemotherapy has no established role.

Astrocytoma (40%)
The most common brain tumour type. Juvenile cerebellar astrocytoma is cystic, often slowly growing, and the results of treatment with surgery are excellent. Non-juvenile astrocytoma occurs at all sites but more frequently in the cerebral hemispheres. They vary from relatively benign to highly malignant *(glioblastoma multiforme)* and, despite surgery and radiotherapy, the outlook, particularly for children with high-grade tumours, is poor. The value of chemotherapy in the treatment of astrocytoma is not yet established but may be used more frequently in future.

Craniopharyngioma (4%)
A developmental tumour arising from the squamous remnant of Rathke's pouch. It is not truly malignant but is locally invasive and grows slowly in the suprasellar region. It presents with raised intracranial pressure, visual field loss and pituitary dysfunction, typically as growth failure. Surgical excision with or without subsequent radiation is required. Although prognosis for survival is good, these children may be visually impaired and often have complex endocrine deficiencies.

Medulloblastoma (20%)
Nearly always arises in the midline of the posterior fossa. Presentation is with ataxia as well as headache and vomiting. The tumour may seed through the CNS via the CSF and up to 20% have spinal metastases at diagnosis. Treatment with whole CNS radiation after maximal surgical resection has produced 5-year survival rates of 50%. Chemotherapy has a place in the treatment of children with a higher than average risk of relapse, e.g. after incomplete surgical excision.

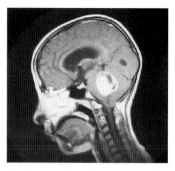

Figure 21.9 Sagittal MRI scan showing a tumour in the posterior fossa and mild ventricular dilatation.

particularly bone pain, bone marrow suppression, weight loss and malaise.

The diagnosis can often be made from characteristic clinical and radiological features and raised urinary catecholamine (VMA, HVA) levels. Confirmatory biopsy is usually obtained and evidence of metastatic disease detected with bone marrow sampling, bone scan and MIBG (metaiodobenzyl guanidine) scan (Case history 21.3). MIBG is a radiolabelled tumour-specific agent, which provides a sensitive radioisotope scan to measure disease extent and monitor response to treatment. Its therapeutic use has been explored but has not found an established role.

The most important clinical prognostic features are age and stage of disease at diagnosis. Unfortunately, the majority of children over 1 year present with advanced disease and have a poor prognosis. Increasingly, information about the biological characteristics of neuroblastoma is being used to guide therapy and prognosis. Over-expression of the N-*myc* oncogene, evidence for deletion of material on chromosome 1 (del 1p) and gain of genetic material on chromosome 17q in tumour cells are associated with a poorer prognosis.

The few children with localised primaries without metastatic disease can often be cured with surgery alone. For the majority with advanced disease, chemotherapy has the central role. Children showing a good initial response may benefit from consolidation with high-dose chemotherapy with peripheral blood stem cell rescue. Unfortunately the risk of relapse is high and the prospect for cure for children with metastatic disease is still little better than 30%.

Screening for raised urinary catecholamines to identify asymptomatic disease in infants is feasible but there is no conclusive evidence that this reduces mortality from the disease and it is not practised within the UK.

Wilms' tumour (nephroblastoma)

Wilms' tumour originates from embryonal renal tissue and is the commonest renal tumour of childhood. There is a Wilms' tumour susceptibility gene which was identified from the rare association between Wilms' tumour and sporadic aniridia which was known to be associated with loss of genetic material from chromosome 11. Over 80% of patients present before 5 years of age and it is very rarely seen after 10 years of age. Most children present with a large abdominal mass, often found incidentally in an otherwise well child (Box 21.1). Occasionally, children have chronic symptoms of poor appetite and poor weight gain. Haemorrhage into the mass may cause abdominal pain and anaemia. Macroscopic haematuria is uncommon but recognised and many children have a degree of hypertension, presumably related to distortion of renal vessels, which normalises with treatment. About 5% have bilateral disease at diagnosis.

Radiological diagnosis from ultrasound or CT/MRI (Fig. 21.12) is usually characteristic, showing an intrinsic renal mass distorting the normal structure. Staging information to assess distant metastases (usually in the lung), initial tumour resectability and function of the contralateral kidney is required. The current treatment protocol in the UK recommends initial chemotherapy for all children over 6 months of age. This is followed by delayed nephrectomy after which the tumour is staged histologically upon which subsequent treatment is planned. All children require chemotherapy, but radiotherapy is restricted to those with more advanced disease.

Overall, the prognosis is good, with more than 80% of all patients cured. The cure rate even for the 15% of patients with metastatic disease at presentation is over 60%, but relapse carries a poor prognosis. Recent clinical trials have shown that it is possible to reduce the intensity of treatment for less advanced disease without compromising survival.

Soft tissue sarcomas

Rhabdomyosarcoma is the most common form of soft tissue sarcoma in childhood. The tumour is thought to originate from primitive mesenchymal tissue and there are a wide variety of primary sites, resulting in varying presentations and prognosis.

Head and neck

These are the most common sites of disease (40%), causing, for example, proptosis, nasal obstruction or bloodstained nasal discharge.

Genitourinary tumours

These are the next most common, and may involve the bladder, paratesticular structures or the female genitourinary tract. Symptoms include dysuria and urinary obstruction, scrotal mass or bloodstained vaginal discharge.

Metastatic disease (lung, liver, bone or bone marrow)

This is present in approximately 15% of patients at diagnosis (Fig. 21.13) and is associated with a particularly poor prognosis.

Treatment depends on the site, size and extent of disease. Staging investigations must provide a

Case History
21.3 Neuroblastoma

Jack, a 2-year-old boy, was taken to his general practitioner by his mother because he had become generally unwell and was not eating as well as usual. Recently he appeared reluctant to walk and sometimes cried when he was picked up. His previously normal sleeping pattern had become disturbed and Jack's grandmother thought he was rather pale and had lost weight. On examination the general practitioner confirmed that he seemed generally miserable and was concerned to note a probable mass in the upper abdomen. Urgent referral to his local hospital was made, where an ultrasound examination confirmed an abdominal mass and he was noted to be hypertensive. An MRI scan confirmed a very large upper abdominal mass in complex relationship with the left kidney and the major vessels, suggestive of neuroblastoma (Fig. 21.10a and b). Subsequent investigations confirmed bone marrow infiltration by tumour cells and a positive MIBG scan showing uptake at the primary and distant sites consistent with metastatic disease (Fig. 21.11).

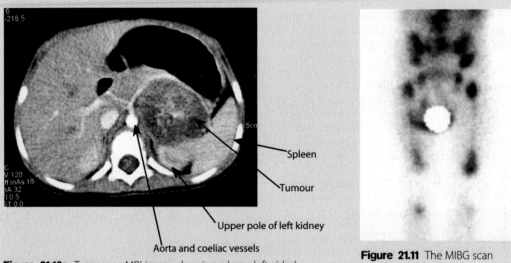

Spleen

Tumour

Upper pole of left kidney

Aorta and coeliac vessels

Figure 21.10a Transverse MRI image showing a large left-sided primary neuroblastoma arising from the adrenal region and distorting coeliac and mesenteric blood vessels.

Figure 21.11 The MIBG scan 'maps' metastatic tumour distribution in bone and bone marrow. This image shows the lower half of the abdomen, pelvis and legs. The dark areas are evidence of high isotope uptake and the pattern is consistent with widespread metastatic disease. (Normal uptake from excretion of isotope into urine in the bladder has been blocked in this exposure.)

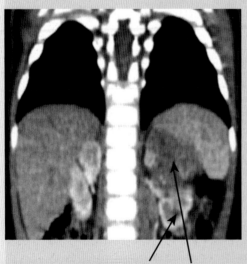

Left kidney   Tumour

Figure 21.10b MRI scan of the abdomen and chest showing the same left adrenal neuroblastoma pushing upwards and medially, distorting and displacing the kidney.

Large tumour, showing the characteristic mixed tissue densities (cystic and solid). It arises within the kidney and envelops a remnant of normal renal tissue

Remnant of left kidney

Liver

Normal kidney

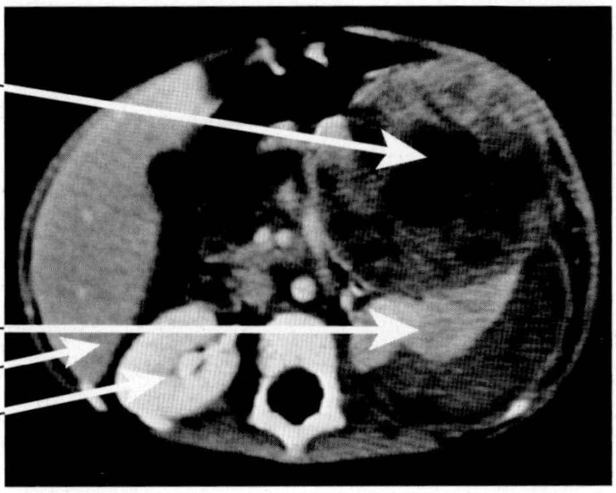

Figure 21.12 Large Wilms' tumour arising within the left kidney showing characteristic cystic and solid tissue densities.

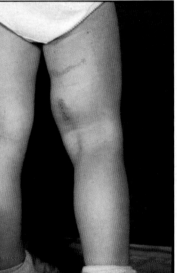

Figure 21.13 Rhabdomyo-sarcoma of lower limb. The scar is from a biopsy.

comprehensive assessment of these factors. The minority (15%) of patients with completely resected local disease require only a short course of chemotherapy to treat presumed micrometastatic disease, and no radiotherapy. The tumour margins are always deceptively ill-defined, and attempts at primary surgical excision are often unsuccessful and should be discouraged unless this can be achieved without mutilation or irreversible organ damage. The majority of patients require aggressive combination chemotherapy and often radiotherapy. Overall cure rates are about 65%.

Bone tumours

Malignant bone tumours are uncommon before puberty. Osteogenic sarcoma is more common than Ewing's sarcoma, but Ewing's sarcoma is seen more often in younger children. Both have a male predominance.

The limbs are the most common site. Persistent localised bone pain is a characteristic symptom, usually preceding the detection of a mass. At diagnosis, most patients are well and even metastatic disease (most common in the lungs) is asymptomatic. A bone X-ray shows destruction and variable periosteal new bone formation. In Ewing's sarcoma there is often a substantial soft tissue mass. Initial evaluation must include careful assessment of the primary site to define the extent of the local disease, particularly if limb-saving surgery is contemplated.

Both tumours are difficult to treat, but the prognosis has improved in recent years. In both tumours, treatment involves the use of combination chemotherapy given before surgery. Whenever possible, amputation is avoided by using en bloc resection of tumours with endoprosthetic resection (Fig. 21.14). In Ewing's sarcoma, radiotherapy is used in the management of local disease, especially when surgical resection is impossible or incomplete, e.g. in the pelvis or axial skeleton.

Retinoblastoma

Retinoblastoma is a malignant tumour of retinal cells and, although rare, it accounts for about 5% of severe visual impairment in children (Fig. 21.15). It may affect one or both eyes. All bilateral tumours are hereditary, as are about 15% of unilateral cases. The retinoblastoma susceptibility gene has now been identified on chromosome 13. The pattern of inheritance is dominant but with incomplete penetrance. Most cases present within the first 3 years of life. Children from families with the hereditary form of the disease should be screened regularly from birth. The most common presentation of unsuspected disease is when a white pupillary reflex is noted to replace the normal red one or with a squint (Fig. 21.16).

The aim of treatment is to cure yet preserve vision. Enucleation of the eye may be necessary for

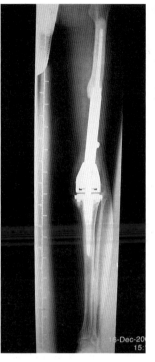

Figure 21.14 To preserve the leg, an endoprosthetic replacement of the femur has been performed in a child with Ewing's sarcoma. The prosthesis can be extended for growth.

disease, but it is more often reserved for the treatment of recurrence. Most patients are cured, although many are visually impaired. There is a significant risk of second malignancy (especially sarcoma) among the survivors of hereditary retinoblastoma.

Liver tumours

Liver tumours are rare. Primary liver tumours in the newborn are more likely to be benign (haemangioma). Primary malignant liver tumours are mostly hepatoblastoma (65%) or hepatocellular carcinoma (25%). Hepatocellular carcinoma may arise in children with pre-existing liver disease.

Initial presentation is with abdominal distension or with a mass. Pain and jaundice are rare. Investigation with ultrasound or CT/MRI scan confirms a large intrinsic liver mass, occasionally with calcification. Elevated serum alphafetoprotein (AFP) is detected in nearly all cases of hepatoblastoma and in some cases of hepatocellular carcinoma. AFP is a sensitive marker for determining response to therapy and can be a sensitive means of postoperative follow-up when a rise in the serum level may be the first indication of relapse. Most hepatoblastomas show a good response to chemotherapy after which surgical resection can usually be achieved. Liver transplantation is a possibility for a minority of patients with unresectable disease confined to the liver. The majority of children with hepatoblastoma can now be cured. The prognosis for children with hepatocellular carcinoma is less satisfactory.

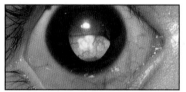

Figure 21.15 Retinoblastoma presenting as a white mass behind the pupil.

Germ cell tumours

Germ cell tumours (GCTs) are rare and may be benign or malignant. They arise from the primitive germ cells which migrate from yolk sac endoderm to form gonads in the embryo. Benign tumours are most common in the sacrococcygeal region and most malignant germ cell tumours are found in the gonads. Serum markers (AFP and β-HCG) are invaluable in confirming the diagnosis and in monitoring response to treatment.

Malignant germ cell tumours are very sensitive to chemotherapy, and a very good outcome can be expected for disease at most sites.

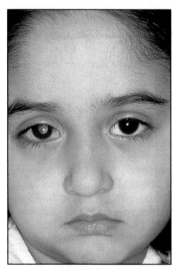

Figure 21.16 White pupillary reflex in retinoblastoma.

Langerhans cell histiocytosis

Langerhans cell histiocytosis (LCH) is a rare disorder characterised by an abnormal proliferation of histiocytes. It is no longer believed to be a truly malignant condition and is classified as a disorder of dendritic (antigen presenting) cells. However, its sometimes aggressive behaviour and response to chemotherapy place it within the practice of oncologists. There is a spectrum of the disorder from localised bone lesions to a systemic presentation, more common in infants.

more advanced disease. Treatment with chemotherapy to shrink the tumour followed by local laser treatment to the retina is being used successfully. Radiotherapy may be used in advanced

Bone lesions

These may present at any age with pain, swelling or even fracture. X-ray reveals a characteristic lytic lesion with a well-defined border. These lesions frequently involve the skull (Fig. 21.17). Biopsy is usually necessary and full skeletal survey is required to identify multiple lesions. Biopsy, with or without curettage, may constitute successful treatment and asymptomatic lesions may justify surveillance and not require specific treatment.

Diabetes insipidus

Diabetes insipidus can occur with other patterns of presentation although the association of skull disease with proptosis and hypothalamic infiltration is recognised. Once established, diabetes insipidus is not usually reversed by successful treatment of the underlying disease and long-term treatment with desmopressin (DDAVP) is usually required.

Systemic LCH

This most aggressive form of LCH tends to present in infancy with a seborrhoeic rash (Fig. 21.18) and soft tissue involvement of the gums, ears, lungs, liver, spleen, lymph nodes and bone marrow. This form of LCH is usually progressive and requires chemotherapy, although spontaneous regression may occur. The prognosis is variable but most patients are cured.

Long-term survivors

Currently, there are over 26 000 adult survivors of childhood cancer in the UK. Over half have at least one residual problem as a consequence of either the disease or its treatment (Table 21.1). All survivors need regular long-term follow-up to provide appropriate treatment or advice. This need for specialist multidisciplinary follow-up continues into adulthood, and its provision presents a challenge within adult health care services. At present, the majority of survivors have remained under the care of paediatric oncologists, although specialist adult clinics are being established. Some survivors will require specific counselling for problems such as poor growth, infertility and sexual dysfunction, and advances in the use of adult growth hormone and assisted conception techniques have enhanced the lives of many

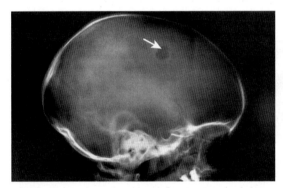

Figure 21.17 Lytic bone lesions on a skull X-ray in Langerhans cell histiocytosis.

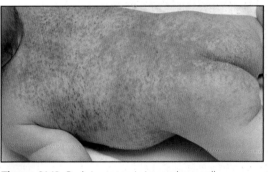

Figure 21.18 Rash in systemic Langerhans cell histiocytosis. It is often mistaken for seborrhoeic dermatitis or eczema.

Table 21.1 Some problems which may occur following cure of childhood cancer

Problem	Cause
Specific organ dysfunction	Nephrectomy for Wilms' tumour
	Toxicity from chemotherapy, e.g. renal from cisplatin or ifosfamide, cardiac from doxorubicin or mediastinal radiotherapy
Growth/endocrine problems	Growth hormone deficiency from pituitary irradiation
	Bone growth retardation at sites of irradiation
Infertility	Gonadal irradiation
	Alkylating agent chemotherapy (cyclophosphamide, ifosfamide)
Neuropsychological problems	Cranial irradiation (particularly at age <5 years)
	Brain surgery
Second malignancy	Irradiation
	Alkylating agent chemotherapy
Social/educational disadvantage	Chronic ill health
	Absence from school

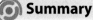

Summary

Presentation of malignant disease in children

Preschool

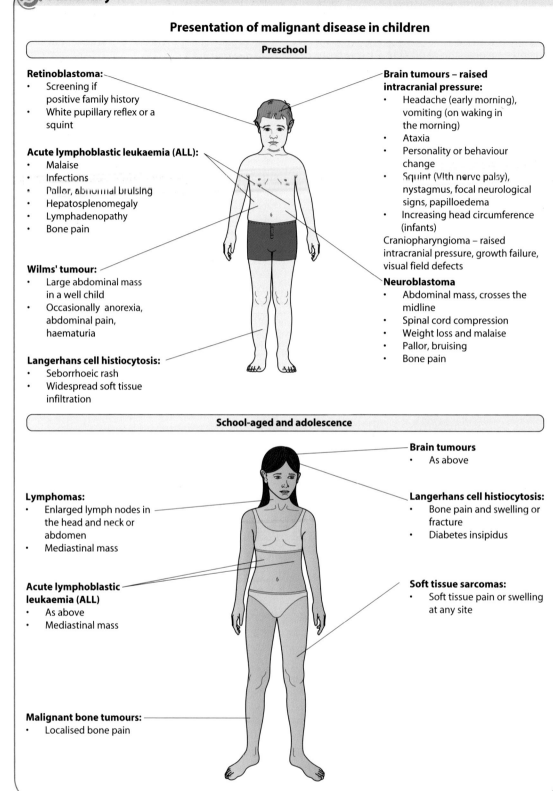

Retinoblastoma:
* Screening if positive family history
* White pupillary reflex or a squint

Acute lymphoblastic leukaemia (ALL):
* Malaise
* Infections
* Pallor, abnormal bruising
* Hepatosplenomegaly
* Lymphadenopathy
* Bone pain

Wilms' tumour:
* Large abdominal mass in a well child
* Occasionally anorexia, abdominal pain, haematuria

Langerhans cell histiocytosis:
* Seborrhoeic rash
* Widespread soft tissue infiltration

Brain tumours – raised intracranial pressure:
* Headache (early morning), vomiting (on waking in the morning)
* Ataxia
* Personality or behaviour change
* Squint (VIth nerve palsy), nystagmus, focal neurological signs, papilloedema
* Increasing head circumference (infants)

Craniopharyngioma – raised intracranial pressure, growth failure, visual field defects

Neuroblastoma
* Abdominal mass, crosses the midline
* Spinal cord compression
* Weight loss and malaise
* Pallor, bruising
* Bone pain

School-aged and adolescence

Lymphomas:
* Enlarged lymph nodes in the head and neck or abdomen
* Mediastinal mass

Acute lymphoblastic leukaemia (ALL)
* As above
* Mediastinal mass

Malignant bone tumours:
* Localised bone pain

Brain tumours
* As above

Langerhans cell histiocytosis:
* Bone pain and swelling or fracture
* Diabetes insipidus

Soft tissue sarcomas:
* Soft tissue pain or swelling at any site

patients. The risk of second tumours is small but may rise with increasing survival rates. When new treatment protocols for childhood cancers are developed, there is now a need to reduce, whenever possible, the toxicity of treatment to spare the children adverse short- and long-term effects.

Terminal care

When a child relapses, further treatment may be considered. A small number can still be cured and others may have a further significant remission with good quality life. However, for some children a time comes when death is inevitable and the staff and family must make the decision to concentrate on palliative care.

Most parents prefer to care for their terminally ill child at home, but will need practical help and emotional support. Pain control and symptom relief are a serious source of anxiety for parents, but they can often be achieved successfully at home. Health professionals with experience in palliative care for children can work with the family and local health care workers. After the child's death, families should be offered continuing contact with an appropriate member of the team who looked after their child, and be given support through their bereavement.

> **With adequate support from health professionals, palliative care for children can usually be provided at home.**

Further reading

Pinkerton C R, Plowman P N, Pieters R (eds) 2004 Paediatric oncology. Oxford University Press, Oxford. *Definitive, major textbook*

Stiller C A 2004 Epidemiology and genetics of childhood cancer. Oncogene 23(38):6429–6444. *Comprehensive review of the incidence and causes of cancer in children*

Voute P A, Barrett A, Caron H, Stevens M C G (eds) 2005 Cancer in children: clinical management, 5th edn. Oxford University Press, Oxford. *Short textbook*

Haematological disorders

Haemopoiesis is the process which maintains lifelong production of haemopoietic blood cells. The main site of haemopoiesis in fetal life is the liver, whereas throughout postnatal life it is the bone marrow. All haemopoietic cells are derived from *pluripotent haemopoietic stem cells*, which are crucial for normal blood production; deficiency causes bone marrow failure because stem cells are required for the ongoing replacement of dying cells. The number of pluripotent stem cells stays relatively constant throughout life because the pool of stem cells is maintained by a balance between stem cell proliferation and differentiation into more mature haemopoietic cells of all the haemopoietic lineages. Haemopoietic stem cells from healthy donors can be used to treat children with bone marrow failure (*stem cell transplantation*).

Haemoglobin production in the fetus and newborn

The most important difference between haemopoiesis in the fetus compared to postnatal life is the changing pattern of haemoglobin (Hb) production at each stage of development. The composition and names of these haemoglobins are shown in Table 22.1. The first globin chain produced is ε-globin followed almost immediately by α- and γ-globin, which are expressed from 4–5 weeks' gestation. Fetal Hb (HbF) is made up of 2 α chains and 2 γ chains (α2γ2) and is the main Hb during fetal life. It has a higher affinity for oxygen than adult Hb, which allows it to extract and hold on to oxygen, an advantage in the relatively hypoxic environment of the fetus (Fig. 22.1). At birth, the types of Hb in the term infant are: HbF, HbA and HbA2. Fetal Hb is gradually replaced by adult haemoglobin during the first year of life. These fetal and embryonic haemoglobins are not normally detectable after infancy but they are produced in children with inherited disorders of haemoglobin production (haemoglobinopathies) and their detection helps in the diagnosis of these disorders.

Haematological values at birth and the first few weeks of life

Features are:

* At birth, the Hb in term infants is high, 14–21.5 g/dl, to compensate for the low oxygen concentration in the fetus. The Hb falls over the first few weeks, mainly due to reduced erythropoiesis, reaching a nadir of just below

Table 22.1 Embryonic, fetal and adult haemoglobins

Haemoglobin type	Globin chains	
	α-gene cluster	β-gene cluster
Embryonic		
Hb Gower 1	ξ2	ε2
Hb Gower 2	α2	ε2
Hb Portland	ξ2	γ2
Fetal		
HbF	α2	γ2
Adult		
Hb A	α2	β2
HbA2	α2	δ2
Proportion of haemoglobin types		
Birth	HbF 70–80%, HbA 25–30%, HbA$_2$ 1–3%	
Adults	HbA 97%, HbA$_2$ 2%	

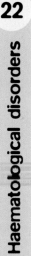

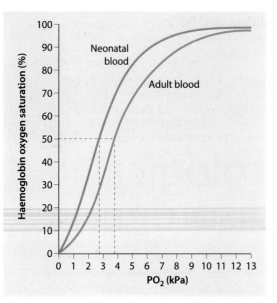

Figure 22.1 Oxygen dissociation curve showing the left shift of fetal haemoglobin compared with adult haemoglobin. Fetal haemoglobin has a higher affinity for oxygen.

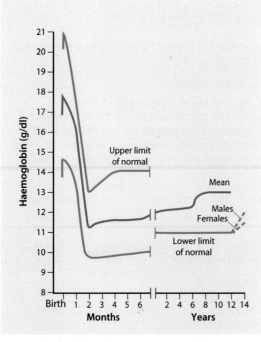

Figure 22.2 Changes in haemoglobin concentration with age, showing that the haemoglobin is high at birth, falling to its lowest concentration at 2–3 months of age.

10 g/dl at 2 months of age (Fig. 22.2). Normal haematological values at birth and during childhood are shown in the Appendix.
- Preterm babies have a steeper fall in Hb to a mean of 6.5–9 g/dl at 4–8 weeks chronological age.
- Normal blood volume at birth varies with gestational age. In healthy term infants the

average blood volume is 80 ml/kg; in preterm infants the average blood volume is 100 ml/kg.
- Stores of iron, folic acid and vitamin B_{12} in term and preterm babies are adequate at birth. However, in preterm infants, stores of iron and folic acid are lower and are depleted more quickly, leading to deficiency after 2–4 months if the recommended daily intakes are not maintained.
- White blood cell counts in neonates are higher than in older children ($10–25 \times 10^9$/L).
- Platelet counts at birth are within the normal adult range ($150–400 \times 10^9$/L).

> **Summary**
>
> **Haemoglobin at birth:**
> - The Hb concentration is high at birth (>14 g/dl) but falls to its lowest level at 2 months of age
> - Fetal Hb (HbF) is gradually replaced by adult Hb during infancy.

Anaemia

Anaemia is defined as an Hb level below the normal range. The normal range varies with age, so anaemia can be defined as:

- Neonate: Hb <14 g/dl
- 1–12 months: Hb <10 g/dl
- 1–12 years: Hb <11 g/dl.

Anaemia results from one or more of the following mechanisms:

- reduced red cell production – either due to ineffective erythropoiesis (e.g. iron deficiency, the commonest cause of anaemia) or due to red cell *aplasia*
- increased red cell destruction (*haemolysis*)
- blood loss – relatively uncommon cause in children.

There may be a combination of these three mechanisms, e.g. *anaemia of prematurity*.

Using this approach the principal causes of anaemia are shown in Figure 22.3 and a diagnostic approach to identifying their causes is shown in Figure 22.4.

> 🌼 **The definition of anaemia varies with age – Hb <10 g/dl in infants (post-neonatal), Hb <11 g/dl from 1 to 12 years old.**

Anaemia due to reduced red cell production

Reduced red cell production may be due to:

1. 'ineffective erythropoiesis'– here red cell production occurs at a normal or increased rate but differentiation or survival of the red cells is defective (e.g. iron deficiency).

Causes of anaemia in infants & children

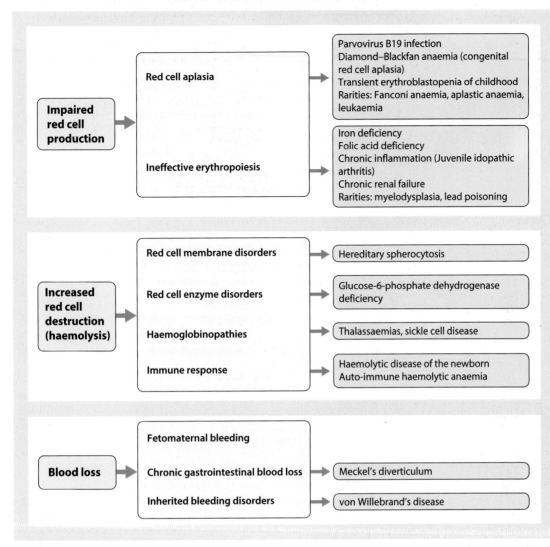

Figure 22.3 Causes of anaemia in infants and children.

2. complete absence of red cell production (red cell aplasia).

Diagnostic clues to ineffective erythropoiesis are:

- normal reticulocyte count
- abnormal mean cell volume (MCV) of the red cells: low in iron deficiency and raised in folic acid deficiency or myelodysplasia.

Iron deficiency

The main causes of iron deficiency are:

- inadequate intake
- malabsorption
- blood loss.

Inadequate intake of iron is common in infants because additional iron is required for the increase in blood volume accompanying growth and to build up the child's iron stores (Fig. 22.5). A 1-year-old infant requires an intake of iron of about 8 mg/day, which is about the same as his father (9 mg/day) but only half that of his mother (15 mg/day).

Iron may come from:

- breast milk (low iron content but 50% of the iron is absorbed)
- infant formula (supplemented with adequate amounts of iron)
- cow's milk (higher iron content than breast milk but only 10% is absorbed)
- solids introduced at weaning, e.g. cereals (cereals are supplemented with iron but only 1% is absorbed).

Iron deficiency may develop because of a delay in the introduction of mixed feeding beyond 4–6 months of age or to a diet with insufficient iron-rich foods, especially if it contains a large amount of cow's milk (Box 22.1). Iron absorption is markedly

Simple diagnostic approach to anaemia in children

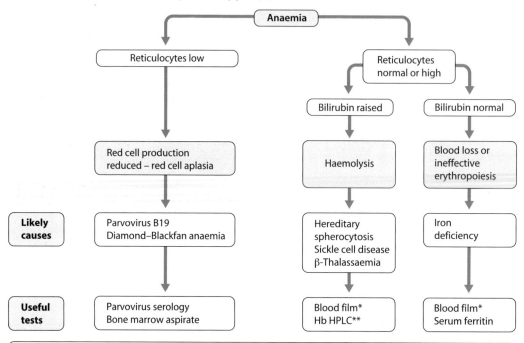

Figure 22.4 Diagnostic approach to anaemia.

increased when eaten with food rich in vitamin C (fresh fruit and vegetables) and is inhibited by tannin in tea.

> Infants should not be fed unmodified cow's milk as its iron content is low and poorly absorbed.

Clinical features

Most infants and children are asymptomatic until the Hb drops below 6–7 g/dl. As the anaemia worsens, children tire easily and young infants feed more slowly than usual. They may appear pale but pallor is an unreliable sign unless confirmed by pallor of the conjunctivae, tongue or palmar creases. Some children have 'pica', a term which describes the inappropriate eating of non-food materials such as soil, chalk, gravel or foam rubber (see Case history 22.1). There is evidence that iron deficiency anaemia may be detrimental to behaviour and intellectual function. The history should include asking about blood loss and symptoms or signs suggesting malabsorption.

Box 22.1 Dietary sources of iron

High in iron
Red meat – beef, lamb
Liver, kidney
Oily fish – pilchards, sardines, etc.

Average iron
Pulses, beans and peas
Fortified breakfast cereals with added vitamin C
Wholemeal products
Dark green vegetables – broccoli, spinach, etc.
Dried fruit – raisins, sultanas
Nuts and seeds – cashews, peanut butter, etc.

Foods to avoid in excess in toddlers
Cow's milk
Tea – tannin inhibits iron uptake
High-fibre foods – phytates inhibit iron absorption

Iron requirements during childhood

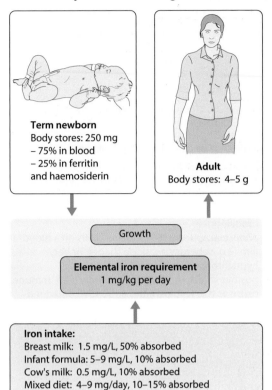

Term newborn
Body stores: 250 mg
– 75% in blood
– 25% in ferritin and haemosiderin

Adult
Body stores: 4–5 g

Growth

Elemental iron requirement
1 mg/kg per day

Iron intake:
Breast milk: 1.5 mg/L, 50% absorbed
Infant formula: 5–9 mg/L, 10% absorbed
Cow's milk: 0.5 mg/L, 10% absorbed
Mixed diet: 4–9 mg/day, 10–15% absorbed

Figure 22.5 Iron requirements during childhood.

Diagnosis

The diagnostic clues are:

* microcytic, hypochromic anaemia (low MCV and MCH)
* low serum ferritin.

The other main causes of microcytic anaemia are:

* β-thalassaemia trait (usually children of Asian, Arabic or Mediterranean origin)
* α-thalassaemia trait (usually children of African or Far Eastern origin)
* anaemia of chronic disease (e.g. due to renal failure).

Management

For most children management involves *dietary advice* and supplementation with *oral iron*. The best tolerated preparations are Sytron (sodium iron edetate) or Niferex (polysaccharide iron complex) – unlike some other preparations these do not stain the teeth. Iron supplementation should be continued for a minimum of 3 months to restore the Hb to normal and also to replenish the iron stores. With good compliance, the Hb will rise by about 1 g/dl per week. Failure to respond to oral iron usually means the child is not getting the treatment. However, investigation for other causes, in particular malabsorption (e.g. due to coeliac disease) or chronic blood loss (e.g. due to Meckel's diverticulum) is advisable if the history or examination

Case History
22.1 Iron deficiency anaemia

Ayesha, aged 2 years, was noted to look pale when she attended her general practitioner for an upper respiratory tract infection. A blood count showed Hb 5.0 g/dl, MCV 54 fl (normal 72–85 fl) and MCH 16 (normal 24–39 pg). She was drinking 3 pints of cow's milk per day and was a very fussy eater, refusing meat. She had started eating soil when playing in the garden.

Because of the inappropriately large volume of milk she was drinking, she was not sufficiently hungry to eat solid food. Replacing some of the milk with iron-rich food and treatment with oral iron produced a rise in the Hb to 7.5 g/dl within 4 weeks. Her pica (eating non-food materials) stopped.

suggests a non-dietary cause or if there is failure to respond to therapy in compliant patients. Blood transfusion should never be necessary for dietary iron deficiency. Even children with an Hb as low as 2–3 g/dl have arrived at this low level over a prolonged period and can tolerate it.

Treatment of iron deficiency with normal Hb

Whether children who have a normal Hb but biochemical evidence of iron deficiency (e.g. low serum ferritin) should be treated with oral iron is controversial. In favour of treatment is the knowledge that iron is required for normal brain development and there is evidence that iron deficiency anaemia is associated with behavioural and intellectual deficiencies which may be reversible with iron therapy. However, it is not yet clear whether treatment of subclinical iron deficiency confers significant benefit. Treatment also carries a risk of accidental poisoning with oral iron, which is very toxic. A simple strategy is to provide dietary advice to increase oral iron and its absorption in all children with subclinical deficiency and to offer parents the option of additional treatment with oral iron supplements.

> Treatment of iron deficiency anaemia is with dietary advice and oral iron therapy for several months

Red cell aplasia

There are three main causes of red cell aplasia in children:

* congenital red cell aplasia ('Diamond–Blackfan anaemia')
* transient erythroblastopenia of childhood
* parvovirus B19 infection: this infection only causes red cell aplasia in children with inherited haemolytic anaemias and not in healthy children.

The diagnostic clues to red cell aplasia are:

- low reticulocyte count despite low Hb
- normal bilirubin
- negative direct antiglobulin test (Coombs' test)
- absent red cell precursors on bone marrow examination.

Diamond–Blackfan anaemia (DBA) is a rare disease (5–7 cases/million live births). There is a family history in 20% of cases; the remaining 80% are sporadic. A specific gene mutation (RPS19) is implicated in some cases. Most cases present at 2–3 months of age but 25% present at birth. Affected infants have symptoms of anaemia; some have other congenital anomalies, such as short stature or abnormal thumbs. Treatment is by oral steroids; monthly red blood cell transfusions are given to children who are steroid unresponsive.

Transient erythroblastopenia of childhood (TEC) is usually triggered by viral infections and has the same haematological features as DBA. The main differences between them is that TEC always recovers, usually within several weeks, there is no family history or RPS19 mutation and there are no congenital anomalies.

Increased red cell destruction (haemolytic anaemia)

Haemolytic anaemia is characterised by reduced red cell lifespan due to increased red cell destruction in the circulation (intravascular haemolysis) or liver or spleen (extravascular haemolysis). The lifespan of a normal red cell is 120 days and the bone marrow produces 173 000 million red cells per day. In haemolysis, red cell survival may be reduced to a few days but bone marrow production can increase about eightfold, so haemolysis only leads to anaemia when the bone marrow is no longer able to compensate for the premature destruction of red cells.

In children, unlike neonates, immune haemolytic anaemias are uncommon. The main cause of haemolysis in children is *intrinsic* abnormalities of the red blood cells:

- red cell membrane disorders (e.g. hereditary spherocytosis)
- red cell enzyme disorders (e.g. glucose-6-phosphate dehydrogenase deficiency)

- haemoglobinopathies (abnormal haemoglobins, e.g. β-thalassaemia major, sickle cell disease).

Haemolysis from increased red cell breakdown leads to:

- anaemia
- reticuloendothelial hyperplasia – hepatomegaly and splenomegaly
- elevated unconjugated bilirubin
- excess urinary urobilinogen.

The diagnostic clues to haemolysis are:

- raised reticulocyte count (on the blood film this is called 'polychromasia' as the reticulocytes have a characteristic lilac colour)
- unconjugated bilirubinaemia and increased urinary urobilinogen
- abnormal appearance of the red cells on a blood film (e.g. spherocytes, sickle shaped or very hypochromic) (Fig. 22.6)
- positive direct antiglobulin test (only if an immune cause as this test identifies antibody-coated red blood cells)
- increased erythropoiesis in the bone marrow.

Hereditary spherocytosis (HS)

Occurs in 1 in 5000 births in Caucasians. It usually has an autosomal dominant inheritance, but in 25% there is no family history and it is caused by new mutations. The disease is caused by mutations in genes for the skeletal proteins of the red cell membrane (mainly spectrin, ankyrin or band 3). This results in the red cell losing part of its membrane when it passes through the spleen. This reduction in its surface–to–volume ratio causes the cells to become spheroidal, making them less deformable than normal red blood cells and leads to their destruction in the microvasculature of the spleen.

Clinical features

The disorder is often suspected because of a positive family history. Even within the same family, the clinical manifestations are highly variable. It may be completely asymptomatic. The clinical features include:

- jaundice – usually develops during childhood but may be intermittent; may cause severe haemolytic jaundice in the first few days of life

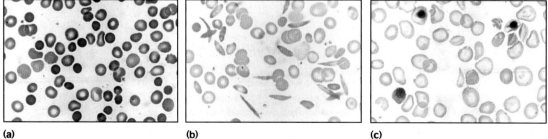

(a)　　　　　　　　(b)　　　　　　　　(c)

Figure 22.6 Abnormally shaped red blood cells help make the diagnosis in haemolytic anaemias. **(a)** Spherocytes in hereditary spherocytosis. **(b)** Sickle cells in sickle cell disease. **(c)** Hypochromic cells in thalassaemia.

- anaemia – presents in childhood with mild anaemia (haemoglobin 9–11 g/dl), but the haemoglobin level may fall with an intercurrent infection; many children have 'compensated' haemolysis with a normal haemoglobin
- mild to moderate splenomegaly – depends on the rate of haemolysis; this may be the mode of presentation in the first year of life
- aplastic crisis – uncommon, associated with parvovirus B19 infection
- gallstones – due to increased bilirubin excretion.

Diagnosis

The blood film is usually diagnostic but more specific tests are available (e.g. osmotic fragility, dye binding tests) though seldom required. Antibody-induced anaemia is also associated with sphero-cytes and this should be excluded with a direct antibody test in the absence of a family history of hereditary spherocytosis.

Management

Most children have mild chronic haemolytic anaemia and the only treatment they require is oral folic acid as they have a raised folic acid requirement secondary to their increased red blood cell production. Splenectomy is beneficial but is only indicated for poor growth or troublesome symptoms of anaemia (e.g. severe tiredness, loss of vigour) and is usually deferred until after 7 years of age because of the risks of post-splenectomy sepsis. Prior to splenectomy all patients should be checked that they have been vaccinated against *Haemophilus influenzae* (Hib), meningitis C and *Streptococcus pneumoniae* and lifelong daily oral penicillin prophylaxis is advised. Aplastic crisis from parvovirus B19 infection usually requires one or two blood transfusions over 3–4 weeks when no red blood cells are produced. If gallstones are symptomatic cholecystectomy may be necessary.

Glucose-6-phosphate dehydrogenase (G6PD) deficiency

G6PD deficiency is the commonest red cell enzymo-pathy, affecting over 100 million people worldwide. It has a high prevalence (10–20%) in individuals originating from central Africa, the Mediterranean, the Middle East and the Far East. Many different mutations of the gene have been described, leading to different clinical features in different populations.

G6PD is the rate-limiting enzyme in the pentose phosphate pathway and is essential for preventing oxidative damage to red cells. Red cells lacking G6PD are susceptible to oxidant-induced haemo-lysis. G6PD deficiency is X-linked and therefore predominantly affects males. Females who are heterozygotes are usually clinically normal as they have about half the normal G6PD activity. Females may be affected either if they are homozygous or, more commonly, when by chance more of the normal than the abnormal X chromosomes have been inactivated (extreme Lyonisation – the Lyon hypothesis is that, in every XX cell, one of the X chromosomes is inactivated and that this is random). In Mediterranean, Middle Eastern and Oriental populations, affected males have very low or absent enzyme activity in their red cells. Affected Afro-Caribbeans have 10–15% normal enzyme activity. Young red blood cells may have normal enzyme activity whilst older cells are deficient.

Clinical manifestations

Children usually present clinically with:

- *neonatal jaundice* – onset is usually in the first 3 days of life. Worldwide it is the most common cause of severe neonatal jaundice requiring exchange transfusion.
- *acute haemolysis* – precipitated by:
  - infection, the most common precipitating factor
  - certain drugs (Box 22.2)
  - fava beans (broad beans)
  - naphthalene in mothballs

Intravascular haemolysis is associated with fever, malaise and the passage of dark urine, as it contains haemoglobin as well as urobilinogen. The haemo-globin level falls rapidly.

Diagnosis

Between episodes almost all patients have a completely normal blood picture. The diagnosis is made by measuring G6PD activity in red blood cells. During a haemolytic crisis, G6PD levels may be misleadingly elevated due to the higher enzyme concentration in reticulocytes, which are produced in increased numbers in response to the destruction of mature red cells. A repeat assay is then required in the steady state to confirm the diagnosis.

• •

Box 22.2 Drugs and chemicals which can cause haemolysis in children with G6PD deficiency

Antimalarials
Primaquine
Quinine
Chloroquine

Antibiotics
Sulphonamides
Quinolones

Analgesics
Aspirin (in high doses)

Chemicals
Naphthalene (mothballs)
Divicine (fava beans – also called broad beans)

Adapted from: Mehta A, Mason P J, Vulliamy T J. Glucose-6-phosphate dehydrogenase deficiency. *Baillière's Best Practice & Research. Clinical Haematology* 2000;13:21–38.

Management

The parents should be given advice about the signs of acute haemolysis (jaundice, pallor and dark urine) and provided with a list of drugs, chemicals and food to avoid (see Box 22.2). Transfusions are rarely required, even for acute episodes.

Haemoglobinopathies

These are red blood cell disorders which cause haemolytic anaemia because of reduced or absent production of HbA (α- and β-thalassaemias) or because of the production of an abnormal Hb (e.g. sickle cell disease). α-Thalassaemias are caused by deletions (occasionally mutations) in the α-globin gene. β-Thalassaemia and sickle cell disease are caused by mutations of the β-globin gene. Clinical manifestations of the haemoglobinopathies affecting the β-chain are delayed until after 6 months of age when most of the HbF present at birth has been replaced by adult HbA (Figs 22.7 and 22.8).

Sickle cell disease

This is now the commonest genetic disorder in children in many European countries, including the UK (prevalence 1 in 2000 live births). Sickle cell disease is the collective name given to haemoglobinopathies in which HbS is inherited. HbS forms as a result of a point mutation in codon 6 of the β-globin gene which causes a change in the amino acid encoded from glutamine to valine. Sickle cell disease is most common in patients whose parents are black and originate from tropical Africa or the Caribbean but it is also found in the Middle East and in low prevalence in most other parts of the world except for northern Europeans.

There are three main forms of sickle cell disease:

- sickle cell anaemia
- SC disease
- sickle β-thalassaemia

In:

- *Sickle cell anaemia (HbSS)* – patients are homozygous for HbS, i.e. virtually all their Hb is HbS; they have *no* HbA because they have no normal β-globin genes.
- *SC disease (HbSC)* – affected children inherit HbS from one parent and HbC from the other parent (HbC is formed as a result of a different point mutation in β-globin), so they also have *no* HbA because they have no normal β-globin genes.
- *Sickle β-thalassaemia* – affected children inherit HbS from one parent and β-thalassaemia trait from the other. They have no normal β-globin genes and most patients can make no HbA and therefore have similar symptoms to those with sickle cell anaemia.
- *Sickle trait* – Inheritance of HbS from one parent and a normal β-globin gene from the other parent, so approximately 40% of the haemoglobin is HbS. They do not have sickle cell disease but are carriers of HbS, so can transmit HbS to their offspring. They are asymptomatic and are only identified as a result of blood tests.

Pathogenesis

In HbSS, the haemoglobin molecule becomes deformed (insoluble) in the deoxygenated state. HbS polymerises within red blood cells forming rigid tubular spiral bodies which deform the red cells into a sickle shape. Irreversibly sickled red cells have a reduced lifespan and may be trapped in the microcirculation, resulting in thrombosis and therefore ischaemia in an organ or bone (Fig. 22.9). This is exacerbated by low oxygen tension, dehydration and cold.

The clinical manifestations of sickle cell disease vary widely between different individuals. Disease severity is also dependent upon the inheritance of other coexisting haemoglobinopathies, e.g. HbS/β-thalassaemia results in severe disease, HbS/β+-thalassaemia in mild disease. Disease severity is greatly reduced by a high HbF level (common in Arab variants).

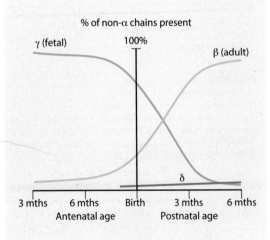

Figure 22.7 Changes in haemoglobin chains in the fetus and infancy.

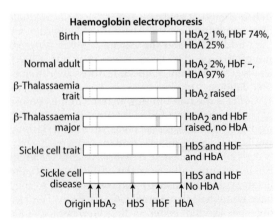

Figure 22.8 Haemoglobins in sickle cell disease.

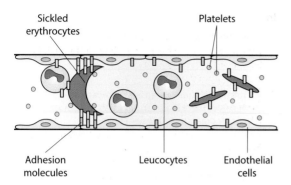

Figure 22.9 Pathogenesis of painful vaso-occlusive crises in sickle cell disease. In sickle cell disease HbS polymerises within erythrocytes causing them to deform into a sickle shape. During sickle cell crises sickle erythrocytes express a number of adhesion molecules, which cause them to adhere abnormally to the vascular endothelium and obstruct blood flow in the microcirculation. Leucocytes and platelets are also frequently activated during sickle cell crises and contribute to the microvascular obstruction leading to ischaemia in an organ or bone. This process is exacerbated by low oxygen tension, dehydration and cold.

Clinical features

These are listed in Figure 22.10.

Management

Prophylaxis In order to prevent pneumococcal infection, all patients should receive twice daily penicillin throughout childhood and be immunised against pneumococcus. The child should be fully immunised, including against *Haemophilus influenzae* type b. All patients should receive once daily oral folic acid because of the increased demand for folic acid caused by the chronic haemolytic anaemia. Vaso-occlusive crises should be minimised by avoiding exposure to cold, dehydration, excessive exercise, undue stress or hypoxia. This requires common sense measures – dressing children warmly, giving drink especially before exercise and taking extra care to keep children warm after swimming or when playing outside in the winter.

Treatment of acute crises Painful crises should be treated with oral or intravenous analgesia according to need (may require opiates) and good hydration (oral or intravenous as required); infection should be treated with antibiotics; oxygen should be given if the oxygen saturation is reduced. Exchange transfusion is indicated for acute chest syndrome, stroke and priapism.

Treatment of chronic problems Children who have recurrent hospital admissions for painful vaso-occlusive crises or acute chest syndrome (see Case history 22.2) may benefit from hydroxyurea, a drug which increases their HbF production and helps protect against further crises. It requires

monitoring for side-effects. The most severely affected children (1–5%) who have had a stroke or who do not respond to hydroxyurea may be offered a bone marrow transplant. This is the only cure for sickle cell disease but can only be safely carried out if the child has an HLA-identical sibling who can donate their bone marrow – the cure rate is 90% but there is a 5% risk of fatal transplant-related complications.

Prognosis

Sickle cell disease is a cause of premature death due to one or more of these severe complications; around 50% of patients with the most severe form of sickle cell disease die before the age of 40 years. However, the mortality rate during childhood is around 3%, usually from bacterial infection.

Prenatal diagnosis and screening

Many countries with a high prevalence of haemo-globinopathies, including the UK, perform neonatal screening using the biochemical screening test (Guthrie test). Early diagnosis of sickle cell disease allows penicillin prophylaxis to be started in early infancy instead of awaiting clinical presentation, possibly due to a severe infection. Prenatal diagnosis can be carried out by chorionic villus sampling at the end of the first trimester if parents wish to choose this option to prevent the birth of an affected child.

Sickle cell trait (AS)

This is asymptomatic and rarely causes problems except under conditions of low oxygen tension. General anaesthesia does not constitute a risk in this population as long as they have been identified and hypoxia avoided.

SC disease

Children with SC disease usually have a nearly normal haemoglobin level and fewer painful crises than those with sickle cell disease, but they may develop proliferative retinopathy in adolescence. Their eyes should be checked periodically.

β-Thalassaemias

The β-thalassaemias occur most often in people from the Indian subcontinent, Mediterranean and Middle East (Fig. 22.14). In the UK, most affected children are born to parents from the Indian subcontinent; in the past, many were born to Greek Cypriots, but this has become uncommon through active counselling within their community.

As there is a deficiency of β-chains, γ-chain synthesis continues beyond the neonatal period, producing an increased proportion of HbF, and δ-chain production increases the amount of HbA_2. This results in precipitation of globin chains within the red cell membrane, bringing about cell death within the bone marrow (ineffective erythropoiesis) and premature removal of circulating red cells by

Clinical manifestations of sickle cell disease

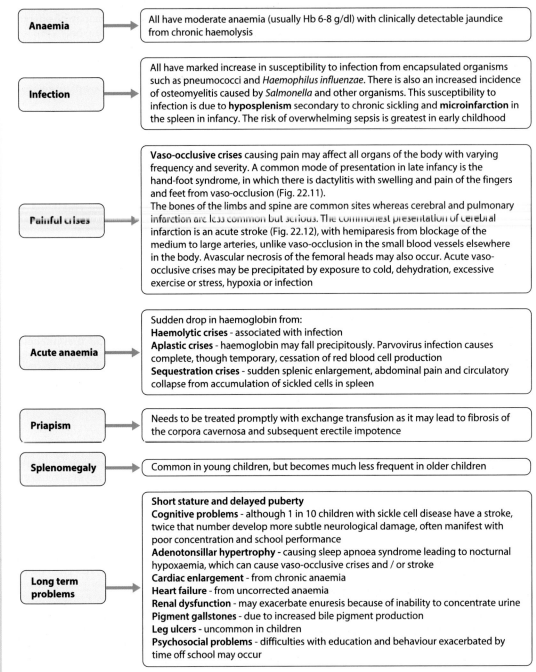

Anaemia	All have moderate anaemia (usually Hb 6-8 g/dl) with clinically detectable jaundice from chronic haemolysis
Infection	All have marked increase in susceptibility to infection from encapsulated organisms such as pneumococci and *Haemophilus influenzae*. There is also an increased incidence of osteomyelitis caused by *Salmonella* and other organisms. This susceptibility to infection is due to **hyposplenism** secondary to chronic sickling and **microinfarction** in the spleen in infancy. The risk of overwhelming sepsis is greatest in early childhood
Painful crises	**Vaso-occlusive crises** causing pain may affect all organs of the body with varying frequency and severity. A common mode of presentation in late infancy is the hand-foot syndrome, in which there is dactylitis with swelling and pain of the fingers and feet from vaso-occlusion (Fig. 22.11). The bones of the limbs and spine are common sites whereas cerebral and pulmonary infarction are less common but serious. The commonest presentation of cerebral infarction is an acute stroke (Fig. 22.12), with hemiparesis from blockage of the medium to large arteries, unlike vaso-occlusion in the small blood vessels elsewhere in the body. Avascular necrosis of the femoral heads may also occur. Acute vaso-occlusive crises may be precipitated by exposure to cold, dehydration, excessive exercise or stress, hypoxia or infection
Acute anaemia	Sudden drop in haemoglobin from: **Haemolytic crises** - associated with infection **Aplastic crises** - haemoglobin may fall precipitously. Parvovirus infection causes complete, though temporary, cessation of red blood cell production **Sequestration crises** - sudden splenic enlargement, abdominal pain and circulatory collapse from accumulation of sickled cells in spleen
Priapism	Needs to be treated promptly with exchange transfusion as it may lead to fibrosis of the corpora cavernosa and subsequent erectile impotence
Splenomegaly	Common in young children, but becomes much less frequent in older children
Long term problems	**Short stature and delayed puberty** **Cognitive problems** - although 1 in 10 children with sickle cell disease have a stroke, twice that number develop more subtle neurological damage, often manifest with poor concentration and school performance **Adenotonsillar hypertrophy** - causing sleep apnoea syndrome leading to nocturnal hypoxaemia, which can cause vaso-occlusive crises and / or stroke **Cardiac enlargement** - from chronic anaemia **Heart failure** - from uncorrected anaemia **Renal dysfunction** - may exacerbate enuresis because of inability to concentrate urine **Pigment gallstones** - due to increased bile pigment production **Leg ulcers** - uncommon in children **Psychosocial problems** - difficulties with education and behaviour exacerbated by time off school may occur

Figure 22.10 Clinical manifestations of sickle cell disease.

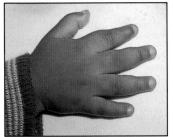

Figure 22.11
Dactylitis in sickle cell disease.

the spleen. The disease severity of β-thalassaemia depends on the amount of HbA and HbF present:

- β-*Thalassaemia major* – HbA (α2β2) cannot be produced because of the abnormal β-globin gene. The most severe form.
- β-*Thalassaemia intermedia* – the β-globin mutations allow a small amount of HbA and/or a large amount of HbF to be produced. Milder, variable.

- β-*Thalassaemia trait* – one normal and one abnormal β-globin gene. Asymptomatic carrier.

β-Thalassaemia major

Autosomal recessive inheritance of mutations in each of the two β-globin genes (one from each parent).

Clinical features (Fig. 22.15)

These are:

- severe anaemia and jaundice from 3–6 months of age
- failure to thrive/growth failure
- extramedullary haemopoiesis, causing bone marrow expansion which leads to the classical facies with maxillary overgrowth and skull bossing; there is marked hepatosplenomegaly (not seen in appropriately transfused children).

Management

The condition is uniformly fatal without regular blood transfusions, so all patients are given lifelong monthly transfusions of red blood cells. The aim is to maintain the haemoglobin concentration above 10 g/dl in order to reduce growth failure and prevent bone deformation. Repeated blood transfusion causes chronic iron overload, which causes cardiac failure, liver cirrhosis, diabetes, infertility and growth failure. To minimise the risk, iron chelation therapy with subcutaneous desferrioxamine, given overnight, is started from 2 to 3 years of age. Patients who comply well with transfusion and chelation have a 90% chance of living into their forties and beyond. However, compliance is

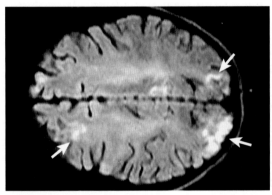

Figure 22.12 MRI of the brain in sickle cell disease showing multiple cerebral infarcts.

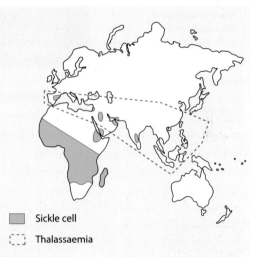

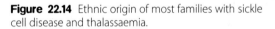

Figure 22.14 Ethnic origin of most families with sickle cell disease and thalassaemia.

Case History
22.2 Acute sickle chest syndrome

Princess, a 9-year-old girl with known homozygous sickle cell disease, presented with increasing chest pain for 6 hours. She had a non-productive cough. On examination she had a fever of 39.7°C. Her breathing was laboured, respiratory rate increased and there was reduced air entry at both bases.

Investigations
- Haemoglobin 6 g/dl, WBC 14 × 10⁹/L, platelets 350 × 10⁹/L
- Chest X-ray – see Figure 22.13
- Oxygen saturation – 89% in air
- Arterial PO$_2$ – 9.3 kPa (70 mmHg) breathing face mask oxygen
- Blood cultures were taken and viral titres performed.

A diagnosis of acute sickle chest syndrome was made, a potentially fatal condition. She was given oxygen by CPAP (continuous positive airways pressure). An exchange transfusion was performed. Broad-spectrum antibiotics were commenced. She responded well to treatment.

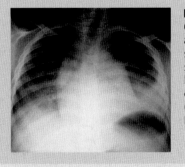

Figure 22.13 Chest X-ray in acute sickle chest syndrome showing bilateral lower zone consolidation. (Courtesy of Dr Parviz Habibi.)

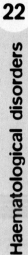
Clinical features and complications of β-thalassaemia major

Pallor

Jaundice

Bossing of the skull
Maxillary overgrowth

Splenomegaly

Need for repeated
blood transfusions
Complications shown in
Box 22.3

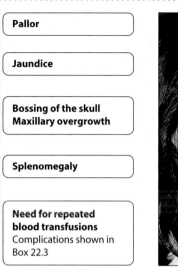

Figure 22.15 Facies in β-thalassaemia showing maxillary overgrowth and skull bossing in a child who has not been adequately transfused.

Box 22.3 Complications of long-term blood transfusion in children

Iron deposition – the most important (all patients)
Heart – cardiomyopathy
Liver – cirrhosis
Pancreas – diabetes
Pituitary gland – delayed growth and sexual maturation
Skin – hyperpigmentation

Antibody formation (10% of children)
Allo-antibodies in the patient make finding compatible blood very difficult

Infection – now uncommon (<10% of children)
Hepatitis A, B, C
HIV
Malaria
Prions (e.g. new variant CJD)

Venous access (common problem)
Often traumatic in young children
Central venous access device (e.g. Portacath) may be required; these predispose to infection

difficult. Those who cannot comply have a high mortality in early adulthood from iron overload. The complications of multiple transfusions are shown in Box 22.3. An alternative treatment for β-thalassaemia major is bone marrow transplantation, which is currently the only cure. It is generally reserved for children with an HLA-identical sibling as there is then a 90% chance of success (i.e. transfusion independence and long-term cure) but a 5% chance of transplant-related mortality.

Prenatal diagnosis

For parents who are both heterozygous for β-thalassaemia, there is a 1 in 4 risk of having an affected child. Prenatal diagnosis of β-thalassaemia (DNA analysis of a chorionic villus sample) should be offered together with genetic counselling to help parents to make informed decisions about whether or not to continue the pregnancy.

β-Thalassaemia trait

Heterozygotes are usually asymptomatic. The red cells are usually hypochromic and microcytic. Anaemia is mild or absent, with a disproportionate reduction in MCH (18–22 fl) and MCV (60–70 fl). The red blood cell count is therefore usually increased (>5.5 × 10^{12}/L). The most important diagnostic feature is the raised HbA$_2$ (and in about half there is a mild elevation of HbF level of 1–3%) on haemoglobin electrophoresis. β-Thalassaemia trait can cause confusion with mild iron deficiency and lead to unnecessary iron therapy.

α-Thalassaemias

Healthy individuals have four α-globin genes. The manifestation of α-thalassaemia syndromes depends on the number of functional α-globin genes.

The most severe α-thalassaemia, *α-thalassaemia major* (also known as Hb Barts hydrops fetalis), is caused by deletion of all four α-globin genes, so no HbA (α2β2) can be produced. It occurs mainly in families of south-east Asian origin and presents in mid-trimester with fetal hydrops (oedema and ascites) from fetal anaemia, which is always fatal in utero or within hours of delivery. The only long-term survivors of α-thalassaemia major are those who have received monthly intrauterine transfusions until delivery followed by lifelong monthly transfusions after birth. The diagnosis is made by Hb electrophoresis or Hb HPLC (high performance liquid chromatography), which shows only Hb Barts.

When only three of the α-globin genes are deleted (*HbH disease*), affected children have mild–moderate anaemia but occasional patients are transfusion-dependent.

Deletion of one or two α-globin genes (known as α-thalassaemia trait) is usually asymptomatic and anaemia is mild or absent. The red cells may be hypochromic and microcytic, which may cause confusion with iron deficiency.

Anaemia in the newborn

1. Reduced red blood cell production

There are two main but rare causes in the newborn and both cause red cell aplasia:

- congenital infection with parvovirus B19
- congenital red cell aplasia (Diamond–Blackfan anaemia).

In this situation the Hb is low and the red blood cells look normal. The diagnostic clue is that the reticulocyte count is low and the bilirubin is normal.

2. Increased red cell destruction (haemolytic anaemia)

This occurs either because of an antibody destroying the red blood cells (i.e. an extrinsic cause) or because there is an intrinsic abnormality of the surface or intracellular contents of the red blood cell. The main causes of haemolytic anaemia in neonates are:

- immune (e.g. haemolytic disease of the newborn)
- red cell membrane disorders (e.g. hereditary spherocytosis)
- red cell enzyme disorders (e.g. glucose-6-phosphate dehydrogenase deficiency)
- abnormal haemoglobins (e.g. α-thalassaemia major).

The diagnostic clues to a haemolytic anaemia are an increased reticulocyte count (due to increased red cell production to compensate for the anaemia) and increased unconjugated bilirubin (due to increased red cell destruction with release of this bile pigment into the plasma).

Haemolytic disease of the newborn (immune haemolytic anaemia of the newborn) is due to antibodies against blood group antigens. The most important are: anti-D (a 'Rhesus' antigen), anti-A or anti-B (ABO blood group antigens) and anti-Kell. The mother is always negative for the relevant antigen (e.g. rhesus D-negative) and the baby is always positive; the mother then makes antibodies

against the baby's blood group and these antibodies cross the placenta into the baby's circulation causing fetal or neonatal haemolytic anaemia. The diagnostic clue to this type of haemolytic anaemia is a positive direct anti-globulin test (Coombs test). This test is only positive in antibody-mediated anaemias and so is negative in all the other types of haemolytic anaemia. These conditions are considered further in Chapter 10.

The most common causes of non-immune haemolytic anaemia in neonates are: G6PD (glucose-6-phosphate dehydrogenase) deficiency and hereditary spherocytosis. Haemoglobinopathies, apart from α-thalassaemia, rarely present with clinical features in the neonatal period but are detected on neonatal biochemical screening (Guthrie test).

3. Blood loss

The main causes are:

- feto-maternal haemorrhage (occult bleeding into the mother)
- twin-to-twin transfusion (bleeding from one twin into the other one)
- blood loss around the time of delivery (e.g. placental abruption).

The main diagnostic clue is severe anaemia with a raised reticulocyte count and normal bilirubin.

4. Anaemia of prematurity

The main causes are:

- inadequate erythropoietin production
- reduced red cell lifespan
- frequent blood sampling whilst in hospital
- iron and folic acid deficiency (after 2–3 months).

Bone marrow failure syndromes

Bone marrow failure (also known as aplastic anaemia) is a rare condition characterised by a reduction or absence of all three main lineages in the bone marrow leading to peripheral blood pancytopenia. It may be inherited or acquired. The acquired cases may be due to viruses (especially hepatitis viruses), drugs (such as sulphonamides, chemotherapy) or toxins (such as benzene, glue); however, many cases are labelled as 'idiopathic' because a specific cause cannot be identified.

The condition may be partial or complete. It may start as failure of a single lineage but progress to involve all three cell lines.

The clinical presentation is with:

- anaemia due to reduced red cell numbers
- infection due to reduced white cell numbers (especially neutrophils)
- bruising and bleeding due to thrombocytopenia.

Inherited aplastic anaemia

These disorders are all rare.

⊚ Summary

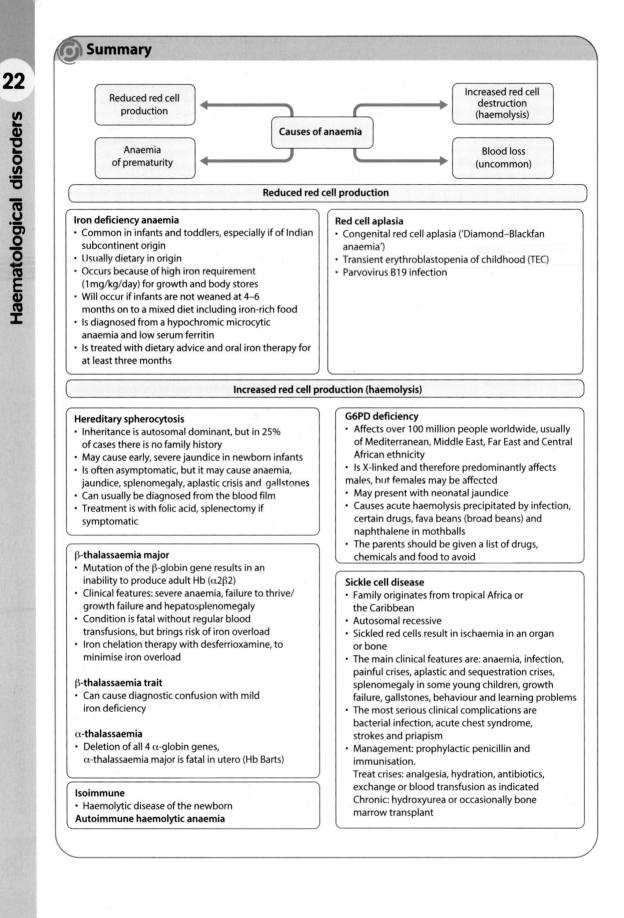

```
                    Reduced red cell          ⟷          ⟷        Increased red cell
                       production                                     destruction
                                          Causes of anaemia          (haemolysis)
                      Anaemia            ⟷          ⟷          Blood loss
                   of prematurity                                   (uncommon)
```

Reduced red cell production

Iron deficiency anaemia
- Common in infants and toddlers, especially if of Indian subcontinent origin
- Usually dietary in origin
- Occurs because of high iron requirement (1mg/kg/day) for growth and body stores
- Will occur if infants are not weaned at 4–6 months on to a mixed diet including iron-rich food
- Is diagnosed from a hypochromic microcytic anaemia and low serum ferritin
- Is treated with dietary advice and oral iron therapy for at least three months

Red cell aplasia
- Congenital red cell aplasia ('Diamond–Blackfan anaemia')
- Transient erythroblastopenia of childhood (TEC)
- Parvovirus B19 infection

Increased red cell production (haemolysis)

Hereditary spherocytosis
- Inheritance is autosomal dominant, but in 25% of cases there is no family history
- May cause early, severe jaundice in newborn infants
- Is often asymptomatic, but it may cause anaemia, jaundice, splenomegaly, aplastic crisis and gallstones
- Can usually be diagnosed from the blood film
- Treatment is with folic acid, splenectomy if symptomatic

β-thalassaemia major
- Mutation of the β-globin gene results in an inability to produce adult Hb (α2β2)
- Clinical features: severe anaemia, failure to thrive/growth failure and hepatosplenomegaly
- Condition is fatal without regular blood transfusions, but brings risk of iron overload
- Iron chelation therapy with desferrioxamine, to minimise iron overload

β-thalassaemia trait
- Can cause diagnostic confusion with mild iron deficiency

α-thalassaemia
- Deletion of all 4 α-globin genes, α-thalassaemia major is fatal in utero (Hb Barts)

Isoimmune
- Haemolytic disease of the newborn
Autoimmune haemolytic anaemia

G6PD deficiency
- Affects over 100 million people worldwide, usually of Mediterranean, Middle East, Far East and Central African ethnicity
- Is X-linked and therefore predominantly affects males, but females may be affected
- May present with neonatal jaundice
- Causes acute haemolysis precipitated by infection, certain drugs, fava beans (broad beans) and naphthalene in mothballs
- The parents should be given a list of drugs, chemicals and food to avoid

Sickle cell disease
- Family originates from tropical Africa or the Caribbean
- Autosomal recessive
- Sickled red cells result in ischaemia in an organ or bone
- The main clinical features are: anaemia, infection, painful crises, aplastic and sequestration crises, splenomegaly in some young children, growth failure, gallstones, behaviour and learning problems
- The most serious clinical complications are bacterial infection, acute chest syndrome, strokes and priapism
- Management: prophylactic penicillin and immunisation.
  Treat crises: analgesia, hydration, antibiotics, exchange or blood transfusion as indicated
  Chronic: hydroxyurea or occasionally bone marrow transplant

Fanconi anaemia

This is the most common inherited form of aplastic anaemia. It is an autosomal recessive condition. The majority of children have congenital anomalies, including short stature, abnormal radii and thumbs, renal malformations, microphthalmia and pigmented skin lesions. Children may present with one or more of these anomalies or with signs of bone marrow failure which do not usually become apparent until the age of 5 or 6 years. Neonates with Fanconi anaemia nearly always have a normal blood count but it can be diagnosed by demonstrating increased chromosomal breakage of peripheral blood lymphocytes. This test can be used to identify affected family members or for prenatal diagnosis. Affected children are at high risk of death from bone marrow failure or transformation to acute leukaemia. The recommended treatment is bone marrow transplantation using normal donor marrow from an unaffected sibling or matched unrelated marrow donor.

Schwachman–Diamond syndrome

This rare autosomal recessive disorder is characterised by bone marrow failure together with signs of pancreatic exocrine failure and skeletal abnormalities. Most are caused by mutations in the SBDS gene, which can be used for identifying unusual cases or prenatal diagnosis. The most common haematological problem is an isolated neutropenia or mild pancytopenia. Like Fanconi anaemia, there is an increased risk of transforming to acute leukaemia.

Bleeding disorders

Normal haemostasis

Haemostasis describes the normal process of blood clotting. It takes place via a series of complex, tightly regulated interactions involving cellular and plasma factors.

There are five main components:

- *Blood vessels* – both initiate and limit coagulation. Intact vascular endothelium secretes prostaglandin I_2 and nitric oxide (which promote vasodilatation and inhibit platelet aggregation). Damaged endothelium releases tissue factor and procoagulants (e.g. collagen and von Willebrand factor) and there are inhibitors of coagulation on the endothelial surface (thrombomodulin, antithrombin and protein S) to modulate coagulation.
- *Platelets* – are vital for haemostasis as they aggregate at sites of vessel injury to form the primary haemostatic plug which is then stabilised by fibrin.
- *Coagulation factors* – are produced (mainly by the liver) in an inactive form and are activated when coagulation is initiated (usually by tissue factor which is released by vessel injury).
- *Coagulation inhibitors* – these either circulate in plasma or are bound to endothelium and are necessary to prevent widespread coagulation throughout the body once coagulation has been initiated.
- *Fibrinolysis* – this process limits fibrin deposition at the site of injury due to activity of the key enzyme plasmin.

The end point of the coagulation cascade is generation of thrombin. A simplified model is shown in Figure 22.16a and b. The two main pathways for thrombin generation were identified many years ago – the intrinsic and extrinsic pathways. Important components of these pathways are still being discovered. In recent years, the crucial role of tissue factor (TF) in haemostasis has been recognised and it is now thought that the extrinsic pathway is the one primarily responsible for initiating both normal haemostasis and thrombotic disease.

Diagnostic approach

Defects in the coagulation factors, in platelet number or function or in the fibrinolytic pathway

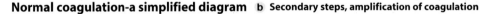

Normal coagulation-a simplified diagram   b **Secondary steps, amplification of coagulation**

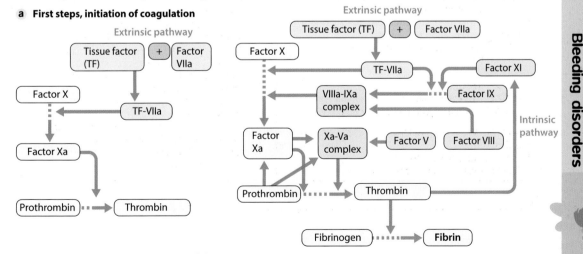

Figure 22.16 Schematic representation of the coagulation pathway. **(a)** First steps (shown in *blue*). **(b)** Secondary steps (shown in *red*).

are associated with an increased risk of bleeding. In contrast, defects in the naturally occurring inhibitors of coagulation (e.g. protein C) or in the vessel wall (e.g. damage from vascular catheters) are associated with thrombosis. In some cases, both pro- and anticoagulant abnormalities can occur at the same time, as seen in disseminated intravascular coagulation (DIC).

The diagnostic evaluation of an infant or child for a possible bleeding disorder includes:

- identifying features in the clinical presentation that suggest the underlying diagnosis and further investigation, as indicated in Box 22.4
- initial laboratory screening tests to determine the most likely diagnosis (Table 22.2)
- specialist investigation to characterise a deficiency or exclude important conditions that can present with normal initial investigations, e.g. mild von Willebrand's disease, factor XIII deficiency and platelet function disorders.

The most useful initial screening tests are:

- full blood count and blood film
- prothrombin time (PT) – measures the activity of factors II, V, VII and X

- activated partial thromboplastin time (APTT) – measures the activity of factors II, V, VIII, IX, X, XI and XII
- if PT or APTT is prolonged, a 50 : 50 mix with normal plasma will distinguish between possible factor deficiency or presence of inhibitor
- thrombin time – tests for deficiency or dysfunction of fibrinogen
- quantitative fibrinogen assay
- D-dimers
- biochemical screen including renal and liver function tests.

The 'bleeding time' is no longer used to investigate platelet disorders as it is unreliable. It has been replaced by in vitro tests of platelet function on a platelet function analyser, which can be performed on a peripheral blood sample.

In the neonate the levels of all clotting factors except factor VIII (FVIII) and fibrinogen are lower in term infants at birth; preterm infants have even lower levels. Therefore the results have to be compared with normal values in infants of a similar gestational and postnatal age. In view of this, and since it is often difficult to obtain good quality neonatal samples, it is sometimes necessary to exclude

---

Box 22.4 Helpful clinical features in evaluating bleeding disorders

Age of onset
Neonate – Haemophilias with intracranial haemorrhage or bleeding after circumcision
Toddler – Haemophilias when starting to walk
Adolescent – von Willebrand's disease with menorrhagia

Family history
Family tree – detailed family tree required
Gender of affected relatives (if all boys, suggests haemophilia)

Bleeding history
Previous surgical procedures and dental extractions – if uncomplicated, suggests bleeding tendency is acquired rather then inherited

Presence of systemic disorders
Drug history
Unusual pattern or inconsistent history – consider non-accidental injury

Pattern of bleeding
Mucous membrane bleeding and skin haemorrhage – characteristic of platelet disorders or von Willebrand's disease
Bleeding into muscles or into joints – characteristic of haemophilia
Scarring and delayed haemorrhage – suggestive of disorders of connective tissue, e.g. Marfan's syndrome, osteogenesis imperfecta or factor XIII deficiency

---

Table 22.2 Investigations in haemophilia A and von Willebrand's disease

	Haemophilia A	**von Willebrand's disease**
PT	Normal	Normal
APTT	↑↑	↑ or normal
Factor VIII:C	↓↓	↓ or normal
vWF Ag	Normal	↓
RiCoF (activity)	Normal	↓
Ristocetin-induced platelet aggregation	Normal	Abnormal
vWF multimers	Normal	Variable

PT: prothrombin time; APTT: activated partial thromboplastin time; RiCoF: ristocetin co-factor, measures vWD activity.

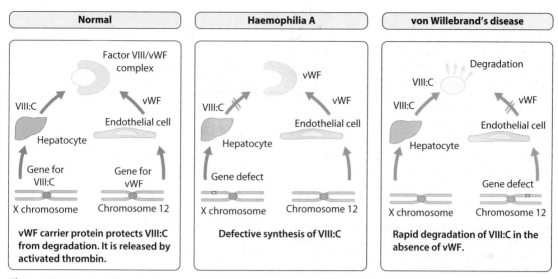

Normal	Haemophilia A	von Willebrand's disease

Factor VIII/vWF complex

VIII:C — vWF

Hepatocyte — Endothelial cell

Gene for VIII:C — Gene for vWF

X chromosome — Chromosome 12

vWF carrier protein protects VIII:C from degradation. It is released by activated thrombin.

vWF

VIII:C — vWF

Hepatocyte — Endothelial cell

Gene defect

X chromosome — Chromosome 12

Defective synthesis of VIII:C

Degradation

VIII:C — vWF

Hepatocyte — Endothelial cell

Gene defect

X chromosome — Chromosome 12

Rapid degradation of VIII:C in the absence of vWF.

Figure 22.17 Factor VIII synthesis: normal, haemophilia A and von Willebrand's disease.

an inherited coagulation factor deficiency by testing the coagulation of both parents.

Haemophilia

The commonest severe inherited coagulation disorders are haemophilia A and haemophilia B. Both have X-linked recessive inheritance. In haemophila A, there is FVIII deficiency (Fig. 22.17); it has a frequency of 1 in 5000 male births. Haemophilia B (FIX deficiency) has a frequency of 1 in 30 000 male births. Two-thirds of newly diagnosed infants have a family history of haemophilia, whereas one-third are sporadic. Identifying female carriers requires a detailed family history, analysis of coagulation factors and DNA analysis. Prenatal diagnosis is available using DNA analysis.

Clinical features

The disorder is graded as severe, moderate or mild depending on the FVIII:C (or IX:C in haemophilia B) level (Table 22.3). The hallmark of severe disease is recurrent spontaneous bleeding into joints and muscles, which can lead to crippling arthritis if not properly treated (Fig. 22.18). Most children present towards the end of the first year of life, when they start to crawl then walk (and fall over). Bleeding episodes are most frequent in joints and muscles. Where there is no family history, non-accidental injury may initially be suspected. Almost 40% of cases present in the neonatal period, particularly with intracranial haemorrhage, bleeding post-circumcision or prolonged oozing from heel stick and venepuncture sites. The severity remains constant within a family.

Management

Recombinant FVIII concentrate for haemophilia A or recombinant FIX concentrate for haemophilia B is given by prompt intravenous infusion whenever

Table 22.3 Severity of haemophilia

Factor VIII:C	Severity	Bleeding tendency
<1%	Severe	Spontaneous joint/muscle bleeds
1–5%	Moderate	Bleed after minor trauma
>5–40%	Mild	Bleed after surgery

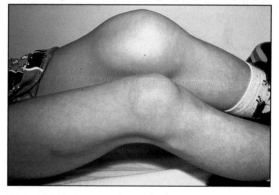

Figure 22.18 Severe arthropathy from recurrent joint bleeds in haemophilia. The aim of modern management is to prevent this from occurring.

there is any bleeding. If recombinant products are unavailable, highly purified, virally inactivated plasma-derived products should be used. The quantity required depends on the site and nature of the bleed. In general, raising the circulating level to 30% of normal is sufficient to treat minor bleeds and simple joint bleeds. Major surgery or life-threatening bleeds require the level to be raised to 100% and then maintained at 30–50% for up to 2 weeks to prevent secondary haemorrhage. This can only be achieved by regular infusion of factor concentrate (usually 8- to 12-hourly for FVIII, 12- to 24-hourly for FIX, or by continuous infusion) and by closely monitoring plasma levels. *Intramuscular injections, aspirin and non-steroidal anti-inflammatory drugs should be avoided in all patients with haemophilia.*

Complications are listed in Box 22.5.

Home treatment is encouraged to avoid delay in treatment which increases the risk of permanent damage, e.g. progressive arthropathy. Parents are usually taught to give replacement therapy at home when the child is 2–3 years of age and many children are able to administer their own treatment from 7–8 years of age.

Prophylactic FVIII/IX is given to all children with severe haemophilia to further reduce the risk of chronic joint damage by raising the baseline level above 2%. Primary prophylaxis usually begins at age 2–3 years, and is given two to three times per week. If peripheral venous access is poor, a central venous access device (e.g. Portacath) may be required. Prophylaxis has been shown to result in better joint function in adult life.

Desmopressin (DDAVP) may allow mild haemophilia A to be managed without the use of blood products. It is given by infusion and stimulates endogenous release of FVIII:C and von Willebrand factor. Adequate levels can be achieved to enable minor surgery and dental extraction to be undertaken. DDAVP is ineffective in haemophila B.

Haemophilia centres should supervise the management of children with bleeding disorders. They provide a multidisciplinary approach with expert medical, nursing and laboratory input. Specialised physiotherapy is needed to preserve muscle strength and avoid damage from immobilisation. Psychosocial support is an integral part of maintaining compliance.

Self-help groups such as the Haemophilia Society may provide families with helpful information and support.

• •
Box 22.5 Complications of treatment of haemophilia

Inhibitors, i.e. antibodies to FVIII or FIX
Develop in 5–20%
Reduce or completely inhibit the effect of treatment
Require the use of very high doses of factor VIII or bypassing agents (e.g. FVIIa) for treating bleeding
May be amenable to immune tolerance induction

Transfusion-transmitted infections
Hepatitis A, B and C
HIV
?Prions

Vascular access
Peripheral veins – may be difficult to cannulate
Central venous access devices may become infected or thrombosed

von Willebrand's disease (vWD)

Von Willebrand factor (vWF) has two major roles:

- it facilitates platelet adhesion to damaged endothelium
- it acts as the carrier protein for FVIII:C, protecting it from inactivation and clearance.

Von Willebrand's disease (vWD) results from either a quantitative or qualitative deficiency of von Willebrand factor (vWF). This causes defective platelet plug formation and, since vWF is a carrier protein for FVIII:C, patients with vWD also are deficient in FVIII:C (see Fig. 22.17).

There are many different mutations in the vWF gene and many different types of vWD. The inheritance is usually autosomal dominant. The commonest subtype, type 1 (60–80%), is usually fairly mild and is often not diagnosed until puberty or adulthood.

Clinical features

These are:

- bruising
- excessive, prolonged bleeding after surgery
- mucosal bleeding such as epistaxis and menorrhagia.

In contrast to haemophilia, spontaneous soft tissue bleeding such as large haematomas and haemarthroses are rare.

Management

Treatment depends on the type and severity of the disorder. Type 1 vWD can usually be treated with DDAVP, which causes secretion of both FVIII and vWF into plasma. DDAVP should be used with caution in children <1 year of age as it can cause hyponatraemia due to water retention and may cause seizures, particularly after repeated doses and if fluid intake is not strictly regulated. More severe types of vWD have to be treated with *plasma-derived* FVIII concentrate as DDAVP is ineffective and recombinant FVIII concentrate contains no vWF. Cryoprecipitate is no longer used to treat vWD as it has not undergone viral inactivation. *Intramuscular injections, aspirin and non-steroidal anti-inflammatory drugs should be avoided in all patients with vWD.*

Acquired disorders of coagulation

The main acquired disorders of coagulation affecting children are those secondary to:

- haemorrhagic disease of the newborn due to vitamin K deficiency (see Ch. 10)
- liver disease
- ITP (immune thrombocytopenia)
- DIC (disseminated intravascular coagulation).

Vitamin K is essential for the production of active forms of factors II, VII, IX, X and protein C and S.

Summary

The child with abnormal bleeding – into soft tissues, mucocutaneous or following surgery

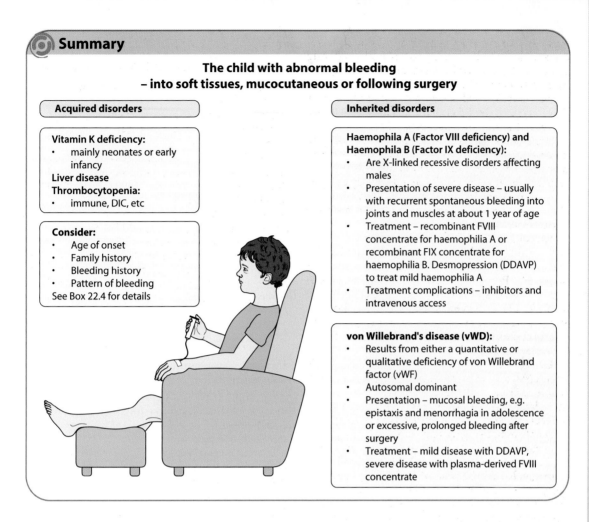

Acquired disorders

Vitamin K deficiency:
- mainly neonates or early infancy

Liver disease

Thrombocytopenia:
- immune, DIC, etc

Consider:
- Age of onset
- Family history
- Bleeding history
- Pattern of bleeding

See Box 22.4 for details

Inherited disorders

Haemophila A (Factor VIII deficiency) and Haemophila B (Factor IX deficiency):
- Are X-linked recessive disorders affecting males
- Presentation of severe disease – usually with recurrent spontaneous bleeding into joints and muscles at about 1 year of age
- Treatment – recombinant FVIII concentrate for haemophilia A or recombinant FIX concentrate for haemophilia B. Desmopression (DDAVP) to treat mild haemophilia A
- Treatment complications – inhibitors and intravenous access

von Willebrand's disease (vWD):
- Results from either a quantitative or qualitative deficiency of von Willebrand factor (vWF)
- Autosomal dominant
- Presentation – mucosal bleeding, e.g. epistaxis and menorrhagia in adolescence or excessive, prolonged bleeding after surgery
- Treatment – mild disease with DDAVP, severe disease with plasma-derived FVIII concentrate

Vitamin K deficiency therefore causes reduced levels of all of these factors. The main clinical consequence of this is a prolonged prothrombin time and an increased risk of bleeding. Children may become deficient in vitamin K due to:

- inadequate intake (e.g. neonates, long-term chronic illness with poor intake)
- malabsorption (e.g. coeliac disease, cystic fibrosis, obstructive jaundice)
- vitamin K antagonists (e.g. warfarin).

Thrombocytopenia

Thrombocytopenia is a platelet count $<150 \times 10^9$/L. The risk of bleeding depends on the level of the platelet count:

- severe thrombocytopenia (platelets $<20 \times 10^9$/L – risk of spontaneous bleeding
- moderate thrombocytopenia (platelets $20–50 \times 10^9$/L) – at risk of excess bleeding during operations or trauma but low risk of spontaneous bleeding
- mild thrombocytopenia (platelets $50–150 \times 10^9$/L) – low risk of bleeding during operations or trauma.

Thrombocytopenia may result in bruising, petechiae, purpura and mucosal bleeding (e.g. epistaxis, bleeding from gums when brushing teeth). Major haemorrhage in the form of severe gastrointestinal haemorrhage, haematuria and intracranial bleeding is much less common. The causes of easy bruising and purpura are listed in Table 22.4. While purpura may signify thrombocytopenia, it also occurs with a normal platelet count from platelet dysfunction and vascular disorders.

Immune thrombocytopenia (ITP)

Immune thrombocytopenia (also called idiopathic thrombocytopenic purpura) is the commonest cause of thrombocytopenia in childhood. It has an incidence of around 4 per 100 000 children per year. It is caused by immune-mediated destruction of circulating platelets due to anti-platelet autoantibodies. The reduced platelet count is accompanied by a compensatory increase of megakaryocytes in the bone marrow.

Clinical features

Most children present between the ages of 2 and 10 years, with onset often 1–2 weeks after a viral

Table 22.4 Causes of purpura or easy bruising

Platelet count reduced, i.e. thrombocytopenia

Increased platelet destruction or consumption

Immune	ITP (immune thrombocytopenia)
	SLE (systemic lupus erythematosus)
	Alloimmune neonatal thrombocytopenia
Non-immune	Haemolytic uraemic syndrome
	Thrombotic thrombocytopenic purpura
	DIC (disseminated intravascular coagulation)
	Congenital heart disease
	Giant haemangiomas (Kasabach–Merritt syndrome)
	Hypersplenism

Impaired platelet production

Congenital	Fanconi anaemia
	Wiskott–Aldrich syndrome
	Bernard–Soulier syndrome
Acquired	Aplastic anaemia
	Marrow infiltration (e.g. leukaemia)
	Drug-induced

Platelet count normal

Platelet dysfunction

Congenital	Rare disorders, e.g. Glanzmann's thromboasthenia
Acquired	Uraemia, cardiopulmonary bypass

Vascular disorders

Congenital	Rare disorders, e.g. Ehlers–Danlos, Marfan's syndrome, hereditary haemorrhagic telangiectasia
Acquired	Meningococcal and other severe infections
	Vasculitis, e.g. Henoch–Schönlein purpura, SLE
	Scurvy

infection. There is usually a short history of days or weeks. Affected children develop petechiae and purpura and superficial bruising (see Case history 22.3). It can cause epistaxis and other mucosal bleeding but profuse bleeding is uncommon despite the fact that the platelet count often falls to $< 10 \times 10^9$/L. Intracranial bleeding is a serious but rare complication, occurring in 0.1–0.5%, mainly in those with a long period of severe thrombocytopenia.

Diagnosis

ITP is a diagnosis of exclusion, so careful attention must be paid to the history, clinical features and blood film to ensure that another more sinister diagnosis is not missed. In the younger child a congenital cause (such as Wiskott–Aldrich or Bernard–Soulier syndromes) should be considered. Any atypical clinical features, such as the presence of hepatosplenomegaly or marked lymphadenopathy, should prompt a bone marrow examination to exclude acute leukaemia or aplastic anaemia. A bone marrow examination should also be performed if the child is going to be treated with steroids since this treatment may temporarily mask these diagnoses. SLE (systemic lupus erythematosus) should also be considered. However, if the clinical features are characteristic, with no abnormality in the blood other than a low platelet count and no intention to treat, there is no need to examine the bone marrow.

Management

In about 80% of children, the disease is acute, benign and self-limiting, usually remitting spontaneously within 6–8 weeks. Most children can be managed at home and do not require hospital admission. Treatment is controversial. Most children do not need any therapy even if their platelet count is $<10 \times 10^9$/L but treatment should be given if there is evidence of major bleeding (e.g. intracranial or gastrointestinal haemorrhage) or persistent minor bleeding (e.g. persistent oral bleeding). The treatment options are oral prednisolone or intravenous immunoglobulin, but both have significant side-effects and do not alter the chance of achieving complete remission. Immunoglobulin infusions usually result in a more rapid rise in the platelet count than steroids. Platelet transfusions are reserved for life-threatening haemorrhage as they raise the platelet count only for a few hours. The prednisolone should be given only as a short course, irrespective of the platelet count. The parents need immediate 24-hour access to hospital

Case History

22.3 Immune thrombocytopenic purpura (ITP)

Sian, aged 5 years, developed bruising and a skin rash over 24 hours. She had had an upper respiratory tract infection the previous week. On examination she appeared well but had a purpuric skin rash with some bruises on the trunk and legs (Fig. 22.19). There were three blood blisters on her tongue and buccal mucosa, but no fundal haemorrhages, lymphadeno-pathy or hepatosplenomegly. Urine was normal on stix testing. A full blood count showed Hb 11.5 g/dl with normal indices, WBC and differential normal, platelet count 17×10^9/L. The platelets on the blood film were large; the film was otherwise normal. A diagnosis of ITP was made and she was discharged home. Her parents were counselled and given emergency contact names and telephone numbers. They were also given literature on the condition and advised that she should avoid contact sports but should continue to attend school. Over the next 2 weeks she continued to develop bruising and purpura but was asymptomatic. By the third week she had no new bruises, and her platelet count was 25×10^9/L; the blood count and film showed no new abnormalities. The following week, the platelet count was 74×10^9/L and a week later it was 200×10^9/L. She was discharged from follow-up.

In immune thrombocytopenic purpura, in spite of impressive cutaneous manifestations and extremely low platelet count, the outlook is good and most will remit quickly without any intervention.

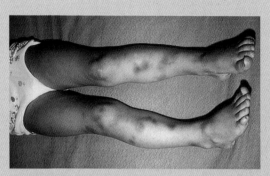

Figure 22.19 Bruising and purpura from immune thrombocytopenic purpura.

treatment, and the child should avoid trauma, as far as possible, and contact sports while the platelet count is a very low.

Chronic ITP

In 20% of children the platelet count remains low 6 months after diagnosis; this is known as chronic ITP. No treatment is given unless there is major bleeding. As for acute ITP, long-term steroid treatment should not be used. Therefore treatment is mainly supportive, the child should avoid contact sports but be encouraged to continue normal activities, including schooling. As with acute ITP, parents need 24-hour access to hospital. The family may benefit from the parent ITP Support Group. Most children remit within 3 years from onset or stabilise with moderate, asymptomatic thrombo-cytopenia. Children with significant bleeding are rare and require specialist care. Splenectomy is probably the most effective treatment for this group, but has significant morbidity and may be unsuccessful in up to 25% of cases. If ITP in a child becomes chronic, regular screening for SLE should be performed, as the thrombocytopenia may predate the development of autoantibodies.

Disseminated intravascular coagulation

Disseminated intravascular coagulation (DIC) describes a disorder characterised by coagulation pathway activation leading to diffuse fibrin deposition in the microvasculature and consumption of coagulation factors and platelets.

The commonest causes of activation of coagul-ation are severe sepsis or shock due to circulatory collapse, e.g. in meningococcal septicaemia, or extensive tissue damage from trauma or burns. DIC may be acute or chronic and is likely to be initiated through the tissue factor pathway. The predominant clinical feature is bruising, purpura and haemorrhage. However, the pathophysio-logical process is characterised by microvascular thrombosis and purpura fulminans may occur.

No single test reliably diagnoses DIC. However, DIC should be suspected when the following abnormalities coexist – thrombocytopenia, pro-longed PT (prothrombin time), prolonged APTT, low fibrinogen, raised fibrinogen degradation products and D-dimers and microangiopathic haemolytic anaemia. There is also usually a marked reduction in the naturally occurring anticoagulants, protein C, S and antithrombin.

The most important aspect of management is to treat the underlying cause of the DIC (usually sepsis) whilst providing intensive care. Supportive care may be provided with fresh frozen plasma (to replace clotting factors), cryoprecipitate and platelets. Antithrombin and protein C concentrates have been used, particularly in severe menin-gococcal septicaemia with purpura fulminans. The use of heparin remains controversial.

Summary

The child with petechiae or purpura

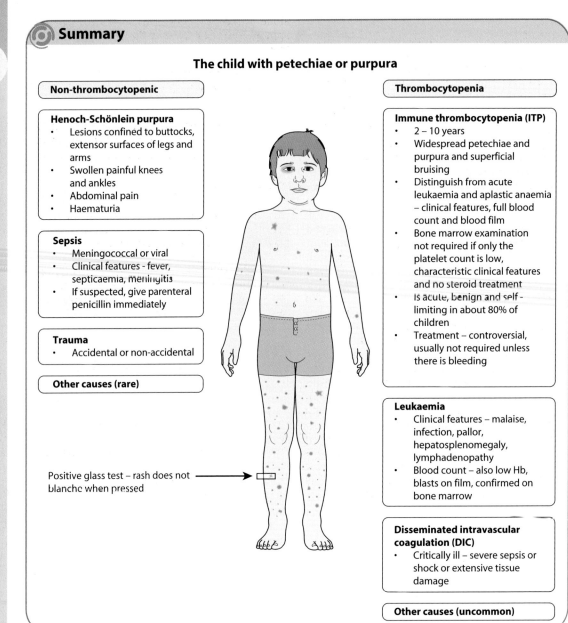

Non-thrombocytopenic

Henoch-Schönlein purpura
- Lesions confined to buttocks, extensor surfaces of legs and arms
- Swollen painful knees and ankles
- Abdominal pain
- Haematuria

Sepsis
- Meningococcal or viral
- Clinical features - fever, septicaemia, meningitis
- If suspected, give parenteral penicillin immediately

Trauma
- Accidental or non-accidental

Other causes (rare)

Positive glass test – rash does not blanche when pressed

Thrombocytopenia

Immune thrombocytopenia (ITP)
- 2 – 10 years
- Widespread petechiae and purpura and superficial bruising
- Distinguish from acute leukaemia and aplastic anaemia – clinical features, full blood count and blood film
- Bone marrow examination not required if only the platelet count is low, characteristic clinical features and no steroid treatment
- Is acute, benign and self-limiting in about 80% of children
- Treatment – controversial, usually not required unless there is bleeding

Leukaemia
- Clinical features – malaise, infection, pallor, hepatosplenomegaly, lymphadenopathy
- Blood count – also low Hb, blasts on film, confirmed on bone marrow

Disseminated intravascular coagulation (DIC)
- Critically ill – severe sepsis or shock or extensive tissue damage

Other causes (uncommon)

Thrombosis in children

Thrombosis is uncommon in children. It may be due to an inherited disorder or acquired secondary to another underlying illness or its treatment. Thrombosis of cerebral vessels usually presents with signs of a stroke. The condition is considered further in Chapter 10 on neonatal medicine and Chapter 27 on neurological disorders.

Inherited disorders (thrombophilias) are:

- protein C deficiency
- protein S deficiency
- antithrombin deficiency.

All of these disorders are autosomal dominant, but even heterozygotes are predisposed to thrombosis, usually venous thrombosis, during the second or third decade of life. Homozygous deficiency of protein C and protein S are uncommon and present with life-threatening thrombosis with widespread haemorrhage and purpura into the skin (known as 'purpura fulminans') in the neonatal period. Homozygous antithrombin deficiency is not seen, probably because it is lethal in the fetus.

Acquired disorders are:

- catheter-related thrombosis
- DIC (disseminated intravascular coagulation)
- hypernatraemia
- polycythaemia (e.g. due to congenital heart disease)
- malignancy
- SLE (systemic lupus erythematosus).

Diagnosis

Although inherited thrombophilia is very uncommon, these disorders predispose to life-threatening thrombosis and so it is important not to miss the diagnosis in any child presenting with an unexplained thrombotic event. Therefore screening tests for the presence of an inherited thrombophilia should be carried out in the following situations:

- any child with unanticipated or extensive venous thrombosis, ischaemic skin lesions or neonatal purpura fulminans
- any child with a positive family history of neonatal purpura fulminans.

The screening tests are assays for protein C and S, antithrombin assay, polymerase chain reaction (PCR) for factor V Leiden (activated protein C resistance) and for the prothrombin^{20210A} gene mutation.

Mutations in factor V (factor V Leiden) and the prothrombin gene respectively are present in 5% and 2% of the northern European population. Both slightly increase the risk of thrombosis but are not currently thought to be powerful risk factors on their own. However, there is some evidence that co-inheritance of one or both mutations with another form of inherited thrombophilia increases the risk of thrombosis. Therefore it is reasonable to screen children who develop thrombosis for all of these factors in order to plan the best management to prevent thrombosis. In the UK, current practice is not to screen asymptomatic children for genetic defects which are not going to affect their medical management, e.g. on the basis of family history alone, until they are old enough to receive appropriate counselling and make decisions for themselves.

Summary

Thrombosis:
- all children with thrombosis should be screened for inherited or acquired predisposing disorders.

Further reading

Lilleyman J S, Hann I M, Blanchette V S (eds) 2005 Pediatric haematology, 3rd edn. Churchill Livingstone, Edinburgh. *A single volume, comprehensive textbook*

Nathan D G, Orkin S H (eds) 2003 Nathan and Oski's Hematology of infancy and childhood, 6th edn. Saunders, Philadelphia. *Comprehensive, two volume textbook*

Internet

British Committee for Standards in Haematology guidelines – www.bcshguidelines.com
Diamond–Blackfan syndrome – www.diamondblackfan.org
Haemophilia – www.haemophilia.org.uk or www.wfh.org
Shwachman–Diamond syndrome – www.shwachman-diamondsupport.org
Sickle cell disease – www.sicklecellsociety.org
Thalassaemia – www.ukts.org

Emotions and behaviour

Knowledge of children's emotions and behaviour is important in order to:

- know what constitutes the normal range
- understand common, innocent minor deviations and responses to stress, physical illness and injuries
- recognise and manage emotional and behavioural disorders.

Principles of normal development

Normal parenting

A child's behaviour, emotional responses and personality are the end result of an interplay between genetic predisposition and environmental influences. The environment provides experience from which stems knowledge, learned behaviour or emotional responses and attitudes to oneself and the world. Personal relationships are the major environmental factor in promoting psychosocial development and the child's family is the principal source of these. Within the family, children should be protected, nurtured, educated and contained so that their development is supported optimally. With the rising number of single parents and divorces, the form of the family is no longer predictable, but it is possible to make statements about what constitutes competent parenting (Box 23.1). Beyond this, the parents' attitude towards their children and how they handle their individual children help to determine how their personalities develop.

Normal early relationships

In the first 2 months of a baby's life, infants are not fussy about who responds to their needs. From 3 to 6 months they become more selective, demanding comfort from one or two caregivers. By 6–8 months they are particular about who responds to their needs or holds them, especially when distressed, and show tearful *separation anxiety* if their main caregiver, usually the mother, is not there. If tired, tearful, unhappy or in pain, they will cling to her

Box 23.1 Competent parents

- Are there when needed
- Protect their children from harm
- Love their children – provide affection, support, comfort, food and shelter
- Use their authority so that they are in charge of their children (rather than vice versa)
- Respect their children's immature status and judge it accurately
- Keep adult business (sex, marital conflict, etc.) away from their children
- Set reasonable limits of tolerance on their children's behaviour
- Establish a moderate amount of justifiable household rules
- Have their own lives and do not live through their children
- Maintain their own self-esteem and personal development

and be comforted by her presence as an *attachment figure*. At this time the child learns to crawl, and so is able to leave a primary caregiver and possibly encounter danger. The development of attachment behaviour allows the infant to keep track of his parent's whereabouts and resist separation. This close attachment relationship derives from social interaction and the mother's sensitive responsiveness to the baby's needs, not from any blood tie. It need not be with the biological mother, although it usually is. Its importance lies in it being:

- a particularly close relationship within which the child's development of trust, empathy, conscience and ideals is promoted, forming a prototype for future close relationships
- the child's primary source of comfort, providing his principal method of coping with stress (fear, anxiety, pain, etc.).

This underscores the importance of having a young child's parent 'rooming in' if he has to be admitted to hospital. He would otherwise be doubly distressed both by the absence of his attachment figure as well as by the threat of strange surroundings or procedures and by the stress of pain or illness.

If a young child is placed in strange, impersonal surroundings and separated from his mother for more than several hours, a *triphasic acute separation* reaction may set in (Fig. 23.1):

- mounting anxiety about the fact that his mother fails to reappear produces distressed, irritable tearfulness (*protest*) which is hard to comfort
- after a day or two, this turns into a withdrawn state with no play, no interest in food, and little speech or willingness for personal contact (*despair*)
- the child gradually cheers up from this but the close contact with his mother has been lost and he is relatively indifferent to her when she reappears (*detachment*).

Recreating the original closeness can take weeks and is accompanied by a phase of irritability, misbehaviour and clinging. This can sometimes be seen when children who have been admitted to hospital as an emergency return home.

Children who have never had the opportunity for a close, secure attachment relationship in their early years are at risk of growing up as self-centred individuals who seek the affection and attention of others but have difficulty with close personal relationships and with learning to conform with social rules of conduct.

The selective clinging of early attachment behaviour diminishes over time so that in the second year of life children extend their emotional attachments to their father or other family members. By school age, they can tolerate separations from their parents for several hours. Children vary in their ability to do this; a child who is constitutionally apprehensive, who has an exceptionally anxious mother, or who has parents who fight or utter threats of abandonment will continue to cling to his mother for protection and comfort. A series of frightening events will tend to perpetuate clinging, which may persist well into middle childhood (age 5–12 years). This interferes with children's capacity to learn how to cope with anxiety on their own (Fig. 23.2).

With entry into school, the importance of teachers and other children in shaping psychosocial development increases and their influence must be taken into account in understanding any schoolchild's development.

Summary

Early relationships
Young children:
- develop a close attachment relationship with their mother (or main caregiver)
- if separated from their mother, may develop separation anxiety
- if admitted to hospital, should be able to have their parents stay with them.

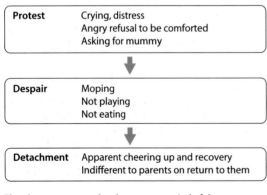

The three stages of the acute separation response in children

Protest	Crying, distress Angry refusal to be comforted Asking for mummy
Despair	Moping Not playing Not eating
Detachment	Apparent cheering up and recovery Indifferent to parents on return to them

The above sequence develops over a period of days, but with considerable variation between children.

Figure 23.1 The three stages of the acute separation response in young children.

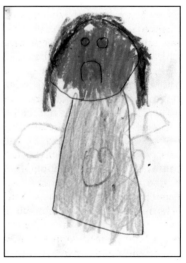

Figure 23.2 A 6-year-old with separation anxiety showing what it feels like to leave her mother to go to school.

Temperament

Children differ from each other in personality from birth, just as they do in physical appearance. This individuality in behavioural style or temperament is partly genetically determined. It is not fixed but changes slowly in the light of experience. It affects how other people deal with them.

A child born with a *difficult temperament* is prone to:

- predominantly negative mood – whinging, moaning, crying
- intense emotional reactions – screaming rather than whimpering, jumping for joy rather than smiling
- irregular biological functions – a lack of rhythm in sleeping, hunger or toileting
- negative initial responses to novel situations, e.g. pushing a new toy away
- protracted adjustment to new situations – taking weeks or months to settle into a new playgroup.

Such a pattern is a vulnerability factor for future emotional and behaviour problems. It may be hard for parents to maintain an affectionate relationship with a child who has a difficult temperament. Their self-confidence falters as they feel guilty that they have failed as parents. They need support to maintain a positive, loving relationship with their child who will, if this can be done, soften and become easier to handle over a period of months. If parents lapse into irritable intolerance themselves, this is likely to maintain the child's grouchy and unsatisfied manner and may lead eventually to low self-esteem or the development of behaviour problems.

Self-esteem

Children develop views and make attributions about themselves. Most children experience praise and success in enough areas of their lives to develop a sense of inner self-confidence and self-worth. Those who do not are at increased risk of developing emotional and behaviour disorders which in turn may breed further shame and failure. A child who does not consider himself worthwhile and valued by others will play safe and not attempt new activities or explore new situations because of a fear of failure. This restricts his development of coping skills and knowledge of the world generally. It may also be a vulnerability factor for depression and anxiety disorders. Children who lack a belief in their own worth may adopt extraordinary and problematic behaviours in order to attract the attention and acclaim of others. For instance, one child took to openly eating dog faeces because it attracted a crowd of amazed children around her. Repeated failure, academically or socially, will undermine self-esteem, as will some disorders themselves (dyspraxia, enuresis and faecal soiling in particular). The most important source of low self-esteem, though, is the child's parents, either because of their own low self-esteem or because of abuse (emotional, sexual or physical) and neglect.

Box 23.2 The quality of preschool thought

- The child is at the centre of his world ('I'm tired so it's getting dark')
- Everything has a purpose ('The sea is there for us to swim in')
- Inanimate objects are alive ('Naughty table hurt me') and have feelings and motives
- Poor categorisation (all men are Daddies)
- Use of magical thinking ('If I close my eyes, she'll go away')
- Use of sequences or routines rather than a sense of time
- The use of toys and other aspects of imaginative play as aids to thought (particularly in making sense of experience and social relationships)

Cognitive style

As children grow older, their thinking styles evolve from one that is concrete to one that is able to cope with abstract thought. Below the age of about 5 years, thought is fundamentally egocentric, with the child being at the centre of his world (Box 23.2). During middle childhood the dominant mode of thought is practical and orderly but tied to immediate circumstances and specific experiences rather than hypothetical possibilities or metaphors. Not until the mid-teens does the adult style of abstract thought begin to appear.

> **Adjust the way you talk to children to be compatible with their thinking style.**

Coping with chronic or serious illness or adversities in childhood

Children can respond to adversity including illness in a number of ways:

- *Cognitive response* – can lie anywhere along the spectrum of over-acceptance to denial, with fluctuation over time. In over-acceptance the child may allow the illness to overtake their life resulting in high levels of anxiety about the slightest symptom. With denial, symptoms and warning signs may be ignored and treatment poorly adhered to.
- *Emotional response* – to diagnosis of illness and at times of relapse may have similarities to a bereavement reaction or reaction to loss, with shock, denial, anger, followed by acceptance and adjustment (Fig. 23.3). Such responses to a serious illness are normal as long as the child proceeds through the phases.
- *Behavioural response* – young children tend to regress when stressed and behave as younger than they actually are. A toddler may become overactive or clingy and display sleep and feeding difficulties.

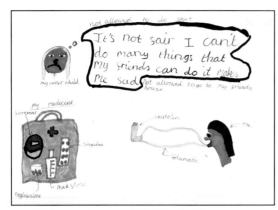

Figure 23.3 Drawing by 10-year-old girl with asthma showing how she felt about her illness. She was struggling to take her medicines and had multiple hospital admissions. Family therapy helped her to come to terms with her illness and take her medications.

Regressive responses in older children predominantly manifest as problems with toileting, academic performance and peer relationships.

- *Somatic response* – can include expression of worry and distress through bodily symptoms such as recurrent abdominal pain.

Children suffering from chronic or serious illness are more vulnerable to mental health problems. This is related to:

- *Nature of illness* – this includes severity, chronicity, presence of constant discomfort and demands of treatment. Children with neurological disorders involving the brain, e.g. epilepsy, are at increased risk.
- *Stage of illness* – for example diagnosis, deteriorations signalled by the need for new demanding treatments or by admissions to hospital.
- *Age of the child* – in infancy illness may affect attachment and developmental milestones such as autonomy and mobility. Over 5 years of age there is a greater impact on educational progress, athletic activities and achievement. In adolescence, social adjustment, individual identity, independence from the family and poor adherence to treatment become more of an issue. Prolonged separation from parents resulting from illness will have a particularly negative impact between the age of 6 months and 3 years.
- *Personality features* – a child who is more adaptable to new situations will fare better. In contrast, a child who from early life has been difficult to soothe will fare worse
- *Intellectual capacity* – brighter children generally cope better.
- *Family factors* – the illness can have detrimental effects on the family and family difficulties can aggravate adaptation to illness.

Summary

Responses of children to illness or adversity include:

- over-acceptance or refusal to accept the situation
- the sequence of shock, denial, anger, followed by acceptance and adjustment
- regression of behaviour
- somatic symptoms.

Adversities in the family

Family relationships are, for most children, the source of their most powerful emotions. Similarly, parents have more effect than anyone else on children's social learning and behaviour. It follows that families are generally the most potent environmental influence on a child's mental health. They are not all-powerful, since a predisposition to particular childhood emotional and behavioural problems can be inherited, but family influences interact with this so that overt disorder may or may not emerge. Not all disorders have their origin in family adversities: hyperkinetic disorder, tics and autism arise independently of them. Nevertheless, the non-genetic contribution of family interactions to emotional and behavioural disorders is often substantial and the mechanisms whereby they produce disorder are various. The following are some of the known risk factors:

- angry discord between family members
- parental mental ill health, especially maternal depression
- divorce (Boxes 23.3 and 23.4) and bereavement
- intrusive overprotection
- lack of parental authority
- physical and sexual abuse
- emotional rejection or unremitting criticism
- use of violence, terror, threats of abandonment or excessive guilt as disciplinary devices
- taunting or belittlement of the child
- inconsistent, unpredictable discipline
- using the child to fulfil the unreasonable personal emotional needs of a parent
- inappropriate responsibilities or expectations for the child's level of maturity.

Many of these can be aggravated by a difficult or unrewarding child who creates an adverse environment for himself. It is unwise to blame the parents for causing their child's problem without examining how much the child contributes to the situation.

Adversities may also arise outside the family. Experiences with other children are increasingly recognised as highly significant in psychosocial development. Bullying is a known adversity, a specific instance of peer rejection in which a child is actively persecuted by others. Merely being left out of things (as opposed to being driven away) is

---

Box 23.3 Reactions to parental divorce

Preschool
Fear of further abandonment:
– intensified clinging at threatened separations
– sleep disturbances
– tearful, irritable and demanding
– desultory play

Middle childhood
Miserable at loss of parent, pining for restitution of family
Self-blame in younger (age 6–8) age group
Angry blaming of one parent for divorce in older (age 9–12) age group
Loyalty conflicts
Anxiety and jealousy at parents' new partners
Educational underachievement

Adolescents
Wide variation in response
Various attempts to master the situation:
– detachment from family
– rapid maturation
– moral idealism
– critical of parents
Educational underachievement
Depression in some

much less pernicious. Conversely, having a number of steady, good-quality peer relationships is a marker for good prognosis in an emotional or behaviour problem which has resulted from environmental influences.

Box 23.4 Adjustment tasks facing children of divorced parents

1. Acknowledgement of parental separation
2. Regaining sense of direction in life activities
3. Dealing with sense of loss and rejection
4. Forgiving parents for break-up
5. Accepting permanence of divorce, relinquishing wish for the previously intact family
6. Feeling able to enter into new emotional relationships

Summary

Regarding adversities:
- the child's family is the most potent influence in the child's mental health
- many but not all mental health problems originate from adversities in the family
- the child's personality and adversities outside the family, e.g. bullying, may aggravate the situation.

Problems of the preschool years

Meal refusal

A common scenario is a mother complaining that her child refuses to eat any or much of what she provides; mealtimes have become a battleground. Examination reveals a healthy, well-nourished child whose height and weight are securely within normal limits on a centile growth chart, or a small and thin child with normal growth.

An account of what goes on at a typical mealtime may reveal:

- a past history of force-feeding
- irregular meals so that the child is not predictably hungry
- unsuitable meals
- unreasonably large portions
- multiple opportunities for distraction, e.g. TV.

Most importantly, how much does the child eat between meals? A well-nourished child is getting food from somewhere. Not all parents regard sweets and crisps as being food. Some mothers, whilst concerned about their child's apparently poor food intake, provide little variety in the child's diet. For strategies for dealing with meal refusal see Box 23.5.

Box 23.5 Strategy for meal refusal

Mealtime history

What is the parent most concerned about?
Nutrition?
– refer to growth chart
Discipline and parenting?
– family history of eating problems
– parenting style
– what do others say?
– is it part of a broader problem?

How much food is eaten between meals?
– food diary to record child's intake over number of days

Advice
As long as offered wholesome food, children are remarkably good at eating a constant and appropriate quantity of food when allowed a free choice
As it is impossible to force a child to eat, avoid confrontation at mealtimes
Develop a relaxed atmosphere
Use favourite foods as a reward
Reduce eating between meals if necessary, though many young children prefer small, frequent snacks

Sleep-related problems

Difficulty in settling to sleep at bedtime

This is a common problem in the toddler years. The child will not go to sleep unless the parent is present. Most instances are normal expressions of separation anxiety, but there may be other obvious reasons for it which can be explored in taking a history (Box 23.6), supplemented if necessary by the parents keeping a prospective sleep diary. Many cases will respond to common-sense advice:

- creating a bedtime and a bedtime routine which cues the child to what is required
- telling the child to lie quietly in bed until he falls asleep, recognising that children cannot fall asleep to order (although that is what everyone tells them to do).

More refractory cases may merit a couple of nights of respite sedation (with trimeprazine) to enable parents to catch up on lost sleep themselves. Once they are feeling more on top of things, they can impose a graded pattern of lengthening periods between tucking their child up in bed and coming back after a few minutes to visit him, but leaving the room before the child falls asleep. The object is to provide the opportunity for the child to learn how to fall sleep alone, a skill he has not yet developed.

Waking at night

This is normal, but some children cry because they cannot settle themselves back to sleep without their parent's presence. This is often associated with difficulty settling in the evenings, which should be treated first. Some children who can settle in the evening may be unable to settle when they wake in the night because the circumstances are different – it is quieter, darker, etc. The graded approach described above for evening settling can also be used in the middle of the night. Parents will find it helpful to take alternate nights on duty to share the burden. Sedative medication is less likely to be effective than with evening settling problems.

Nightmares

These are bad dreams which can be recalled by the child. They are common, rarely requiring professional attention unless they occur frequently or are stereotyped in content, indicating a morbid preoccupation. Reassuring the child will usually suffice.

Night (sleep) terrors

These are different from nightmares, occurring about $1^1/_2$ hours after settling. The parents find the child sitting up in bed, eyes open, seemingly awake but obviously disorientated, confused and distressed and unresponsive to their questions and reassurances. The child settles back to sleep after a few minutes and has no recollection of the episode in the morning. A night terror is a *parasomnia*, a disturbance of the structure of sleep wherein a very rapid emergence from the first period of deep slow-wave sleep produces a state of high arousal and confusion. Sleepwalking has similar origins and the two may be combined. Most night terrors need little more than reassurance directed towards the parents. If necessary, they can sometimes be stopped by keeping a record of their timing and then briefly waking the child 15 minutes before the terror is expected each night for about a week.

Disobedience, defiance and tantrums

Normal toddlers often go through a phase of refusing to comply with parents' demands, sometimes angrily ('the terrible 2s'). This is an understandable reaction to the discovery that the world is not organised around them. They also become confused and angered by the fact that the parent who provides them with comfort when they are distressed is also the person who is making them do things they do not wish to do. This seems exceptionally unfair to them. That is one reason why children play their parents up but may be fine with others. All this can exhaust and demoralise parents, not least because many people offer advice or criticism (everyone thinks themselves an expert in the area of children's development and behaviour). The points listed in Box 23.7 can be made.

Box 23.6 Reasons for a child not settling at night

Too much sleep in the late afternoon
Displaced sleep/wake cycle – not waking child in morning because did not settle until late on the previous night
Separation anxiety
Overstimulated or overwrought in evening
Kept awake by siblings or noisy neighbours or TV in the bedroom
Erratic parental practices: no bedtime or routine to cue child into sleep readiness, sudden removal from play to go to bed without prior warning
Use of bedroom as punishment
Dislike of darkness and silence – night light and playing story tapes can be helpful

---

Box 23.7 Managing toddler disobedience

Ensure your demand is reasonable for the developmental stage of the child
Tell the child what you want him to do rather than nagging about what you don't want him to do
Praise for compliance, especially when it is spontaneous (catch him doing the right thing)
Use simple incentives to reward good behaviour
Frame deals along the lines of 'If you (do this or that) … then we/I can do such and such' (not the other way round)
Avoid threats that cannot be carried out
Carry out threats that are made
Ignore defiance as much as possible

•••••••••••••••••••••••••••••••••

Box 23.8 Analysing a tantrum

Antecedents – what happened in the minutes before the episode
Behaviour – exactly what the episode consisted of
Consequences – what happened as a result

•••••••••••••••••••••••••••••••••

Box 23.9 Tantrums: management strategies

Affection and attention
Distraction
Avoiding antecedents
Ignoring:
– Effective but can be difficult
– No surrender
Time out from positive reinforcement:
– Walk away, returning when quietens down
– Separate from siblings
– Put on a 'naughty chair' for a short time
Cuddling tightly
Star chart

Temper tantrums are ordinary responses to frustration, especially at not being allowed to have or do something. They are common and normal in young preschool children. If asked for advice, a sensible first move is to take a history, analysing a couple of tantrums according to the ABC paradigm (Box 23.8). Next, examine the child to identify potential medical or psychological factors. Medical factors include global or language delay, hearing impairment (e.g. glue ear) and medication with bronchodilators or anticonvulsants. If none are present, there are management strategies that can be adopted, some of which are shown in Box 23.9.

The easiest course of action is to distract the child or, if this cannot be done, to let the tantrum burn itself out while the parent leaves the room, returning a few minutes later when things quieten down. Obviously this should be done in a calm, neutral manner and certainly not accompanied by threats of abandonment. Tantrums which are essentially coercive (when a child is demanding something from a parent) must be met by a refusal to give in. They can often be forestalled by the simple expedient of making rules which the child can be reminded of before the situation presents itself. An alternative course is to use 'time out', which is a form of structured ignoring. The child in a tantrum is placed somewhere such as the hallway where no-one will talk to him for a short time, e.g. 1 minute per year of age. During this period they are ignored completely. Parents often expect this manoeuvre to produce a contrite child, complaining if it does not do so immediately. In fact, it works according to different principles (not as a response to punishment but to the withdrawal of attention) and often takes several weeks to effect a gradual improvement. It may help to ask the mother to keep records to document this.

Disobedience can be dealt with by using a star chart to reward the child for complying with parental requests. The chart needs to be where the child can see it and it must be the case that the child knows what he has to do in order to get a star. It is wisest not to 'fine' the child by taking stars away once they have been earned. If the parent who is rewarding compliance by the child praises at the same time as giving the star, there is not usually any need to tie stars in with a material reward; praise suffices.

For temper tantrums:
- **analyse according to antecedents, behaviour and consequences**
- **consider distraction, avoiding antecedents, ignoring, timeout.**

Aggressive behaviour

Small children can be aggressive for a host of reasons, ranging from spite to exuberance. Much aggressive behaviour is learned, either by being rewarded (often inadvertently) or by copying parents or siblings. For example, many instances of aggressive, demanding behaviour are provoked or intensified by a parent shouting at or hitting their child. In such cases it is the parent's behaviour which needs to change. In most instances, the same principles as apply to tantrums are valid: make rules, stick to them, keep cool, don't give in and use timeout if necessary. The latter can often be used on a 1–2–3 principle (Fig. 23.4). A tired or stressed child will be irritable and prone to angry outbursts, as will children whose communication skills are compromised by deafness or a developmental language disorder so that they are frustrated and exasperated. Optimistic reassurance that the child will spontaneously grow out of a pattern of aggressive behaviour is mistaken; once established, an aggressive behavioural style is remarkably persistent over a period of years.

Autism

This is considered in Chapter 4.

The 1–2–3 principle for tantrums or aggressive behaviour

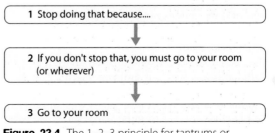

Figure 23.4 The 1–2–3 principle for tantrums or aggressive behaviour.

Problems of middle childhood

Nocturnal enuresis

Children can wet themselves by day or night, but in colloquial speech, 'enuresis' is synonymous with bedwetting. It is quite common: about 6% of 5-year-olds and 3% of 10-year-olds are not dry at night. Boys outnumber girls by nearly 2 to 1. There is a genetically determined delay in acquiring sphincter competence, with two-thirds of children with enuresis having an affected first-degree relative. There may also be interference in learning to become dry at night. Small children need reasonable freedom from stress and a measure of parental approval in order to learn night-time continence. It is well recognised that emotional stress can interfere and cause secondary enuresis (relapse after a period of dryness). Most children with enuresis are psychologically normal and the treatment of secondary enuresis still relies mainly on the symptomatic approach described below, although any underlying stress or emotional disorder must be addressed.

Organic causes of enuresis are uncommon but include:

- urinary tract infection
- faecal retention severe enough to reduce bladder volume and cause bladder neck dysfunction
- polyuria from osmotic diuresis, e.g. diabetes mellitus, or renal concentrating disorders, e.g. chronic renal failure.

A urine sample should always be tested for glucose and protein and checked for infection. Daytime and secondary enuresis are considered in Chapter 18.

The management of nocturnal enuresis is straightforward but needs to be painstaking to succeed. After the age of 4 years, enuresis resolves spontaneously in only 5% of affected children each year. In practice, treatment is rarely undertaken before 6 years of age.

1. Explanation

The first step is to explain to both child and parent that the problem is common and beyond conscious control. The parents should stop punitive procedures, as these are counterproductive.

2. Star chart

The child earns praise and a star each morning if his bed is dry. Wet beds are treated in a matter-of-fact way and the child is not blamed for them.

3. Enuresis alarm

If a child does not respond to a star chart, it may be supplemented with an enuresis alarm. This is a sensor, usually placed in the child's pants, which sounds an alarm when it becomes wet. In order to be effective, the alarm must wake the child, who gets out of bed, goes to pass urine, returns and helps to remake a wet bed before going back to sleep. It is not necessary to reset the alarm that night. Parental help can be enlisted in the night using a baby alarm to transmit the noise of the alarm to the parents' bedroom.

The alarm method takes several weeks to achieve dryness but is effective in most cases so long as the child is motivated and the procedure is fully explained. About one-third relapse after a few months, in which case repeat treatment with the alarm usually produces lasting dryness.

4. Desmopressin

Short-term relief from bedwetting, e.g. for holidays or sleepovers, can be achieved by the use of the synthetic analogue of antidiuretic hormone, desmopressin, taken as tablets or sublingually. This achieves a suppressant effect rather than a lasting cure.

5. Self-help groups, e.g. Enuresis Resource and Information Centre (ERIC)

These provide advice and assistance to parents and health professionals.

> ### Summary
>
> **Nocturnal enuresis:**
> - common, males more than females
> - most affected children are psychologically and physically normal
> - treatment usually considered only at >6 years of age
> - management – explanation, star charts, enuresis alarm, sometimes desmopressin.

Faecal soiling

It is abnormal for a child to soil after the age of 4 years. Thereafter, children who soil fall into two broad groups – those with and those without a rectum loaded with faeces. Because of this, it is important to ascertain whether there is faecal retention by abdominal palpation and by digital anorectal examination if necessary. Faeces in the rectum are always an abnormal finding. The reasons why a child's rectum should become loaded are various and commonly involve an interplay between constitutional factors and experience. Some children have a rectum that only empties occasionally, perhaps because of poor coordination with anal sphincter relaxation, and are thus more prone to developing retention. Superimposed upon this are a number of other factors:

- constipation, possibly following dehydration during an illness
- inhibition of defecation because of pain from a fissure
- inhibition because of fear of punishment for incontinence
- anxieties about using the toilet.

Once established, a huge bolus of hard faeces may be beyond the capacity of the child to shift. Furthermore, a rectum loaded with hard or soft faeces (both are found) dilates and habituates to distension so that the child becomes unaware of the need to empty it. The loaded rectum inhibits the anus via the rectoanal reflex and stool may seep out with spontaneous rectal contractions beyond the child's control. Soiling occurs in the child's pants, which may then be removed and hidden out of shame.

Any reasons for faecal retention, such as an anal fissure, should be identified and treated, but the most important thing is to empty the rectum as soon as possible. The child and parents need to understand that retention is present and how it leads to incontinence.

A stool softener (macrogol, docusate or lactulose) is given for a couple of weeks, followed, if necessary, by oral laxatives (sodium picosulphate or senna) and high volumes of oral macrogol solution. Sometimes an enema is required. Once the child has an empty rectum, he can be encouraged to defecate regularly in the toilet, which earns stars on a star chart. Such retraining may take a number of weeks while the distended rectum shrinks to normal size. Throughout this period a regular laxative is usually needed. The stars may therefore need to be cashed in for tangible rewards such as extra pocket money in order to maintain the incentive.

In some cases, repeated soiling will have been such a humiliating experience for the child that they psychologically deny there is a problem and cooperation is doubtful. Others find that their involuntary soiling allows them a measure of revenge against hostile parents and are reluctant to surrender a useful weapon. Such cases will need psychiatric referral.

Soiling may occur in conjunction with an empty rectum on examination for various other uncommon reasons. Some children have an urgency of defecation for apparently constitutional reasons and can only postpone defecation for a few minutes; they can be taken by surprise. Some children have neuropathic bowel secondary to occult spinal abnormality, usually associated with urinary incontinence. Similarly, diarrhoea can overwhelm bowel control. The child may have a general learning disability with a mental age below 4 years, so that expectations of social bowel control

need to be revised accordingly. Lastly, the child may defecate intentionally as a hostile act. Such children are entrenched in distorted relationships with their parents and require psychiatric referral.

Recurrent unexplained somatic symptoms/somatisation

Recurrent medically unexplained (functional somatic) symptoms are common in childhood and adolescence. In many cases they are aggravated by some kind of stress and they can be the expression of an anxiety or depressive disorder. Somatisation is the term used for the communication of emotional distress, troubled relationships and personal predicaments through bodily symptoms. The prepubertal child may experience affective distress as recurrent abdominal pain (this symptom peaking at age 9 years) and headaches (peaking at age 12 years). With increasing age, limb pain, aching muscles, fatigue and neurological symptoms become more prominent.

Recurrent central abdominal pain, often sharp and colicky, affects about 10% of school-age children. The causes are considered in Chapter 13. In the majority of cases, no organic cause can be objectively demonstrated, yet the child is obviously in pain. Some will have an emotional cause for their pain, but in many, no aetiology, medical or psychiatric, can be demonstrated.

The history must attend to possible sources of stress and the child should be interviewed about school, friends and family, noting the general level of anxiety and ability to communicate. This should be an integral part of the interview and not done as an afterthought when organic causes have been excluded. A thorough physical examination is important to reassure the child and family that there is no underlying organic cause. It also provides an opportunity to gain further information about the nature of the pain and the child's reaction to it. When examining the child, it is sensible to ask him to point to where the pain is. In general, the further the pain is from the umbilicus, the more likely it is being caused by organic pathology (Apley's rule).

The pain may be limited to school days or coincide with upsetting events in the home, such as parental conflict, or other specific situations. A short interview with the child on his own can reveal sources of stress which may be otherwise unrecognised by parents or which the child is wary of mentioning in front of them. Problems at school, particularly bullying and teasing, or difficulties with a teacher or classwork may only be known by the child. A report from the school may be helpful. A joint interview with both parents and the child is a good arena for explaining to the child and family how organic disease has been ruled out and, if appropriate, how tension can give rise to pain using familiar examples such as headache. It is often necessary to promote communication between family members to avoid any tendency for somatic

Summary

Faecal retention:
- is present in most children who soil
- may be due to constipation or reluctance to open the bowels because of pain or reluctance to use the toilet
- when present, the rectum needs to be emptied, initially with a stool softener and laxative followed by retraining.

symptoms to replace verbal communication of distress. Learning pain coping skills such as relaxation may be helpful, especially for headaches. Referral to child and adolescent mental health services is indicated if any identified stressors cannot be relieved by straightforward means, if there is serious family dysfunction, or if the pain impairs the child's general functioning at home or school.

Summary

Somatic symptoms:

- may be a means of communicating emotional distress
- sources of stress should be identified, and ameliorated if possible
- in many children with unexplained recurrent abdominal pain or headaches, no significant sources of stress are identified.

Tics

A tic is a quick, sudden, coordinated movement which is apparently purposeful, recurs in the same part of the child's body and can often be re-produced by the child on request. It is not entirely involuntary in that it can be purposefully suppressed to some extent. About 1 in 10 children develop a tic at some stage, typically around the face and head – blinking, frowning, head-flicking, sniffing, throat clearing and grunting being the commonest. They are most likely to occur when the child is inactive (watching TV or on long car journeys) and often disappear when actively concentrating. They may worsen with anxiety but they are not themselves an emotional reaction. In most cases, there is a family history. These simple, *transient childhood tics* clear up over the next few months, though they may recur from time to time. They should be treated with reassurance in the first place.

Less commonly, the child has tics from which he is hardly ever free. They may be multiple, though there is fluctuation in the predominance of any particular tic and in overall severity. This is a chronic tic disorder which, if it includes both multiple motor tics and vocal tics such as hooting, yelping or swearing, is known as *Gilles de la Tourette's* syndrome. These conditions tend to be persistent in the medium term, requiring medica-tion (such as clonidine, haloperidol or sulpiride) and specialist supervision.

Hyperactivity

Young children are characteristically lively, some more than others, by virtue of their immaturity. When their level of motor activity exceeds that regarded as normal, they may be termed 'hyper-active' by their parents. This is a judgement which depends upon the parents' standards and expec-

tations. The term can thus incorrectly be used as a complaint about a child who is normally active in overall terms but who can be cheeky and boisterous at times. Such a child is *not* hyperactive, but the parents need advice about how to handle unwanted behaviour.

In the true *hyperkinetic disorder*, the child is undoubtedly overactive in most situations and has impaired concentration with a short attention span or distractibility. Because of the latter, the term *attention deficit hyperactivity disorder* (ADHD) has become widely used. Differences in diagnostic criteria mean that prevalence rates among pre-pubertal schoolchildren are variously estimated as between 10 and 50 per 1000 children, boys exceed-ing girls threefold. There is a powerful genetic predisposition and the underlying problem is a dysfunction of brain neuron circuits that rely on dopamine as a neurotransmitter and which control self-monitoring and self-regulation.

Affected children are unable to sustain attention or persist with tasks. They cannot control their impulses – they manifest disorganised, poorly regulated and excessive activity, have difficulty with taking turns, sharing, are socially disinhibited and butt into other people's conversations and play. Their inattention and hyperactivity are worst in familiar or uninteresting situations. They also cannot regulate their activity according to the situation – they are fidgety, have excessive move-ments inappropriate to task completion, lose possessions and are generally disorganised. Typically they have short tempers and form poor relationships with other children, who find them exasperating.

The children do poorly in school and lose self-esteem. They may drift into antisocial activities for a variety of reasons, partly because their behaviour drives parents, teachers and peers to use coercion and punishment which are ineffectual or breed resentment.

The child will usually need to be assessed by an educational psychologist.

First-line management, particularly in preschool children, is the active promotion of behavioural and educational progress by specific advice to parents and teachers to build concentration skills, encourage quiet self-occupation, increase self-esteem and moderate extreme behaviour. Behav-iour modification programmes are used which involve having clear rules and expectations, being consistent and rewarding concentration.

For those children in whom this is insufficient, hyperactivity responds symptomatically to several types of medication, although this is usually reserved for children older than 6 years of age. Stimulants such as methylphenidate or dexamphet-amine channel attention and promote on-task, focused behaviour. The usual approach is not to put the child on medication until behavioural and educational progress is actively promoted by the specific measures mentioned above. It may then be necessary to continue medication for several years, sometimes until the mid-teens. Specialist supervision is mandatory. Close liaison with the school is required throughout the years of treatment.

The role of diet in the cause and management of hyperactivity is controversial. Current evidence indicates that the sort of diet which aims blindly to reduce sugar, artificial additives or colourants has no effect. A few children display an idiosyncratic behavioural reaction such as excitability or irritability to particular foods. If this seems likely, putting the child on an exclusion diet may be useful. Individual foods can be reintroduced while examining for a worsening of behaviour, so that incriminated foods can subsequently be excluded from the child's diet. This is an arduous activity, best implemented by a specialist clinic with supervision from a dietician.

⊙ Summary

Attention deficit hyperactivity disorder (ADHD):
- usually affects preschool children, males more than females
- clinical features – cannot sustain attention, excessively active, socially disinhibited, poor at relationships, prone to temper tantrums, poor school performance
- management – educational psychologist assessment, behaviour modification programmes by parents and teachers, stimulant medication if necessary.

Antisocial behaviour

Children steal, lie, disobey, light fires, destroy things and pick fights for various reasons:

- failure to learn when to exercise social restraint
- lack of social skills, such as the ability to negotiate a disagreement
- they may be responding to the challenges of their peers in spite of their parents' prohibitions
- they may be chronically angry and resentful
- they may find their own notions of good behaviour overwhelmed by emotion such as sadness or temptation.

When serious antisocial behaviour which infringes the rights of others is the dominant feature of the clinical picture and is so severe as to represent a handicap to general functioning, a diagnosis of *conduct disorder* is made. Children with conduct disorder have not necessarily broken the law, although their behaviour excites strong social disapproval. They typically come from homes in which there is considerable discord between family members, especially between the child and his parents. A milder form, characterised by angry, defiant behaviour to authority figures such as parents and teachers, is known as *oppositional-defiant disorder (ODD)*.

Treating conduct disorder can be difficult, not least because parental cooperation is often minimal. It involves a combination of training techniques for parents, family therapy and behaviour therapy and is a task for a mental health professional. Medication has little part to play. The most promising way of helping is by early intervention through intensive parenting programmes for parents of preschool children with oppositional defiant disorder.

Anxiety

Pathological anxiety exists in two forms: specific and general. In phobias there is fear of a specific object or situation which is excessive and handicapping and cannot be dealt with by reassurance. Most children have a number of irrational fears (the dark, ghosts, kidnappers, dogs, spiders, bats, snakes) which are common and do not usually handicap the child's ordinary life. Some of these persist into adulthood. If they are so severe that the child's ability to lead an ordinary life is affected, then treatment by behavioural therapy with exposure to the feared event may be indicated and is usually successful.

More diffuse general anxiety presents indirectly in childhood and it is rare for a child to complain directly about anxiety. Often, it is first manifest as physical complaints: nausea, headache or pain. It may take the form of hypochondriasis and the child repeatedly asks for reassurance that he is not going to die. Some children with generalised anxiety are strikingly manipulative, attempting to gain control over their parents and the world in general so that they can feel less fearful. It may be a justifiable reaction to an event or situation, or be disproportionate. If the condition follows a recognisable precipitant such as a parental illness and the parents can be directed to provide comfort and support, prognosis is good. If it arises insidiously, specialist mental health referral is indicated.

🌼 **Children rarely say spontaneously that they are anxious – instead they tend to complain of aches and pains or behave manipulatively.**

School refusal

During the years of compulsory school attendance, a child may be absent from school because of illness, because his parents keep him off school or because of truancy in which the child chooses to do something else rather than attend school. In truancy a child leaves to go to school but never arrives or leaves early. It is often accompanied by other behavioural difficulties. A few non-attenders at school suffer from *school refusal*, an inability to attend school on account of overwhelming anxiety. Such children may not complain of anxiety but of its physical concomitants or the consequences of hyperventilation. Anxiety may present as complaints of nausea, headache or otherwise not being well, which are confined to weekday, term-time mornings, clearing up by midday. It may

Box 23.10 Treatment of school refusal

Advise and support parents and school about the condition

Treat any underlying emotional disorder

Plan and facilitate an early and graded return to school at a pace tolerable for the child with all involved (child, family, teachers, educational psychologist and educational welfare officers)

Help the parents make it more rewarding for the child to return to school than stay at home

Address bullying or educational difficulties if present

Box 23.11 Causes of underachievement at school

Long-standing problem
Visual problems
Hearing problems
Dyslexia
Generalised specific learning problems
Hyperactivity
Anti-education family background
Chaotic family background

Recent onset of problem
Preoccupations (parental divorce, bullying, etc.)
Fatigue
Depression
Rebellion against teacher, parents or 'swot' label
Unsuspected poor attendance at school
Sexual abuse
Drug abuse
Schizophrenia (rare)
Degenerative brain condition, rare but important

be rational, as when the child is being bullied or there is educational underachievement. If it is disproportionate to stresses at school, it is termed school refusal, an anxiety problem with two common causes – separation anxiety from parents persisting beyond the toddler years and anxiety provoked by some aspect of school, true school phobia. These can coexist.

School refusal based on separation anxiety is typical of children under the age of about 11 years. It may be provoked by an adverse life event such as illness, a death in the family or a move of house. The child is unable to tolerate separation from his attachment figure without whom he cannot go anywhere, including school. Treatment is aimed at gently promoting increasing separations from the parents (e.g. staying overnight with relatives or friends) whilst arranging an early return to school. Some adolescents with school refusal have a depressive disorder, but more usually there is an interaction between an anxiety disorder and long-standing personality issues such as intolerance of uncertainty.

True school phobia is seen in slightly older, anxious children who are frequently uncommunicative and stubborn.

The management of school refusal is shown in Box 23.10.

Educational underachievement

Children who achieve less well in school than expected are sometimes brought to doctors. It is important to evaluate parents' and teachers' expectations and ensure the child is actually able to rise to them. The services of an educational psychologist are indispensable. Core medical responsibilities include testing sight and hearing and attempting to elicit the cause of underachievement according to the list in Box 23.11. The topic is considered further in Chapter 4.

Adolescence

Although a popular image of adolescence is one of angry, rebellious teenagers, alienated from their parents and embroiled in emotional turmoil, studies show that most adolescents maintain good relationships with their parents. They do, though, tend to bicker with them about minor domestic matters and what they are allowed to do. Minor psychological symptoms such as moodiness or social sensitivity are quite common (as they are in adults), but serious psychiatric problems are no more prevalent than in adult life. Family relationships are often influenced by teenagers' negotiation of their own autonomy, the emergence of their own sense of themselves and the first moves towards a personal identity. At the same time their parents may be experiencing mid-life crises of confidence in career, physical appearance or sexuality, so that parental and teenage preoccupations coincide, not always helpfully.

Cognitive style

The style of thought specifically associated with adolescence is formal operational (abstract) thought (Box 23.12), but this is acquired at various ages by different individuals during the teenage years, and a substantial minority seem never to develop it at all. Doctors are at a disadvantage here as they have been selected by a series of examinations for excellence of their ability to manipulate abstractions and compare hypothetical predictions; they have often forgotten what it is like to think otherwise and communicate poorly with patients who still think concretely and practically (school-age children, about half of all teenagers and perhaps 1 in 5 adults). When interviewing adolescents, the skill is to avoid being patronising while being sensitive as to whether abstract and reflective thought is solidly achieved. Using practical examples (not metaphors) and checking whether you have been understood will help to avoid the common problem of being faced with an adolescent who responds to ques-

Box 23.12 Formal operational thought

The ability to form abstract thoughts
Comparing implications of hypotheses
Thinking about one's own thinking
Testing the logic that links propositions
Manipulating interactive abstract concepts

tions with a sullen 'don't know'. This is considered further in Chapter 28.

Anorexia nervosa

Dieting to slim is endemic among teenage girls. Part of the reason for this is the contemporary equation between thinness and attractiveness, an assumption prevalent in advertising and fashion. Resonant with this is the finding that most teenage girls (but very few boys) overestimate their body width and depth, perceiving and judging themselves as fatter than they actually are.

Slimming through self-imposed calorie restriction is usually self-limiting because the goal is achieved or because the girl gives up; hunger wins through. In some girls, however, the slimming process takes over and there supervenes what has been called a 'relentless pursuit of thinness', typically with a phobic horror of normal body weight and shape. This is *anorexia nervosa*, and the features are:

- A distorted perception of her body which increases with weight loss.
- A determined attempt to lose weight or avoid weight gain, by either restricting food intake, self-induced vomiting, laxative abuse, excessive exercising or using a combination of these methods.
- When body weight falls below a critical point (about 48 kg) pubertal development is halted and reversed so that menstruation ceases and the girl effectively becomes a prepubertal child. This may spare her some of the challenges of adolescence, particularly those related to sexuality.
- The discovery by a girl who has felt powerless that through self-starvation she can control her shape and development and thus increase her sense of self-worth and self-effectiveness.
- Preoccupations and dreams of food and cooking which come to dominate mental life as a response to starvation. There ensues a tremendous mental struggle not to give in and eat, which assumes prime importance in the girl's mental life.
- The dramatic and visible effects of self-starvation on the girl which can unite some parents in caring for their daughter and save a discordant marriage from divorce, something which she may fear is imminent.

An affected girl will often deny hunger, reassure everyone that she is in the peak of health, exercise to lose weight and disagree fervently that she is too thin. She will be careless of her own emaciation and seem unconcerned that she is starving herself to death. To the bewilderment of her parents, she may cook for others and read cookery books avidly. She may well be deceitful to anyone she perceives as thwarting her in her quest. Thus she will conceal her poor eating by secretly disposing of her meals or lying about her weight. Both before and during her illness she will show obsessional, perfectionistic character traits; without these she would not have the capacity to establish herself as a persistent dieter. Indeed, she is likely to be described as having been quiet, compliant and hard-working, 'the last person to develop anorexia nervosa'. Her parents will often present as nice people who avoid conflict.

As a result of starvation, her body develops a low metabolic rate with slow-to-relax tendon reflexes, reduced peripheral circulation, bradycardia and amenorrhoea. Fine lanugo hair appears over her trunk and limbs. She does not lose pubic or axillary hair, although incompletely established puberty is delayed. Serum T3 may be low, giving rise to a false suspicion of hypothyroidism. Plasma proteins are sometimes low and ankle oedema not uncommon. Blood and urine levels of luteinising hormone and follicle-stimulating hormone are low and non-cyclical.

Some girls discover that self-restraint in carbohydrate intake can be bypassed by self-induced vomiting following repeated bouts of over-eating and that weight can be lost through diuretics. Some take laxatives in the belief that these will remove the food they have eaten. This can cause wide fluctuations in weight and metabolic abnormalities such as hypokalaemia and alkalosis. This condition is *bulimia* which can occur at normal body weight or in association with low body weight as an ominous complication of anorexia nervosa. It tends to affect older rather than younger teenagers. Bulimia at normal body weight can be managed by encouraging a regular diet, monitoring this by a diary and providing individual or group psychotherapy.

The prevalence rate among teenagers for anorexia nervosa is a little less than 1%, but the incidence rate may have increasing over the last 50 years. The peak age of onset is 14 and girls outnumber boys by about 10 : 1. Bulimia is commoner, although prevalence rates vary widely depending on the degree of severity. It also shows a markedly female preponderance and may also be becoming more frequent.

Management

The initial management of anorexia nervosa is to restore near-normal body weight by refeeding. The corner stone of treatment is parental counselling, often as part of family therapy, in which the seriousness of the situation is explained. The parents are helped to take complete responsibility for their child's health until she is ready to take more responsibility for herself. Management is preferably as an outpatient. The girl's weight, not

Adolescence

399

her eating, is monitored and a gain of about 500 g a week is required. Failure to meet this target results in admission to hospital for refeeding with no appeal or bargaining accepted. Good nursing is the key to this, but a small number of girls continue to lose weight in hospital so that tube-feeding may be required. An initial daily dietary intake of about 2000 calories is adopted, as trying to enforce large meals is usually unsuccessful. A more psycho-therapeutic approach may be introduced when her weight has reached the level it was before dieting started. It is aimed at counselling the girl and her family in more constructive ways of confronting developmental demands, including handling conflict, maintaining self-esteem, personal autonomy and relationships.

The prognosis for children and adolescents is unsatisfactory, with as many as 50% failing to make a full recovery. Factors predicting a better outcome include a good parental relationship and an ability on the child's part to express previously suppressed negative emotions. Approximately 5% die by suicide, malnutrition or infection, though usually not until later in life.

Summary

In anorexia nervosa:
- female : male ratio is 10 : 1
- peak age of onset – 14 years
- affected girls have a distorted body image, so seldom agree that they are too thin and may deceive everyone by pretending to eat
- features include – determined efforts to lose weight, arrest of puberty, cessation of periods
- may be accompanied by bulimia – overeating followed by self-induced vomiting
- management is parental counselling to restore body weight
- some require hospitalisation; prognosis is variable, but has a mortality from suicide, malnutrition and infection

Chronic fatigue syndrome

Chronic fatigue syndrome (CFS) refers to persisting high levels of subjective fatigue leading to rapid exhaustion on minimal physical or mental exertion. The term is broader and more neutral than the specific pathology or aetiology implied by myalgic encephalomyelitis (ME) or postviral fatigue syndrome, which follows an apparently viral febrile illness. There is sometimes serological evidence of recent infection with coxsackie B or Epstein–Barr virus (EBV) or a hepatitis virus. Some cases have no history or evidence of a precipitating infection and there are no specific diagnostic tests. The clinical picture is somewhat diffuse and there are no pathognomonic symptoms. Myalgia, migratory arthralgia, headache, difficulty getting off to sleep, poor concentration and irritability are virtually universal. Stomach pains, scalp tenderness, eye pain and photophobia, and tender cervical lymph-adenopathy are frequently encountered. Depressive symptoms are common and there is continuing debate as to how much of the clinical picture is physical and how much psychological. Usually parents insist on there being a physical cause and there is a risk that the doctor will carry out excessive unprofitable investigations. Most experienced doctors now regard the final clinical picture as resulting from both physical and psychological factors.

The majority of cases will remit spontaneously with time, but this takes months or sometimes years. Earlier recommendations of continuous rest have been shown to be unhelpful and can lead to secondary complications. The preferred approach is to adopt gentle rehabilitation, possibly involving physiotherapy, so that exercise tolerance is gradually increased. If too much pressure is put upon the child, tantrums or mute withdrawal can occur. Argument about how much of the condition is physical and how much psychological is unhelpful. The parents and the child need continuing support to maintain as much of a normal life as possible, including school attendance. The mood of children with depressive symptoms may respond to antidepressant medication, but this is a treatment only for depressive symptoms and it is unlikely to result in alleviation of the fatigability.

Summary

In chronic fatigue syndrome:
- there is exhaustion on minimal exertion
- there is thought to be a combination of physical and psychological factors
- management is with gradual rehabilitation, but may take months or years.

Depression

Low mood can arise secondary to adverse circumstances or sometimes spontaneously. Depression as a clinical condition is more than sadness and misery; it extends to affect motivation, judgement, the ability to experience pleasure and provokes emotions of guilt and despair. It may disturb sleep, appetite and weight. It leads to social withdrawal; an important sign. Such a state is well recognised among adolescents, particularly girls, but occasionally affects prepubertal children. The general picture is comparable to depression in adults but there are differences (Box 23.13).

A diagnosis of depression depends crucially upon interviewing the adolescent on his own as well as taking a history from the parents. Teenagers will, out of loyalty, often pretend to their parents that things are all right if interviewed in their presence. It is necessary to ask about feelings directly and to ask specifically about suicidal ideas and plans.

Treatment depends upon the relationship between low mood and causal circumstances.

Adversity such as bullying should be reversed if possible. If this cannot be done, as in the case of impending parental divorce, then counselling using cognitive behavioural approaches where links are made between feelings, thoughts and behaviour have been shown to help. If therapy is insufficient and the depression is severe, then an SSRI (selective serotonin reuptake inhibitor antidepressant), fluoxetine, is indicated. Suicidal teenagers need admission to a psychiatric in-patient unit.

Deliberate self-harm

Like adults, teenagers who take overdoses do so for a variety of motives, of which suicide is only one. For a high proportion, the overdose is a blind and desperate gesture which may draw attention to a predicament perceived by them as irresolvable. Issues such as bullying or abuse should be considered. About half of teenagers who overdose are clinically depressed. Episodes of deliberate self-harm must be taken seriously as they carry significant risk of recurrence.

A useful aid to assess suicide risk is the PATHOS score shown in Box 23.14.

Drug misuse

Most teenagers are exposed to illicit drugs at some stage. A number will then experiment with them, some becoming habitual users. Usually this is for recreational purposes, but a few use them to avoid unpleasant feelings or memories. A very small number become dependent, psychologically or physically. What is taken varies with culture and opportunity but alcohol and cannabis are common; solvents, LSD, ecstasy and amphetamine derivatives somewhat less so; and cocaine or heroin currently least prevalent though their use is increasing. The addictive potential of the last two is the greatest and their dangers are well known.

Abuse implies heavy misuse. The signs vary with the agent but include:

- intoxication
- unexplained absences from home or school
- mixing with known users
- high rates of spending or stealing money
- possession of the equipment required for ingestion
- medical complications associated with use.

Doctors may be asked by worried parents whether an adolescent is abusing and the question can often only be resolved by interviewing the adolescent, possibly combined with taking a urine sample for drug screening. Medical involvement is predominantly focused on solitary users, who usually have other psychopathology including depression, or with the physical consequences of intoxication or injection when these threaten health. Solvent abuse (mainly glue and aerosol sniffing) is quite widespread as a group activity of young adolescents in some areas and is usually of no more consequence than under-age drinking. It can occasionally give rise to cardiac dysrhythmias, bone marrow suppression or renal failure, and any of these can cause death, as may a fall when intoxicated. Cannabis and LSD use is usually not dangerous, but in a few adolescents they trigger anxiety or psychotic disorders. Ecstasy taken at dances or raves can cause dangerous hyperthermia and dehydration.

Doctors need to ensure that any adolescent known to them who is thought to be using drugs knows the specific risks to health. Dependence is rare among teenagers and most likely to involve alcohol. The few who are using illicit drugs for respite from psychological distress need referral to a psychiatrist.

Psychosis

Psychosis is a breakdown in the appreciation of reality and a lack of insight that anything is wrong. This can effect ideas and beliefs resulting in delusional thinking where abnormal beliefs are held with an unshakeable quality and lead to odd behaviour. The connectedness and coherence of thoughts may break down, so that speech is hard to follow, leading to thought disorder. Perceptual abnormalities lead to hallucinations where a perception is experienced in the absence of a stimulus.

Psychotic disorders include:

* schizophrenia, where no specific medical cause is identified and there is generally no major disturbance of mood other than blunting or flattening of affect
* bipolar affective disorder, where the psychosis is associated with a mood disorder be it lowered mood as in depression or elevation in mood as in mania.
* organic psychosis including delirium, substance-induced disorders and dementia.

Both schizophrenia and bipolar affective disorder are rare before puberty but increase in frequency of presentation during adolescence. In these disorders the psychotic symptoms occur in clear consciousness.

Investigations should include a urine drug screen, exclusion of medication-induced psychosis (e.g. high-dose stimulants or anticholinergic drugs), exclusion of medical causes (i.e. infection, seizures, thyroid abnormalities and sleep disorders) and dementia.

Where schizophrenia, bipolar disorder or organic psychosis is suspected, referral to a psychiatrist is needed for comprehensive treatment with antipsychotic medication, psychoeducation, family therapy and where appropriate individual therapy.

> **Psychosis:**
> * **may present during adolescence**
> * **may be precipitated by or be a consequence of substance abuse.**

Management of emotional and behavioural problems

For most emotional and behavioural problems, there is an interplay between adversities in the family, peer group and school, and strengths or vulnerabilities in the child. Sometimes these are referred to as risk (predisposing) factors: things that do not in themselves produce a disorder but will do so when interacting with other adversities. Conversely, they are less likely to do so if there is a compensating strength (such as high intelligence, good self-esteem, secure attachment, good peer relations or an emotionally warm relationship with a parent). An environmental adversity may be acute (a life event) or chronic. It challenges the coping skills of the child, and a resulting emotional or behavioural problem results if these are overwhelmed. The problem may resolve spontaneously or persist.

With this in mind, it is possible to talk about the three Ps of causation:

* predisposition (vulnerability)
* precipitation
* perpetuation.

In clinical practice, a precipitant is what many people call the 'cause', but it is often the factors that perpetuate or maintain the problem that one has to deal with.

Assessment

It is best to interview both parents if possible. While doing so, consider the quality of their marriage and the parents' mental state. Ask open questions where possible and feel able to ask directly about feelings. Assess the attitudes of the parents to the child. Obtain examples of the problem and estimate its frequency, severity, duration and the impact it has on both the child and family.

Interview the child alone if it seems appropriate. Explain to the parents that you always like to have a few words with children on their own as you are their doctor too. Assess the extent of the child's suffering (they may be somewhat brazen and minimise this). Keep your questions very simple and specific, making sure the child understands what it is you want to know. This also applies to teenagers. Consider whether reports from school or other involved agencies might help. In many instances, it is worth asking the parents to keep a prospective record of the problem by means of a diary or chart which you can inspect in a few days' time. Tell them what headings you want this under (such as 'antecedents, behaviour and consequences' for temper tantrums).

Management

Figure 23.5 shows an approach to managing a child displaying an emotional or behavioural problem. The process of making a referral to a child and adolescent mental health service (CAMHS) is most likely to succeed if the referrer has already taken some of the history and engaged the parents and child in an attempt to alleviate the problem. Many doctors, general practitioners and paediatricians, in particular, are good generalists in child mental health issues and the mental health specialist should be seen as a specialist extension of their expertise, rather than a completely different sort of person.

In general, the management of children's emotional and behavioural problems:

* is psychological rather than pharmacological
* does not need the child to be admitted to hospital
* involves parents as key participants
* may involve a variety of health and social service professionals.

Often more than one intervention is required so that treatments are combined and several professionals

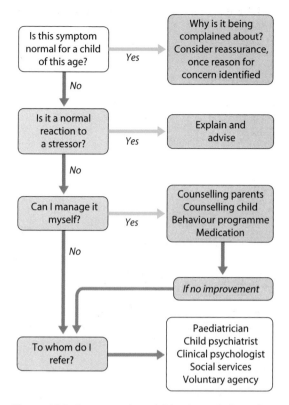

Figure 23.5 An approach to children's psychological problems.

become involved. The main treatment interventions employed are described in Box 23.15.

Medication plays a comparatively small role, although particular instances for which there is evidence for their efficacy are the use of stimulant drugs in hyperkinetic disorder (ADHD) and antidepressants for depressed adolescents. There is sometimes a temptation to sedate a child who is causing a problem but this is rarely effective and ethically questionable.

Further reading

Garralda M E, Hyde C (eds) 2003 Managing children with psychiatric problems, 2nd edn. BMJ, London.

Lask B, Taylor S, Nunn K 2003 Practical child psychiatry. BMJ Books, London.

Spender Q, Salt N, Dawkins J, Kendrick T, Hill P 2001 Child mental health in primary care. Radcliffe Medical Press, Oxford.

Box 23.15 Main psychological treatment interventions employed for emotional and behaviour problems.

Explanation and reassurance
Suitable for mild problems with a good prognosis arising in children from supportive families who can work out for themselves a sensible way of managing the problem until it subsides.

Counselling of child or parents
Used to modify attitudes and habits of thought. A child with a difficult temperament would be an indication for parental counselling; adolescents who are anxiously hypochondriacal could be counselled themselves.

In parental counselling the aim is to enhance parental coping not by telling the parent what to do but by helping them to find their own solutions, so increasing their confidence and effectiveness.

Parenting groups
Recently parenting groups have become popular where a number of parents are seen together and given tools on how to play as well as respond to their children's challenging behaviour. Various approaches are rehearsed using role play and the facilitation of a therapist.

Behaviour therapy
Uses a pragmatic approach to problems which alters the environmental factors which trigger or maintain behaviours. It is particularly effective in the management of behaviour problems in young children.

Family therapy
Has become widely used by child mental health professionals. It uses a series of interviews with the entire household to alter dysfunctional patterns of relationships between family members on the basis that many children's problems are perpetuated by the ways in which family members live with and deal with each other.

Cognitive therapy
Used by specialists to explore the way thinking affects feelings and behaviour in order to alter the way teenagers judge themselves in relation to a situation. Good evidence for efficacy in a range of disorders including depression.

Individual or group dynamic psychotherapy
More structured and intense extension of counselling which can help children who, for example, have emotional conflicts which are manifest as relationship difficulties with a parent. Once the mainstay of child psychiatry, it is now more sparingly used.

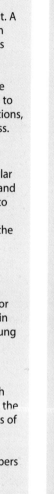

Management of emotional and behavioural problems

Skin

The newborn

The skin at birth is covered with vernix caseosa. This whitish greasy coat is produced by epithelial cell breakdown and, in utero, protects the skin from the amniotic fluid. In the preterm infant, the skin is thin, poorly keratinised and lacks subcutaneous fat. Transepidermal water loss is markedly increased when compared with a term infant. The preterm infant is also unable to sweat until a few weeks old, whereas the term infant can sweat from birth.

Common birthmarks and rashes in the newborn period are described under the examination of the newborn infant (see Ch. 9). Some less common skin conditions presenting in the newborn period are described in this chapter.

Bullous impetigo

This is an uncommon but potentially serious blistering form of impetigo, seen particularly in the newborn (Fig. 24.1). It is most often caused by phage group II strains of *Staphylococcus*

aureus. Treatment is with systemic antibiotics, e.g. penicillinase-resistant penicillin (see also Ch. 14).

Melanocytic naevi (moles)

Congenital moles occur in up to 3% of neonates and any that are present are usually small. Melanocytic naevi become increasingly common as children get older and the presence of large numbers in an adult may be indicative of childhood sun exposure. Prolonged exposure to sunlight should be avoided and sunscreen preparations with a sun protection factor exceeding 20 should be applied liberally to exposed skin in bright weather and reapplied every few hours.

Congenital pigmented naevi involving extensive areas of skin (i.e. naevi more than 9 cm in diameter) are rare but disfiguring (Fig. 24.2) and carry a 4–6% lifetime risk of subsequent malignant melanoma. They require prompt referral to a paediatric dermatologist and plastic surgeon to assess the feasibility of removal. Malignant melanoma is rare before puberty except in such giant naevi. However, in adults, the incidence of malignant melan-

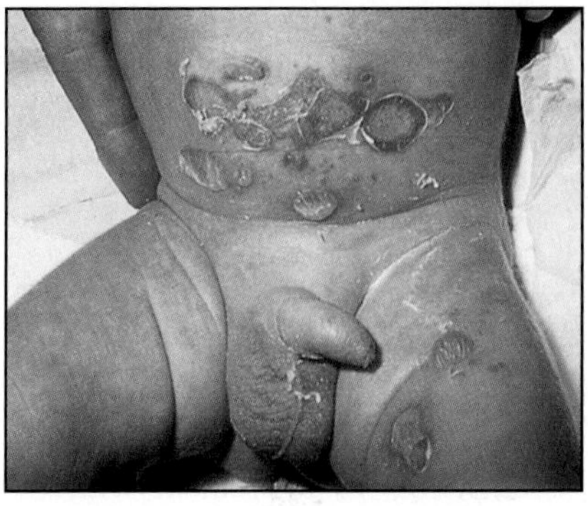

Figure 24.1 Bullous impetigo in a newborn infant.

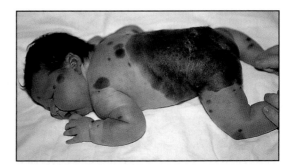

Figure 24.2 A large (giant) congenital pigmented hairy naevus. Many other smaller naevi are also visible.

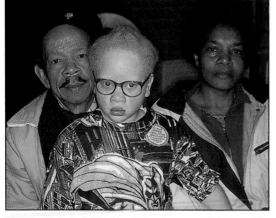

Figure 24.3 A child with oculocutaneous albinism with her parents.

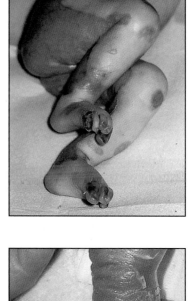

Figure 24.4
Severe, autosomal recessive form of epidermolysis bullosa.

Figure 24.5
Collodion membrane peeling in a newborn infant.

oma has increased dramatically over the past 30 years. Risk factors for melanoma include a positive family history, having a large number of melanocytic naevi, fair skin, repeated episodes of sunburn, and living in a hot climate with chronic skin exposure to the sun.

Parents should prevent their children becoming sunburnt.

Albinism

This is due to a defect in biosynthesis and distribution of melanin. The albinism may be oculo-cutaneous, ocular or partial, depending on the distribution of depigmentation in the skin and eye (Fig. 24.3). The lack of pigment in the iris, retina, eyelids and eyebrows results in failure to develop a fixation reflex. There is pendular nystagmus and photophobia, which causes a constant frowning. No treatment is available, but correction of refractive errors and tinted lenses may be helpful. In a few children, the fitting of tinted contact lenses from early infancy allows the development of normal fixation. The disorder is an important cause of severe visual impairment. The pale skin is prone to sunburn and skin cancer. In sunlight, a hat should be worn and high factor barrier cream applied to the skin.

Epidermolysis bullosa

This is a rare group of conditions with over 20 subtypes, characterised by blistering of the skin and mucous membranes. Autosomal dominant variants tend to be milder; autosomal recessive variants may be severe and even fatal. Blisters occur spontaneously or following minor trauma (Fig. 24.4). They need to be differentiated from scalds. Management is directed to avoiding injury from even minor skin trauma and treating secondary infection. In the severe forms, the fingers and toes may become fused, and contractures of the limbs develop from repeated blistering and healing. Mucous membrane involvement may result in oral ulceration and

stenosis from oesophageal erosions. Management, including maintenance of adequate nutrition, should be by a multidisciplinary team including a paediatric dermatologist, paediatrician, plastic surgeon and dietician.

Collodion baby

This is a rare manifestation of the inherited ichthyoses, a group of conditions in which the skin is dry and scaly. Infants are born with a taut parchment-like or collodion-like membrane (Fig. 24.5). Emollients are usually applied to moisturise and soften the skin. The membrane becomes fissured and separates within a few weeks, leaving either normal or ichthyotic skin.

Rashes of infancy

Napkin rashes

Napkin rashes are common, although irritant reactions are much less of a problem with the widespread use of disposable nappies, as they are

Box **24.1** Causes of napkin rashes

Common	Rare
Irritant (contact) dermatitis	Acrodermatitis enteropathica (see p. 221)
Infantile seborrhoeic dermatitis	Langerhans cell histiocytosis (Letterer–Siwe disease) (see p. 359)
Candida infection	Wiskott–Aldrich syndrome (see p. 259)
Atopic eczema	

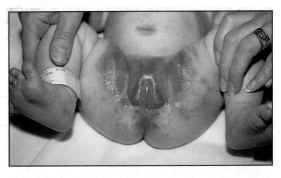

Figure 24.6 Napkin rash due to *Candida* infection. The skin flexures are involved and there may be satellite pustules.

more absorbent. Some causes are listed in Box 24.1. Irritant dermatitis, the most common napkin rash, may occur if nappies are not changed frequently enough or if the infant has diarrhoea. However, irritant dermatitis can occur even when the napkin area is cleaned regularly. The rash is due to the irritant effect of urine on the skin of susceptible infants. Urea-splitting organisms in faeces increase the alkalinity and likelihood of a rash.

The irritant eruption affects the convex surfaces of the buttocks, perineal region, lower abdomen and top of thighs. Characteristically, the flexures are spared, which differentiates it from other causes of napkin rash. The rash is erythematous and may have a scalded appearance. More severe forms are associated with erosions and ulcer formation. Mild cases respond to the use of a protective emollient, whereas more severe cases may require mild topical corticosteroids. While leaving the child without a napkin will accelerate resolution, it is rarely practical at home.

Candida infection may cause and often complicates napkin rashes. The rash is erythematous, includes the skin flexures and there may be satellite lesions (Fig. 24.6). Treatment is with a topical antifungal agent.

Infantile seborrhoeic dermatitis

This eruption of unknown cause presents in the first 2 months of life. It starts on the scalp as an erythematous scaly eruption. The scales form a thick yellow adherent layer, commonly called cradle-cap (Fig. 24.7a). The scaly rash may spread to

the face, behind the ears and then extend to the flexures and napkin area (Fig. 24.7b). In contrast to atopic eczema, it is not itchy and the child is unperturbed by it. However, it is associated with an increased risk of subsequently developing atopic eczema. Mild cases will resolve with emollients. The scales on the scalp can be cleared with an ointment containing low concentration sulphur and salicylic acid applied to the scalp daily for a few hours and then washed off. Widespread body eruption will clear with a mild topical corticosteroid, either alone or mixed with an antibacterial and antifungal agent if appropriate.

Atopic eczema

The prevalence of atopic eczema in children is 12–20%. Its onset is usually in the first year of life. It is, however, uncommon in the first 2 months, unlike infantile seborrhoeic dermatitis, which is relatively common at this age. There is often a family history of atopic disorders – eczema, asthma, allergic rhinitis (e.g. hay fever). Up to 50% of children with atopic eczema will develop asthma or hay fever. Exclusive breast-feeding may delay the onset of eczema in predisposed children but does not alter the natural history of the disorder. Atopic eczema is mainly a disease of childhood, being most severe and troublesome in the first year of life and resolving in 50% by 12 years of age, and in 75% by 16 years.

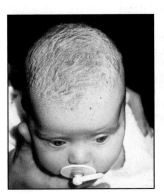

(a)

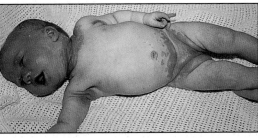

(b)

Figure 24.7 Infantile seborrhoeic dermatitis. **(a)** Cradle cap. **(b)** Distribution on the scalp and face, behind the ears, flexures and nappy area.

Itching

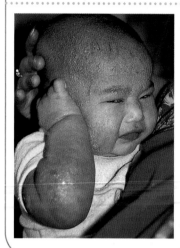

Figure 24.8 Excoriation of the skin from scratching. Itch is the key clinical feature in eczema at all ages, leading to an 'itch–scratch–itch' cycle. It is 'the itch that rashes' in atopic eczema.

Box 24.2 Some causes of itchy rashes

Atopic eczema
Chickenpox
Urticaria/allergic reactions
Contact dermatitis
Insect bites/papular urticaria
Scabies
Fungal infections
Pityriasis rosea

No itch? – then it's not eczema.

Diagnosis

The diagnosis is made clinically. If tested, most affected children have an elevated total plasma IgE level. If there is a history to suggest a particular allergic cause, skin prick and radioallergosorbent (RAST) tests may be helpful in the older child. If the disease is unusually severe, atypical or associated with unusual infections or failure to thrive, an immune deficiency disorder should be excluded.

Clinical features

Rashes may itch in many conditions (Box 24.2), but in atopic eczema (Fig. 24.8) itching is the main symptom at all ages and this results in scratching and exacerbation of the rash. The excoriated areas become erythematous, weeping and crusted. Distribution of the eruption tends to change with age, as indicated in Figure 24.9. Atopic skin is usually dry, and prolonged scratching and rubbing of the skin may lead to lichenification, in which there is accentuation of the normal skin markings (Fig. 24.10).

Complications

Causes of exacerbations of eczema are listed in Box 24.3. However, flare-ups are common, often for no obvious reason. Eczematous skin can readily become infected, usually with *Staphylococcus* or *Streptococcus*. Inflammation increases the avidity of skin for *Staph. aureus* and reduces the expression of antimicrobial peptides which are needed to control microbial infections. *Staph. aureus* thrives on atopic skin and releases superantigens which seem to maintain and worsen eczema. Herpes simplex virus infection, although less frequent, is potentially very serious as it can spread rapidly on atopic skin, causing an extensive vesicular reaction, eczema herpeticum (see Ch. 14). Lymphadeno-pathy is common with active eczema and usually resolves when the skin improves.

Management

A number of treatment modalities are available.

Avoiding irritants and precipitants

It is advisable to avoid soap and biological detergents. Clothing next to the skin should be of pure cotton where possible, avoiding nylon and pure woollen garments. Nails need to be cut short to reduce skin damage from scratching, and mittens at night may be helpful in the very young. When an allergen such as cow's milk has been proven to be a precipitant, it should be avoided.

Emollients

These are the mainstay of management, moisturising and softening the skin. They should be applied liberally two or more times a day and after a bath. They include aqueous cream BP or ointments such as one containing equal parts of white soft paraffin and liquid paraffin. Ointments are preferable to creams when the skin is very dry. A daily bath using an emollient oil as a soap substitute is also beneficial.

Topical corticosteroids

These are an effective treatment for eczema, but must be used with care. Mildly potent corticosteroids, such as 1% hydrocortisone ointment, can be applied to the eczematous areas twice daily. Moderately potent topical steroids play a pivotal role in the management of acute exacerbations, but their use must be kept to a minimum and use on the face generally avoided. Excessive use of topical steroids may cause thinning of the skin as well as systemic side-effects. However, fear of these side-

Eczema

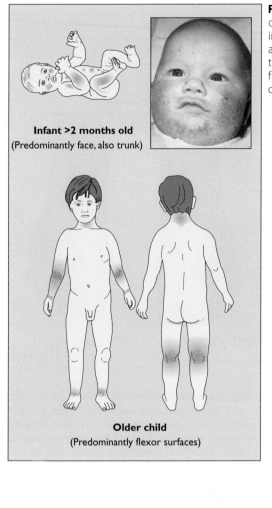

Infant >2 months old
(Predominantly face, also trunk)

Older child
(Predominantly flexor surfaces)

Figure 24.9 Distribution of atopic eczema. The distribution of eczema tends to change with age. In infants, the face and scalp are prominently affected, although the trunk may be involved. In older children, the skin flexures (cubital and popliteal fossae) and frictional areas, such as the neck, wrists and ankles, are characteristically involved.

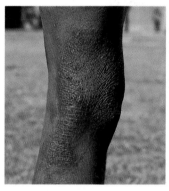

Figure 24.10 Lichenification. Thickening of the skin with accentuation of skin creases from persistent scratching.

Box 24.3 Causes of exacerbation of eczema

Bacterial infection, e.g. *Staphylococcus*, *Streptococcus* spp
Viral infection, e.g. herpes simplex virus
Ingestion of an allergen, e.g. egg
Contact with an irritant or allergen
Environment – heat, humidity
Change or reduction in medication
Psychological stress
Unexplained

---

effects should not deter their use in controlling exacerbations.

Immunomodulators

In children over 2 years old, short-term topical use of tacrolimus or pimecrolimus may be indicated to avoid or reduce use of topical corticosteroids.

Occlusive bandages

These are helpful over limbs when scratching and lichenification are a problem. They may be impregnated with zinc paste or zinc and tar paste. The bandages are worn overnight or for 2–3 days at a time until the skin has improved. For widespread itching in young children, wet stockinette wraps may be helpful; diluted topical steroids mixed with emollient are applied to the skin and damp wraps fashioned for trunk and limbs are then applied with overlying dry wraps or clothes.

Antibiotics or antiviral agents

Antibiotics with hydrocortisone can be applied topically for mildly infected eczema. Systemic antibiotics are indicated for more widespread or severe infection. Eczema herpeticum is treated with systemic aciclovir.

H_1 histamine antagonists

Itch suppression is with an oral antihistamine. The newer antihistamines are not sedative.

Dietary elimination

Food allergy may occur in some infants with eczema. Food allergens include cow's milk, egg and soya. However, any food may be implicated in an eczema flare-up. Dietary elimination should be considered if there is a strong suggestive history and skin and blood tests are positive. Dietary elimination for 4–6 weeks is usually required to detect a response. This should be carried out with

Summary

Assessment of the child with eczema

Condition of the skin
Distribution of the eczema, is the skin excoriated, weeping, crusted, lichenified?
How troublesome is the itching?
Worse or better than usual?
What causes exacerbation - food or other allergens, irritants, medications, stress?
Does it disturb sleep?
Does it interfere with life?
Family knowledgeable about condition and its management?

Management
Avoiding soap, frequently using emollients?
Avoiding nylon and wool clothes?
Is there a need to give or change medications:
• Topical corticosteroids
• Occlusive bandages
• Antibiotics or antiviral agents
• Antihistamines
On dietary elimination or is it indicated? If so, dietician supervision?
Need for psychosocial support?

Check:
• Any evidence of infection - bacterial or herpes simplex virus?
• Problems from other allergic disorders?
• Is growth normal?

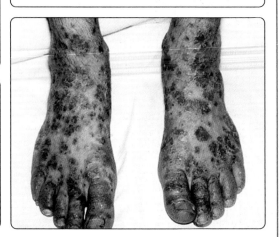

Figure 24.11 Exacerbation of eczema.

the advice of a dietician to ensure complete avoidance of specific food constituents and that the diet remains nutritionally adequate. A food challenge is required to be fully objective, but is usually reserved for older children. Children can usually tolerate the offending foods when they are older.

Psychosocial support

In most children, eczema is mild and can be controlled with emollients and mildly potent topical steroids, and additional psychological support is not required. However, eczema can be sufficiently severe to be disrupting both to the child and to the whole family. The parents and the child need considerable advice, help and support from health professionals, other affected families or fellow sufferers. In the UK, the National Eczema Society provides support and education about the disorder.

Infections and infestations

Bullous impetigo has been considered earlier in this chapter and acute bacterial and viral infections of the skin are considered in Chapter 14.

Viral infections

Viral warts

These are caused by the human papillomavirus, of which there are well over 100 types. Warts are common in children, usually on the fingers and soles (verrucae). Most disappear spontaneously over a few months or years and treatment is only indicated if the lesions are painful or are a cosmetic problem. They can be difficult to treat, but daily application of a proprietary salicylic acid and lactic acid paint or glutaraldehyde (10%) lotion can be used. Cryotherapy with liquid nitrogen is effective treatment but can be painful and often needs repeated application, and its use should be reserved for older children.

Molluscum contagiosum

This is caused by a poxvirus. The lesions are small, skin-coloured, pearly papules with central umbilication (Fig. 24.12). They may be single but are usually multiple. Lesions are often widespread but tend to disappear spontaneously within a year. If necessary, a topical antibacterial can be applied to prevent or treat secondary bacterial infection, and cryotherapy (2–3 seconds only) can be used in older children, away from the face, to hasten the disappearance of more chronic lesions.

Fungal infections

Ringworm

Dermatophyte fungi invade dead keratinous structures, such as the horny layer of skin, nails and hair. The term ringworm is used because of the often ringed (annular) appearance of skin lesions. A severe inflammatory pustular ringworm patch is called a kerion (Fig. 24.13).

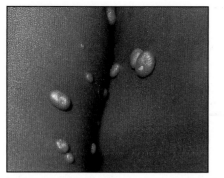

Figure 24.12 Molluscum contagiosum on the chest and upper arm showing the pearly papules with central umbilication through which the infectious central core is eventually shed.

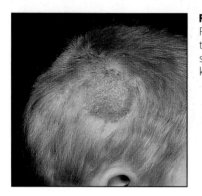

Figure 24.13 Ringworm of the scalp showing a kerion.

Tinea capitis (scalp ringworm), sometimes acquired from dogs and cats, causes scaling and patchy alopecia with broken hairs. Examination under filtered ultraviolet (Wood's) light may show bright greenish/yellow fluorescence of the infected hairs with some fungal species.

Rapid diagnosis can be made by microscopic examination of skin scrapings for fungal hyphae. Definitive identification of the fungus is by culture. Treatment of mild infections is with topical antifungal preparations, but more severe infections require systemic antifungal treatment for several weeks. Any animal source of infection also needs to be treated.

Summary

Tinea capitis (scalp ringworm):
- annular scaling scalp lesion with patchy alopecia with broken hairs
- fungal hyphae on skin scrapings
- treated with topical or systemic antifungal
- treat the dog or cat, if infected.

Parasitic infestations

Scabies

Scabies is caused by an infestation with the eight-legged mite *Sarcoptes scabiei*, which burrows down

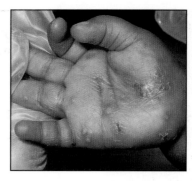

Figure 24.14 Scabies in a young child affecting the palm.

the epidermis along the stratum corneum. Severe itching occurs 2–6 weeks after infestation and is worse in warm conditions and at night.

In older children, burrows, papules and vesicles involve the skin between the fingers and toes, axillae, flexor aspects of the wrists, belt line and around the nipples, penis and buttocks. In infants and young children, the distribution often includes the palms, soles and trunk (Fig. 24.14). The presence of lesions on the soles can be helpful in making the diagnosis. The head, neck and face can be involved in babies but is uncommon.

Diagnosis is made on clinical grounds with the history of itching and characteristic lesions. Although burrows are considered pathognomonic, they may be hard to identify because of secondary infection due to scratching. Itching in other family members is a helpful clinical indicator. Confirmation can be made by microscopic examination of skin scrapings from the lesions to identify mite, eggs and mite faeces.

Complications

The skin becomes excoriated due to scratching and there may be a secondary eczematous or urticarial reaction masking the true diagnosis. Secondary bacterial infection is common, giving crusted, pustular lesions. Sometimes slowly resolving nodular lesions are visible.

Treatment

As it is spread by close bodily contact, the child and whole family should be treated whether or not they have evidence of infestation. Permethrin cream (5%) should be applied below the neck to all areas and washed off after 8–12 hours. In babies, the face and scalp should be included, avoiding the eyes. Benzyl benzoate emulsion (25%) applied below the neck only (diluted according to age) and left on for 12 hours is also effective but smells and has an irritant action. Malathion lotion (0.5% aqueous) is another effective preparation applied below the neck and left on for 12 hours.

If a child and other members of the family are itching, suspect scabies.

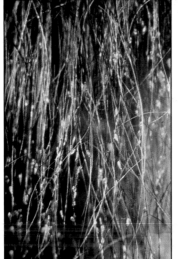

Figure 24.15
Head lice. Profuse nits (egg capsules) are visible on these scalp hairs. Live lice were also visible on the scalp.

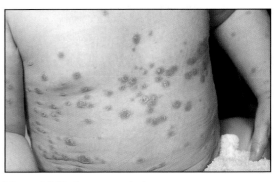

Figure 24.16 Guttate psoriasis.

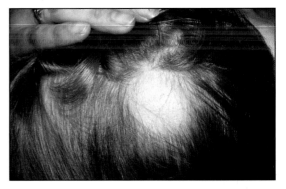

Figure 24.17 Alopecia areata. Smooth non-inflamed patch of hair fall.

Pediculosis

Pediculosis capitis (head lice infestation) is the most common form of lice infestation in children. It is widespread and troublesome among primary school children. Presentation may be itching of the scalp and nape or from identifying live lice on the scalp or nits (empty egg cases) on hairs (Fig. 24.15). Louse eggs are cemented to hair close to the scalp and the nits (small whitish oval capsules) remain attached to the hair shaft as the hair grows. There may be secondary bacterial infection leading to a misdiagnosis of impetigo. Post-occipital lymphadenopathy is common. Once infestation is confirmed by finding live lice, treatment is by applying a solution of 0.5% malathion to the hair and leaving it on overnight. The hair is then shampooed and the lice and nits removed with a fine-tooth comb. Treatment should be repeated a week later. Permethrin (1%) as a cream rinse would be an alternative application; it is left on for 10 minutes only. Flammability of alcohol-based lotions should be noted.

> ### ⓘ Summary
>
> **Scabies:**
> - very itchy burrows, papules and vesicles – distribution varies with age
> - scratching leads to excoriation, secondary eczematous or urticarial reaction often with secondary bacterial infection
> - not only the child but the whole family need treatment.

Other childhood skin disorders

Psoriasis

This familial disorder rarely presents before the age of 2 years. The guttate type (Fig. 24.16) is common in children and often follows a streptococcal or viral sore throat or ear infection. Lesions are small, raindrop-like, round or oval erythematous scaly patches on the trunk and upper limbs, and an attack usually resolves over 3–4 months. Chronic psoriasis with plaques or annular lesions is less common. Fine pitting of the nails may be seen in chronic disease but is unusual in children. Treatment for guttate psoriasis is with bland ointments. Coal tar preparations are useful for plaque psoriasis and scalp involvement. Dithranol preparations are very effective in resistant plaque psoriasis. Calcipotriol, a vitamin D analogue, can also be useful for plaque psoriasis in those over 6 years old. Occasionally, children with chronic psoriasis develop arthritis.

Pityriasis rosea

This acute, benign self-limiting condition is thought to be of viral origin. It usually begins with a single round or oval scaly macule, the herald patch, 2–5 cm in diameter, on the trunk, upper arm, neck or thigh. After a few days, numerous smaller dull pink macules develop on the trunk, upper arms and thighs. The rash tends to follow the line of the ribs posteriorly, described as the 'fir tree pattern'. Sometimes the lesions are itchy. No treatment is required and the rash resolves within 4–6 weeks.

Alopecia areata (Fig. 24.17)

This is a common form of hair loss in children and, understandably, a cause of much family distress.

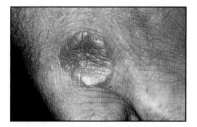

Figure 24.18 Granuloma annulare Ringed lesion with non-inflamed raised edge.

Hairless, single or multiple non-inflamed smooth areas of skin, usually over the scalp, are visible; remnants of broken-off hairs, visible as 'exclamation mark' hairs may be seen at the edge of active patches of hair fall. The more extensive the hair loss the poorer the prognosis but regrowth often occurs within 6–12 months. Prognosis should be more guarded in children with atopic disorders.

Granuloma annulare (Fig. 24.18)

Lesions are typically ringed (annular) with a raised flesh-coloured non-scaling edge (unlike ringworm). They may occur anywhere but usually over bony prominences, especially over hands and feet. Lesions may be single or multiple, are usually 1–3 cm in diameter and tend to disappear spontaneously but may take years to do so.

Acne vulgaris

Acne may begin 1–2 years before the onset of puberty following androgenic stimulation of the sebaceous glands and an increased sebum excretion rate. Obstruction to the flow of sebum in the sebaceous follicle initiates the process of acne. There are a variety of lesions, initially open comedones (blackheads) or closed comedones (whiteheads) progressing to papules, pustules, nodules and cysts. Lesions occur mainly on the face, back, chest and shoulders. The more severe cystic and nodular lesions often produce scarring. Menstruation and emotional stress may be associated with exacerba-

tions. The condition usually resolves in the late teens, although it may persist.

Topical treatment is directed at encouraging the skin to peel using a keratolytic agent, such as benzoyl peroxide, applied once or twice daily after washing. Sunshine in moderation, topical antibiotics or topical retinoids may be helpful. For more severe acne, oral antibiotic therapy with tetracyclines (only when over 12 years old, because they may discolour the teeth in younger children) or erythromycin is indicated. The retinoid isotretinoin is reserved for severe acne in teenagers unresponsive to other treatments.

Rashes and systemic disease

Skin rashes may be a sign of systemic disease. Examples are:

- Facial rash in systemic lupus erythematosus (SLE) or dermatomyositis.
- Purpura over the buttocks, lower limbs and elbows in Henoch–Schönlein purpura.
- Erythema nodosum (Fig. 24.19, Box 24.4).
- Erythema multiforme (Fig. 24.20, Box 24.5), which may be associated with a systemic disorder, but often no cause is identified.
- Stevens–Johnson syndrome, a severe bullous form of erythema multiforme also involving the mucous membranes (Fig. 24.21). The eye involvement may include conjunctivitis, corneal ulceration and uveitis, and ophthalmological assessment is required. It may be caused by drug sensitivity or infection, with morbidity and sometimes even mortality from infection, toxaemia or renal damage.
- Urticaria.

Urticaria

Urticaria (hives or weals) is described in Chapter 15 and the management of anaphylaxis in Chapter 6.

Papular urticaria is a delayed hypersensitivity reaction most commonly seen on the legs, following a bite from a flea, bedbug, or animal or bird mite. Irritation, vesicles, papules and weals appear

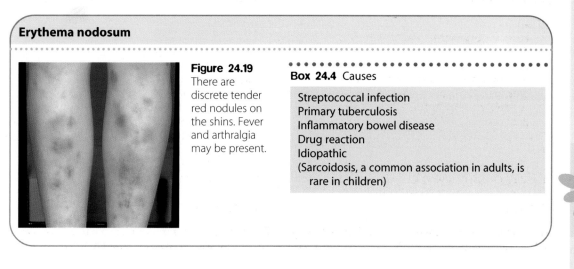

Erythema nodosum

Figure 24.19 There are discrete tender red nodules on the shins. Fever and arthralgia may be present.

Box 24.4 Causes

Streptococcal infection
Primary tuberculosis
Inflammatory bowel disease
Drug reaction
Idiopathic
(Sarcoidosis, a common association in adults, is rare in children)

Erythema multiforme

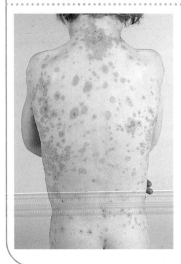

Figure 24.20
There are target lesions with a central papule surrounded by an erythematous ring. Lesions may also be vesicular or bullous.

Box 24.5 Causes

Herpes simplex infection
Mycoplasma pneumoniae infection
Other infections
Drug reaction
Idiopathic

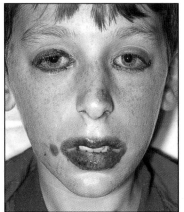

Figure 24.21
Stevens–Johnson syndrome showing severe conjunctivitis and ulceration of the mouth. (Courtesy of Dr Rob Primhak.)

and secondary infection due to scratching is common. It may last for weeks or months and may be recurrent.

Hereditary angioedema is a rare autosomal dominant disorder caused by a deficiency or dysfunction of C1-esterase inhibitor. There is no urticaria, but subcutaneous swellings occur, often accompanied by abdominal pain. The trigger is usually trauma. Angioedema may cause respiratory obstruction. Treatment of a severe acute attack is with a purified preparation of the inhibitor, but replacement therapy with fresh frozen plasma can be used as a short-term measure.

Further reading

Verbov J 2002 Handbook of paediatric dermatology. Martin Dunitz, London

Endocrine and metabolic disorders

Features of endocrine and metabolic disorders in children are:

- Almost all diabetes mellitus is insulin-dependent.
- Hypoglycaemia must be excluded whenever children become suddenly ill.
- Congenital hypothyroidism is relatively common and is detected on routine biochemical screening (Guthrie test).
- Inborn errors of metabolism are individually rare but are considered in a wide range of differential diagnoses.

Diabetes mellitus

The incidence of diabetes in children has increased steadily over the last 20 years and now affects around 2 per 1000 children by 16 years of age. This is most likely to be a result of changes in environmental risk factors. There is considerable racial and geographical variation – the condition is more common in northern countries, with the highest incidence in Finland. Almost all children are insulin-dependent (type 1 diabetes). Type 2 non-insulin-dependent diabetes due to insulin resistance is starting to occur in childhood as severe obesity becomes more common. The causes of diabetes are listed in Box 25.1.

 Almost all children have insulin-dependent (type 1) diabetes, although type 2 diabetes is starting to be seen.

Aetiology

Both genetic predisposition and environmental precipitants play a role. Inherited susceptibility is demonstrated by:

Box 25.1 Classification of diabetes according to aetiology (adapted from American Diabetes Association, Report of Expert Committee on the diagnosis and classification of diabetes mellitus. *Diabetes Care* 22 (Suppl. 1), 1999)

Type 1. Insulin-dependent
Most childhood diabetes

Type 2. Non-insulin-dependent
Usually older children, obesity-related, positive family history, not prone to ketosis, commoner in some ethnic groups

Type 3. Other specific types
Genetic defects in β-cell function (maturity-onset diabetes of the young, MODY, several subtypes)
Genetic defects in insulin action
Infections, e.g. congenital rubella
Drugs, e.g. corticosteroids
Pancreatic exocrine insufficiency, e.g. cystic fibrosis
Endocrine diseases, e.g. Cushing's syndrome
Genetic/chromosomal syndromes, e.g. Down's and Turner's

Type 4. Gestational diabetes (GDM)

415

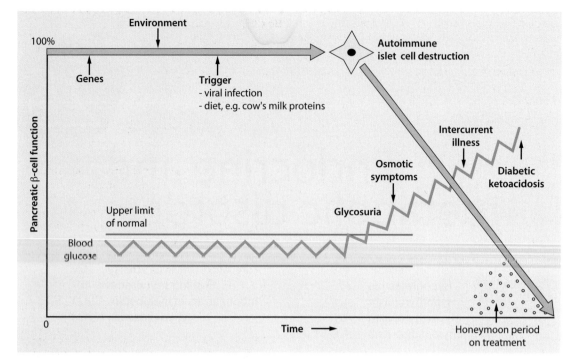

Figure 25.1 Stages in the development of diabetes.

- an identical twin of a diabetic having a 30–50% chance of developing the disease
- the increased risk of a child developing diabetes if a parent has insulin-dependent diabetes (1 in 20–40 if the father is affected, 1 in 40–80 if it is the mother)
- the increased risk of diabetes amongst those who are HLA-DR3 or HLA-DR4 and a reduced risk with DR2 and DR5.

Molecular mimicry probably occurs between an environmental trigger and an antigen on the surface of β-cells of the pancreas. Triggers which may contribute are viral infections, accounting for the more frequent presentation in spring and autumn, and diet, possibly cow's milk proteins (Fig. 25.1). This results in an autoimmune process which damages the pancreatic β-cells and leads to an absolute insulin deficiency. Markers of β-cell destruction include islet cell antibodies and antibodies to glutamic acid decarboxylase (GAD). There is an association with other autoimmune disorders such as hypothyroidism.

Clinical features

The age at presentation is shown in Figure 25.2. It is uncommon before the age of 1 year, but the incidence rises steadily during the early school years to reach a peak at 12–13 years of age. In contrast to adults, children usually present with only a few weeks of polyuria, excessive thirst (polydipsia) and weight loss; young children may also develop secondary nocturnal enuresis. Most children are diagnosed at this early stage of the illness (Box 25.2). Advanced diabetic ketoacidosis

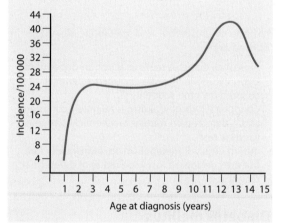

Figure 25.2 Age at presentation. Diabetes occurs even in young children, but its incidence increases with age. (Data from Metcalfe M A, Baum J D, Incidence of insulin dependent diabetes in children aged under 15 years in the British Isles during 1988. *British Medical Journal* 1991; 302: 443–447.)

has become an uncommon presentation (<10% in some areas of the UK), but requires urgent recognition and treatment. Diabetic ketoacidosis may be misdiagnosed if the hyperventilation is mistaken for pneumonia or the abdominal pain for appendicitis.

Diagnosis

The diagnosis is usually confirmed in a symptomatic child by finding a markedly raised random blood glucose (>11.1 mmol/L by the current WHO

Box 25.2 Symptoms and signs of diabetes

Early

Most common – the 'classical triad':
Excessive drinking (polydipsia)
Polyuria
Weight loss

Less common:
Enuresis (secondary)
Skin sepsis
Candida and other infections

Late – diabetic ketoacidosis

Smell of acetone on breath
Vomiting
Dehydration
Abdominal pain
Hyperventilation due to acidosis (Kussmaul
  breathing)
Hypovolaemic shock
Drowsiness
Coma

Box 25.3 The diabetes team

Consultant paediatrician(s) with a special interest
  in diabetes
Paediatric diabetes specialist nurse(s)
Paediatric dietician
Clinical psychologist
Social worker
Adult diabetologist for joint adolescent clinics

- matching of food intake with insulin and exercise
- 'sick-day rules' during illness to prevent
  ketoacidosis
- blood glucose (fingerprick) monitoring
- the recognition and treatment of hypoglycaemia
- where to get advice 24 hours a day
- the help available from voluntary groups, i.e. local
  groups and, in the UK, 'Diabetes UK'
- the psychological impact of a lifelong condition
  with potentially serious short- and long-term
  complications.

A considerable period of time needs to be spent with the family to provide this information and psychological support. The information provided for the child must be appropriate for age and updated regularly. The specialist nurse should liaise with the school (teachers, those who prepare school meals, physical education teachers) and the primary care team.

definition), glycosuria and ketonuria. Where there is any doubt, a fasting blood glucose (>7 mmol/L) or a raised glycosylated haemoglobin (HbA_{1C}) are helpful. A diagnostic glucose tolerance test is rarely required in children. Type 2 diabetes should be suspected if there is a family history, in children from the Asian subcontinent and in severely obese children with signs of insulin resistance (acanthosis nigricans – velvety dark skin on the neck or armpits, skin tags or the polycystic ovary phenotype in teenage girls).

Initial management of type 1 diabetes

Even type 1 diabetes in childhood is uncommon and much of the initial and routine care is delivered by specialist teams (Box 25.3).

The initial management will depend on the child's clinical condition. Those in advanced diabetic ketoacidosis require urgent hospital admission and treatment (see section on 'Diabetic ketoacidosis'). Most newly presenting children are alert and able to eat and drink and can be managed with subcutaneous insulin alone. Intravenous fluid is required if the child is vomiting or dehydrated. In some centres, children newly presenting with diabetes who do not require intravenous therapy are not admitted to hospital but are managed entirely at home.

An intensive educational programme is needed for the parents and child to cover:

- a basic understanding of the pathophysiology of
  diabetes
- injection of insulin – technique and sites
- diet – regular meals and snacks, reduced refined
  carbohydrate; healthy diet with no more than 30%
  fat intake

Insulin

Insulin is made chemically identical to human insulin by recombinant DNA technology or by chemical modification of pork insulin. All insulin that is used in the UK in children is human and in concentrations of 100 U/ml (U-100). The types of insulin include:

1. Human insulin analogues. Rapid-acting insulin analogues, e.g. insulin lispro or insulin aspart (Humalog and NovoRapid) – faster onset and shorter duration of action than soluble insulin. There are also very long-acting insulin analogues, e.g. insulin detemir (Levemir) or glargine (Lantus).
2. Short-acting soluble insulin. Onset of action (30–60 minutes), peak 2–4 hours, duration up to 8 hours. Given 15–30 minutes before meals. Examples are Actrapid and Humulin S.
3. Intermediate-acting insulin. Onset 1–2 hours, peak 4–12 hours. Isophane insulin is insulin with protamine, e.g. Insulatard and Humulin I.
4. Predetermined preparations of mixed short- and intermediate-acting isophane insulins. Examples are Mixtard 30/70 and Humulin M3 (contain 30% soluble and 70% isophane insulin).

Insulin can be given by injections using a variety of syringe and needle sizes, pen-like devices with insulin-containing cartridges, and jet injectors that inject insulin as a fine stream into the skin.

Insulin may be injected into the subcutaneous tissue of the upper arm, the anterior and lateral

Diabetes mellitus

417

aspects of the thigh, the buttocks and the abdomen. Rotation of the injection sites is essential to prevent lipohypertrophy or, more rarely, lipoatrophy. The skin should be pinched up and the insulin injected at a 45° angle. Using a long needle or an injection technique that is 'too vertical' causes a painful, bruised intramuscular injection. Shallow intra-dermal injections can also cause scarring and should be avoided.

In young children, insulin is usually given twice a day, before breakfast and evening meals, as a mixture of short-acting (approximately 30%) and medium- or long-acting insulin (approximately 70%) (Fig. 25.3). In general, about two-thirds of the daily dose is given before breakfast and one-third before the evening meal. Short-acting analogues may be used as needed in between routine injections to cover unexpected high sugars, espe-cially during ill-health. In toddlers with food refusal a very short-acting analogue may be given after each meal on a background of a single long-acting insulin rather than an inflexible twice-daily injection.

Teenagers, and now even younger children, are increasingly using a 3–4 times/day injection regimen ('basal-bolus') with short-acting insulin (Lispro or Insulin Aspart) being given before each meal and long-acting insulin (Glargine or Detemir) in the late evening or before breakfast to provide insulin background. This allows greater flexibility by relating the insulin more closely to food intake and exercise (see Fig. 25.3).

Continuous subcutaneous insulin infusion (CSII) delivered by a micro-processor controlled pump can approximate insulin delivery to physiological requirements but requires the use of an indwelling plastic needle and multiple tests to achieve optimum control and so is not suitable for all patients.

Shortly after presentation, when some pancreatic function is preserved, insulin requirements often become minimal, the so-called 'honeymoon period'. Requirements subsequently increase to 0.5–1 or even up to 2 units/kg per day during puberty.

Diet

The diet and insulin regimen need to be matched (Fig. 25.4). The aim is to optimise metabolic control whilst maintaining normal growth. On the standard twice-daily regimen, food intake is divided into three main meals with snacks between meals and before going to bed. The snacks are required to avoid hypoglycaemia. Children on a basal-bolus regimen or with CSII can eat more flexibly and need not take snacks other than before planned exercise and before bed if they are prone to nocturnal hypoglycaemia. A healthy diet is recommended,

Insulin regimens

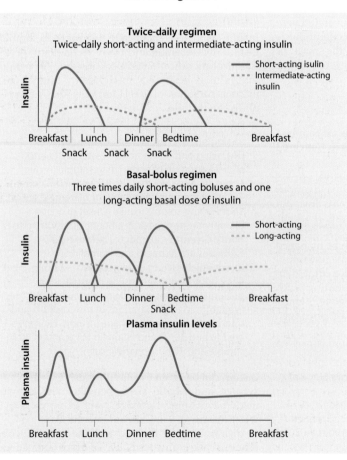

Figure 25.3 Twice daily and basal-bolus insulin regimens and plasma insulin levels on continuous pump insulin.

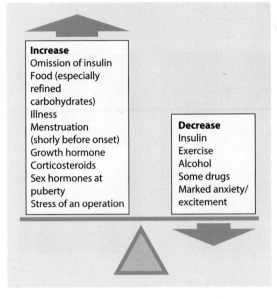

Increase
Omission of insulin
Food (especially refined carbohydrates)
Illness
Menstruation (shorly before onset)
Growth hormone
Corticosteroids
Sex hormones at puberty
Stress of an operation

Decrease
Insulin
Exercise
Alcohol
Some drugs
Marked anxiety/excitement

Figure 25.4 Factors affecting blood glucose levels.

with a high complex carbohydrate and relatively low fat content (<30% of total calories). The diet should be high in fibre, which will provide a sustained release of glucose, rather than refined carbohydrate, which causes rapid swings in glucose levels.

Blood glucose monitoring

Regular blood glucose profiles and blood glucose measurements, when a low or high level is suspected, are required to adjust the insulin regimen and learn how changes in lifestyle, food and exercise affect control. A record should be kept in a diary or transferred from the memory of the blood glucose meter. The aim is to maintain blood glucose as near to normal (4–6 mmol/L) as possible. In practice, in order also to avoid hypoglycaemic episodes, this means levels of 4–10 mmol/L in children and 4–8 mmol/L in adolescents for as much of the time as possible. As children usually dislike having fingerpricks, this limits the frequency of their use. Realistic goals need to be agreed, with compromises reached about the frequency of monitoring. During changes in lifestyle (e.g. holidays) or illness, it is not unreasonable to ask for three or four tests per day. Many adolescents test less than once per week, if at all.

Transcutaneous sensors and indwelling plastic needles giving a continuous reading of blood glucose are becoming more widely available and less obtrusive but still require calibration with a blood test several times a day.

Urine glucose testing may rarely be substituted in the very young or timid. Urine or blood ketone testing is mandatory during infections or when control is poor to try to avoid severe ketoacidosis.

The measurement of glycosylated haemoglobin (HbA$_{1C}$) is particularly helpful as a guide of overall control over the previous 6 weeks and should be checked regularly. The level is directly related to the risk of later complications, but may be misleading if the red blood cell lifespan is reduced, such as in sickle cell trait or if the HbA molecule is abnormal, as in thalassaemia. A level of less than 7% is an often stated but rarely achievable target.

Hypoglycaemia in diabetes

Most children develop well-defined symptoms when their blood glucose falls below about 4 mmol/L. The symptoms are highly individual and change with age, but most complain of hunger, sweatiness, feeling faint or dizzy or of a 'wobbly feeling' in their legs. If unrecognised or untreated, hypoglycaemia may progress to seizures and coma. Parents can often detect hypoglycaemia in young children by their pallor and irritability, sometimes presenting as unreasonable behaviour. If there is any doubt, the blood glucose concentration should be checked or food given.

Treating a 'hypo' at an early stage requires the administration of easily absorbed glucose in the form of glucose tablets (e.g. Dextrosol or similar) or a sugary drink. Children should always have easy access to their hypo remedy, although young children quickly learn to complain of hypo symptoms in order to leave class or obtain a sweet drink! Oral glucose gels (e.g. Hypostop) are easily and quickly absorbed from the buccal mucosa and so are helpful if the child is unwilling or unable to cooperate to eat. It can be administered by teachers or other helpers. Parents and school should be provided with a glucagon injection kit for the treatment of severe hypoglycaemia and taught how to administer it intramuscularly to terminate severe hypos. Severe hypoglycaemia can usually be predicted (or explained in retrospect – missed meal, heavy exercise). The aim is anticipation and prevention. Hypoglycaemia in an unconscious child brought to hospital is treated with glucose given intravenously.

Diabetic ketoacidosis

Presentation is described in Box 25.2, essential investigations in Box 25.4 and management in Figure 25.5.

Long-term management

The aims of long-term management are:

- normal growth and development
- maintaining as normal a home and school life as possible
- good diabetic control through knowledge and good technique
- encouraging children to become self-reliant, but with adult supervision until they are able to take responsibility
- avoidance of hypoglycaemia
- the prevention of long-term complications and an HbA$_{1C}$ of 7% or less.

These aims are extremely difficult to achieve!

Diabetic ketoacidosis

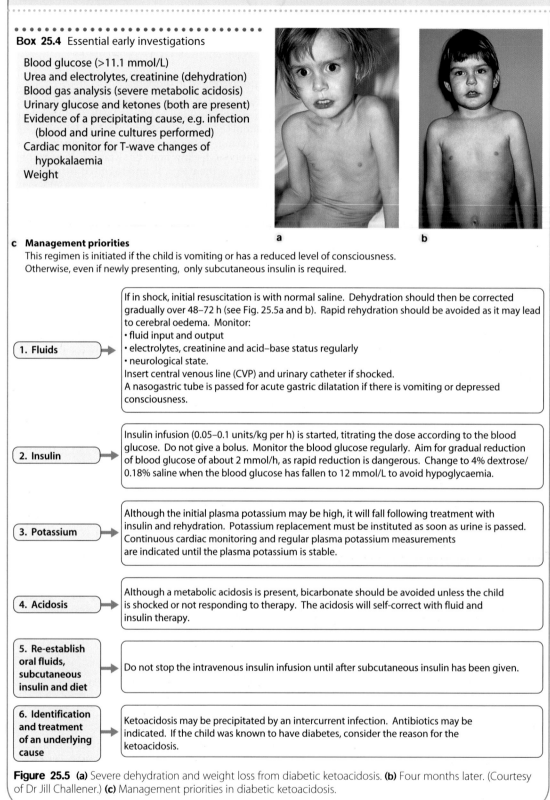

Box 25.4 Essential early investigations

Blood glucose (>11.1 mmol/L)
Urea and electrolytes, creatinine (dehydration)
Blood gas analysis (severe metabolic acidosis)
Urinary glucose and ketones (both are present)
Evidence of a precipitating cause, e.g. infection
  (blood and urine cultures performed)
Cardiac monitor for T-wave changes of
  hypokalaemia
Weight

a   b

c Management priorities

This regimen is initiated if the child is vomiting or has a reduced level of consciousness.
Otherwise, even if newly presenting, only subcutaneous insulin is required.

1. Fluids

If in shock, initial resuscitation is with normal saline. Dehydration should then be corrected gradually over 48–72 h (see Fig. 25.5a and b). Rapid rehydration should be avoided as it may lead to cerebral oedema. Monitor:
• fluid input and output
• electrolytes, creatinine and acid–base status regularly
• neurological state.
Insert central venous line (CVP) and urinary catheter if shocked.
A nasogastric tube is passed for acute gastric dilatation if there is vomiting or depressed consciousness.

2. Insulin

Insulin infusion (0.05–0.1 units/kg per h) is started, titrating the dose according to the blood glucose. Do not give a bolus. Monitor the blood glucose regularly. Aim for gradual reduction of blood glucose of about 2 mmol/h, as rapid reduction is dangerous. Change to 4% dextrose/0.18% saline when the blood glucose has fallen to 12 mmol/L to avoid hypoglycaemia.

3. Potassium

Although the initial plasma potassium may be high, it will fall following treatment with insulin and rehydration. Potassium replacement must be instituted as soon as urine is passed. Continuous cardiac monitoring and regular plasma potassium measurements are indicated until the plasma potassium is stable.

4. Acidosis

Although a metabolic acidosis is present, bicarbonate should be avoided unless the child is shocked or not responding to therapy. The acidosis will self-correct with fluid and insulin therapy.

5. Re-establish oral fluids, subcutaneous insulin and diet

Do not stop the intravenous insulin infusion until after subcutaneous insulin has been given.

6. Identification and treatment of an underlying cause

Ketoacidosis may be precipitated by an intercurrent infection. Antibiotics may be indicated. If the child was known to have diabetes, consider the reason for the ketoacidosis.

Figure 25.5 **(a)** Severe dehydration and weight loss from diabetic ketoacidosis. **(b)** Four months later. (Courtesy of Dr Jill Challener.) **(c)** Management priorities in diabetic ketoacidosis.

Problems in diabetic control

Good blood glucose control is particularly difficult in the following circumstances:

- Eating too many sugary foods, such as sweets taken at odd times, at parties or on the way home from school.
- Infrequent or unreliable blood glucose testing. 'Perfect' results are often invented and written down just before clinic to please the diabetes team.
- Illness – viral illnesses are common in the young and although it is usually stated that infections cause insulin requirements to increase, in practice the insulin dose required is variable, partly because of reduced food intake. The dose of insulin should be adjusted according to regular blood glucose monitoring. Insulin *must* be continued during times of illness and the urine or blood tested for ketones. If ketosis is increasing along with a rising blood sugar, the family should know how to seek immediate advice to ensure that they increase the soluble insulin dose appropriately or seek medical help for possible intravenous therapy.
- Exercise – vigorous or prolonged planned exercise (cross-country running, long-distance hiking, skiing) requires reduction of the insulin dose and increase in dietary intake. Late hypoglycaemia may occur during the night or even the next day, but may be avoided by taking an extra bedtime snack, including slow-acting carbohydrate such as cereal or bread. Less vigorous exercise such as sports lessons in school and spontaneous outdoor play can be managed with an extra snack or a reduction in short-acting insulin before the exercise.
- Family disturbance such as divorce or separation.
- Inadequate family motivation, support or understanding. As children can never have a 'holiday' from their diabetes, they need a great deal of encouragement to continuously maintain good control. Educational programmes for children and families need to be arranged regularly and matched to their current level of education. Special courses and holiday camps are available; in the UK they are organised by Diabetes UK and local groups.

Management of diabetes at school

An individualised care plan should be developed by the parents, diabetes team and the school to address the specific needs of the child. This will include the child's dietary needs, requirements to have snacks at specified times and what to do if the child becomes hypoglycaemic or loses consciousness.

Puberty and adolescence

The rapid growth spurt in early puberty is governed by a complex interaction of hormonal changes, some of which involve insulin and insulin-like growth factors. Growth hormone, oestrogen and testosterone all antagonise insulin action and there is thus an increase in the insulin requirement from the usual 0.5–1.0 units/kg per day of early childhood up to 2 or more units/kg per day. The psychological changes accompanying adolescence may make this a time of rebellion where adherence to insulin and dietary regimens is minimal. Diabetic teenagers know that they will not become ill immediately if they cheat with their diet or miss an injection. Some will inevitably test the degree to which the rules can be broken, choosing to ignore the uncomfortable facts of diabetes provided that they 'feel OK'. This usually results in avoidance of blood testing and a tendency to work on the false assumption that feeling well equates with good control. Many teenage girls experiment with crash diets at some time, which are likely to cause major problems in diabetic control. They also learn that glycosuria can be used as an 'aid' to losing weight.

Battles with parents may concentrate on diabetic management instead of the more usual teenage concerns (Table 25.1). Conflict may also extend to involve the professionals of the diabetic team,

Table 25.1 How diabetes interferes with normal adolescence

Aims and problems of normal adolescence	How diabetes interferes
Physical and sexual maturation	Delayed sexual maturation
	Invasion of privacy with frequent medical examinations
Conformity with peer group	Meals must be eaten on time
	Frequent injections and blood tests
Self-image	Hypoglycaemic attacks show that they are different
Self-esteem	Impaired body image
Independence from parents	Parental over-protection and reluctance to allow their child to be away from home
	Battles over diabetes
Economic independence	Loading of insurance premiums
	Discrimination by employers
	Statutory rules against becoming a pilot or driving heavy goods or public service vehicles

because of intense anger against the disease which marks them out as different from their peers. Many parents are very protective at this time, while teenagers should be encouraged to take responsibility for their diabetes. Health education about smoking, alcohol and contraception may need to be provided. Liaison with a psychologist or child psychiatrist may be helpful. The professionals of the diabetic team may need to encourage diabetic teenagers to take better care of themselves. It is usually unhelpful to give lectures about the long-term risks to health, as these are likely to be seen as irrelevant by the teenagers. However, they may be helped if:

- there are clear short-term goals agreed by the patient
- their efforts to improve their diabetic control, e.g. an improving or satisfactory HbA$_{1c}$ level, are communicated promptly and enthusiastically
- there is a united team approach, with agreement between professionals of the essentials they wish to promote and clear, unambiguous guidelines for health and diabetic management
- peer group pressure is used to promote health.

Activities such as holidays, etc., that allow teenagers to participate while learning about their diabetic management are encouraged. They may also benefit by being used as teachers of younger children.

Successful long-term diabetic management depends on education and increasing self-reliance and responsibility.

Prevention of long-term complications

It has been shown that meticulous diabetic control delays or prevents diabetic retinopathy and nephropathy and, if retinopathy occurs, it can slow the progression (American Multicentre Diabetes Control and Complications Trial – DCCT). Levels of glycosylated haemoglobin above 7.5% are related to risk of later complications in an almost exponential fashion and so the ideal is to keep this level as close to normal as possible (7% or less). In reality, this is only achieved by intensive management with three or four injections of insulin daily, four or more blood glucose estimations each day and frequent clinic check-ups. However, intensive treatment

---

Summary

Assessment of the child with diabetes

Assessment of diabetic control:
- Any episodes of hypoglycaemia, diabetic ketoacidosis, hospital admission?
- Absence from school
- Interference with normal life
- HbA$_{1c}$ results
- Diary of blood glucose results – if monitoring, is he reacting to results?
- Insulin regimen – appropriate?
- Diet – healthy diet, manipulating food intake and insulin to maintain good control?

General overview (periodic):
- Normal growth and pubertal development, avoiding obesity
- Blood pressure check for hypertension
- Renal disease – screening for microalbuminuria
- Eyes – for retinopathy or cataracts
- Feet – maintaining good care
- Screening for coeliac and thyroid disease
- Annual reminder to have flu vaccination

Knowledge and psychosocial aspects:
- Good understanding of diabetes, would participation/ holidays with other diabetic children be beneficial? Member of Diabetes UK?
- Becoming self-reliant, but appropriate supervision at home, school, diabetic team?
- Taking exercise, sport? Diabetes not interfering with it?
- Leading as normal life as possible?
- Smoking, alcohol?
- Is 'hypo' treatment readily available?
- Are there short-term goals to improve control?

Injection sites – check for lipohypertrophy or lipoatrophy

results in an increased risk of severe hypoglycaemia and weight gain. The intensive regimen is probably not suitable for all very young children because of the increased risk of hypoglycaemia, with its detrimental effect on the growing brain, and the unpopularity of multiple injections (including a lunchtime injection at school) and frequent blood tests.

Although long-term health problems are uncommon during childhood, there needs to be regular review for long-term complications and associated illnesses:

- *Growth and pubertal development*. Some delay in the onset of puberty may occur. Obesity is common, especially in females, if their insulin dose is not reduced towards the end of puberty.
- *Blood pressure* – must be checked at least once a year for evidence of hypertension.
- *Renal disease* – the detection of microalbuminuria is an early sign of nephropathy and should be screened annually in teenagers.
- *Eyes* – retinopathy or cataracts requiring treatment are rare in children but should be monitored annually after 5 years of diabetes or from the onset of puberty.
- *Feet* – children should be encouraged to take good care of their feet from an early age, to avoid tight shoes and treat any infections early.
- *Other associated illnesses* – coeliac disease and thyroid disease are more common in type 1 diabetes and easily missed clinically, so screening for them is recommended annually. Good diabetes control in childhood reduces the risk of long-term complications.

Hypoglycaemia

Hypoglycaemia is a common problem in neonates but is seen much less often beyond this period. It is often defined as a plasma glucose less than 2.6 mmol/L, although the development of clinical features will depend on whether other energy substrates can be utilised. Clinical features include:

- sweating
- pallor
- central nervous system signs of irritability, headache, seizures and coma.

The neurological sequelae may be permanent if hypoglycaemia persists and include epilepsy, severe learning difficulties and microcephaly. This risk is greatest in early childhood during the period of most rapid brain growth.

Infants have high energy requirements and relatively poor reserves of glucose from gluconeogenesis and glycogenesis. They are at risk of hypoglycaemia with fasting. Infants should never be starved for more than 4 hours, e.g. preoperatively. A blood glucose should be checked in any child who:

- becomes septicaemic or appears seriously ill
- has a prolonged seizure
- develops an altered state of consciousness.

This is often done at the bedside using glucose-sensitive strips, whose accuracy is improved by use of a meter. However, the strips only indicate that the glucose is within a low range of values and any low reading must always be confirmed by laboratory measurement.

If the cause of the hypoglycaemia is unknown, *it is vital that blood is collected at the time of the hypoglycaemia* and the first available urine sent for analysis so that a valuable opportunity for making the diagnosis is not missed (Box 25.5).

Causes

These are listed in Box 25.6.

Box 25.5 Tests to perform when hypoglycaemia is present

Blood
1. Confirm hypoglycaemia with laboratory blood glucose
2. Growth hormone, cortisol, insulin, C-peptide, fatty acids, acetoacetate, 3-hydroxybutyrate, glycerol, branched-chain amino acids, acylcarnitine profile, lactate, pyruvate

First urine after hypoglycaemia
Organic acids
Consider saving blood and urine for toxicology, e.g. salicylate, sulphonylurea

---

Box 25.6 Causes of hypoglycaemia beyond the neonatal period

Fasting
Insulin excess
Excess exogenous insulin, e.g. in diabetes mellitus/ insulin given surreptitiously
β-cell tumours/disorders – persistent hypoglycaemic hyperinsulinism of infancy (PHHI, previously called nesidioblastosis), insulinoma
Drug-induced (sulphonylurea)
Autoimmune (insulin receptor antibodies)
Beckwith syndrome

Without hyperinsulinaemia
Liver disease
Ketotic hypoglycaemia of childhood
Inborn errors of metabolism, e.g. glycogen storage disorders
Hormonal deficiency: GH↓, ACTH↓, Addison's disease, congenital adrenal hyperplasia

Reactive/non-fasting
Galactosaemia
Leucine sensitivity
Fructose intolerance
Maternal diabetes
Hormonal deficiency
Aspirin/alcohol poisoning

Ketotic hypoglycaemia is a poorly defined entity in which young children readily become hypoglycaemic following a short period of starvation, probably due to limited reserves for gluconeogenesis. The child is often short and thin and the insulin levels are low. Regular snacks and extra glucose drinks when ill will usually prevent hypoglycaemia. The condition resolves spontaneously in later life. A number of rare endocrine and metabolic disorders may present with hypoglycaemia at almost any age in childhood. Hepatomegaly would suggest the possibility of an inherited glycogen storage disorder, in which hypoglycaemia can be profound. Persistent hypoglycaemic hyperinsulinism of infancy (PHHI, which used to be called nesidioblastosis) is a rare problem of infancy where there is a mutation of ion channels causing dysregulation of insulin release by the islet cells of the pancreas, leading to profound non-ketotic hypoglycaemia.

Treatment

Hypoglycaemia can usually be corrected with an intravenous infusion of glucose (2–4 ml/kg of 10% dextrose). Care must be taken to avoid giving an excess volume as the solution is hypertonic. If there is delay in establishing an infusion or failure to respond, glucagon is given intramuscularly (0.5–1 mg).

Corticosteroids may also be used if there is a possibility of hypopituitarism or hypoadrenalism. The correction of hypoglycaemia must always be documented with satisfactory laboratory glucose measurements.

Summary

Hypoglycaemia:
- should be excluded in any child with septicaemia, who is seriously ill, has a prolonged seizure or altered state of consciousness
- low blood glucose on bedside testing must be confirmed by laboratory measurement
- if the cause is unknown, diagnostic blood and urine samples should if possible be taken at the time.

Hypothyroidism

There is only a small amount of thyroxine transfer from the mother to the fetus, although severe maternal hypothyroidism can affect the developing brain. The fetal thyroid predominantly produces 'reverse T_3', a derivative of T_3 which is largely inactive. After birth there is a surge in the level of thyroid-stimulating hormone (TSH) which is accompanied by a marked rise in T_4 and T_3 levels. The TSH declines to the normal adult range within a week. Preterm infants may have very low levels of T_4 for the first few weeks of life whilst the TSH is within the normal range; under these circumstances, additional thyroxine is not required.

Congenital hypothyroidism

Detection of congenital hypothyroidism is important, as it is:

- relatively common, occurring in 1 in 4000 births
- one of the few preventable causes of severe learning difficulties.

Causes of congenital hypothyroidism are:

- *Maldescent of the thyroid and athyrosis* – the commonest cause of sporadic congenital hypothyroidism. In early fetal life, the thyroid migrates from a position at the base of the tongue (sublingual) to its normal site below the larynx. The thyroid may fail to develop completely or partially. In maldescent, the thyroid remains as a lingual mass or a unilobular small gland. The reason for this failure of formation or migration is not well understood.
- *Dyshormonogenesis*, an inborn error of thyroid hormone synthesis, in about 5–10% of cases, although commoner in some ethnic groups with consanguineous marriage.
- *Iodine deficiency*, the commonest cause of congenital hypothyroidism worldwide but rare in the UK. It can be prevented by iodination of salt in the maternal diet.
- Hypothyroidism due to *TSH deficiency* – isolated TSH deficiency is rare (<1% of cases) and is usually associated with panhypopituitarism, which usually manifests with growth hormone and adrenocorticotropic hormone (ACTH) deficiency before the hypothyroidism becomes evident.

The clinical features (Box 25.7 and Fig. 25.6) are difficult to differentiate from normal in the first month of life but become more prominent with age. Fortunately, most affected infants are now identified by routine neonatal biochemical screening (Guthrie test) for raised TSH levels in the blood (some countries also measure T_4) and treatment is usually started before 3 weeks of age. There is a slight excess of other congenital abnormalities, especially heart defects.

Early treatment is essential to prevent learning difficulties. With neonatal screening the results of long-term intellectual development have been satisfactory and intelligence should be in the normal range for the majority of children. Treatment is lifelong with oral replacement of thyroxine, titrating the dose to maintain normal growth, TSH and T_4 levels.

Juvenile hypothyroidism

This is usually caused by autoimmune thyroiditis. Other autoimmune disorders, e.g. diabetes mellitus, may develop, particularly in children with Down's or Turner's syndrome. In some families, Addison's disease may also occur.

Congenital	Acquired
Failure to thrive	Short stature/growth failure
Feeding problems	Cold intolerance
Prolonged jaundice	Dry skin
Constipation	Cold peripheries
Pale, cold, mottled dry skin	Bradycardia
Coarse facies	Thin, dry hair
Large tongue	Pale, puffy eyes with loss
Hoarse cry	of eyebrows
Goitre (occasionally)	Goitre
Umbilical hernia	Slow-relaxing reflexes
Delayed development	Constipation
	Delayed puberty
	Obesity
	Slipped upper femoral epiphysis
	Deterioration in school work
	Learning difficulties

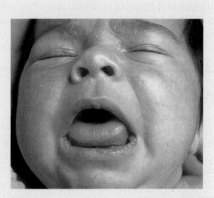

Figure 25.6 Untreated congenital hypothyroidism.

The clinical features are listed in Box 25.7. It is commoner in females. There is growth failure accompanied by delayed bone age. A goitre is often present but this may also be physiological in pubertal girls. Treatment is with thyroxine.

Summary

Congenital hypothyroidism:
- is identified on routine neonatal biochemical screening (Guthrie test)
- although present antenatally, treatment started soon after birth results in satisfactory intellectual development.

Hyperthyroidism

This usually results from Graves' disease (autoimmune thyroiditis) secondary to the production of thyroid-stimulating immunoglobulins (TSIs). The clinical features are similar to those in adults, although eye signs are less common (Box 25.8 and Fig. 25.7). It is most often seen in teenage girls. The levels of thyroxine (T_4) and/or triiodothyronine (T_3) are elevated, TSH levels are suppressed to very low levels. Antithyroid peroxisomal antibodies may also be present which may eventually result in spontaneous resolution of the thyrotoxicosis but subsequently cause hypothyroidism.

The first line of treatment is medical, with drugs such as carbimazole or propylthiouracil which interfere with thyroid hormone synthesis. Initially, beta-blockers can be added for symptomatic relief of anxiety, tremor and tachycardia. Medical treatment is given for about 2 years, which should control the thyrotoxicosis, but the eye signs may not resolve. When medical treatment is stopped, 40–75% relapse. A second course of drugs may then

Systemic	Eye signs (uncommon in children)
Anxiety, restlessness	Exophthalmos
Increased appetite	Ophthalmoplegia
Sweating	Lid retraction
Diarrhoea	Lid lag
Weight loss	
Rapid growth in height	
Advanced bone maturity	
Tremor	
Tachycardia, wide pulse pressure	
Warm, vasodilated peripheries	
Goitre (bruit)	
Learning difficulties/ behaviour problems	
Psychosis	

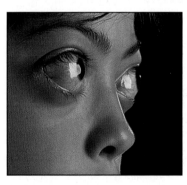

Figure 25.7 Exophthalmos in Graves' disease.

be given or surgery in the form of subtotal thyroidectomy will usually result in permanent remission. Radioiodine treatment is simple and is no longer considered to result in later neoplasia. Follow-up is always required as thyroxine replacement is often needed for subsequent hypothyroidism.

Neonatal hyperthyroidism may occur in infants of mothers with Graves' disease from the transplacental transfer of TSIs. Treatment is required as it is potentially fatal but it resolves spontaneously with time.

Parathyroid disorders

Hypoparathyroidism is rare in childhood. Parathormone (PTH) plays a key role in the mobilisation of calcium by osteoclasts and the excretion of phosphate in the urine. In addition to a low serum calcium, there is a raised serum phosphate and a normal alkaline phosphatase. The parathormone level is very low.

Hypoparathyroidism in infants is usually due to a congenital deficiency (DiGeorge syndrome), associated with thymic aplasia, defective immunity, cardiac defects and facial abnormalities. In older children, hypoparathyroidism is usually an autoimmune disorder associated with Addison's disease.

In *pseudohypoparathyroidism* there is end-organ resistance to the action of parathormone caused by a mutation in a signalling molecule. Serum calcium and phosphate levels are abnormal but the parathormone levels are normal or high. Other abnormalities are short stature, obesity, subcutaneous nodules, short fourth metacarpals and mild learning difficulties. There may be teeth enamel hypoplasia and calcification of the basal ganglia. A related state, in which there are the physical characteristics of pseudohypoparathyroidism but the calcium, phosphate and PTH are all normal, is called *pseudopseudohypoparathyroidism*. There may be a positive family history of both disorders in the same kindred.

Treatment of acute symptomatic hypocalcaemia is with an intravenous infusion of calcium gluconate. The 10% solution of calcium gluconate must be diluted as extravasation of the infusion will result in severe skin damage. Chronic hypocalcaemia is treated with oral calcium and high doses of vitamin D analogues, adjusting the dose to maintain the plasma calcium concentration just below the normal range. Hypercalciuria is to be avoided as it may cause nephrocalcinosis and so the urinary calcium excretion should be monitored.

Adrenal cortical insufficiency

Congenital adrenal hyperplasia is the commonest non-iatrogenic cause of insufficient cortisol and mineralocorticoid secretion (see Ch. 10).

Primary adrenal cortical insufficiency (known as Addison's disease) is rare in children. It may result from:

- an autoimmune process, sometimes in association with other autoimmune endocrine disorders, e.g. diabetes mellitus, hypothyroidism, hypoparathyroidism
- haemorrhage/infarction – neonatal, meningococcal septicaemia (usually fatal)
- adrenoleucodystrophy, a rare neurodegenerative disorder
- tuberculosis, now rare.

Adrenal insufficiency may also be secondary to hypopituitarism from hypothalamic–pituitary disease or from hypothalamic–pituitary–adrenal suppression following long-term corticosteroid therapy.

Presentation

Infants present acutely (Box 25.9) with a salt-losing crisis, hypotension and/or hypoglycaemia. Dehydration may follow a gastroenteritis-like illness, from which the child recovers until the next episode. In older children, presentation is usually with chronic ill health and pigmentation (Fig. 25.8).

Diagnosis

This is made by finding hyponatraemia and hyperkalaemia, often associated with a metabolic acidosis and hypoglycaemia. The plasma cortisol is low or normal and the plasma ACTH concentration high (except in hypopituitarism). With an ACTH (Synacthen) test, plasma cortisol concentrations remain low in both primary adrenal failure and in long-standing pituitary/hypothalamic Addison's disease. A normal response excludes adrenal cortical insufficiency.

• •

Box 25.9 Features of adrenal cortical insufficiency

Acute	Chronic
Hyponatraemia	Vomiting
Hyperkalaemia	Lethargy
Hypoglycaemia	Brown pigmentation
Dehydration	(gums, scars, skin creases)
Hypotension	Growth failure
Circulatory collapse	

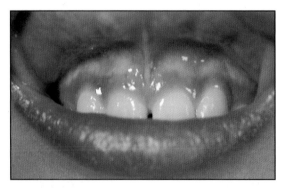

Figure 25.8 Buccal pigmentation in adrenal cortical insufficiency (Addison's disease). This 9-year-old boy presented with salt craving and pigmentation. (Courtesy of Dr Steven Robinson.)

Management

An adrenal crisis requires urgent treatment with intravenous saline, glucose and hydrocortisone. Long-term treatment is with glucocorticoid and mineralocorticoid replacement. The dose of glucocorticoid needs to be increased three- to five-fold at times of illness or for an operation. Parents are taught how to inject intramuscular hydrocortisone in an emergency. All children at risk of an adrenal crisis should wear a MedicAlert bracelet.

Summary

Adrenal cortical insufficiency:
* is usually due to corticosteroid therapy, congenital adrenal hyperplasia or, rarely, Addison's disease
* may result in an adrenal crisis requiring urgent treatment.

Cushing's syndrome

Glucocorticoid excess in children is usually a side-effect of long-term glucocorticoid treatment (intravenous, oral or, more rarely, inhaled, nasal or topical) for conditions such as the nephrotic syndrome, asthma or bronchopulmonary dysplasia (Box 25.10 and Fig. 25.9). Corticosteroids are potent growth suppressors and prolonged use in high dosage will lead to reduced adult height. This unwanted side-effect of systemic corticosteroids is markedly reduced by taking corticosteroid medication in the morning on alternate days.

Other causes of glucocorticoid excess are rare. It may be ACTH driven, from a pituitary adenoma, usually in older children, or from ectopic ACTH-producing tumours, but these almost never occur in children. ACTH-independent disease is usually from corticosteroid therapy, but may be from adrenocortical tumours (benign or malignant), when there may also be virilisation; these usually occur in young children. A diagnosis of Cushing's syndrome is often questioned in obese children. Most obese children from dietary excess are of above-average height, in contrast to children with Cushing's syndrome, who are short and have growth failure.

Box 25.10 Clinical features of Cushing's syndrome

Growth failure/short stature	Bruising
Face and trunk obesity	Carbohydrate
Red cheeks	intolerance
Hirsutism	Muscle wasting
Striae	Osteoporosis
Hypertension	Psychological problems

If Cushing's syndrome is a possibility then the normal diurnal variation of cortisol (high in the morning, low at midnight) may be shown to be lost – in Cushing's syndrome the midnight concentration is also high. The 24-hour urine free cortisol is also high. After the administration of dexamethasone, there is failure to suppress the plasma 09.00 h cortisol levels. Adrenal tumours are identified on CT or MRI scan of the abdomen and a pituitary adenoma on MRI brain scan. Adrenal tumours are usually unilateral and are treated by adrenalectomy and radiotherapy if indicated. Pituitary adenomas are best treated by transsphenoidal resection, but radiotherapy can be used.

Inborn errors of metabolism

Although individually rare, inborn errors of metabolism are an important cause of paediatric morbidity and mortality. The specialised nature of the diagnostic tests and subsequent management often means that these patients are managed in specialist centres. However, as the prognosis for most patients depends upon the speed of diagnosis, all doctors need to be familiar with their variable presentation and diagnosis. It is often assumed that a precise knowledge of a large number of biochemical pathways is necessary to make a diagnosis but in fact a more than adequate diagnostic approach can be based on the correct use of only a few screening tests.

Presentation

An inborn error of metabolism may be suspected before birth from a positive family history or previous unexplained deaths in the family.

After birth, inborn errors of metabolism usually, but not invariably, present in one of five ways:

* as a result of newborn screening, e.g. phenylketonuria (PKU), or family screening, e.g. familial hypercholesterolaemia

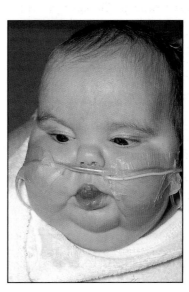

Figure 25.9 Facial obesity from prolonged course of high dose corticosteroids for bronchopulmonary dysplasia in a preterm infant. Such prolonged courses are no longer used. Additional oxygen therapy is being given via nasal cannulae.

- after a short period of apparent normality, with a severe neonatal illness with poor feeding, vomiting, encephalopathy, acidosis, coma and death, e.g. organic acid or urea cycle disorders
- as an infant or older child with an illness similar to that described above but with hypoglycaemia as a prominent feature or as an ALTE (acute life-threatening episode) or near-miss 'cot death', e.g. a fat oxidation defect such as medium-chain acyl-CoA dehydrogenase deficiency (MCADD)
- in a subacute way, after a period of normal development, with regression, organomegaly and coarse facies, e.g. mucopolysaccharide disease or other lysosomal storage disorder or with enlargement of the liver and/or spleen alone, with or without accompanying biochemical upset such as hypoglycaemia, e.g. glycogen storage disease
- as a dysmorphic syndrome.

Newborn screening

The parents of all babies born in the United Kingdom are offered a screening test to detect hypothyroidism and phenylketonuria (PKU). The tests are done on a spot of blood from a heel prick collected onto a filter paper. Although it is technically possible to screen for a much larger group of disorders, this has been resisted in the UK. However, the screening programme has been extended to include cystic fibrosis, haemoglobinopathies and in some regions the metabolic disorder MCADD.

Amino acid disorders

Phenylketonuria

This occurs in 1 in 10 000–15 000 live births in the UK. It is either due to a deficiency of the enzyme phenylalanine hydroxylase (classical PKU) or in the synthesis or recycling of the biopterin cofactor for this enzyme. Untreated, it usually presents with developmental delay at 6–12 months of age. There may be a musty odour due to the metabolite phenylacetic acid. Many affected children are fair-haired and blue-eyed and some develop eczema and seizures. Fortunately, most affected children are detected through the national biochemical screening programme (Guthrie test).

Treatment of classical PKU is with restriction of dietary phenylalanine, whilst ensuring there is sufficient for optimal physical and neurological growth. The blood plasma phenylalanine is monitored regularly. The current recommendation is to maintain the diet throughout life. This is particularly important during pregnancy, when high maternal phenylalanine levels may damage the fetus.

Cofactor defects, which have a much poorer prognosis than classical PKU, are treated with a diet low in phenylalanine and neurotransmitter precursors.

Homocystinuria

This is due to cystathionine synthetase deficiency. Presentation is with developmental delay and eventually subluxation of the ocular lens (ectopia lentis). There is progressive learning difficulty, psychiatric disorders and convulsions. Skeletal manifestations resemble Marfan's syndrome. The complexion is usually fair with brittle hair. Thromboembolic episodes may occur at any age. Almost half respond to large doses of the coenzyme pyridoxine. Those who do not respond are treated with a low-methionine diet supplemented with cysteine and with the addition of the remethylating agent betaine.

Tyrosinaemia

Tyrosinaemia (type 1) is a rare autosomal recessive disorder caused by a deficiency of fumarylaceto-acetase. Accumulation of toxic metabolites results in damage to the liver (leading to liver failure) and renal tubules (resulting in Fanconi syndrome). Untreated the disorder is fatal but effective therapy is now available with a drug called NTBC, which inhibits an enzyme required in the catabolism of tyrosine, together with a diet low in tyrosine and phenylalanine.

Disorders presenting acutely in the neonatal period

This group includes:

- disorders of the catabolic pathways of several essential amino acids (the branched-chain amino acids, leucine, isoleucine and valine, and odd-chain amino acids, e.g. threonine) to cause maple syrup urine disease and other organic acid disorders
- defects in the urea cycle
- a disorder of carbohydrate metabolism – classical galactosaemia.

In these disorders the affected child is normal at birth and after several days develops non-specific signs and symptoms shared with other more common neonatal disorders such as generalised infection. The most common patterns of illness are:

- vomiting, acidosis and circulatory disturbance, followed by depressed consciousness and convulsions – suggestive of one of the organic acidaemias
- neurological features of lethargy, refusal to feed, hypotonia, drowsiness, unconsciousness and apnoea – suggestive of primary defects of the urea cycle. Improvement when given intravenous fluids but relapse if milk feeds are restarted is characteristic of classical galactosaemia.

Diagnosis is with a 'metabolic screen' in addition to the standard investigations for unwell infants The 'metabolic screen' varies between laboratories and should be discussed with the specialist laboratory before collecting samples. The urgency should also be indicated. Both blood and urine samples are likely to be required. A simple bedside test for ketones can be helpful as heavy ketosis and acidosis in an encephalopathic infant is strongly suggestive of an organic acid disorder. In patients with acidosis, calculation of the anion gap (the sum of serum concentrations of sodium and potassium minus the sum of the concentrations of chloride and bicarbonate) can be helpful. Values greater than 25 mmol/L (normal 12–16 mmol/L) are usually secondary to an organic acidaemia. It is good practice to collect all urine passed by the infant for possible future analysis (or until a diagnosis is established) as well as collecting a sample of blood before any blood transfusion in case the latter interferes with the interpretation of laboratory tests.

Both short-term and long-term management depend on the underlying diagnosis. In the immediate emergency situation removal of toxic metabolites and limitation of catabolism have the highest priority. Transfer to a neonatal intensive care unit, mechanical ventilation and haemodialysis are often required. Long-term management involves skilled dietetic support as well as the use of specific medications depending on the underlying diagnosis.

Disorders of carbohydrate metabolism

Galactosaemia

This rare, recessively inherited disorder results from deficiency of the enzyme galactose-1-phosphate uridyl transferase, which is essential for galactose metabolism. When lactose-containing milk feeds such as breast or infant formula are introduced, affected infants feed poorly, vomit and develop jaundice and hepatomegaly and hepatic failure (see Ch. 20). Chronic liver disease, cataracts and developmental delay are inevitable if the condition is untreated. Management is with a lactose- and galactose-free diet for life. Even if treated early, there are usually moderate learning difficulties (adult IQ 60–80).

Glycogen storage disorders

These mostly recessively inherited disorders have specific enzyme defects which prevent mobilisation of glucose from glycogen, resulting in an abnormal storage of glycogen in liver and/or muscle. There are nine main enzyme defects, some of which are shown in Table 25.2. The disorder may predominantly affect muscle (e.g. types II, V), leading to skeletal muscle weakness. In type II (Pompe's disease) there is generalised intralysosomal storage of glycogen. The heart is severely affected, leading to death from cardiomyopathy. In other types (e.g. I, III) the liver is the main organ of storage, and hepatomegaly and hypoglycaemia are prominent (Fig. 25.10). Long-term complications of type I include hyperlipidaemia, hyperuricaemia, the dev-

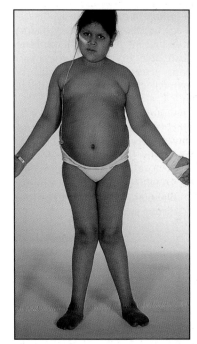

Figure 25.10 Type I glycogen storage disease in a 12-year-old girl. There is truncal obesity with a distended abdomen from an enlarged liver; short stature and hypotrophic muscles; 'doll' facies; nasogastric feeding to maintain blood glucose levels overnight.

Table 25.2 Some of the glycogen storage disorders

Type	Enzyme defect	Onset	Liver	Muscle	Comments
Type I (von Gierke)	Glucose-6-phosphatase	Infant	+++	–	See Fig. 25.10 Enlarged liver and kidneys Growth failure. Hypoglycaemia Good prognosis
Type II (Pompe)	Lysosomal α-glucosidase	Infant	++	+++	Hypotonia and cardiomegaly at several months. Death from heart failure
Type III (Cori)	Amylo-1,6-glucosidase	Infant	++	+	Milder features of type I, but muscles may be affected Good prognosis
Type V (McArdle)	Phosphorylase	Child	–	++	Temporary weakness and cramps muscles after exercise Myoglobinuria in later life

elopment of hepatic adenomas and cardiovascular disease.

Management is to maintain blood glucose by frequent feeds or by carbohydrate infusion via a gastrostomy or nasogastric tube in infancy. In older children, glucose levels can be maintained using slow-release oligosaccharides (corn starch). In type III disorder, a high-protein diet is recommended to prevent growth retardation and myopathy.

Hyperlipidaemia

Hyperlipidaemia is one of the main risk factors for coronary heart disease. Identification and treatment of hyperlipidaemia in childhood may delay the onset of cardiovascular disease in later life.

Children should be screened for hyperlipidaemia if they are at increased risk – if a parent or grandparent has a history of coronary heart disease before 55 years of age or if there is a family history of a lipid disorder. At present, screening all children is not thought justifiable in view of the many uncertainties about selecting who should be treated, what treatment should be given and its effect on outcome.

If the serum cholesterol is high (>5.3 mmol/L) on random testing, fasting serum cholesterol, triglyceride and low-density lipoprotein (LDL) and high-density lipoprotein (HDL) cholesterol are measured. Secondary causes of hypercholesterolaemia should be considered, such as obesity, hypothyroidism, diabetes mellitus, nephrotic syndrome and obstructive jaundice.

Familial hypercholesterolaemia (FH)

This autosomal dominant disorder of lipoprotein metabolism is due to a defect in the LDL receptor. About 1 in 500 of the population are affected. The serum LDL cholesterol concentration is markedly raised (>3.3 mmol/L). The condition is associated with premature coronary heart disease, which occurs in half by 50 years of age in males and by 60 years in females. Skin and tendon xanthomata (Fig. 25.11) may be present, but are uncommon in childhood. Drug therapy is considered in children aged 10 years and older and depends on how high the LDL cholesterol concentration is raised, if there is a family history of premature coronary heart disease (<55 years of age), if there is evidence of tissue lipid deposition (xanthomata or bruits) and

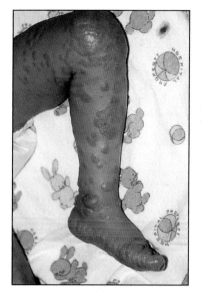

Figure 25.11
Severe skin xanthomata. In this child it was secondary to liver failure and resolved within weeks of liver transplantation.

other non-lipid risk factors, e.g. diabetes. The main drugs used are the non-systemically acting bile acid sequestrants and more recently the HMG-CoA reductase inhibitors, the statins. Although bile acid sequestrants are moderately effective, compliance remains a major problem with them. Statins have been shown to be effective in children, without adverse effects on growth, maturation or endocrine function. The fibrate drug fenofibrate has also been shown to reduce LDL cholesterol and to be well tolerated by children and adolescents.

Homozygous disease is very rare and much more severe, causing xanthomata in childhood and clinical cardiovascular disease in the second decade. Affected children require referral to a specialist centre. Response to drugs is variable depending on the gene mutation. Liver transplantation has been tried.

Further reading

Brook C, Clayton P, Brown R 2005 Brook's Paediatric Endocrinology, 7th edn. Blackwell, Oxford

Lifshitz F (ed) 2002 Pediatric endocrinology, 4th edn. Marcel Dekker, New York

Wales J K H, Rogol A D, Wit J M 2003 Pediatric endocrinology and growth. Saunders, London

Bones, joints and rheumatic disorders

Features in the presentation of musculoskeletal or rheumatic disease in children are:

- musculoskeletal concerns of parents are common and are often variations of normal alignment in the growing skeleton, whereas rheumatic disease is rare but delay in diagnosis may have disastrous long-term consequences (Table 26.1)
- the constitutional features of fever, rash, anorexia, headache, listlessness, weakness or pain are common and are usually associated with transient illness but may herald a chronic inflammatory disease
- combinations of clinical features, especially pivotal features such as peripheral joint swelling, increase the likelihood of a rheumatic diagnosis.

Assessment of the musculoskeletal system

An outline is shown in Fig. 26.1.

Variations of normal posture

These are common and may be noticed by parents or on routine developmental surveillance. Most resolve without any treatment, but any that are severe, persistent, painful or asymmetrical should be referred for a specialist opinion.

Table 26.1 Relative frequency and urgency of diagnosis of conditions which may present with musculoskeletal clinical features

Disease	Relative frequency	Relative urgency of diagnosis
Septic arthritis	Rare	Very urgent
Non-accidental injury	Uncommon	Very urgent
Kawasaki's disease	Rare	Very urgent
Acute lymphoblastic leukaemia	Rare	Urgent
Osteomyelitis	Rare	Urgent
Henoch–Schönlein purpura	Common	Urgent
Connective tissue diseases	Rare	Urgent
Reactive arthritis	Common	Semi urgent
Juvenile idiopathic arthritis	Rare	Semi urgent
Hypermobility	Common	Not urgent
Skeletal dysplasias	Very rare	Not urgent

Bones, joints and rheumatic disorders

Overview:
- Observe walking into room, play, dressing

Key musculoskeletal questions:
- Non-specific/constitutional: fever, anorexia, poor growth, irritability, rash, weakness, sleep disturbance
- Specific: joint pain, stiffness, swelling, instability, muscle weakness, pseudo-paralysis
- Functional activities of daily living

Screening examination: to detect disease
Detailed examination: to define pathology

Examination:
- Always observe active movements before attempting passive movements to avoid causing pain

Patient lying supine:
Lower limbs
1. Inspection
- Note symmetry
- Size – limb length, muscle wasting, joint enlargement
- Skin – scars, colour, warmth, vascular pattern
- Postural deformity – flexion, valgus
2. Palpation:
- Soles of feet, insertion of tendon into bone (enthesitis)
- Joint margins – metatarsal squeeze (take care), anterior ankle, medial knee
- Palpate joint enlargement – is it bony, soft tissue or fluid?
3. Active movement – curl toes, dorsiflex ankles, bend knees and hips, watch for subtle compensatory movements
4. Passive movement - joint range of movement of forefoot and hindfoot inversion/eversion, relaxed passive extension of the knees, internal rotation of hips (knees and hips flexed to 90%) - watch for increased range (hypermobility) and compensatory movements

Examination (Cont'd)
Patient sitting up:
Upper limbs
1. Inspection - symmetry, size, scars, wasting, enlargement, nails
2. Palpation - joint, bony enlargements, warmth
3. Active movement - finger extension, fist, tuck, wrist extension (prayer position), arms straight up then behind head then behind lower back, neck extension and rotation (chin to shoulder)
4. Passive movement - joint range of movement, wrist flexion and extension

Patient standing up:
Axial skeleton
- Inspect symmetry from behind – especially posterior ankles, pelvic position, spine
- Spinal movement – scoliosis, lumbar mobility (lumbar curve on forward flexion, lumbar pain on hyperextension), cervical spine extension and lateral rotation
- Gait - normal, tip-toes, heels
- Muscle power – Gower's test (from supine to standing), gait
- Temporo-mandibular joint – palpation, symmetry and depth of mouth opening
- Sacroiliac joints – direct palpation

Figure 26.1 An outline of the assessment of the musculoskeletal system.

Bow legs (genu varum)

This is bowing of the tibiae causing the knees to be wide apart while standing with the feet together (Fig. 26.2). It is common in toddlers and children up to 3 years of age and seldom needs treatment. Another cause of bow legs is rickets; check for the presence of other clinical features (see Ch. 11). Rickets can be demonstrated on an X-ray of the metaphyses. Marked bow legs may also occur in Blount's disease (infantile tibia vara), an uncommon condition predominantly seen in Afro-Caribbean children. There is beaking of the proximal medial tibial epiphysis on X-ray. Orthoses (splints and special footwear) and surgical correction may be required.

Knock-knees (genu valgum)

In this condition, the feet are wide apart when standing with the knees held together (Fig. 26.3). It is seen in many children between 2 and 7 years of age, resulting in an intermalleolar distance at the ankles of up to 5 cm. It usually resolves.

Flat feet (pes planus)

Toddlers learning to walk usually have flat feet due to flatness of the medial longitudinal arch and the presence of a fat pad which subsequently disappears (Fig. 26.4). Most people develop a medial longitudinal arch; although some do not, this is rarely troublesome. An arch can usually be demonstrated on standing on tiptoe. Marked flat feet can be the presentation of a collagen disorder such as Ehlers–Danlos syndrome or hypermobility. Some children with flat feet develop a prominence of the navicular bone on the medial aspect of the foot which resolves, but modification of the child's shoes or an arch support may be required. This will provide symptomatic relief but does not influence outcome. Surgery for flat feet is rarely indicated, but may be considered in symptomatic adolescents.

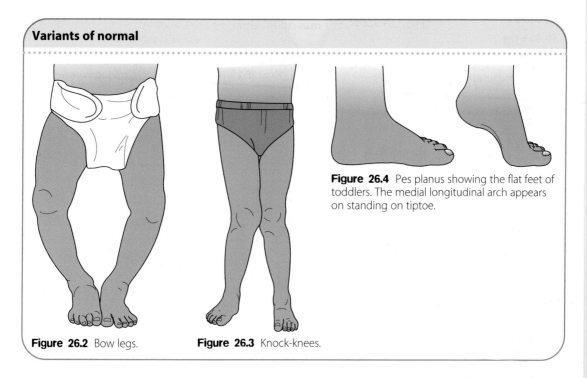

Figure 26.4 Pes planus showing the flat feet of toddlers. The medial longitudinal arch appears on standing on tiptoe.

Figure 26.2 Bow legs.   **Figure 26.3** Knock-knees.

In-toeing

There are three main causes:

- metatarsus varus (Fig. 26.5a) – an adduction deformity of a highly mobile forefoot
- medial tibial torsion (Fig. 26.5b) – at the lower leg, when the tibia is laterally rotated less than normal in relation to the femur
- persistent anteversion of the femoral neck (Fig. 26.5c) – at the hip, when the femoral neck is twisted forward more than normal.

Their clinical features are described in Box 26.1.

Out-toeing

This is uncommon but may occur in infants between 6 and 12 months of age. When bilateral, it is due to lateral rotation of the hips and resolves spontaneously.

Toe walking

This is common in 1- to 3-year-old children. It may become persistent, usually from habit, but may be due to mild cerebral palsy. It may also be due to isolated tightness of the Achilles tendons. In older boys, Duchenne's muscular dystrophy should be excluded.

Disorders of the hip, knee and feet

Limp

Developmental dysplasia of the hip may be detected on routine examination of the newborn infant. Beyond infancy, hip disorders usually present with a limp, which may be painful or painless (Table 26.2). They may also present with referred pain in the knee.

Developmental dysplasia of the hip (DDH) (previously called congenital dislocation of the hip; CDH)

This is a spectrum of disorders ranging from dysplasia to subluxation through to frank dislocation of the hip. Early detection is important as it usually responds to conservative treatment; late diagnosis is usually associated with hip dysplasia which requires complex treatment often including surgery. Neonatal screening is performed as part of the routine examination of the newborn, checking if the hip can be dislocated posteriorly out of the acetabulum (Barlow's manoeuvre) or can be relocated back into the acetabulum on abduction (Ortolani's manoeuvre), as described on page 142. These tests are repeated at routine surveillance at 8 weeks of age. Thereafter, presentation of the condition may be with detection of asymmetry of skinfolds around the hip, limited abduction of the hip, shortening of the affected leg or a limp or abnormal gait.

On neonatal screening, an abnormality of the hip is detected in about 6–10 per 1000 live births. Most will resolve spontaneously. The true birth prevalence of DDH is about 1.5 per 1000 live births. Clinical neonatal screening misses some cases. This may be because of inexperience of the examiner, but in some cases it is not possible to clinically detect dislocation at this stage, e.g. where there is only a mildly shallow acetabulum. To overcome these problems, some centres perform ultrasound screening on all newborn infants. It is highly specific in

433

In-toeing

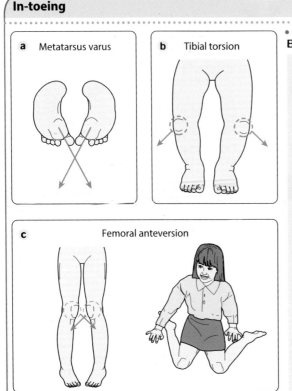

a Metatarsus varus

b Tibial torsion

c Femoral anteversion

Figure 26.5 In-toeing **(a)** at the feet, **(b)** lower leg, **(c)** hip, with 'W' sitting.

• •

Box 26.1 Clinical features of in-toeing in children

Metatarsus varus
- Occurs in infants
- Passively correctable
- Heel is held in the normal position
- No treatment required unless it persists beyond 5 years of age and is symptomatic

Medial tibial torsion
- Occurs in toddlers
- May be associated with bowing of the tibiae
- Self-corrects within about 5 years

Persistent anteversion of the femoral neck
- Presents in childhood
- Usually self-corrects by 8 years of age
- May be associated with hypermobility of the joints
- Children sit between their feet with the hips fully internally rotated ('W' sitting)
- Most do not require treatment but femoral osteotomy may be required for persistent anteversion

---

Summary

Variations of musculoskeletal normality and differential diagnosis:

Perceived disorder	Normal age range	Differential diagnoses to consider
Bow legs	1–3 years	Rickets, osteogenesis imperfecta, Blount's disease
Knock knees	2–7 years	Juvenile idiopathic arthritis
Flat feet	1–2 years	Hypermobility, congenital tarsal fusion
In-toeing	1–2 years	Tibial torsion, femoral anteversion
Out-toeing	6–12 months	Hypermobility, Ehlers–Danlos and Marfan's syndromes
Toe walking	1–3 years	Spastic diplegia, muscular dystrophy

---

detecting DDH but is expensive and has a high rate of false positives, and is not recommended nationally. It is performed in some centres in infants at increased risk (family history, breech presentation).

If developmental dysplasia of the hip is suspected, a specialist orthopaedic opinion should be obtained. An ultrasound examination should be performed and allows detailed assessment of the hip, quantifying the degree of dysplasia and whether there is subluxation or dislocation. This information also helps in planning management and in avoiding unnecessary treatment. If the initial ultrasound is abnormal, the infant may be placed in a positioning device, which puts the hips in abduction (e.g. Craig splint), or in a restraining device (e.g. Pavlik harness (Fig. 26.6)) for several

months. Progress needs to be monitored by ultrasound or X-ray. The splinting must be done expertly, as necrosis of the femoral head is a potential complication.

In most instances, a satisfactory response is obtained. If the hip has not stabilised or the condition is diagnosed late, hip abduction using traction and a further period of splinting (in a plaster hip spica) may be tried. If unsuccessful, an MRI or CT scan of the hip and/or an arthrogram will provide more detailed information of the joint. Weight-bearing on a dislocated hip should be avoided as it causes damage to the femoral head and acetabulum. Open reduction and derotation femoral osteotomy will be required if conservative measures fail.

Table 26.2 Causes of limp

Age	Painful limp	Painless limp
1–3 years	Septic arthritis/osteomyelitis Transient synovitis Trauma – accidental/non-accidental	Developmental dysplasia of the hip Neuromuscular, e.g. cerebral palsy Unequal leg length Juvenile idiopathic arthritis
3–10 years	Transient synovitis Septic arthritis/osteomyelitis Trauma Juvenile idiopathic arthritis (JIA) Perthes disease (acute) Malignant disease, e.g. leukaemia	Perthes disease (chronic) Developmental dysplasia of the hip Neuromuscular disorders, e.g. Duchenne's muscular dystrophy Juvenile idiopathic arthritis
11–16 years	Slipped upper femoral epiphysis (acute) Avascular necrosis of the femoral head Juvenile idiopathic arthritis Trauma Septic arthritis/osteomyelitis Bone tumours	Slipped upper femoral epiphysis (chronic) Juvenile idiopathic arthritis Dysplastic hip

Transient synovitis (TS, irritable hip)

This is the most common cause of acute hip pain in children. It occurs in children aged 2–12 years old. It often follows or is accompanied by a viral infection. Presentation is with sudden onset of pain in the hip or a limp. There is no pain at rest, but there is decreased range of movement, particularly external rotation. The pain may be referred to the knee. The child is afebrile or has a mild fever and does not appear ill.

The neutrophil count and acute-phase reactants are normal or slightly raised. Blood cultures are negative and the X-ray of the joint is normal, but there may be a small joint effusion on ultrasound.

This contrasts with septic arthritis, when the child has a high fever and looks unwell, there is pain at rest and minimal or no movement of the hip. The neutrophil count and acute-phase reactants are markedly raised. If there is any suspicion of septic arthritis, the joint is aspirated under ultrasound guidance. In a small proportion of children, transient synovitis is found to be the presentation of Perthes disease or of slipped upper femoral epiphysis. Management of transient synovitis is with bed rest and, rarely, skin traction. It usually improves within a few days.

Perthes disease

This is due to ischaemia of the femoral epiphysis, resulting in avascular necrosis, followed by revascularisation and reossification over 18–36 months. It mainly affects boys (male : female ratio of 5 : 1) of 5–10 years of age. Presentation is insidious, with the onset of a limp or hip pain. The condition may initially be mistaken for transient synovitis. It is bilateral in 10–20%. X-rays show increased density in the femoral head, which subsequently becomes fragmented and irregular (Fig. 26.7). Even if the initial X-ray is normal, a

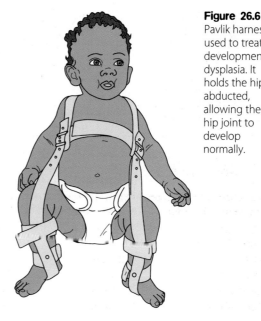

Figure 26.6
Pavlik harness used to treat developmental dysplasia. It holds the hip abducted, allowing the hip joint to develop normally.

repeat may be required if clinical symptoms persist. A bone scan and MRI scan can be helpful in making the diagnosis.

In most children, the prognosis is good, particularly in those below 6 years of age with less than half the epiphysis involved. When over half the epiphysis is affected and the child is over 6 years old, deformity of the femoral head and metaphyseal damage are more likely, resulting in subsequent degenerative arthritis in adult life. If the condition is identified early and less than half the femoral head is affected, only bed rest and traction may be required. In more severe disease, the femoral head needs to be covered by the acetabulum to act as a mould for the reossifying epiphysis. This is achieved by maintaining the hip in abduction with plaster or calipers or by performing femoral or pelvic osteotomy.

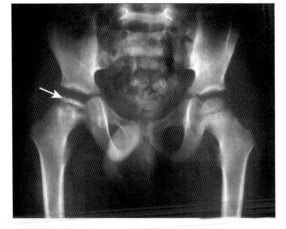

Figure 26.7 Perthes disease, showing flattening with sclerosis and fragmentation of the right femoral capital epiphysis; the left hip is normal.

Slipped upper femoral epiphysis

There is displacement of the epiphysis of the femoral head postero-inferiorly. It is most common at 10–15 years of age during the adolescent growth spurt, particularly in obese boys. Skeletal maturation may be found to be delayed. Presentation is with a limp or hip pain, which may be referred to the knee. There is restricted abduction and internal rotation of the hip. The onset may be acute, following minor trauma. In 20% it is bilateral. The diagnosis is confirmed on X-ray (Fig. 26.8), although a frog lateral view is sometimes required. Management is surgical, usually with pin fixation in situ. Severe slips may require subsequent corrective realignment osteotomy once the epiphysis has fused or, rarely, open reduction of the hip, but this carries a risk of avascular necrosis.

Summary

Regarding hip disorders:
- developmental dysplasia of the hip – may be detected on screening at birth or 8 weeks, detection of asymmetry of skinfolds around the hip, limited abduction of the hip, shortening of the affected leg or a limp or abnormal gait
- transient synovitis – most common cause of acute hip pain or a limp
- Perthes disease – usually school-aged boys with hip pain or limp
- slipped upper femoral epiphysis – usually obese adolescent with a limp or hip pain

The painful knee

When assessing a painful knee, the hip must always be examined, as hip pain is often referred to the knee.

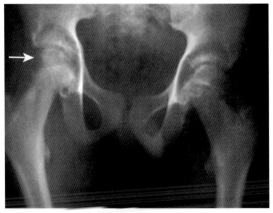

Figure 26.8 Slipped upper femoral epiphysis of the right hip; the left hip is normal.

Osgood–Schlatter disease

This is an overuse syndrome commonly occurring in physically active males around puberty, resulting in a partial avulsion fracture through the ossification centre of the tibial tuberosity (traction apophysitis). There is localised tenderness and swelling over the tibial tubercle. The disease is bilateral in 25–50%. Most resolve with reduced physical activity, trying to avoid over-restriction for a disorder which is self-limiting. A knee immobiliser splint may be helpful. In some patients the disorder fails to resolve over several months; a period of immobilisation may then be required.

Chondromalacia patellae

In this condition there is softening of the articular cartilage of the patella. It most often affects adolescent females, causing pain when the patella is tightly apposed to the femoral condyles, as in standing up from sitting or on walking up stairs. Treatment is with rest and physiotherapy for quadriceps muscle strengthening.

Osteochondritis dissecans

Pain is caused by separation of bone and cartilage from the medial femoral condyle following avascular necrosis. Complete separation of articular fragments may result in loose body formation and symptoms of knee locking or giving way. Treatment is initially with rest and quadriceps exercises; sometimes arthroscopic surgery is required.

Subluxation and dislocation of the patella

Subluxation produces the feeling of instability or giving way of the knee. Treatment is with quadriceps exercises; surgery to realign the pull of the quadriceps on the patellar tendon is occasionally required.

Dislocation of the patella laterally occurs suddenly. Reduction occurs spontaneously or on gentle extension of the knee. An X-ray is required to differentiate loose bodies from bone fracture. Immobilisation, and sometimes surgery, is required.

Injuries

Contact sports usually result in acute injuries to the knee, while non-contact sports with sustained activity tend to result in chronic injury and overuse syndromes. Sporting injuries to the menisci and ligaments are common in adolescents. MRI scans are helpful to determine the extent of damage. Management is usually conservative. In infants and young children, similar injuries are more likely to result in fractures, as their ligaments are relatively stronger than their bones.

Talipes equinovarus (clubfoot)

Positional talipes from intrauterine compression is common. The foot is of normal size and the deformity is mild and can be corrected to the neutral position with passive manipulation. Often the baby's intrauterine posture can be recreated. If the positional deformity is marked, parents can be shown passive exercises by the physiotherapist.

Talipes equinovarus is a complex abnormality (Figs 26.9 and 26.10). The entire foot is inverted and supinated and the forefoot is adducted. The heel is rotated inwards and in plantarflexion. The affected foot is shorter and the calf muscles thinner than normal. The position of the foot is fixed and cannot be corrected completely. It is often bilateral. The birth prevalence is 0.9 per 1000 live births, with a sex ratio of males to females of 2 : 1. It is of multifactorial inheritance, but may also be secondary to oligohydramnios during pregnancy. It may be a feature of a malformation syndrome or of a neuromuscular disorder such as spina bifida. There is an association with developmental dysplasia of the hip (DDH).

Treatment is started promptly, while the tissues are lax, with stretching and strapping or serial plaster casts. If this corrects the disorder, treatment can be discontinued or night splints used. If the condition is severe, corrective surgery is usually necessary. As the results of corrective surgery performed at a few weeks of age have been disappointing, surgery is usually delayed to 6–9 months of age. The condition needs to be differentiated from the rare *congenital vertical talus*, where the foot is stiff and rocker-bottom in shape. Many of these infants have other malformations. The diagnosis can be confirmed on X-ray. Surgery is usually required.

Talipes calcaneovalgus

The foot is dorsiflexed and everted (Fig. 26.11). It usually results from intrauterine moulding and self-corrects. Passive foot exercises are sometimes advised. There is an association with developmental dysplasia of the hip.

Pes cavus

In pes cavus there is a high arched foot. When it presents in older children, it is often associated with neuromuscular disorders, e.g. Friedreich's ataxia and type I hereditary motor sensory neuropathy

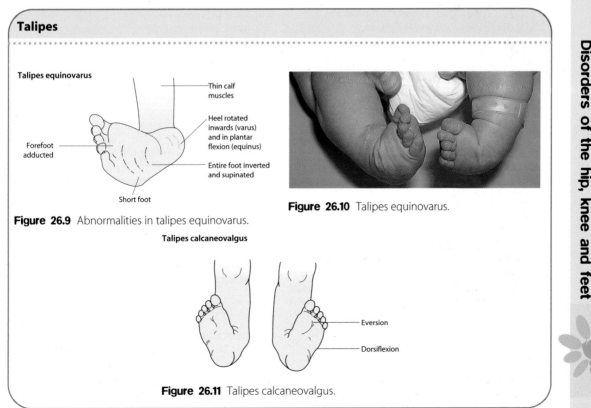

Talipes

Talipes equinovarus

Thin calf muscles

Heel rotated inwards (varus) and in plantar flexion (equinus)

Forefoot adducted

Entire foot inverted and supinated

Short foot

Figure 26.9 Abnormalities in talipes equinovarus.

Figure 26.10 Talipes equinovarus.

Talipes calcaneovalgus

Eversion

Dorsiflexion

Figure 26.11 Talipes calcaneovalgus.

(peroneal muscular atrophy). Treatment is required if the foot becomes stiff or painful.

Summary

Regarding talipes equinovarus:
- needs to be differentiated from positional talipes
- check for neuromuscular disorder or spinal lesion and for developmental dysplasia of the hip (DDH).

Disorders of the back, spine and neck

Back pain

Back pain is uncommon in pre-adolescent children, becoming more common during adolescence. In contrast to adults, a cause can often be identified, and the younger the child, the more likely it is that there will be significant pathology:

- *muscle spasm* or soft tissue pain from injury, often sport-related
- *poor posture* may accompany hypermobility of the joints
- *Scheuermann's disease* – an osteochondritis of the thoracic vertebrae in adolescents resulting in a fixed kyphosis; diagnosed on X-ray
- *spondylolysis/spondylolisthesis* – stress fracture of the pars interarticularis of the vertebra, typically lower lumbar (spondylolysis); if the affected vertebral body moves anteriorly, it produces a spondylolisthesis; diagnosis by X-ray
- *vertebral osteomyelitis/discitis* – often presents in young children with reluctance to walk or bear weight, and tenderness over the affected site; while plain X-rays may show abnormalities suggesting the diagnosis, bone and CT scans are the diagnostic investigations of choice
- *tumours* – may be benign or malignant
- *spinal cord/root compression* – e.g. from a tumour or prolapsed intervertebral disc
- *idiopathic pain syndrome* – diagnosed when no physical cause is found; may be exacerbated by psychological stress.

Scoliosis

Scoliosis is a lateral curvature in the frontal plane of the spine. In structural scoliosis, there is rotation of the vertebral bodies which causes a prominence in the back from rib asymmetry. It is a cosmetic problem, but in severe cases can lead to cardio-respiratory failure from distortion of the chest.

Causes of scoliosis are:

- *Idiopathic.* The most common, either early onset (less than 5 years old) or late onset.
- *Congenital.* From a congenital defect of the spine, e.g. hemivertebra, spina bifida, VACTERL

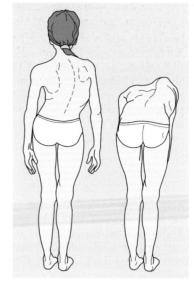

Figure 26.12
Structural scoliosis with vertebral rotation shown by rib rotation on bending forward.

association (vertebral, anorectal, cardiac, tracheo-oesophageal, renal and radial limb anomalies).
- *Secondary.* To other disorders, such as neuromuscular imbalance (e.g. in cerebral palsy, muscular dystrophy, polio) or disorders of bone such as neurofibromatosis or of connective tissues such as Marfan's syndrome. It may be postural in origin, such as secondary to leg length discrepancy.

Early-onset idiopathic scoliosis usually resolves, but a few progress. Late-onset idiopathic scoliosis is the most common type (85%) and mainly affects girls 10–14 years of age during their pubertal growth spurt.

The scoliosis can be identified on examining the child's back when bent forward (Fig. 26.12). This has been used as a screening test, but it identifies many minor degrees of curvature which resolve spontaneously and does not appear to reduce the need for surgery. For these reasons, routine screening is not currently recommended in the UK. If the scoliosis disappears on forward bending, it is postural and resolves, although leg lengths should be checked. The severity of the curvature of the spine can be determined by measuring the angle of curvature on an X-ray of the spine. Mild scoliosis usually resolves spontaneously. Treatment of severe scoliosis is with spinal braces, although their efficacy is questionable, and sometimes with specialist spinal surgery.

Torticollis

The most common cause of torticollis (wry neck) in infants is a sternomastoid tumour (congenital muscular torticollis). Other causes of torticollis to consider are ENT infection, cervical spine arthritis or malformation and posterior fossa tumour. Sternomastoid tumours occur in the first few weeks of life and present with a mobile, non-tender nodule, which can be felt within the body of the sternocleidomastoid muscle. There may be restriction of head turning and tilting of the head. The condition usually resolves in 2–6 months. Passive stretching is advised, but its efficacy is unproven.

The painful limb

Idiopathic pain

Episodes of generalised pain in the lower limbs, referred to as 'growing pains' or nocturnal idiopathic pain, are common in preschool and school-aged children. The pain often wakes the child from sleep and settles with massage or comforting. It occurs less often during the day, the child is otherwise healthy and there is no evidence of musculoskeletal disease.

Older children or adolescents with hypermobility may complain of musculoskeletal pain mainly confined to the lower limbs and back, in the absence of joint swelling. In hypermobilty the thumbs and little fingers can be hyperextended onto the forearms (Fig. 26.13), elbows and knees can be hyperextended beyond 10°, palms can be placed flat on the floor with knees straight. Lower limb findings associated with hypermobility are pes planus, out-toeing gait, over-pronated feet (secondary to ankle hypermobility) and genu recurvatum (hyperextensibility of the knee joint), all of which may be improved by the use of custom-moulded hard insoles aimed at supporting the longitudinal foot arch and stabilising the ankle. The success of such insoles is dependent on specialised assessment and fitting. Most mechanical causes of joint pain tend to be worse after exercise and as the day progresses, but early morning stiffness the day or two after exercise may be a feature.

The most dramatic musculoskeletal pain is encountered in adolescents with idiopathic pain syndromes. These may be localised (complex regional pain syndromes) or generalised (such as fibromyalgia).

Complex regional pain syndrome

Complex regional pain in childhood may begin after trauma (often minor) or without a clear precipitant. The characteristic features include severe pain, hyperaesthesia (increased sensitivity to stimuli), allodynia (pain from a stimulus that does not normally produce pain), immobility of the affected limb even to the extent of adopting a bizarre posture, and occasionally limb swelling and mottling or cool pallor of the skin.

Diffuse musculoskeletal pain syndrome

Diffuse musculoskeletal pain syndromes are characterised by disturbed sleep patterns (initial insomnia, exhausted wakening and napping during the day), tenderness over the soft tissue 'trigger' points with facial grimacing and a sharp intake of breath if touched, and the absence of other findings to suggest organic disease. It may be part of chronic fatigue syndrome.

Stress (including school pressures, bullying or other forms of abuse, and even parental pressure) is often an accompanying feature, although may be unknown to the parents. Meticulous physical examination and judicious investigation is needed to rule out an underlying organic pathology. Occasionally, an idiopathic pain syndrome may complicate a pre-existing organic disease such as juvenile idiopathic arthritis. An individualised, intensive, multi-professional, rehabilitation regimen, either community or inpatient based, is required to restore function.

Acute onset limb pain

Limb pain of acute onset has a number of causes. Trauma is the most common, usually accidental from sports injuries or falls, but occasionally non-accidental. Osteomyelitis and bone tumours are uncommon, but need urgent treatment.

Osteomyelitis

In osteomyelitis, there is infection of the metaphysis of long bones. The most common sites are the distal femur and proximal tibia, but any bone may be affected (Fig. 26.14). It is usually due to haematogenous spread of the pathogen, but may arise by direct spread from an infected wound. The skin is swollen directly over the affected site. Where the joint capsule is inserted distal to the epiphyseal plate, as in the hip, osteomyelitis may spread to cause septic arthritis. Most infections are caused by *Staphylococcus aureus*, but other pathogens include *Streptococcus* and *Haemophilus influenzae*. In sickle cell anaemia, there is an increased risk of staphylococcal and salmonella osteomyelitis. Chronic infection can cause a localised abscess in the bone (Brodie's abscess) but is uncommon. Infection may be from tuberculosis, but this is rare in the UK.

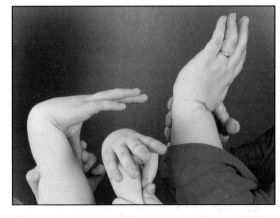

Figure 26.13 Hypermobility syndrome, showing ability to hyperextend the thumb onto the forearm of a mother and two of her children!

Osteomyelitis

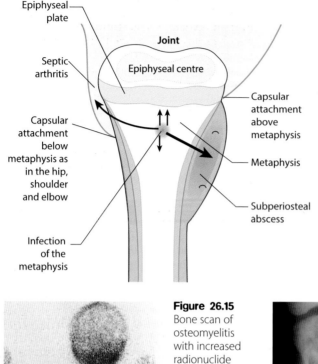

Epiphyseal plate

Joint

Epiphyseal centre

Septic arthritis

Capsular attachment below metaphysis as in the hip, shoulder and elbow

Capsular attachment above metaphysis

Metaphysis

Subperiosteal abscess

Infection of the metaphysis

Figure 26.14 Possible spread of osteomyelitis. In children, the epiphyseal growth plate limits the spread of metaphyseal infection. In infants, before there has been maturation of the growth plate, infection can spread directly to cause joint destruction and arrested growth.

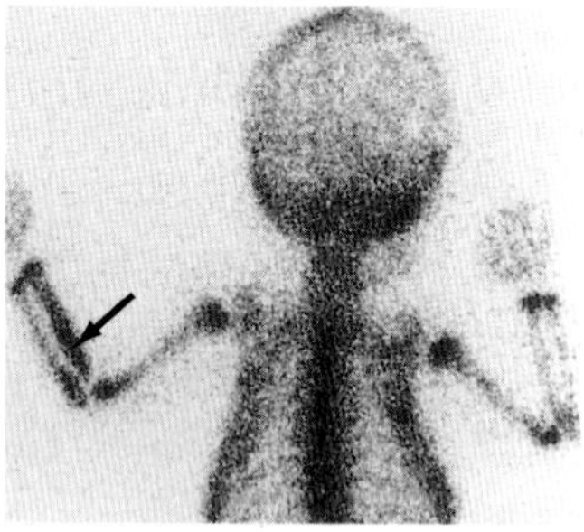

Figure 26.15 Bone scan of osteomyelitis with increased radionuclide uptake of the left radius. (Courtesy of Professor H. Carty.)

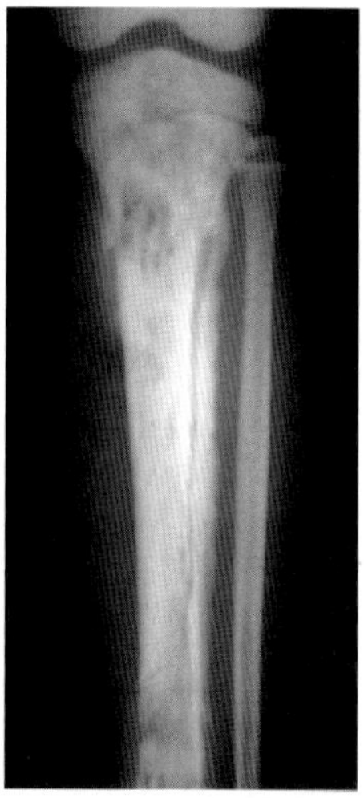

Figure 26.16 Chronic osteomyelitis, showing periosteal reaction along the lateral shaft of the tibia and multiple hypodense areas within the metaphyseal regions.

Presentation

This is usually with a markedly painful, immobile limb (pseudoparesis) in a child with an acute febrile illness. Directly over the infected site there is swelling and exquisite tenderness, and it may be erythematous and warm. Moving the limb causes severe pain. There may be a sterile effusion of an adjacent joint. Presentation may be more insidious in infants, in whom swelling or reduced limb movement is the initial sign. Beyond infancy, presentation may be with back pain in a vertebral infection or with a limp or groin pain in infection of the pelvis. Occasionally, there are multiple foci (e.g. disseminated staphylococcal or *H. influenzae* infection).

Investigation

Blood cultures are usually positive and the white blood count and acute-phase reactants are raised.

X-rays are initially normal, other than showing soft tissue swelling; it takes 7–10 days for subperiosteal new bone formation and localised bone rarefaction to become visible. Earlier changes suggesting altered blood supply may be visible on contrast MRI scanning and ultrasound may show periosteal elevation at presentation. The likely site of infection can be demonstrated using radionuclide bone scan (Fig. 26.15) although the image resolution is poor compared with an MRI. The X-ray changes of chronic osteomyelitis are shown in Figure 26.16.

Treatment

Prompt treatment with parenteral antibiotics is required for several weeks to prevent bone necrosis, chronic infection with a discharging sinus, limb deformity and amyloidosis. Antibiotics are given intravenously until there is clinical recovery and the acute-phase reactants have returned to normal, followed by oral therapy for several weeks. Aspiration or surgical decompression of the subperiosteal space may be performed if the presentation is atypical or is in immunocompromised children. Surgical drainage is performed if the condition does not respond rapidly to antibiotic therapy. The affected limb is initially rested in a splint and subsequently mobilised.

Summary

Osteomyelitis:

- presents with fever, a painful, immobile limb, swelling and extreme tenderness, especially on moving the limb
- blood cultures are usually positive
- parenteral antibiotics must be given immediately
- surgical drainage if unresponsive to antibiotic therapy.

Bone tumours

Malignant tumours – osteogenic sarcoma and Ewing's tumour – are rare. They present with pain or swelling, or occasionally with a pathological fracture (see Ch. 21). Osteoid osteoma is a benign tumour affecting adolescents, especially boys, usually involving the femur or tibia. The pain is more severe at night and improves with salicylate therapy. There may be some localised tenderness. The X-ray is usually diagnostic, with a sharply demarcated radiolucent nidus of osteoid tissue surrounded by sclerotic bone. If the X-ray is normal, a CT or MRI scan is required. Treatment is by surgical removal.

Arthritis

Presentation may be acute when there is a combination of pain, swelling, heat, redness and restricted movement in a joint. It must be distinguished from joint pain (arthralgia). In chronic arthritis there may be insidious onset of early morning stiffness of the joints, 'gelling' after inactivity, the development of a limp or slowness on walking. Initially, there may be only minimal evidence of joint swelling, but subsequently there may be swelling of the joint due to fluid within it (an effusion or pus or blood), inflammation and, in chronic arthritis, proliferation (thickening) of the synovium and swelling of the periarticular soft tissues. Long term, there may be bone expansion from overgrowth, which in the knee may cause leg lengthening and in the wrist advancement of bone age.

In a monoarthritis of acute onset, septic arthritis or osteomyelitis must be diagnosed and treated urgently. Other conditions which need to be considered, using the hip as an example, are listed as causes of a painful limp in Table 26.2. The causes of polyarthritis are listed in Table 26.3.

Reactive arthritis

Reactive arthritis is the most common form of arthritis in childhood. It is characterised by transient joint swelling (usually less than 6 weeks), following (or rarely accompanying) evidence of extra-articular infection. The enteric bacteria (*Salmonella*, *Shigella*, *Campylobacter* and *Yersinia*) are often the cause in children. Other infections include rubella, parvovirus B19, influenza, herpes and coxsackie viruses, *Mycoplasma* and *Borellia burgdorferi* (Lyme disease). Rheumatic fever and post-streptococcal reactive arthritis are rare in developed countries but are frequent in many developing countries.

Septic arthritis

This is a serious infection of the joint space as it can lead to bone destruction. It is most common in children less than 2 years old. It usually results from haematogenous spread, but may also occur following a puncture wound or infected skin lesions, e.g. chickenpox. In young children, it may result from spread from adjacent osteomyelitis

Table 26.3 Causes of polyarthritis

Infection	Bacterial – septicaemia/septic arthritis, TB
	Viral – rubella, mumps, adenovirus, coxsackie B, herpes, hepatitis, parvovirus
	Other – *Mycoplasma*, Lyme disease, rickettsia
	Reactive – gastrointestinal infection, streptococcal infection
	Rheumatic fever
Inflammatory bowel disease	Crohn's disease, ulcerative colitis
Vasculitis	Henoch–Schönlein purpura, Kawasaki's disease
Haematological disorders	Haemophilia, sickle cell disease
Malignant disorders	Leukaemia, neuroblastoma
Connective tissue disorders	Juvenile idiopathic arthritis (JIA), systemic lupus erythematosus (SLE), dermatomyositis, mixed connective tissue disease (MCTD), polyarteritis nodosa (PAN)
Other	Cystic fibrosis

into joints where the capsule inserts below the epiphyseal growth plate. Usually only one joint is affected, with the hip being a particular concern in infants and young children. Beyond the neonatal period, the most common organism is *Staphylococcus aureus*, and usually only one joint is affected. *H. influenzae* was an important cause in young children prior to Hib immunisation and often affected multiple sites. Underlying and predisposing illnesses such as immunodeficiency and sickle cell disease should be considered.

Presentation

This is usually with an erythematous, warm, acutely tender joint, with a reduced range of movement, in an acutely unwell, febrile child. Infants often hold the limb still (pseudoparesis, pseudoparalysis) and cry if it is moved. A joint effusion may be detectable in peripheral joints. In osteomyelitis, although a sympathetic joint effusion may be present, the tenderness is over the bone, but in up to 15% there is coexistent osteomyelitis. The diagnosis of septic arthritis of the hip can be particularly difficult in toddlers, as the joint is well covered by subcutaneous fat (Fig. 26.17). Initial presentation may be with a limp or pain referred to the knee.

Investigation

There is an increased white cell count and acute-phase reactants. Ultrasound of deep joints, such as the hip, is helpful to identify an effusion. X-rays are used to exclude trauma and other bony lesions. However, in septic arthritis, the X-rays are initially normal, apart from widening of the joint space and soft tissue swelling. A bone scan may be helpful

and an MRI scan may demonstrate an adjacent osteomyelitis. Aspiration of the joint space under ultrasound guidance for organisms and culture is the definitive investigation. Intravenous antibiotics should be instituted only after blood cultures. Ideally, a joint aspiration should also be performed, unless this would cause a significant delay in giving antibiotics. A prolonged course of antibiotics is required, initially intravenously (e.g. flucloxacillin, which in young children is combined with a third-generation cephalosporin to cover *H. influenzae*). Washing out of the joint or surgical drainage may be required if resolution does not occur rapidly or if the joint is deep-seated, such as the hip. The joint is initially immobilised in a functional position, but subsequently must be mobilised to prevent permanent deformity.

> Early treatment of septic arthritis is essential to prevent destruction of the articular cartilage and bone.

Juvenile idiopathic arthritis (JIA, juvenile chronic arthritis, juvenile rheumatoid arthritis)

This is the term used for children and adolescents with persistent joint swelling presenting before 16 years of age in the absence of infection or any defined cause. Ninety-five per cent of children with JIA have a disease that is clinically and immuno-genetically distinct from rheumatoid arthritis in adults. Newly presenting JIA is rare; a general practitioner is likely to encounter 1 new case in 20 years. However, it is one of the commonest physically disabling conditions of childhood, with a prevalence of approximately 1 in 1000 children, amounting to over 12 000 affected children in the UK.

There are at least seven different forms of the disease. It is classified according to its onset as systemic, polyarthritis (more than four joints) (Fig. 26.18) and oligoarthritis (up to and including four joints). Psoriatic arthritis and enthesitis are further subtypes. It is further classified according to the presence of rheumatoid factor and HLA B27 tissue type. The subtypes and their clinical features are shown in Table 26.4.

Complications

Chronic anterior uveitis

This is asymptomatic but can lead to severe visual impairment. Regular ophthalmological screening using a slit lamp is indicated, especially for children with oligoarticular disease.

Flexion contractures of the joints

These occur when the joint is held in the most comfortable position, thereby minimising intra-articular pressure (Fig. 26.19). Chronic disease can lead to joint destruction and the need for joint replacement in a few children.

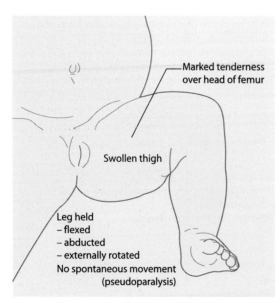

Figure 26.17 Septic arthritis of the hip in infants, showing the characteristic posture to reduce intracapsular pressure. Any leg movement is painful and is resisted.

Marked tenderness over head of femur

Swollen thigh

Leg held
– flexed
– abducted
– externally rotated
No spontaneous movement (pseudoparalysis)

Table 26.4 Classification and clinical features of JIA (juvenile idiopathic arthritis)

JIA subtype (approximate %)	Onset age	Sex ratio (f : m)	Articular pattern	Extra-articular features	Laboratory abnormalities
Oligoarthritis (persistent) (49%)	1–6 years	5 : 1	1–4 (max) joints involved; knee, ankle or wrist most common	Chronic anterior uveitis 20%, leg length discrepancy Prognosis excellent	ANA+
Oligoarthritis (extended) (8%)	1–6 years	5 : 1	> 4 joints involved after first 6 months. Asymmetrical distribution of large and small joints	Chronic anterior uveitis 20%, asymmetrical growth Prognosis moderate	ANA+
Polyarthritis (RF negative) (16%)	1–6 years	5 : 1	Symmetrical large and small joint arthritis, often with marked finger involvement (Fig. 26.18). Cervical spine and temporomandibular joint may be involved.	Low-grade fever, chronic anterior uveitis 5%, late reduction of growth rate Prognosis moderate	
Polyarthritis (RF positive) (3%)	10–16 years	5 : 1	Symmetrical large and small joint arthritis, often with marked finger involvement	Rheumatoid nodules 10% Prognosis poor	RF+ (long-term)
Systemic arthritis (9%)	1–10 years	1 : 1	Oligoarthritis or polyarthritis May have aches and pains in joints and muscles (arthralgia/myalgia) but initially no arthritis	Acute illness, malaise, high daily fever initially, with salmon-pink, macular rash, lymphadenopathy, hepatosplenomegaly, serositis. Prognosis variable to poor	Anaemia, raised neutrophils and platelets, high acute-phase reactants. (see Case history 26.1)
Psoriatic arthritis (7%)	1–16 years	1 : 1	Usually asymmetrical distribution of large and small joints, dactylitis	Psoriasis, nail pitting or dystrophy, chronic anterior uveitis 20% Prognosis moderate	
Enthesitis-related arthritis (7%)	6–16 years	1 : 4	Lower limb, large joint arthritis initially, mild lumbar spine or sacroiliac involvement later on	Enthesitis – localised inflammation at insertion of tendons or ligaments into bone, often in feet, Achilles insertion. Occasional acute uveitis Prognosis moderate	HLA B27+
Undifferentiated arthritis (1%)	1–16 years	2 : 1 (variable)	Overlapping articular and extra-articular patterns between 2 or more subtypes or insufficient criteria for sub-classification	Prognosis variable	

Arthritis

443

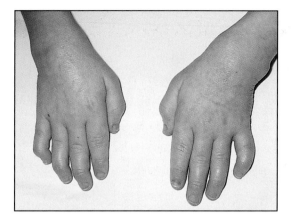

Figure 26.18 Polyarticular juvenile idiopathic arthritis, showing swelling of the wrists, metacarpal and interphalangeal joints and early swan-neck deformities of the fingers.

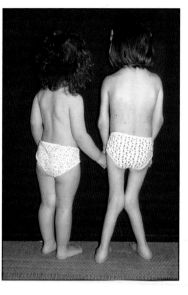

Figure 26.20 Growth failure and marked genu valgum (knock knees) in an 8-year-old girl with juvenile idiopathic arthritis. For comparison, her sister on the left is 4 years old.

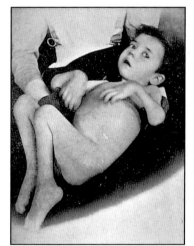

Figure 26.19 Severe untreated polyarthritis or systemic arthritis, from Still's original description in 1897, showing severe misery, fused neck, flexion deformities and wasting of the muscles and subcutaneous tissue.

Growth failure

This may be generalised from anorexia, chronic disease and steroid therapy (Fig. 26.20).

Amyloidosis

This is a rare but serious complication causing proteinuria and subsequent renal failure.

Management

The aim of therapy is to maintain the patient's quality of life and to preserve joint function for as long as the disease is active. Patient education and the support of an experienced paediatric rheumatology team are essential. The team should include a paediatric rheumatologist, and staff with specific paediatric expertise in rehabilitation, disease education, nutrition, drug monitoring, school liaison, family and social support and psychology. In addition, there needs to be ready access to other paediatric specialties including ophthalmology, orthopaedics, maxillo-facial surgery, nephrology, dermatology and psychiatry. Considerable motivation and compliance is required for successful management.

Physiotherapy is essential in order to encourage mobility and maintain a full range of joint movement and muscle strength. Daily exercise is usually required. Hydrotherapy is a helpful adjunct. Resting splints may be used to prevent flexion contractures, and working splints for the wrists to maintain posture while writing.

All children with active arthritis should receive regular non-steroidal anti-inflammatory drugs (NSAIDs) to control pain and suppress inflammation, such as ibuprofen, piroxicam or naproxen. Intra-articular corticosteroid therapy can be helpful; multiple injections may be required. Systemic steroids should be avoided if possible, due to the wide range of adverse side-effects, including growth suppression. However, intravenous methylprednisolone may sometimes be required to gain control of active polyarthritis and may even be life-saving in the face of significant systemic arthritis with pericarditis (see Case history 26.1).

Disease-modifying anti-rheumatic drugs should be considered for any child whose arthritis is not well controlled on NSAIDs and intra-articular steroids alone. Methotrexate is effective in approximately 70% of children with polyarthritis but fewer with systemic disease. It is most effective when given by subcutaneous injection, but can also be given orally. Side-effects should be monitored – the commonest is nausea, but include abdominal pain, elevated liver enzymes and, rarely, mouth ulcers, hair loss and bone marrow suppression. Monitoring should be performed for abnormal liver function and bone-marrow suppression. Anti-TNF (anti-tumour necrosis factor) therapy and other biological agents are increasingly being used for those not adequately controlled on methotrexate or those intolerant of it.

Prognosis

The disease may remit spontaneously, but objective predictors of this outcome are lacking. Long-term follow-up studies have highlighted a rather poorer

Case History
26.1 Juvenile idiopathic arthritis: Systemic arthritis

A 2-year-old boy presented with a high fever (Fig. 26.21a) and malaise. A salmon-coloured rash was present at times of fever (Fig. 26.21b). Investigation showed markedly raised acute-phase reactants. A diagnosis of systemic-onset juvenile idiopathic arthritis was made on the basis of the clinical presentation and exclusion of other disorders (Box 26.2).

Shortly afterwards, he developed polyarthritic joint disease. He required high-dose alternate-day corticosteroid therapy as well as other disease-modifying drugs. He developed marked short stature. In his teens he required bilateral hip replacements. He is now at university, drives his own car and is fiercely independent.

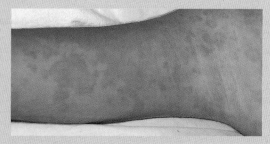

Figure 26.21b Salmon-pink rash.

Box 26.2 Differential diagnosis of systemic arthritis

- Infection – bacterial/viral/protozoal (e.g. malaria), *Mycoplasma* and other (e.g. Lyme disease)
- Kawasaki's disease
- Rheumatic fever
- Reactive arthritis – post-streptococcal, post-enteric, post-viral
- Malignancy – leukaemia, neuroblastoma
- Connective tissue disorders – systemic lupus erythematosus (SLE), polyarteritis nodosa (PAN)

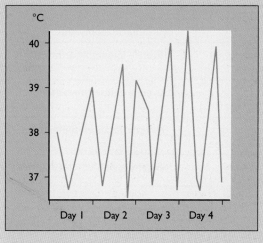

Figure 26.21a Temperature chart.

prognosis for JIA than previously believed. As many as 30% continue to have active arthritis into adulthood, and many more are left with chronic sequelae of restricted joint movement, growth failure and extra-articular abnormalities. This information has resulted in the introduction of more aggressive treatment regimens than previously advocated.

Henoch–Schönlein purpura

This is the most common vasculitis of childhood and presents with a purpuric rash over the lower legs and buttocks, usually associated with arthritis of the ankles or knees. Other features are abdominal pain, haematuria and proteinuria (see Ch. 18).

Systemic lupus erythematosus

Systemic lupus erythematosus is rare in children, but may present in adolescent females. Arthritis is but one of its protean initial manifestations.

Juvenile dermatomyositis

Juvenile dermatomyositis (JDMS) usually begins insidiously with malaise, progressive weakness (which may be mistaken for laziness) and facial rash with erythema over the bridge of the nose and malar areas and a violaceous (heliotropic) discoloration of the eyelids. The skin over the metacarpal and proximal interphalangeal joints may be hypertrophic and pink, and the nailfold capillaries may be dilated and tortuous. Muscle pain is a common, if non-specific, symptom and arthritis is found in 30%. Respiratory failure and aspiration pneumonia may be life-threatening. The condition is described further in Chapter 27.

Malignant disease

Acute lymphoblastic leukaemia may present with bone pain in children (sometimes primarily at night) and even frank arthritis. Neuroblastoma, usually in the young children, may present with

Summary

Diagnostic clues regarding bone and joint and rheumatic disorders		
'Typical' symptom combinations	Pivotal clinical features	Possible diagnoses
Nocturnal wakening with leg pain	Normal child	'Growing pains' Osteoid osteoma
	Anaemia, bruising, irritability, infections	Leukaemia, lymphoma, neuroblastoma (young child)
'Clunk' on hip movement screening, limp in an older infant	Asymmetrical upper leg skin folds, limited hip abduction	Developmental dysplasia of the hip
Febrile, toxic-looking infant, irritability with nappy changing	Restricted joint range (especially hip)	Septic arthritis Osteomyelitis
Sudden limp in a otherwise well young child	Unilateral restricted hip movement	Transient synovitis of the hip
Fever, erythematous rash, red eyes, irritability in infant or young child	Erythema/oedema of hands and feet, oral mucositis, cervical lymphadenopathy.	Kawasaki's disease
Irritability, fever, reluctance to move in an infant or young child	Stiff back, 'tripod' sitting	Discitis Vertebral osteomyelitis
Joint pain, stiffness and restriction Loss of joint function	Persistent joint swelling Loss of joint range	Juvenile idiopathic arthritis
Lethargy, unwilling to do physical activities, irritability, rash	Eyelid erythema Proximal muscle weakness	Juvenile dermatomyositis
Constitutional symptoms, lethargy, arthralgia in an adolescent female	Multi-system abnormalities, haematuria, facial erythema	Systemic lupus erythematosus
Hip pain in an obese adolescent boy	Unilateral hip restriction	Slipped upper femoral epiphysis

systemic arthritis, or bone pain, which may be difficult to localise, from metastases.

Genetic skeletal conditions

These are inherited abnormalities resulting in generalised developmental disorders of bone, of which there are several hundred types. They usually result in reduced growth and abnormality of bone shape rather than impaired strength, except for osteogenesis imperfecta. The bones of the limbs and spine are often affected, resulting in short stature. Intelligence is usually normal. Improved knowledge of the molecular basis of collagen and its disorders is allowing better understanding and delineation of some of these disorders.

Achondroplasia

Inheritance is autosomal dominant, but about 50% are new mutations. Clinical features are short stature from marked shortening of the limbs, a large head, frontal bossing and depression of the nasal bridge (see Fig. 11.10). The hands are short and broad. A marked lumbar lordosis develops. Hydrocephalus sometimes occurs.

Thanatophoric dysplasia

This results in stillbirth. The infants have a large head, extremely short limbs and a small chest. The appearance of the bones on X-ray is characteristic. The importance of the correct diagnosis of this disorder is that, in contrast to achondroplasia, its inheritance is sporadic. It may be identified on antenatal ultrasound.

Cleidocranial dysostosis

In this autosomal dominant disorder, there is absence of part or all of the clavicles and delay in closure of the anterior fontanelle and of ossification of the skull. The child is often able to bring the shoulders together in front of the chest to touch each other as a 'party trick'. Short stature is usually present.

Arthrogryposis

This is a heterogeneous group of congenital disorders in which there is stiffness and contracture of joints. The cause is usually unknown, but there may be an association with oligohydramnios, widespread congenital anomalies or chromosomal

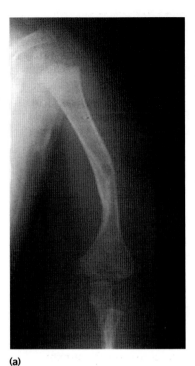

(a)

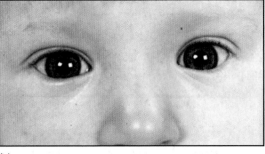

(b)

Figure 26.22 Osteogenesis imperfecta type I, showing **(a)** fracture of the humerus and osteoporotic bones, **(b)** blue sclerae.

> Osteogenesis imperfecta is often considered in the evaluation of unexplained fractures in suspected child abuse.

disorders. It is usually sporadic. Marked flexion contractures of the knees, elbows and wrists, dislocation of the hips and other joints, talipes equinovarus and scoliosis are common, but the disorder may be localised to the upper or lower limbs. The skin is thin, subcutaneous tissue is reduced and there is marked muscle atrophy around the affected joints. Intelligence is usually unaffected. Management is with physiotherapy and correction of deformities, where possible, by splints, plaster casts or surgery. Walking is impaired in the more severe forms of the disorder.

Osteogenesis imperfecta (brittle bone disease)

This is a group of disorders of collagen metabolism causing bone fragility, with bowing and frequent fractures.

In the most common form (type I), which is autosomal dominant, there are fractures during childhood (Fig. 26.22A) and a blue appearance to the sclerae (Fig. 26.22B), and some develop hearing loss. The prognosis is variable. Fractures require splinting to minimise joint deformity.

There is a severe, lethal form (type II) with multiple fractures already present before birth (Fig. 26.23). Many affected infants are stillborn. Inheritance is variable but mostly autosomal dominant or due to new mutations. In other types, scleral discoloration may be minimal.

Osteopetrosis (marble bone disease)

In this rare disorder, the bones are dense but brittle. The severe autosomal recessive disorder presents with failure to thrive, recurrent infection, hypo-

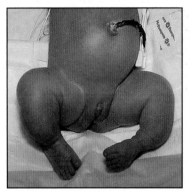

Figure 26.23 Osteogenesis imperfecta (type II) showing shortened, deformed lower limbs from gross deformity of the bones with multiple fractures.

calcaemia, anaemia and thrombocytopenia. Prognosis is poor, but bone marrow transplantation can be curative. A less severe autosomal dominant form may present during childhood with fractures.

Marfan's sydrome

This is an autosomal dominant disorder of connective tissue associated with tall stature, long thin digits (arachnodactyly), hyperextensible joints, a high arched palate, dislocation (usually upwards) of the lenses of the eyes and severe myopia. The body proportions are altered, with long, thin limbs resulting in a greater distance between the pubis and soles (lower segment) than from the crown to the pubis (upper segment). The arm span, measured from the extended fingers, is greater than the height. There may be chest deformity and scoliosis. The major problems are cardiovascular, due to degeneration of the media of vessel walls resulting in a dilated, incompetent aortic root with valvular incompetence and mitral valve prolapse and regurgitation. Aneurysms of the aorta may dissect or rupture. Monitoring by echocardiography is required.

Further reading

Cassidy J, Petty R E, Laxer R, Lindsley C 2005 Textbook of pediatric rheumatology, 5th edn. Elsevier Saunders, Edinburgh

Szer I S, Kimura Y, Malleson P N, Southwood T R (eds) 2006 Arthritis in children and adolescents: juvenile idiopathic arthritis. Oxford University Press, Oxford

Neurological disorders

Headache

Headache in older children and adolescents is a frequent reason for consulting a doctor. The other causes of headache are shown in Box 27.1. The International Headache Society (IHS) has devised a diagnostic classification for headaches. The causes of recurrent headache are considered below.

Tension-type headache

This is a symmetrical headache of gradual onset, often described as tightness, a band or pressure. There are usually no other symptoms, but it may be accompanied by abdominal pain and behaviour problems. It may occur daily.

Migraine

This periodic disorder is characterised by paroxysmal headache, often unilateral, and is characteristically throbbing. It is often accompanied by unpleasant gastrointestinal disturbance such as nausea, vomiting and abdominal pain and by visual disturbance. The visual disturbances include:

- Negative phenomena such as:
  hemianopia (loss of half the visual field)
  scotoma (small areas of visual loss).
- Positive phenomena such as:
  fortification spectra (seeing zigzag lines).

Rarely, there are unilateral sensory or motor symptoms.

Episodes usually last for a few hours, during which time children often prefer to lie down in a quiet, dark place. Sleep often relieves the bout.

Migraine is classified as:

- without aura (formerly called common migraine), affecting approximately 90%
- with aura (formerly called classical migraine) – the headache is preceded by an aura (visual, sensory or motor); this type affects approximately 10% (the aura may occur without a headache)
- complicated – associated with neurological phenomena such as ophthalmoplegia, hemiparesis, paraesthesiae or hemidysaesthesia (altered sensation down one side of the body). It occurs in 1–2% and, rarely, results in permanent neurological deficit. Hemiparetic migraine is linked to a calcium channel defect, often dominantly inherited. Vertebrobasilar migraine gives rise to signs of posterior circulation compromise, such as nystagmus and associated vomiting and dizziness.

Symptoms of tension-type headache and migraine often overlap. They are probably part of the same pathophysiological continuum; there is increasing evidence that both symptom groups result from channelopathies with vascular phenomena being secondary events. Headaches are common in first- and second-degree relatives of children with recurrent headaches. Some cases of cyclical (recurrent) vomiting and recurrent abdominal pain in young children are thought to be due to abdominal migraine. Stress at home or school may trigger headaches and make them more difficult to cope with, although for many, winding down is a trigger. A food diary helps to identify any food triggers, often cheese, chocolate, and caffeine, although they may vary with time. In girls, headaches can be related to menses and the oral contraceptive pill.

Box 27.1 Causes of headache

Causes of recurrent headache

Tension-type headache

Migraine
* without aura
* with aura
* complicated

Raised intracranial pressure and space-occupying lesions

Other causes:
* sinusitis – may cause facial pain, elicited by percussion
* temporomandibular joint discomfort – from dental malocclusion, worse on chewing
* medication – side-effect
* refractive errors – rare cause, but check vision
* head trauma
* solvent, drug and alcohol abuse
* hypertension – uncommon cause, usually with encephalopathy – but blood pressure should always be checked
* benign intracranial hypertension, i.e. no space-occupying lesion or CSF obstruction. Characteristically in overweight adult females but occurs in children.

Causes of acute headache
* Febrile illness
* Migraine
* Stress
* Acute sinusitis
* Meningitis/encephalitis
* Head injury
* Subarachnoid or intracerebral haemorrhage
* Benign intracranial hypertension
* Medications, alcohol, solvent or drug abuse
* Other triggers: ice-cream, from reflex neuralgia

Raised intracranial pressure and space-occupying lesions

Headaches often raise the fear of brain tumours and may be the reason for parents to consult a doctor. Headaches due to a space-occupying lesion are worse when lying down and morning vomiting is characteristic. The headaches may also cause night-time waking. There is often a change in mood, personality or educational performance. Other features suggestive of a space-occupying lesion are:

* visual field defects – from lesions pressing on the optic pathways, e.g. craniopharyngioma (a pituitary tumour)
* cranial nerve abnormalities causing diplopia, new onset squint or facial nerve palsy. The VIth

(abducens) cranial nerve has a long intracranial course and is often affected when there is raised pressure, resulting in a squint with diplopia and inability to abduct the eye beyond the midline. It is a false localising sign. Other nerves are affected depending on the site of lesion, e.g. pontine lesions may affect the VIIth (facial) cranial nerve and cause a facial nerve palsy
* abnormal gait
* torticollis (tilting of the head)
* growth failure, e.g. craniopharyngioma or hypothalamic lesion
* papilloedema – a late feature
* cranial bruits – may be heard in arteriovenous malformations but these lesions are rare.

Other causes

These are listed in Box 27.1.

Management

The mainstay of management is a thorough history and examination with detailed explanation and advice. Imaging is unnecessary in the absence of the symptoms or signs of raised intracranial pressure or abnormal neurological signs. A headache diary can be helpful in pinpointing triggers (usually there are none) and for monitoring management.

Children and parents should be informed that recurrent headaches are common. There are likely to be good and bad patches over months or years but they cause no long-term harm. Written information for the child and parents to take home is helpful. Children should be advised on how to live with and control the headaches, rather than allowing the headaches to dominate their lives. Therapeutic options include:

* psychological support to ameliorate particular causes of stress, e.g. bullying, anxiety over exams or illness in friends or family
* relaxation and other self-regulating techniques
* analgesia – paracetamol and non-steroidal anti-inflammatory drugs (NSAIDs), which should be taken as early as possible if the severity of the headache is increasing
* anti-emetics – prochlorperazine and metoclopramide
* serotonin (5-HT$_1$) agonist, sumatriptan. A nasal preparation of this is licensed for use in children over 12 years of age. Other triptans are not yet licensed in children.

If headaches are frequent, usually greater than one per week, prophylactic agents can be tried. These include:

* pizotifen (5-HT antagonist) – but can cause weight gain and sleepiness
* beta-blockers – propranolol, but contraindicated in asthma.

Systematic reviews show we need further evidence on which to base headache management.

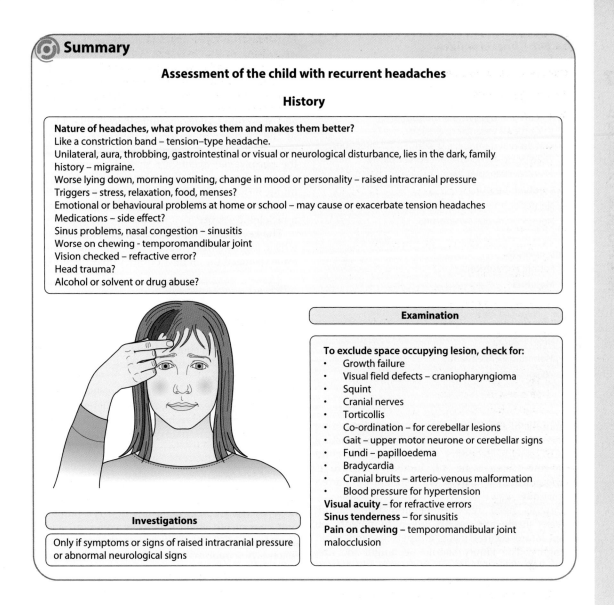

Summary

Assessment of the child with recurrent headaches

History

Nature of headaches, what provokes them and makes them better?
Like a constriction band – tension–type headache.
Unilateral, aura, throbbing, gastrointestinal or visual or neurological disturbance, lies in the dark, family history – migraine.
Worse lying down, morning vomiting, change in mood or personality – raised intracranial pressure
Triggers – stress, relaxation, food, menses?
Emotional or behavioural problems at home or school – may cause or exacerbate tension headaches
Medications – side effect?
Sinus problems, nasal congestion – sinusitis
Worse on chewing - temporomandibular joint
Vision checked – refractive error?
Head trauma?
Alcohol or solvent or drug abuse?

Examination

To exclude space occupying lesion, check for:
- Growth failure
- Visual field defects – craniopharyngioma
- Squint
- Cranial nerves
- Torticollis
- Co-ordination – for cerebellar lesions
- Gait – upper motor neurone or cerebellar signs
- Fundi – papilloedema
- Bradycardia
- Cranial bruits – arterio-venous malformation
- Blood pressure for hypertension

Visual acuity – for refractive errors
Sinus tenderness – for sinusitis
Pain on chewing – temporomandibular joint malocclusion

Investigations

Only if symptoms or signs of raised intracranial pressure or abnormal neurological signs

Seizures

A seizure is a clinical event in which there is a sudden disturbance of neurological function caused by an abnormal or excessive neuronal discharge.

A febrile convulsion is a seizure associated with fever in the absence of another cause and not due to intracranial infection from meningitis or encephalitis.

Epilepsy is recurrent seizures other than febrile convulsions in the absence of an acute cerebral insult.

The causes of seizures are listed in Box 27.2.

Febrile seizures (febrile convulsions)

These occur in 3% of children, between the ages of 6 months and 5 years. There is a genetic predisposition, with a 10% risk if the child has a first-degree relative with febrile seizures. The seizure usually occurs early in a viral infection when the temperature is rising rapidly. The seizures are usually brief, and are generalised tonic-clonic seizures. Thirty to forty per cent will have further febrile seizures. This is more likely the younger the child, the shorter the duration of illness before the seizure, the lower the temperature at the time of seizure and if there is a positive family history.

Simple febrile seizures do not cause brain damage and the child's subsequent intellectual performance is the same as children who do not experience a febrile seizure. There is a 1–2% chance of developing epilepsy, similar to the risk for all children.

However, complex febrile seizures; i.e. those which are focal, prolonged, or repeated in the same illness, have an increased risk of 4–12% of subsequent epilepsy.

The acute management of seizures is described in Chapter 6. Examination should focus on the cause of the fever, which is usually a viral illness but a bacterial infection including meningitis should always be considered. The classical features of meningitis such as neck stiffness and photophobia may not be as apparent in children less than

Box 27.2 Causes of seizures

Epilepsy
- Idiopathic (70–80%)
- Secondary
  - Cerebral dysgenesis/malformation
  - Cerebral vascular occlusion
  - Cerebral damage, e.g. congenital infection, hypoxic–ischaemic encephalopathy, intraventricular haemorrhage/ischaemia
- Cerebral tumour
- Neurodegenerative disorders
- Neurocutaneous syndromes

Non-epileptic
- Febrile convulsions
- Metabolic
  - Hypoglycaemia
  - Hypocalcaemia/hypomagnesaemia
  - Hypo/hypernatraemia
- Head trauma
- Meningitis/encephalitis
- Poisons/toxins

18 months of age, so an infection screen (including blood cultures, urine culture and lumbar puncture for CSF) may be necessary. In the unconscious child (Glasgow Coma Scale <8) lumbar puncture is contraindicated and antibiotics should be started empirically.

Parents need reassurance and information. Advice sheets are usually given to parents on temperature control using antipyretics and tepid sponging. The family should be taught the first aid management of seizures. If there is a history of prolonged seizures (>5 minutes), rescue therapy with rectal diazepam or buccal midazolam can be supplied. Oral prophylactic anti-epileptic drugs are not used as they do not reduce the recurrence rate of seizures or the risk of epilepsy. An EEG is not indicated as it does not serve as a guide for treatment nor does it predict seizure recurrence.

Summary

Febrile seizures:
- affect 3% of children; have a genetic predisposition
- occur between 6 months and 6 years of age
- are usually brief, generalised tonic-clonic seizures occurring with a rapid rise in fever
- if a bacterial infection, especially meningitis, is present, it needs to be identified and treated
- advise family about fever control, management of seizures, consider rescue therapy
- if simple – does not affect intellectual performance or risk of developing epilepsy
- if complex, 4–12% risk of subsequent epilepsy.

Paroxysmal disorders (funny turns) and epilepsy

There is a broad differential diagnosis for children with paroxysmal disorders. Epilepsy is a clinical diagnosis based on the history from eyewitnesses and the child's own account. If available, videos of the seizures or suspected seizures can be of great help. The diagnostic question is whether the paroxysmal events are that of an epilepsy of childhood or one of the many conditions which mimic it (Fig. 27.1). The most common pitfall is that of a syncope leading to an anoxic (non-epileptic) tonic-clonic seizure.

The key to the diagnosis lies in a detailed history, which, together with clinical examination, will determine the need for an EEG or other investigations.

Summary

Breath-holding and reflex anoxic seizures
In toddlers:
- breath-holding attacks – toddler, precipitated by anger, holds breath, goes blue, then limp, rapid recovery
- reflex anoxic seizures – toddler, precipitated by pain, stops breathing, goes pale, brief seizure sometimes, rapid recovery.

Other non-epileptic paroxysmal disorders:
- see Fig. 27.1

The epilepsies of childhood

Epilepsy has an incidence of about 0.05% (after the first year of life when it is more common) and a prevalence of 0.5%. This means that most large secondary schools will have about six children with an epilepsy of childhood or adolescence. Most epilepsy is idiopathic but other causes of seizures are listed in Box 27.2.

An international classification of epilepsy is used. This broadly classifies seizures as either:

- generalised – discharge arises from both hemispheres, or
- focal (also known as localisation-related or partial) – where seizures arise from one or part of one hemisphere.

Generalised seizures may be:

- absence
- myoclonic
- tonic
- tonic-clonic
- astatic.

The manifestations of focal seizures will depend on the part of the brain where the discharge originates:

- *Frontal* seizures – involve the motor cortex. May lead to clonic movements, which may travel proximally (Jacksonian march). Asymmetrical tonic seizures can be seen, which may be bizarre and

Causes of funny turns

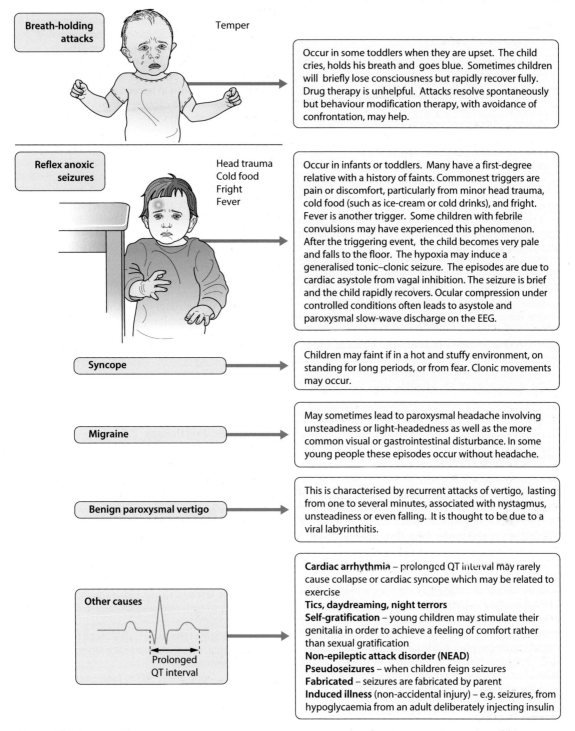

Breath-holding attacks — Temper

Occur in some toddlers when they are upset. The child cries, holds his breath and goes blue. Sometimes children will briefly lose consciousness but rapidly recover fully. Drug therapy is unhelpful. Attacks resolve spontaneously but behaviour modification therapy, with avoidance of confrontation, may help.

Reflex anoxic seizures — Head trauma / Cold food / Fright / Fever

Occur in infants or toddlers. Many have a first-degree relative with a history of faints. Commonest triggers are pain or discomfort, particularly from minor head trauma, cold food (such as ice-cream or cold drinks), and fright. Fever is another trigger. Some children with febrile convulsions may have experienced this phenomenon. After the triggering event, the child becomes very pale and falls to the floor. The hypoxia may induce a generalised tonic–clonic seizure. The episodes are due to cardiac asystole from vagal inhibition. The seizure is brief and the child rapidly recovers. Ocular compression under controlled conditions often leads to asystole and paroxysmal slow-wave discharge on the EEG.

Syncope

Children may faint if in a hot and stuffy environment, on standing for long periods, or from fear. Clonic movements may occur.

Migraine

May sometimes lead to paroxysmal headache involving unsteadiness or light-headedness as well as the more common visual or gastrointestinal disturbance. In some young people these episodes occur without headache.

Benign paroxysmal vertigo

This is characterised by recurrent attacks of vertigo, lasting from one to several minutes, associated with nystagmus, unsteadiness or even falling. It is thought to be due to a viral labyrinthitis.

Other causes — Prolonged QT interval

Cardiac arrhythmia – prolonged QT interval may rarely cause collapse or cardiac syncope which may be related to exercise
Tics, daydreaming, night terrors
Self-gratification – young children may stimulate their genitalia in order to achieve a feeling of comfort rather than sexual gratification
Non-epileptic attack disorder (NEAD)
Pseudoseizures – when children feign seizures
Fabricated – seizures are fabricated by parent
Induced illness (non-accidental injury) – e.g. seizures, from hypoglycaemia from an adult deliberately injecting insulin

Figure 27.1 Causes of funny turns.

hyperkinetic and can be mistakenly dismissed as non-epileptic events.

- *Temporal lobe* seizures, the most common of all the epilepsies – may result in strange warning feelings or aura with smell and taste abnormalities and distortions of sound and shape. Lip-smacking, plucking at one's clothing, and walking in a

non-purposeful manner (automatisms) may be seen, following spread to the pre-motor cortex. Déjà-vu and jamais-vu are described (intense feelings of having been, or never having been, in the same situation before). Consciousness can be impaired and the length of event is longer than a typical absence.

- *Occipital* seizures – cause distortion of vision.
- *Parietal lobe* seizures – cause contralateral dysaesthesias (altered sensation), or distorted body image.

Focal seizures are also delineated according to level of consciousness:

- *simple partial focal* seizures – consciousness is retained
- *complex partial focal* seizures – consciousness is lost. Children with complex partial seizures may, however, retain some memory of the event.
- *partial focal seizures with secondary generalisation* – focal seizure followed by generalised tonic-clonic seizure.

It is often difficult to distinguish simple from complex partial seizures; hence the new term 'dyscognitive seizure'.

The classification of epilepsy into generalised epilepsy, focal epilepsy and epilepsy syndromes is shown in Figure 27.2. Further details of some of the epilepsy syndromes are given in Table 27.1.

The diagnosis is primarily based on a detailed history from the child and eyewitnesses, substantiated by a video if available. Clinical examination should include checking the skin for neurocutaneous markers and a detailed neurological examination to identify any neurological abnormalities. Although epilepsy is usually idiopathic, it may be the presentation or a complication of an underlying neurological disorder.

Investigation of seizures

EEG

An EEG is indicated whenever epilepsy is suspected. It is analysed to identify asymmetry, any focal abnormalities such as sharp waves or slowing that might suggest underlying abnormalities. Many children with epilepsy have a normal initial EEG; and many children who will never have epilepsy have EEG abnormalities. Unless a seizure is actually captured on the EEG it does no more than add supportive evidence (or not) for the diagnosis. If the standard EEG is normal, abnormalities may be better seen during sleep, so a sleep or sleep-deprived record can be helpful. Additional techniques are 24-hour ambulatory EEG or, ideally, video-telemetry. In assessment for surgery more invasive techniques such as subdural electrodes can be used.

Imaging

- *Structural*. MRI and CT brain scans are not required routinely for childhood generalised epilepsies. They are indicated if there are neurological signs between seizures, or if seizures are focal, in order to identify a tumour, vascular lesion, or area of sclerosis which could be treatable. MRI FLAIR (fluid-attenuated inversion recovery) sequences better detect mesial temporal sclerosis in temporal lobe epilepsy.
- *Functional scans*. While it is not always possible to see structural lesions, techniques have advanced to allow functional imaging to detect areas of abnormal metabolism suggestive of seizure foci. These include PET (positron emission tomography) and SPECT (single positron emission computed tomograpy), which use isotopes and ligands, injected and taken up by metabolically active cells. Both can be used between seizures to detect areas of hypometabolism in epileptogenic lesions. SPECT can also be used to capture seizures and areas of hypermetabolism.

Other investigations

Blood tests and metabolic investigations may be warranted when there is developmental regression or seizures are related to feeds or fasting. Genetic studies will become increasingly helpful as certain epilepsy syndromes are now known to be due to genetic deletions causing abnormalities of sodium and other ion channels, the channelopathies.

Management

Management begins with explanation and advice to help adjust to the diagnosis. A specialist epilepsy nurse may assist families by providing education and continuing care. It is common practice not to institute treatment after a single unprovoked seizure. There is around a 50% risk of a further seizure after a single unprovoked seizure and this must be discussed with the family. The diagnosis of epilepsy requires two or recurrent unprovoked seizures.

Anti-epileptic drug therapy

This is the mainstay in managing epileptic seizures. Principles governing their use are:

- Not all seizures require anti-epileptic drug therapy. This decision should be based on the seizure type, frequency and the social and educational consequences of the seizures against the possible unwanted effects of the drugs.
- Choose the appropriate drug for the seizure. Inappropriate antiepileptics may be detrimental, e.g. carbamazepine can make absence and myoclonic seizures worse. However, the evidence base for anti-epileptic drug therapy in children is poor.
- Monotherapy at the minimum dosage is the desired goal, although in practice several drugs may be required.
- All anti-epileptic drugs (AEDs) have potential unwanted effects and these should be discussed with the child and parent.
- Drug levels are not measured routinely but may be useful to check compliance or for some drugs with erratic pharmacokinetics, e.g. phenytoin.
- Patients who have had prolonged seizures are given rescue therapy to have with them. This is usually a benzodiazepine, e.g. rectal diazepam or buccal midazolam.
- Anti-epileptic drug therapy can usually be discontinued after 2 years free of seizures.

Guidance regarding treatment options for different seizure types are shown in Table 27.2. Common

Classification of epilepsy

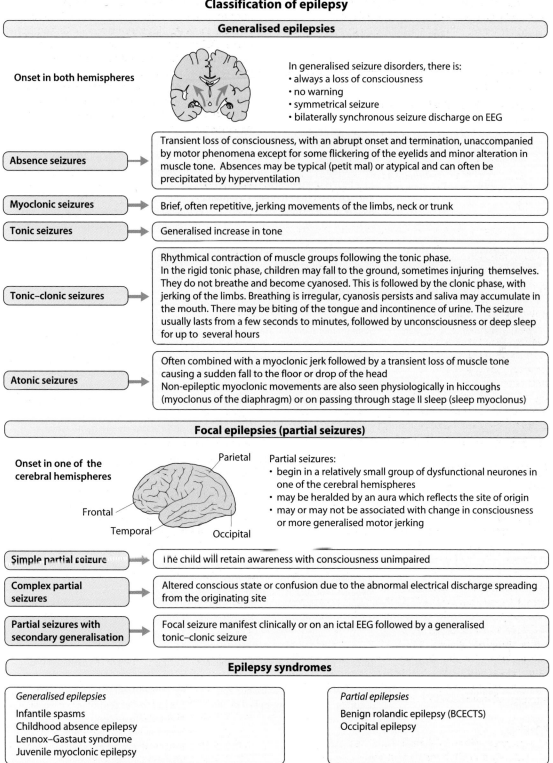

Generalised epilepsies

Onset in both hemispheres

In generalised seizure disorders, there is:
• always a loss of consciousness
• no warning
• symmetrical seizure
• bilaterally synchronous seizure discharge on EEG

Absence seizures → Transient loss of consciousness, with an abrupt onset and termination, unaccompanied by motor phenomena except for some flickering of the eyelids and minor alteration in muscle tone. Absences may be typical (petit mal) or atypical and can often be precipitated by hyperventilation

Myoclonic seizures → Brief, often repetitive, jerking movements of the limbs, neck or trunk

Tonic seizures → Generalised increase in tone

Tonic–clonic seizures → Rhythmical contraction of muscle groups following the tonic phase.
In the rigid tonic phase, children may fall to the ground, sometimes injuring themselves. They do not breathe and become cyanosed. This is followed by the clonic phase, with jerking of the limbs. Breathing is irregular, cyanosis persists and saliva may accumulate in the mouth. There may be biting of the tongue and incontinence of urine. The seizure usually lasts from a few seconds to minutes, followed by unconsciousness or deep sleep for up to several hours

Atonic seizures → Often combined with a myoclonic jerk followed by a transient loss of muscle tone causing a sudden fall to the floor or drop of the head
Non-epileptic myoclonic movements are also seen physiologically in hiccoughs (myoclonus of the diaphragm) or on passing through stage II sleep (sleep myoclonus)

Focal epilepsies (partial seizures)

Onset in one of the cerebral hemispheres

Parietal
Frontal
Temporal
Occipital

Partial seizures:
• begin in a relatively small group of dysfunctional neurones in one of the cerebral hemispheres
• may be heralded by an aura which reflects the site of origin
• may or may not be associated with change in consciousness or more generalised motor jerking

Simple partial seizure → The child will retain awareness with consciousness unimpaired

Complex partial seizures → Altered conscious state or confusion due to the abnormal electrical discharge spreading from the originating site

Partial seizures with secondary generalisation → Focal seizure manifest clinically or on an ictal EEG followed by a generalised tonic–clonic seizure

Epilepsy syndromes

Generalised epilepsies

Infantile spasms
Childhood absence epilepsy
Lennox–Gastaut syndrome
Juvenile myoclonic epilepsy

Partial epilepsies

Benign rolandic epilepsy (BCECTS)
Occipital epilepsy

Figure 27.2 Classification of epilepsy. The term 'dyscognitive seizure' is used for both simple and complex partial seizures as it is often difficult to distinguish between them.

Table 27.1 Some epilepsy syndromes

Name	Age	Seizure pattern	Comments
Generalised epilepsies			
Infantile spasms	4–6 months	Violent flexor spasms of the head, trunk and limbs followed by extension of the arms (so-called 'salaam spasms'). Flexor spasms last 1–2 seconds, often multiple bursts of 20–30 spasms, often on waking, but may occur many times a day. May be misinterpreted as colic. Social interaction often deteriorates – a useful marker in the history.	Many causes, two-thirds have underlying neurological cause. The EEG shows hypsarrhythmia, a chaotic pattern of high-voltage slow waves, and multi-focal sharp wave discharges (Fig. 27.3). Treatment is with vigabatrin or corticosteroids, Good response in 30–40%, but side-effects are common. Most will subsequently lose skills and develop learning disability or epilepsy.
Lennox–Gastaut syndrome	1–3 years	Multiple seizure types, but mostly drop attacks (astatic seizures), tonic seizures and atypical absences. Also neurodevelopmental arrest or regression and behaviour disorder.	Often other complex neurological problems or history of infantile spasms. Prognosis is poor.
Typical (petit mal) absence seizures	4–12 years	Stare momentarily and stop moving, may twitch their eyelids or a hand minimally. Lasts only a few seconds and certainly not longer than 30 seconds. Child has no recall except realises they have missed something and may look puzzled or say 'pardon' on regaining consciousness. Developmentally normal but can interfere with schooling. Accounts for only 2% of childhood epilepsy.	Two-thirds are female. The episodes can be induced by hyperventilation, the child being asked to blow on a piece of paper or windmill for 2–3 minutes, a useful test in the outpatient clinic. The EEG shows generalised 3 per second spike and wave discharge, which is bilaterally synchronous during and sometimes between attacks (Fig. 27.4). Prognosis is good with 95% remission in adolescence. 5–10% may develop tonic-clonic seizures in adult life.
Juvenile myoclonic epilepsy	Adolescence–adulthood	Myoclonic seizures, but generalised tonic-clonic seizures and absences may occur, mostly shortly after waking. A typical history is throwing drinks or cornflakes about in the morning as myoclonus occurs at this time. Learning is unimpaired.	Characteristic EEG. Response to treatment is usually good but lifelong. A genetic linkage has been identified.
Focal epilepsies			
Benign rolandic epilepsy, also known as benign childhood epilepsy with centrotemporal spikes (BCECTS)	4–10 years	Tonic-clonic seizures in sleep, or simple partial seizures with awareness of abnormal feelings in the tongue and distortion of the face (supplied by the rolandic area of the brain).	Comprises 15% of all childhood epilepsies. EEG shows focal sharp waves from the rolandic or centrotemporal area. Important to recognise as it is benign and does not always require treatment. Almost all remit in adolescence.
Benign occipital epilepsy	1–14 years	Younger children – periods of unresponsiveness, eye deviation, vomiting and autonomic features. Older children – headache and visual disturbance including distortion of images and hallucinations.	Uncommon. EEG shows occipital discharges. Remit in childhood.

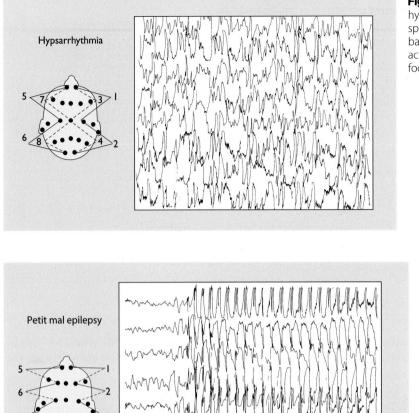

Figure 27.3 EEG of hypsarrhythmia in infantile spasms. There is a chaotic background of slow-wave activity with sharp multi-focal components.

Figure 27.4 EEG in a typical absence seizure in childhood absence epilepsy. There is three per second spike and wave discharge which is bilaterally synchronous during, and sometimes between, attacks.

Table 27.2 Choice of antiepileptic drugs (NICE, National Institute of Clinical Evidence, 2004)

Seizure type	First line	Second line
Generalised epilepsies		
Tonic-clonic	Valproate, carbamazepine	Lamotrigine, topiramate
Absence	Valproate, ethosuximide	Lamotrigine
Myoclonic	Valproate	Lamotrigine
Focal epilepsies	Carbamazepine, valproate	Topiramate, lamotrigine, levetiracetam, oxcarbazepine, gabapentin, tiagabine, vigabatrin

side-effects of anti-epileptic drugs are shown in Table 27.3.

Other treatment options

In children with intractable seizures there are a number of radical treatment options.

- *Ketogenic (fat based) diets* may be helpful in some children. Its mechanism of action is poorly understood.
- *Vagal nerve stimulation*, delivered using externally programmable stimulation of a wire implanted around the vagal nerve, may possibly be useful for focal seizures; trials are being conducted.
- *Surgery*. Cessation of seizures and drug therapy may be achieved in some children whose clinical are localised to a specific location in the brain as demonstrated on the EEG and functional imaging. The main procedure is temporal lobectomy for mesial temporal sclerosis but other procedures include hemispherectomy or hemispherotomy (does not involve hemisphere removal and problems with shifts in space) and

Table 27.3 Common or important side-effects of anti-epileptic drugs

Drug	Side-effects
Valproate	Weight gain, hair loss Rare idiosyncratic liver failure
Carbamazepine/oxcarbazepine	Rash, neutropenia, hyponatraemia, ataxia Liver enzyme induction, can interfere with other medication
Vigabatrin	Restriction of visual fields, which has limited its use. Sedation
Lamotrigine	Rash
Ethosuximide	Nausea and vomiting
Topiramate	Drowsiness, withdrawal and weight loss
Gabapentin	Insomnia
Levetiracetam	Sedation
Benzodiazepines – clobazam, clonazepam, diazepam, nitrazepam	Sedation, tolerance to effect, increased secretions

All the above may cause drowsiness and occasional skin rashes.

focal resections. Detailed assessment is required to ensure that the benefits outweigh the risks.

Advice and prognosis

The aim is to promote independence and confidence. Some children with epilepsy and their families need psychological help to adjust to the condition. The school needs to be aware of the child's problem and teachers advised on the management of seizures. Unrecognised absences may interfere with learning, which is an indication for being vigilant about 'odd episodes' which may represent seizures. Relatively few restrictions are required, but situations where having a seizure could lead to injury or be fatal should be avoided. This includes avoiding deep baths (showers are preferable) and not swimming alone in deep water. Those with photosensitivity should sit at a distance from televisions, can cover one eye, and check that TVs and VDUs in use are acceptable (Epilepsy Action consider most modern TVs and VDUs to be suitable and can provide advice). For adolescents there may be issues to discuss around driving (only after 1 year free of seizures), contraception and pregnancy. There may also be issues with compliance and precipitation of seizures by alcohol and poor sleep routines. Sudden unexpected death in epilepsy, SUDEP, needs to be discussed, and its low risks emphasised. Information is available from self-help groups and organisations such as Epilepsy Action. Children with epilepsy do less well educationally, with social outcomes and with future employment than those with other chronic illnesses such as diabetes. Two-thirds of children with epilepsy go to a mainstream school, but some require educational help for associated learning difficulties. One-third attend a special school, but they often have multiple disabilities and their epilepsy is part of a severe brain disorder. A few children require residential schooling where there are facilities and expertise in monitoring and treating intractable seizures.

Status epilepticus

Status epilepticus, a seizure lasting 30 minutes or repeated seizures for 30 minutes without recovery of consciousness in between, is described in Chapter 6.

> **Summary**
>
> **Epilepsy:**
> * affects 1 in 200 children
> * is classified as generalised or focal (partial) or an epilepsy syndrome of childhood
> * if suspected, an EEG is indicated
> * most but not all seizures require antiepileptic drug therapy, which should be appropriate for the seizure, comprise as few drugs and with the least potential for unwanted effects as possible
> * requires liaison with the school about the management of seizures and avoiding situations which could lead to injury.

Cerebral palsy

This is described in Chapter 4.

Ataxia

Ataxia, from the Greek word for 'without order', describes incoordination of movement, speech and posture. This can be due to cerebellar or posterior sensory pathway problems. Cerebellar causes are more common in children. In cerebellar ataxia there is an unsteady wide-based gait, difficulty in performing repetitive and alternating movements (dysdiadochokinesis), overshooting of target-directed movement (dysmetria) and an intention tremor which becomes more pronounced when the child puts more effort into trying to hold a posture. The gait has a wide base to provide stability to compensate for the truncal ataxia. There may be associated wobble of the head, nystagmus and speech impairment with a scanning dysarthria. Cerebellar ataxia may be caused by various insults to the cerebellum:

- acute, from medication and drugs, including alcohol and solvent abuse
- post-viral, particularly after varicella infection
- posterior fossa lesions or tumours, e.g. medulloblastoma
- genetic and degenerative disorders, e.g. ataxic cerebral palsy, Friedreich's ataxia and ataxia-telangiectasia.

Friedreich's ataxia

This is an autosomal recessive condition The gene mutation (Frataxin) is an example of a trinucleotide repeat disorder. It presents with worsening ataxia, distal wasting in the legs, absent lower limb reflexes but extensor plantar responses because of pyramidal involvement, pes cavus and dysarthria. This is similar to the hereditary motor sensory neuropathies, but in Friedreich's ataxia there is impairment of joint position and vibration sense, extensor plantars and there is often optic atrophy. The cerebellar component becomes more apparent with age. Evolving kyphoscoliosis and cardiomyopathy can cause cardiorespiratory compromise and death at 40–50 years.

Ataxia telangiectasia

This disorder of DNA repair is an autosomal recessive condition. The gene (ATM) has been identified. There may be mild delay in motor development in infancy and oculomotor problems with incoordination and delay in ocular pursuit of objects (oculomotor dyspraxia), with difficulty with balance and coordination becoming evident at school age. There is subsequent deterioration, with a mixture of dystonia and cerebellar signs. Many children require a wheelchair for mobility in early adolescence. Telangiectasia develop in the conjunctiva (Fig. 27.5), neck and shoulders from about 4 years of age. These children:

- have an increased susceptibility to infection, principally from an IgA surface antibody defect
- develop malignant disorders, principally acute lymphoblastic leukaemia (about 10%)
- have a raised serum alphafetoprotein
- have an increased white cell sensitivity to irradiation, which can be used diagnostically, but the ATM gene test is now mostly used.

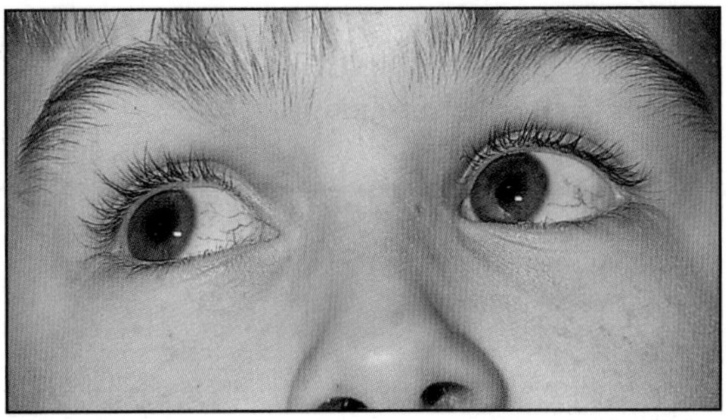

Figure 27.5 Telangiectasia of the conjunctiva are present from about 4 years of age in ataxia telangiectasia.

⟳ Summary

Ataxia:
- cerebellar is more common than posterior sensory pathway problems
- cerebellar causes – medication and drugs, varicella infection, posterior fossa lesions or tumours, genetic and degenerative disorders such as ataxic cerebral palsy, Friedreich's ataxia and ataxia-telangiectasia.

Cerebrovascular disease

Cerebral haemorrhage

Extradural haemorrhage

This usually results from arterial or venous bleeding into the extradural space following direct head trauma. It is usually associated with a skull fracture. In young children there is often a lucid interval until the conscious level deteriorates and seizures occur due to the enlarging haematoma acting as a space-occupying lesion. There may be focal neurological signs with dilatation of the ipsilateral pupil, paresis of the contralateral limbs and a false localising uni- or bilateral VIth nerve paresis. In young children, initial presentation may be with anaemia and shock. The diagnosis is confirmed with a CT scan. Management is to correct hypovolaemia. Surgical evacuation of the haematoma and arrest of the bleeding may be required and can be urgent in some situations.

Subdural haematoma

This results from tearing of the veins as they cross the subdural space. It is a characteristic lesion in non-accidental injury caused by shaking or direct trauma in infants or toddlers. Retinal haemorrhages are usually present. There has been recent controversy surrounding the relative contributions of direct trauma, shearing injury and hypoxia. Subdural haematomas are occasionally seen following a fall from a considerable height.

Summary

Regarding cerebral haemorrhage:
- history of significant head injury – an extradural haemorrhage may be present even if lucid afterwards
- subdural haematoma and retinal haemorrhages – consider non-accidental injury caused by shaking or direct trauma.

Subarachnoid haemorrhage

This is much more common in adults. Presentation is usually with acute onset of head pain, neck stiffness and occasionally fever. Retinal haemorrhage is usually present. Seizures and coma may develop. A CT scan of the head usually identifies blood in the CSF. A lumbar puncture in the acute situation is best avoided as haemorrhage may extend following the release of intracranial pressure. The cause is often an aneurysm or arteriovenous malformation (AVM). It can be identified on MR angiography (MRA) or CT or conventional angiography. Treatment can be neurosurgical or with interventional radiography.

Stroke in childhood

Strokes occur not only in adults but also in infants (see Ch. 10), and children. They originate from vascular, thromboembolic and haemorrhagic pathology. The clinical signs such as hemiplegia or speech or visual disturbance depend on the vascular territory compromised. Compromise of the anterior circulation (internal carotid, anterior and middle cerebral arteries) is more common than of the posterior circulation (vertebrobasilar arteries).

Causes include:

- cardiac – congenital cyanotic heart disease, e.g. Fallot's tetralogy, endocarditis
- haematological – sickle cell disease; deficiencies of anti-thrombotic factors, e.g. protein C
- inflammatory – damage to vessels in autoimmune disease, e.g. SLE (systemic lupus erythematosus)
- metabolic – homocystinuria, mitochondrial disorders, e.g. MELAS (myoclonic epilepsy, lactic acidosis and stroke)
- vascular malformations – moyamoya disease. These children have abnormal vasculature. Moyamoya comes from the Japanese for 'puff of smoke', similar to the blurred appearance seen on angiography.
- post varicella or other viral infections.

Investigations include brain imaging with CT and MRI, and haematological tests for thrombophilia and metabolic tests. Cardiological tests include echocardiography and carotid Doppler studies. Vasculature can be assessed with CT and MR angiography. More subtle vascular changes still require formal angiography. Often no cause can be identified. Long-term rehabilitation, with multi-collaborative working, may be required. Prophylaxis with aspirin may be given but further evidence is needed on the advisability of anti-thrombolytic agents.

Summary

Strokes:
- occur in infants and children
- occurring in the perinatal period may present in late infancy with a hemiplegia
- are a significant cause of morbidity and mortality in patients with sickle cell disease.

Neural tube defects and hydrocephalus

Neural tube defects

Neural tube defects result from failure of normal fusion of the neural plate to form the neural tube during the first 28 days following conception. Their birth prevalence in the UK has fallen dramatically from 4 per 1000 live births in the 1970s to 0.15 per 1000 live births in 1998 and to 0.11 per 1000 live births in 2005 (Fig. 27.6). This is mainly because of a natural decline, as well as antenatal screening.

The reason for the natural decline is uncertain but may be associated with improved maternal nutrition. It is well recognised that mothers of a fetus with a neural tube defect have a 10-fold increase in risk of having a second affected fetus. It has been shown that supplementing these mothers' diet with high doses of folic acid markedly reduces this risk. It is now recommended that women who have had a previously affected infant and are planning a pregnancy should take high-dose folic acid periconceptually. Low-dose periconceptual folic acid supplementation is recommended for all pregnancies.

Anencephaly

This is failure of development of most of the cranium and brain. Affected infants are stillborn or die shortly after birth. It is detected on antenatal ultrasound screening and termination of pregnancy is usually performed.

Encephalocele

There is extrusion of brain and meninges through a midline skull defect, which can be corrected surgically. However, there are often underlying associated cerebral malformations.

Spina bifida occulta

This failure of fusion of the vertebral arch (Fig. 27.7a) is often an incidental finding on X-ray, but there may be an associated overlying skin lesion such as a tuft of hair, lipoma, birth mark or small dermal sinus, usually in the lumbar region. There may be underlying tethering of the cord (diastematomyelia) which, with growth, may cause neurological deficits of bladder function and lower limbs. The extent of the underlying lesion can be delineated using ultrasound and/or MRI scans. Neurosurgical relief of tethering is usually indicated.

Meningocele and myelomeningocele

Meningoceles (Fig. 27.7b) usually have a good prognosis following surgical repair.

Myelomeningoceles (Figs 27.7c and 27.8) can cause a wide range of problems including:

- variable paralysis of the legs
- muscle imbalance which may cause dislocation of the hip and talipes
- sensory loss
- bladder denervation (neuropathic bladder)
- bowel denervation (neuropathic bowel)
- scoliosis
- hydrocephalus from the Arnold–Chiari malformation (herniation of the cerebellar tonsils through the foramen magnum), leading to disruption of CSF flow.

Neural tube defects

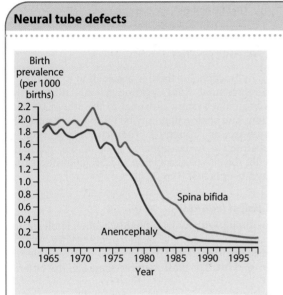

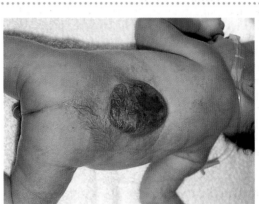

Figure 27.8 Myelomeningocele showing the exposed neural tissue and the patulous anus from neuropathic bowel.

Figure 27.6 The decline in the number of babies born with neural tube defects. This has resulted from a natural decrease together with antenatal diagnosis and termination of pregnancy.

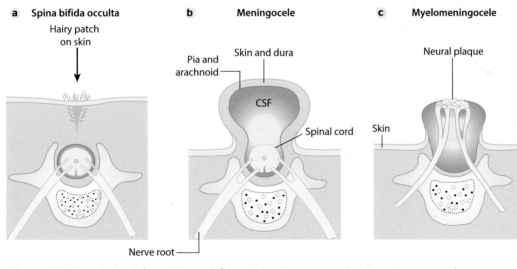

Figure 27.7 Neural tube defects: **(a)** spina bifida occulta; **(b)** meningocele; **(c)** myelomeningocele.

Physiotherapy is required to prevent joint contractures and strengthen paralysed muscles. Walking aids or a wheelchair may be required to permit mobility. With sensory loss, skin care is required to avoid the development of skin damage and ulcers.

An indwelling catheter may be required for bladder denervation, or intermittent urinary catheterisation may be performed by parents or by older children themselves. Urine samples should be checked regularly for infection. Continuous prophylactic antibiotics may be necessary. The child should be monitored for early evidence of hypertension and renal failure. Medication (such as ephedrine or oxybutinin) may improve bladder function and improve urinary dribbling. Bowel denervation requires regular toileting, and laxatives and suppositories are likely to be necessary with a low roughage diet for lesions above L3.

Scoliosis is monitored and may require surgical treatment. Ventricular dilatation from Arnold–Chiari malformation is often present at birth and 80% of affected infants require a shunt for progressive hydrocephalus during the first few weeks of life.

Those children destined to be the most severely disabled have a spinal lesion above L3 at birth. They are unable to walk, have a scoliosis, neuropathic bladder, hydronephrosis and frequently develop hydrocephalus.

Modern medical care has improved the quality of life for severely affected children. Most affected infants are now treated with closure of the lesion of the back soon after birth. Their care is best managed by a specialist multidisciplinary team.

◉ Summary

Neural tube defects:
- include anencephaly, encephalocele, spina bifida occulta, meningocele and myelomeningocele
- the birth prevalence in the UK has fallen dramatically, mainly owing to a natural decline but also to antenatal screening
- the birth prevalence is reduced by periconceptual folic acid
- myelomeningoceles can cause paralysis of the legs, dislocation of the hip and talipes, sensory loss, neuropathic bladder and bowel, scoliosis and hydrocephalus from the Arnold–Chiari malformation.

Hydrocephalus

In hydrocephalus there is obstruction to the flow of cerebrospinal fluid, leading to dilatation of the ventricular system proximal to the site of obstruction. The obstruction may be within the ventricular system or aqueduct (non-communicating or obstructive hydrocephalus), or at the arachnoid villi, the site of absorption of CSF (communicating hydrocephalus) (Box 27.3).

Clinical features

In infants with hydrocephalus, as their skull sutures have not fused, the head circumference may be disproportionately large or show an excessive rate of growth. The skull sutures separate, the anterior

Hydrocephalus

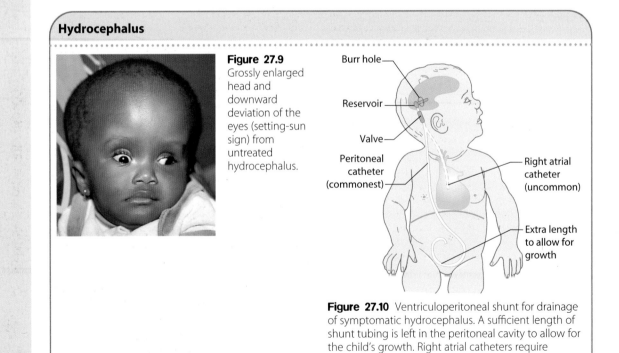

Figure 27.9 Grossly enlarged head and downward deviation of the eyes (setting-sun sign) from untreated hydrocephalus.

Burr hole
Reservoir
Valve
Peritoneal catheter (commonest)
Right atrial catheter (uncommon)
Extra length to allow for growth

Figure 27.10 Ventriculoperitoneal shunt for drainage of symptomatic hydrocephalus. A sufficient length of shunt tubing is left in the peritoneal cavity to allow for the child's growth. Right atrial catheters require revision with growth.

Box 27.3 Causes of hydrocephalus

Non-communicating (obstruction in the ventricular system)

Congenital malformation
    Aqueduct stenosis
    Atresia of the outflow foramina of the fourth
    ventricle (Dandy–Walker malformation)
    Arnold–Chiari malformation
Posterior fossa neoplasm or vascular malformation
Intraventricular haemorrhage in preterm infant

Communicating (failure to reabsorb CSF)

Subarachnoid haemorrhage
Meningitis: e.g. pneumococcal, tuberculous

Some can cause both non-communicating and communicating
hydrocephalus.

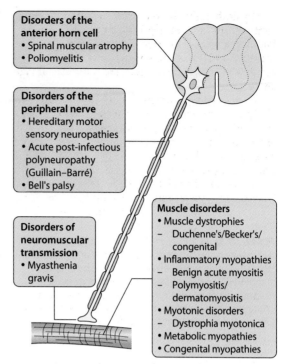

Figure 27.11 Neuromuscular disorders.

fontanelle bulges and the scalp veins become distended. An advanced sign is fixed downward gaze or sun setting of the eyes (Fig. 27.9). Older children will develop signs and symptoms of raised intracranial pressure.

Hydrocephalus may be diagnosed on antenatal ultrasound screening or in preterm infants on routine cranial ultrasound scanning. For suspected hydrocephalus initial assessment is with cranial ultrasound (in infants) or CT and MRI scan. Head circumference should be monitored over time on centile charts.

Treatment is required for symptomatic relief of raised intracranial pressure and to minimise the risk of neurological damage. The mainstay is the insertion of a ventricular shunt (Fig. 27.10), but endoscopic treatment and ventriculostomy can now be performed. Shunts can malfunction due to blockage or infection (usually with coagulase-negative staphylococci). They then need replacing or revising. Overdrainage of fluid can cause low-pressure headaches but the insertion of regulatory valves can help avoid this.

Summary

Hydrocephalus:

- in infants presents with excessive increase in head circumference, separation of skull sutures, bulging of the anterior fontanelle, distension of scalp veins and sun setting of the eyes
- older children present with raised intracranial pressure
- treatment is usually with a ventricular shunt.

Neuromuscular disorders

Any part of the lower motor pathway can be affected in a neuromuscular disorder, so that anterior horn cell disorders, peripheral neuropathies, disorders of neuromuscular transmission and

primary muscle diseases can all occur. The causes of neuromuscular disorders are shown in Figure 27.11. The key clinical feature of a neuromuscular disorder is weakness, which may be progressive or static. Affected children may present with:

- floppiness
- delayed motor milestones
- muscle weakness
- unsteady/abnormal gait
- fatiguability.

The first step is to decide on the site of the lesion. History and examination provide useful clues. Children with myopathy often show the waddling gait suggestive of proximal muscle weakness. More severe weakness results in Gowers' sign. This is the need to turn prone to rise to a standing from a supine position. This is normal until the age of 3 years. It is only when children have become very weak that they 'climb up the legs with the hands' to gain the standing position (Fig. 27.12). A pattern of more distal wasting and weakness, particularly in the presence of pes cavus, suggests an hereditary motor sensory neuropathy. Increasing fatiguability through the day, often with ophthalmoplegia and ptosis, would be more consistent with depletion at the motor end-plate and a diagnosis of myasthenia gravis.

It is usually difficult to differentiate a myopathy from a neuropathy on clinical grounds but there are some broad points to look for:

- Anterior horn cell – there are signs of denervation: weakness, loss of reflexes, fasciculation and wasting as the nerve supply to the muscle fails.

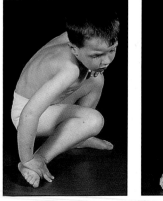
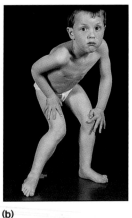

(a)   (b)

Figure 27.12 (a, b) Gowers' sign. The child needs to turn prone to rise (the key, early feature of Gowers' sign), then uses his hands to climb up on his knees before standing (late feature), because of poor hip girdle fixation and/or proximal muscle weakness. Any child continuing to turn prone to rise after 3 years of age is likely to have a neuromuscular condition.

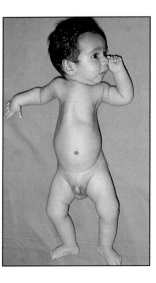

Figure 27.13 Spinal muscular atrophy (Werdnig–Hoffmann disease) showing proximal muscle wasting, chest deformity from weakness of the intercostal muscles and thighs held abducted because of hypotonia.

- Neuropathy – often distal nerves affected. There is weakness, loss of reflexes, sensory loss and temperature change as nerve supply fails.
- Myopathy – there is weakness, wasting, gait changes as muscle structure is affected. Reflexes initially intact. Often more proximal weakness.
- Neuromuscular junction – as end-plate acetylcholine stores become depleted, there is diurnal worsening through the day leading to fatiguability.

Investigations

These depend on the clinical decision regarding the site of lesion.

Myopathy:

- serum creatine phosphokinase – markedly elevated in Duchenne's and Becker's muscular dystrophy
- muscle biopsy, needle or open – modern histochemical techniques often enable a definitive diagnosis
- ultrasound and MRI of muscles – used in specialist centres to diagnose and monitor progress
- DNA testing – to identify abnormal genes.

Neuropathy:

- nerve conduction studies – to identify delayed motor and sensory nerve conduction velocities seen in neuropathy
- DNA testing – for abnormal genes
- nerve biopsy – rarely performed
- EMG (electromyography) helps in differentiating myopathic from neuropathic disorders, e.g. fatiguability on repetitive nerve stimulation in myasthenia. However, it should be used selectively in children, as the nerve conduction studies cause a tingling sensation and electromyography requires insertion of fine needle electrodes.

Diagnosis of neuromuscular disorders has been made easier by the advances made in confirmatory DNA tests for many of them, e.g. spinal muscular atrophy (SMA), Duchenne's muscular dystrophy, myotonic dystrophy, hereditary neuropathies. This also allows antenatal testing and genetic counselling and often obviates the need for the discomfort of peripheral neurophysiology.

Disorders of the anterior horn cell

Presentation is with weakness, wasting and absent reflexes. The features of poliomyelitis are described in Chapter 14.

Spinal muscular atrophy

This disorder is usually autosomal recessive, and due to degeneration of the anterior horn cells, leading to progressive weakness and wasting of skeletal muscles. This is the second most common cause of neuromuscular disease in the UK after Duchenne's muscular dystrophy.

Spinal muscular atrophy type 1 (Werdnig–Hoffmann disease)

A very severe progressive disorder presenting in early infancy (Fig. 27.13). Diminished fetal movements are often noticed during pregnancy and there may be arthrogryposis (positional deformities of the limbs with contractures of at least two joints) at birth. Typical signs include:

- lack of antigravity power in hip flexors
- absent deep tendon reflexes
- intercostal recession
- fasciculation of the tongue.

These children never sit unaided. Death is from respiratory failure by about 12 months of age. There are milder forms of the disorder with a later onset. Children with type 2 spinal muscular atrophy can sit, but never walk independently. Those with type 3 (Kugelberg–Welander) do walk and can present later in life.

Peripheral neuropathies

The hereditary motor sensory neuropathies (HMSN)

This group of disorders typically leads to symmetrical, slowly progressive muscular wasting which is distal rather than proximal. Type I, formerly known as peroneal muscular atrophy (Charcot–Marie–Tooth disease), is usually dominantly inherited and the most common. Affected nerves may be hypertrophic due to demyelination followed by attempts at remyelination. Nerve biopsy typically shows 'onion bulb formation' due to these two processes. Onset is in the first decade with distal atrophy and pes cavus, the legs being affected more than the arms. Rarely, there may be distal sensory loss and the reflexes are diminished. The disease is chronic and only rarely do those affected lose the ability to walk. The initial presentation of Friedreich's ataxia can be similar.

Acute post-infectious polyneuropathy (Guillain–Barré syndrome)

Presentation is typically 2–3 weeks after an upper respiratory tract infection or campylobacter gastroenteritis. There may be fleeting abnormal sensory symptoms in the legs, but the prominent feature is an ascending symmetrical weakness with loss of reflexes and autonomic involvement. Sensory symptoms, usually in the distal limbs, are less striking than the paresis but can be unpleasant. Involvement of bulbar muscles leads to difficulty with chewing and swallowing and the risk of aspiration. Respiratory depression may require artificial ventilation. The maximum muscle weakness may occur only 2–4 weeks after the onset of illness. Although full recovery may be expected in 95% of cases, this may take up to 2 years.

The CSF protein is characteristically markedly raised, but this may not be seen until the second week of illness. The CSF white cell count is not raised. Nerve conduction velocities are reduced.

Management of post-infectious polyneuropathy is supportive, particularly of respiration. Corticosteroids have been shown to have no beneficial effect or may even delay recovery. The disorder is probably due to the formation of antibody attaching itself to protein components of myelin. Controlled trials have shown that the ventilator-dependent period can be significantly reduced by immunoglobulin infusion. If this is not successful, consider using plasma exchange.

Bell's palsy and facial nerve palsies

Bell's palsy is an isolated lower motor neuron paresis of the VIIth cranial nerve leading to facial weakness (Fig. 27.14). Although the aetiology is unclear in Bell's palsy, it is probably post-infectious with an association with herpes simplex virus in adults. Corticosteroids may be of value in reducing oedema in the facial canal during the first week. Recovery is complete in the majority of cases but may take several months. The main complication is

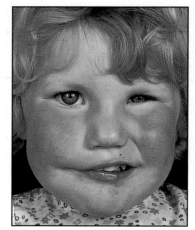

Figure 27.14
Bell's palsy. There is right facial weakness of both the upper and lower face.

conjunctival infection due to incomplete eye closure on blinking. This may require the eye to be protected with a patch or even tarsorrhaphy.

There are several other causes of facial nerve palsy. If symptoms of an VIIIth nerve paresis are also present then the most likely diagnosis is a compressive lesion in the cerebellopontine angle. The herpes virus may invade the geniculate ganglion and give painful vesicles on the tonsillar fauces and external ear, along with a facial nerve paresis. Treatment for this is with aciclovir. Hypertension should be excluded, as there is an association between Bell's palsy and coarctation of the aorta. If the facial weakness is bilateral, sarcoidosis should be suspected, but this is also seen in Lyme disease.

Disorders of neuromuscular transmission

Myasthenia gravis

This presents as abnormal muscle fatiguability which improves with rest or anticholinesterase drugs.

Transient neonatal myasthenia

This is described in Chapter 9.

Juvenile myasthenia

This is similar to adult autoimmune myasthenia and is due to binding of antibody to acetylcholine receptors on the post-junctional synaptic membrane. This gives a reduction of the number of functional receptors. Presentation is usually after 10 years of age with ophthalmoplegia and ptosis, loss of facial expression and difficulty chewing (Fig. 27.15). Generalised, especially proximal, weakness may be seen.

Diagnosis is made by observing improvement following the administration of intravenous edrophonium and can be further confirmed by testing for acetylcholine receptor antibodies (seen in 60–80%). Treatment is with the use of anticholinesterases such as neostigmine or pyridostigmine. In the longer term, immunosuppressive therapy with prednisolone or azathioprine has been

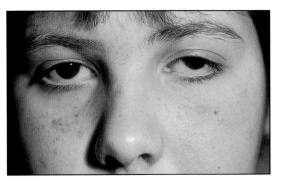

Figure 27.15 Myasthenia gravis showing ptosis from ocular muscle fatigue which improved with edrophonium.

shown to be of value. Plasma exchange is used for crises. Thymectomy is considered if a thymoma is present or if the response to medical therapy is unsatisfactory. About a quarter will show remission post thymectomy and up to half show some improvement.

Muscle disorders

The muscular dystrophies

This is a group of inherited disorders with muscle degeneration, often progressive.

Duchenne's muscular dystrophy

This is the most common muscular dystrophy, affecting 1 in 4000 male infants. It is inherited as an X-linked recessive disorder, although about a third are new mutations. It results from a deletion of chromosome material on the short arm of the X chromosome (at the Xp21 site). This site is now known to code for a protein called dystrophin which maintains the integrity of the muscle cell wall. Where it is deficient, there is an influx of calcium ions, a breakdown of the calcium calmodulin complex and an excess of free radicals. These lead eventually to irreversible destruction of the muscle cells. The serum creatine phosphokinase (CPK) is markedly elevated. Some countries, e.g. Wales, have introduced neonatal screening for Duchenne's dystrophy so that affected children are detected in the neonatal screening test by an elevated CPK.

Children present with a waddling gait or language delay and have to mount stairs one by one. Although the average age of diagnosis remains 5.5 years, children often become symptomatic much earlier.

There may be selective atrophy of muscle, in particular of the sternal head of the pectoralis major and brachioradialis. There is pseudohypertrophy of the calves because of replacement of muscle fibres by fat and fibrous tissue.

In the early school years, affected boys just tend to be slower and more clumsy than their peers. The progressive muscle atrophy and weakness means that they are no longer ambulant by the age of about 10–14 years. Death ensues in the late teens or

twenties from respiratory failure or the associated cardiomyopathy. About a third of affected children have learning difficulties. Scoliosis is a common complication.

Management Appropriate exercise helps to maintain muscle power and mobility and delays the onset of scoliosis. Contractures, particularly at the ankles, should be prevented by passive stretching and the provision of night splints. Walking can be prolonged with the provision of orthoses, in particular those which allow ambulation by the child leaning from side to side. Lengthening of the Achilles tendon may be required to facilitate ambulation. Attention to maintaining a good sitting posture helps to minimise the risk of scoliosis. Scoliosis is managed with a truncal brace, a moulded seat and occasionally surgical insertion of a metal rod into the spine. Later in the illness, episodes of nocturnal hypoxia secondary to weakness of the intercostal muscles may present with lassitude or irritability. Respiratory aids, particularly overnight CPAP (continuous positive airway pressure) or non-invasive positive pressure ventilation (NIPPV), may be provided to improve the quality of life. As with all chronic disabling conditions, parent self-help groups are a useful continuing source of information and support for families. Affected children should be reviewed periodically at a specialist regional centre. Ambulant children with Duchenne's dystrophy are increasingly treated with corticosteroids (prednisolone for 10 days per month) to preserve mobility and prevent scoliosis. The precise mechanism by which glucocorticoids may increase strength in Duchenne's dystrophy is not known but their potential beneficial effects include inhibition of muscle proteolysis, a stimulatory effect on myoblast proliferation, an increase in myogenic repair, an anti-inflammatory/immunosuppressive effect, reduction of cytosolic calcium concentrations and upregulation of utrophin, and alteration in skeletal muscle gene expression.

It may be possible to identify female carriers if they have a mildly raised CPK or if the gene deletion can be detected on DNA analysis. Antenatal diagnosis is then possible.

Becker's muscular dystrophy

In Becker's dystrophy some functional dystrophin is produced. The features are similar to those of Duchenne's dystrophy but clinically the disease progresses more slowly. The average age of onset is 11 years, inability to walk in the late twenties, with death in the early forties, although this is very variable. Some staining for dystrophin is seen on muscle biopsy compared to biopsies from children with Duchenne's, where there is none.

Congenital muscular dystrophies

This is a heterogeneous group of disorders, most with recessive inheritance, which present with muscle weakness at birth or early infancy. Typically

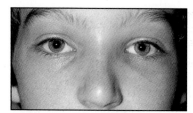

Figure 27.16
Heliotrope rash in dermatomyositis.

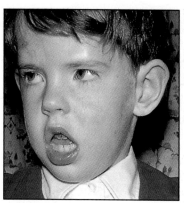

Figure 27.17
Dystrophia myotonica in an 8-year-old who has marked facial weakness and moderately severe learning difficulties.

the proximal weakness is slowly progressive with a tendency to contracture when the ability to walk is lost. Some may run a more static course. Biopsy shows dystrophic features with a reduction of specific proteins such as merosin. These dystrophies may be linked with central nervous abnormalities which may result in learning difficulties.

The inflammatory myopathies

Benign acute myositis

This is assumed to be a post-viral phenomenon as it often follows an upper respiratory tract infection and runs a self-limiting course. Pain and weakness occur in affected muscles. CPK is usually raised.

Dermatomyositis

This is a systemic illness, probably due to an angiopathy. Usual onset is between 5 and 10 years. This can be acute, but more typically is insidious with fever, misery, and eventually symmetrical muscle weakness, which is mainly proximal. Sometimes pharyngeal muscle involvement affects swallowing. There is also a characteristic violaceous (heliotrope) rash to the eyelids, and peri-orbital oedema (Fig. 27.16). The rash may also affect the extensor surfaces of joints, e.g. elbow, and with time subcutaneous calcification can appear. Inflammatory markers (CRP, ESR) can be raised but not invariably. Muscle biopsy shows an inflammatory cell infiltrate and atrophy. Physiotherapy is needed to prevent contractures. Corticosteroids are the standard treatment, and continue at a tailored dose for 2 years. Other immunosuppressants, e.g. methotrexate, ciclosporin, may be needed. Mortality is 5–10%.

Myotonic disorders

Myotonia is delayed relaxation after sustained muscle contraction. It can be identified clinically and on electromyography.

Dystrophia myotonica

This relatively common illness is dominantly inherited and caused by a nucleotide triplet repeat expansion, so this means there can be anticipation through generations, especially when maternally transmitted (see Ch. 8). Newborns can present with hypotonia and feeding and respiratory difficulties due to muscle weakness. It is then useful to examine the mother for myotonia. This manifests as slow release of handshake or difficulty releasing the tightly clasped fist. This may be mild and not have been appreciated. Sensitivity is required as

diagnosis in the neonate may have repercussions for the family. Older children can present with myopathic facies (Fig. 27.17), learning difficulties and myotonia. Adults develop cataracts and males develop baldness and testicular atrophy. Death is usually due to cardiomyopathy.

Metabolic myopathies

Metabolic conditions can affect muscles, due either to the deposition of storage material or to energy-depleting enzyme deficiencies. Presentation is as a floppy infant or, in older children, with muscle weakness or cramps on exercise. The main causes are:

- Glycogen storage disorders (see Ch. 25).
- Disorders of lipid metabolism. Fatty acids are important muscle fuel. Fatty acid oxidation occurs in the mitochondria and defects in this pathway can result in weakness. Carnitine is essential to supply long-chain fatty acids to the mitochondria for breakdown, and carnitine deficiency causes weakness.
- Mitochondrial cytopathies – rare disorders which are coded as maternally inherited mitochondrial DNA. Myopathy may be the major manifestation or the disorder may be multisystem, with lactic acidosis and encephalopathy. Mitochondrial DNA testing is available.

Congenital myopathies

These present at birth or in infancy with generalised hypotonia and muscle weakness. The names describe the changes seen on muscle biopsy or electron microscopy. They include:

- nemaline rod myopathy
- central core disease
- congenital fibre-type disproportion.

Creatine phosphokinase levels are normal or only mildly elevated.

The 'floppy infant'

Persisting hypotonia in infants can be readily felt on picking up the infant, who tends to slip through the fingers or hang like a rag-doll when suspended

Summary

Neuromuscular disorders:

- include disorders of the anterior horn cell, peripheral nerve, neuromuscular transmission and muscle
- present with muscle weakness, which may manifest with floppiness, delayed motor milestones, unsteady gait or muscle fatiguability
- in **spinal muscular atrophy** there is degeneration of the anterior horn cells leading to progressive weakness and wasting of skeletal muscles; tongue fasciculation may aid diagnosis
- in the **hereditary motor sensory neuropathies** (HMSN) there is slowly progressive, symmetrical wasting of the distal muscles
- in **acute post-infectious polyneuropathy** (Guillain–Barré syndrome) there is ascending symmetrical weakness with loss of reflexes and autonomic and sensory involvement; there may be bulbar palsy and respiratory depression
- in **facial nerve palsies**, lower motor neurone lesions cause weakness of lower and upper

facial muscles, whereas upper motor neurone lesions spare the upper forehead muscles
- in **juvenile myasthenia**, presentation is usually after 10 years of age with ophthalmoplegia and ptosis, loss of facial expression and difficulty chewing
- **Duchenne's muscular dystrophy** is X-linked recessive and presents with a waddling gait and difficulty climbing stairs
- **dermatomyositis** usually presents at 5–10 years with malaise and symmetrical proximal muscle weakness, a violaceous (heliotrope) rash to the eyelids
- **dystrophia myotonica** is dominantly inherited; it presents in newborns with hypotonia and feeding and respiratory difficulties due to muscle weakness, in older children with myopathic facies, learning difficulties and myotonia, delayed relaxation after sustained muscle contraction.

Box 27.4 Causes of the floppy infant

Cortical
Hypoxic-ischaemic encephalopathy
Cortical malformations

Genetic
Down's syndrome
Prader–Willi syndrome

Metabolic
Hypothyroidism
Hypocalcaemia

Neuromuscular
Spinal muscular atrophy
Myopathy
Myotonia
Myasthenia gravis

prone. There will be marked head lag when the head is lifted by the arms from supine. The causes are listed in Box 27.4. The clinical examination can help determine the site of the lesion, whether cortical or neuromuscular. Central hypotonia is associated with poor truncal tone but preserved limb tone. Dysmorphic features suggest a genetic cause. Lower motor neurone lesions are suggested by a frog-like posture (see Fig. 27.13), poor anti-gravity movements and absent reflexes.

The neurocutaneous syndromes

The nervous system and the skin have a common ectodermal origin. Embryological disruption causes syndromes involving abnormalities to both systems – the neurocutaneous syndromes.

Neurofibromatosis type 1 (NF1)

This affects 1 in 3000 live births. It is an autosomal dominant, highly penetrant condition. One third are new mutations. The gene has been identified.

In order to make the diagnosis, two or more of these criteria need to be present:

- six or more café-au-lait spots >5 mm in size before puberty, >15 mm after puberty (Fig. 27.18)
- more than one neurofibroma, an unsightly firm nodular overgrowth of any nerve
- axillary freckles (see Fig. 27.18)
- optic glioma which may cause visual impairment
- one Lisch nodule, a hamartoma of the iris seen on slit-lamp examination
- bony lesions from sphenoid dysplasia which can cause eye protrusion
- first-degree relative with NF1.

The cutaneous features tend to become more evident after puberty, and there is a wide spectrum of involvement from mild to severe. Neurofibromata appear in the course of any peripheral nerve, including cranial nerves. They may look unsightly or cause neurological signs if they occur at a site where a peripheral nerve passes through a bony foramen. Visual or auditory impairment may result if there is compression of the IInd or VIIIth cranial nerve. Megalencephaly with learning difficulties and epilepsy are sometimes seen.

Neurofibromatosis type 2 (NF2; bilateral, acoustic or central) is less common and presents in adolescence. Bilateral acoustic neuromata are the predominant feature and present with deafness and

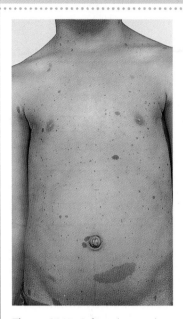

Figure 27.18 Café-au-lait patches and axillary freckling in neurofibromatosis.

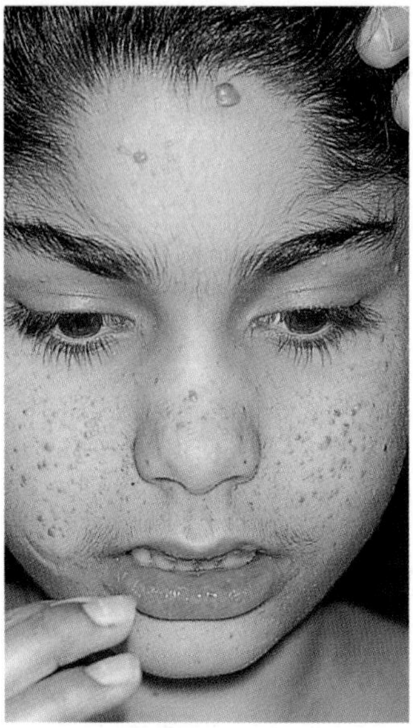

Figure 27.19 Adenoma sebaceum in tuberous sclerosis.

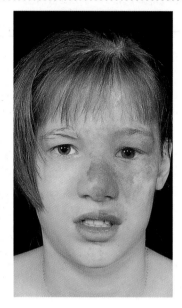

Figure 27.20 Sturge–Weber syndrome. There is a port-wine stain in the distribution of the trigeminal nerve.

sometimes a cerebellopontine angle syndrome with a facial (VIIth) nerve paresis and cerebellar ataxia.

There may be an overlap between the features of NF1 and NF2. Both NF1 and NF2 can be associated with endocrinological disorders, the multiple endocrine neoplasia syndromes (MENS).

Other associations are phaeochromocytoma, pulmonary hypertension, renal artery stenosis with hypertension and gliomatous change, particularly in central nervous system lesions. Rarely, the benign tumours undergo sarcomatous change. However, most people with the disorder carry no features other than the cutaneous stigmata.

Tuberous sclerosis

This disorder is a dominantly inherited disorder but up to 70% are new mutations. Prevalence is 1 in 9000 live births.

The cutaneous features consist of:

- depigmented 'ash leaf'-shaped patches which fluoresce under ultraviolet light (Wood's light)
- roughened patches of skin (shagreen patches) usually over the lumbar spine
- adenoma sebaceum (angiofibromata) in a butterfly distribution over the bridge of the nose and cheeks, which are unusual before the age of 3 years (Fig. 27.19).

Neurological features are:

- infantile spasms and developmental delay
- epilepsy – often focal
- intellectual impairment.

These children have severe learning difficulties and often have autistic features to their behaviour when older. Other features are:

- fibromata beneath the nails (subungual fibromata)
- dense white areas on the retina (phakomata) from local degeneration
- rhabdomyomata of the heart which are identifiable in the early weeks on echocardiography but often resolve
- polycystic kidneys.

As with neurofibromatosis, gliomatous change can occur in the brain lesions. Many people who carry the gene have no stigmata other than the cutaneous features and no associated neurological features.

CT scans will detect the calcified subependymal nodules and tubers from the second year of life. MRI is more sensitive and more clearly identifies other tubers and lesions.

Sturge–Weber syndrome

This is a sporadic disorder with a haemangiomatous facial lesion (a port-wine stain) in the

Summary

The neurocutaneous syndromes:
- include neurofibromatosis, tuberous sclerosis and Sturge–Weber syndrome.

The neurocutaneous syndromes

469

Table 27.4 Lipid storage disorders

Disorder	Enzyme defect	Clinical features
Tay–Sachs disease	Hexosaminidase A	Autosomal recessive disorder Most common among Ashkenazi Jews Developmental regression in late infancy, exaggerated startle response to noise, visual inattention and social unresponsiveness Severe hypotonia, enlarging head Cherry red spot at the macula Death by 2–5 years Diagnosis – measurement of the specific enzyme activity Carrier detection of high-risk couples is practised Prenatal detection is possible
Gaucher's disease	Beta glucosidase	Occurs in 1 in 500 Ashkenazi Jews Chronic childhood form – splenomegaly, bone marrow suppression, bone involvement, normal IQ Splenectomy may alleviate hypersplenism Enzyme replacement therapy is available, but is expensive Acute infantile form – splenomegaly, neurological degeneration with seizures Carrier detection and prenatal diagnosis are possible
Niemann–Pick disease	Sphingomyelinase	At 3–4 months, feeding difficulties and failure to thrive, hepatosplenomegaly, developmental delay, hypotonia and deterioration of hearing and vision Cherry red spot in macula affects 50% Death by 4 years

distribution of the trigeminal nerve associated with a similar lesion intracranially. The ophthalmic division of the trigeminal nerve is always involved (Fig. 27.20). Calcification of the gyri causes characteristic 'rail-road track' calcification on skull X-ray.

In the most severe form, it may present with epilepsy, learning disability and hemiplegia. Children presenting with intractable epilepsy in early infancy may benefit from hemispherectomy. For children who are less severely affected, deterioration is unusual after the age of 5 years, although there may still be seizures and learning difficulties. There is a risk of glaucoma.

Neurodegenerative disorders

These are disorders that cause a deterioration in motor and intellectual function. Abnormal neurological features develop including seizures, spasticity, abnormal head circumference (macro- or microcephaly), involuntary movement disorders, visual and hearing loss and behaviour change. While individually rare, they are numerous and include:

- Lysosomal storage disorders, e.g. lipid storage disorders and mucopolysaccharidoses in which absence of an enzyme leads to accumulation of a harmful metabolite.
- Peroxisomal enzyme defects, e.g. X-linked adrenoleucodystrophy. Peroxisomes are catalase- and oxidase-containing organelles involved in long-chain fatty acid oxidation.

Enzyme deficiencies can lead to accumulation of very long-chain fatty acids (VLCFAs).
- Heredodegenerative disorders, e.g. Huntington's disease, which presents with progressive dystonia, dementia, seizures and corticospinal tract signs.
- Wilson's disease, from the accumulation of copper, may cause changes in behaviour and additional involuntary movements or a mixture of neurological and hepatic symptoms.
- Subacute sclerosing panencephalitis (SSPE), a delayed response in adolescence to previous measles infection causing neurological regression with a characteristic EEG, but has become rare since measles immunisation.

Lysosomal storage disorders

In metachromatic leucodystrophy, a sulfatidosis, accumulation of sulphatides causes demyelination. It is diagnosed on testing white cell enzymes.

In lipid storage disorders (Table 27.4), which are sphingolipidoses, there is an accumulation of sphingolipids, essential components of CNS membranes. They are diagnosed on testing white cell enzymes.

The mucopolysaccharidoses are progressive multisystem disorders which may affect the neurological, ocular, cardiac and skeletal systems (Table 27.5). Hepatosplenomegaly is usually present. Most children present with developmental delay following a period of essentially normal growth and development up to 6–12 months of age. Developmental attainment then slows and children may

Mucopolysaccharidoses

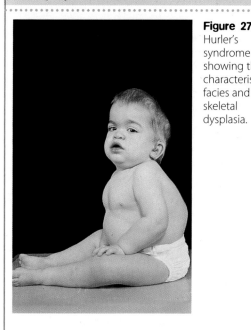

Figure 27.21 Hurler's syndrome showing the characteristic facies and skeletal dysplasia.

Table 27.5 Clinical features of mucopolysaccharidoses

Eyes	Corneal clouding
	Retinal degeneration
	Glaucoma
Skin	Thickened skin
	Coarse facies
Heart	Valvular lesions
	Cardiac failure
Neurology	Developmental regression
Skeletal	Thickened skull
	Broad ribs
	Claw hand
	Thoracic kyphosis
	Lumbar lordosis
Other	Hepatosplenomegaly
	Carpal tunnel syndrome
	Conductive deafness
	Umbilical and inguinal hernias

Table 27.6 Types of mucopolysaccharidoses

Type	Inheritance	Cornea	Heart	Brain	Skeletal
MPS I (Hurler)	AR	+++	++	+++	++
MPS II (Hunter)	X-linked	–	+	++	+
MPS III (Sanfilippo)	AR	+/–	–	+	+
MPS IV (Morquio)	AR	+	+	–	+++
MPS VI (Morateaux–Lamy)	AR	+++	++	–	++

AR, autosomal recessive.

show some loss of skills. It is only in the second 6 months of life that the characteristic facies begin to emerge, with coarsening of the facial features and prominent forehead due to frontal bossing (Fig. 27.21).

The characteristics of five of the varieties are shown in Table 27.6. The diagnosis is made by identifying the enzyme defect and the excretion in the urine of the major storage substances, the glycosaminoglycans (GAGs). Treatment is supportive according to the child's needs. Successful enzyme replacement by bone marrow transplantation has been performed but cannot reverse any established neurological abnormality.

Summary

In neurodegenerative disorders:
- there is developmental regression with the evolution of abnormal neurological signs.

Further reading

Forsyth R, Newton R 2007 Paediatric neurology. Oxford specialist handbook in paediatrics. Oxford University Press, Oxford

Newton R W 1995 Colour atlas of pediatric neurology. Mosby-Wolfe, London. *A well-illustrated textbook*

Useful websites

British Paediatric Neurology Association: http://www.bpna.org.uk
Child Neurology Home page: http://www.waisman.wisc.edu/child-neuro/index.html (provides 'family village' library with information on many neurological diagnoses)
International League Against Epilepsy (ILAE): http://www.ilae.org/ (useful information on epilepsy syndromes)
Neuromuscular homepage (Washington University

School of Medicine): http://www.neuro.wustl.edu/
neuromuscular/
Online Mendelian Inheritance in Man:
www.ncbi.nlm.nih.gov/omim
Systematic reviews of migraine treatment in children,
steroids for facial palsy and treatment of Guillain–
Barré syndrome can be found in the Cochrane library:
http://www.nelh.nhs.uk/cochrane.asp

28

Adolescent medicine

Adolescence is the transition from childhood to adulthood. There is no clearly defined age range, but it is usually considered to be from puberty until 18 years of age. There are 7 million adolescents in the UK, 12–13% of the population.

The transition from being a child to an adult involves many biological, psychological and social changes (Table 28.1). Difficulties may arise if the pubertal changes are early or delayed.

Table 28.1 Developmental changes of adolescence

	Biological	Psychological	Social
Early adolescence	Early puberty Females – breast bud, pubic hair development, start of growth spurt Males– testicular enlargement, start of genital growth	Concrete thinking (Fig. 28.1) but begin to develop moral concepts and awareness of their sexual identity	The early emotional separation from parents, start of a strong peer identification, early exploratory behaviours, e.g. may start smoking
Mid-adolescence	Females – end of growth spurt, menarche, change in body shape Males – sperm production, voice breaks, start of growth spurt Acne Blushing Need for more sleep	Abstract thinking, but still seen as 'bulletproof', increasing verbal dexterity, may develop a fervent ideology (religious, political)	Continuing emotional separation from parents, heterosexual peer interest, early vocational plans
Late adolescence	Males – end of puberty, continued growth in height, strength and body hair	Complex abstract thinking (Fig. 28.1), identification of difference between law and morality, increased impulse control, further development of personal identity, further development or rejection of ideologies	Social autonomy, may develop intimate relationships, further education or employment, may begin or develop financial independence

Adapted from Christie D, Viner R 2005 Adolescent development. In: Viner R (ed.) *ABC of Adolescence*. BMJ books, Blackwell; McIntosh N, Helms P, Smyth R (eds) 2003 *Forfar and Arneil's Textbook of Paediatrics*, 6th edn. Churchill Livingstone, Edinburgh: 1757–1768.

Whilst general practitioners will see all adolescent medical problems, difficulties may arise when obtaining specialist medical care. Those less than 16 years old are looked after by paediatricians over 16 years old by adult physicians and surgeons. However, paediatric facilities, e.g. children's wards, may be geared to the needs of young children rather than adolescents, whilst older adolescents may be overwhelmed by the medical conditions encountered on adult wards and the independence expected of them. Adolescent females with gynaecological problems are often cared for by gynaecologists, usually in adult facilities. Some paediatricians are now specialising in adolescent medicine.

Communicating with adolescents

The adolescent consultation differs from the paediatric consultation for young children in that the adolescent has a larger role in the consultation.

It may be appropriate to see adolescents by themselves as well as with their parents. The principle is that the parents should not be seen alone after the adolescent has spent time with the doctor so that the adolescent can trust that whatever confidences have been disclosed to the doctor have been kept.

Some practical points about communicating and working with adolescents are:

- Make the adolescent the central person in the consultation.
- Be yourself. When establishing rapport, it may be appropriate to engage the adolescent by talking about their interests, e.g. football, clothes or music, but do not try to be cool, false or patronising; your relationship should be as their doctor, not their friend.
- Consider the family dynamics. Is the mother or father answering for the adolescent? Does the adolescent seem to want this or resent being interrupted?

- Avoid being judgemental or lecturing. A frank and direct approach works best. Your role should be that of a knowledgeable, trusted adult from whom they can get advice if they so choose.
- An authoritarian approach is likely to result in a rebellious stance. Working things out together in a practical way has the best chance of success.
- Frame difficult questions so they are less threatening and judgemental, e.g. 'Lots of teenagers drink alcohol, how much do you drink in a week?'
- Confidentiality is important and must be respected. Explain that you will keep everything you are told confidential, unless somebody is at risk of harm.
- Bear in mind proxy presentations, e.g. abdominal pain, when the real reason is anxiety about the possibility of pregnancy or sexually transmitted disease or the result of recreational drug use.
- If a full adolescent psychosocial history is required, the HEADSS acronym may be helpful (Table 28.2), although questions must be tailored to stage of development.
- If they need to have a physical examination, consider their privacy and personal integrity – should a parent or chaperone be present, and would they prefer a doctor of the same sex?
- Communicate and explain concepts appropriate to their cognitive development. For young adolescents, use concrete examples (here and now) rather than abstract concepts ('if … then').

Range of health problems

Adolescence is a healthy stage of life compared with early childhood or old age. The range of health problems affecting adolescents include:

- Common illnesses – respiratory disorders, skin conditions, musculoskeletal problems including sports injuries and somatic complaints. Acute serious illness has become rare, with mortality predominantly from trauma.
- Chronic illness and disability e.g. asthma, epilepsy, diabetes, cerebral palsy. The prevalence of some of the common chronic disorders in adolescence is

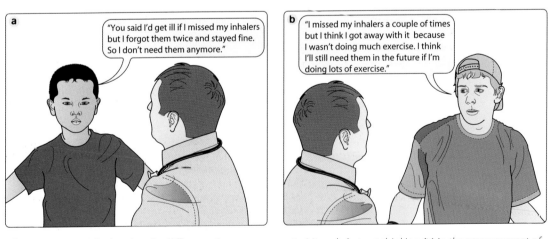

Figure 28.1 Example showing the difference between concrete (**a**) and abstract thinking (**b**) in the management of asthma in an older child and an adolescent.

Table 28.2 HEADSS acronym for psychosocial history in adolescents

H	Home life	Relationships, social support, household chores
E	Education	School, exams, work experience, career, university, financial issues
A	Activities	Exercise and sport
		Social relationships, friends, peers, who can they rely on?
	Affect	Mood
D	Driving	Aged 16 if disabled
	Drugs	Drug use, cigarettes, alcohol, how much? How often?
	Diet	Weight, caffeine (diet drinks), binges/vomits, adequate calcium, vitamin D?
S	Sex	Concerns, periods, contraception (and in relation to medication)
	Sleep	How much? Hard to get to sleep? Wake often? Early waking?
	Suicide	Depression, self-harm

shown in Table 28.3. There is also a range of uncommon disorders with serious chronic morbidity such as malignant disease, juvenile idiopathic arthritis, connective tissue disorders. In addition, children with many congenital disorders which often used to be fatal in childhood now survive into adolescence or adult life, e.g. cystic fibrosis, Duchenne's muscular dystrophy, complex congenital heart disease, metabolic disorders, etc.

- High prevalence of somatic symptoms – fatigue, headaches, backache, etc.
- Mental health problems including suicide and deliberate self-harm.
- Eating disorders and weight problems.
- Those associated with health risk behaviours such as smoking, drinking, drug abuse and sexual health, contraception and teenage pregnancy.

Table 28.3 Prevalence per 1000 adolescents 12–18 years of some chronic illnesses

Disease	Prevalence per 1000 adolescents
Musculoskeletal conditions	41
Skin conditions	32
Significant mental health problems	120
Diabetes	
Type 1	2
Type 2	1–2
Respiratory conditions	150
Asthma	100
Cystic fibrosis	0.1
Epilepsy	4
Ear/Hearing problems	18
Cerebral palsy	1.5

Mortality

The dramatic improvement in the mortality of young children seen since the 1960s has not been matched in adolescents, who now have a higher mortality rate than that of 1- to 4-year-olds (Fig. 28.2). Although deaths in adolescents from communicable diseases have declined markedly, this has not been matched by mortality from road traffic accidents, other injuries and suicide, and these now predominate (Fig. 28.3). Alcohol is thought to be a contributing factor in a third of these deaths.

Impact of chronic conditions

Chronic illness may disrupt biological, psychological and social development. In addition, these developmental changes may affect the control and management of the disorder (Table 28.4). The impact of chronic illness on children and their families is considered in Chapter 23.

Adherence

Poor adherence is a problem for many adolescents as they are beginning to take over management of their illness, wish to avoid parental supervision and may give the management of their illness a lower priority than social and recreational activities. They may not believe that taking the medication really matters, especially if it is preventative or of long-term rather than short term benefit.

Peer relationships and self-image are very important, and therefore, for example, it may be more important for an adolescent with diabetes to lunch promptly so he can sit with his friends rather than go to the school nurse first for his insulin injection. Side-effects are also important, particularly those that may affect well-being or appearance. They may assess risk differently from adults, so that the risk of not being one of their crowd because of having to adhere to a certain

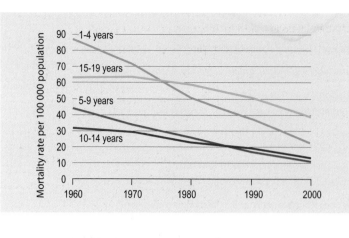

Figure 28.2 Mortality by age group in England and Wales 1960–2003, showing that the mortality rate is now greater at 15–19 years than at 1–4 years. (Source: ONS.)

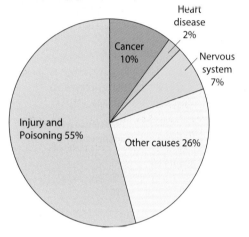

Figure 28.3 Causes of death, 15–19 years of age, in the UK. (Source: ONS, 2005).

treatment may appear to be more important than the risks attached to not taking any medication.

Adherence may be influenced by lack of knowledge and poor recall of previous disease education. The disorder may have presented when the child was much younger, so that the original consultation will have taken place primarily between the doctor and parents. If this communication has not been updated with increasing age, the adolescent's knowledge may be poor, with little understanding about her illness, what medications she is taking and why. As the responsibility for management moves to the young person, information needs to be provided about medications and treatment appropriate for her development. Other ways to maximise adherence are summarised in Table 28.5.

Transition to adult services

The young person with a chronic condition must eventually leave paediatric and adolescent services for adult services. This often involves changing from a treatment model based around close contact between the adolescent and health care professionals (unlimited telephone advice from clinical nurse specialists, possibly home visits, frequent appointments) and involvement with parents and other family members to one where they are likely to be seen infrequently in a busy adult clinic where parental involvement may be minimal or discouraged.

Young people and their parents need both information about the transition process and time to prepare. Parents are often concerned that the adult team will not address their teenager's health care needs. It is helpful if an identified health care professional, often a nurse specialist, is responsible for transition arrangements.

Some flexibility in age of transition is desirable, so that it can occur when the young person is developmentally ready and has the necessary maturity to cope with adult services.

Transfer may be via an adolescent or young adult service with clinics run by both adolescent and adult teams together. Such bridging arrangements have many advantages, but require a sufficient number of patients and medical staff able and willing to provide this service. These clinics are usually for specialist conditions, e.g. diabetes, cystic fibrosis or congenital heart disease. Alternatively, transfer may be successfully accomplished if there is good communication between teams, although it usually involves a radical change in ethos for the adolescent and family. The general practitioner can also provide an important source of continuity between changing specialty practitioners.

Consent and confidentiality

Consent

In England, Wales and Northern Ireland, young people can give consent if they are sufficiently informed and either over 16 years old or under 16 years and competent to make decisions for themselves. Conflict rarely arises about a treatment, as usually the adolescent, their parents and doctors agree that it is necessary. Handling of disagreement over consent is considered in Chapter 5.

Confidentiality

Confidentiality is regarded by adolescents as of crucial importance in their medical care. They want

Table 28.4 Some of the ways in which chronic illness and development interact with each other

	Effect of chronic illness on development	Effect of development on chronic illness
Biological	Delayed puberty Short stature Reduced bone mass accretion Malnutrition secondary to inadequate intake due to increased caloric requirement of disease or anorexia	Pubertal hormones may impact on disease, e.g. growth hormone worsens diabetes and increases insulin requirements; females with cystic fibrosis may have deterioration in lung function Increased caloric requirement may worsen disease control or result in undernutrition–may need dietary supplements or overnight feeding with nasogastric tube or gastrostomy Growth may cause scoliosis
Psychological	Regression to less mature behaviour Adopt sick role Impaired development of sense of attractive/sexual self Parental stress, depression, financial problems in providing care; siblings may suffer	Deny that their health may suffer from their actions Poor adherence and disease control Reject medics like parents
Social	Reduced independence when should be separating Failure of peer relationships Social isolation – unable to participate in sports or social events School absence and decline in school performance, may lower self-esteem Vocational failure	Risk behaviour may adversely affect disease, e.g. smoking and asthma or cystic fibrosis, alcohol and diabetic control, sleep deprivation and epilepsy Chaotic eating habits lead to malnutrition or obesity

Table 28.5 Ways to maximise adherence

Assess the size of the problem and be non-judgemental	Ask: 'Most people have trouble taking their medication. How often do you remember yours?'
Take time to explore practicalities	Try to put yourself in the adolescent's shoes and think through the detail of their regimen with them. Make regimen as simple as possible. Don't forget practical issues – poor adherence may be as simple as not having anywhere private at school to take the treatment.
Explore beliefs	May harbour strange or incorrect beliefs about medications, e.g. falsely attribute a side-effect and therefore refuse to take the medication.
Use daily routines to 'anchor' adherence	Find daily activities to anchor taking the medication, e.g. brushing teeth, or 'with breakfast and dinner' instead of 'twice a day'. Find the least chaotic time of day, often mornings. Let the suggestions come from the adolescent.
Motivation	Negotiate short-term treatment goals. Search for factors that motivate young people, e.g. puberty or growth
Involve and contract	Plan the regimen with the adolescent. Some may respond to a written contract that both sides agree to stick to.
Written instructions	Most of what is said has been shown to be forgotten once they leave the room!
Take time to explain	Check level of knowledge on each occasion.
Solution focused approach	Find out what has been going well and why. Use this information, e.g. 'How have you managed to remain out of hospital for 3 weeks this month?'

to know that information they have disclosed to their doctor is not revealed to others, whether parents, school or police, without their permission. In most circumstances their confidentiality should be kept unless there is a risk of harm, either to themselves from physical or sexual abuse or from suicidal thoughts or to others from homicidal intent. Difficulties relating to confidentiality for adolescents are usually about contraception, abortion, sexually transmitted infections, substance abuse or mental health. It is usually desirable for the parents to be informed and involved in the management of these situations and the adolescent should be encouraged to tell them or allow the doctor to, but if the young person is competent to make these decisions for herself, the courts have supported medical management of these situations without parental knowledge or consent.

Fatigue, headache and other somatic symptoms

Fatigue, headache, abdominal pain, backache and dizziness are common in adolescence. International surveys of adolescents in Europe reveal that two-thirds report morning fatigue more than once a week, 25% have a headache and 15% stomach ache, backache or sleep problems more than once a week. In many, these symptoms appear to be a feature of adolescence, although organic disease must be excluded by history, examination and occasionally investigation. For a minority, they may be a physical manifestation of psychological problems, and are precipitated by or maintained by factors such as bullying or parental discord.

Occasionally the symptoms are so severe and persistent that they considerably affect quality of life, with impairment of school attendance, academic results and peer relationships. This may be from chronic fatigue syndrome or chronic pain syndromes. Further investigation and assessment will be required and multidisciplinary rehabilitation and cognitive behaviour therapy within the family may be beneficial. The management of somatic symptoms and chronic fatigue syndrome are considered further in Chapter 23.

Mental health problems

The prevalence of mental health problems in adolescents is estimated to be about 11%. The main problems are listed in Table 28.6.

Deliberate self-harm varies from little actual harm, where there is a wish to communicate

Table 28.6 Main mental health problems and disorders in adolescents

Problem or disorder	Prevalence (%)
Depression	3–5
Anxiety	4–6
Attention deficit/hyperactivity disorder	2–4
Eating disorders	1–2
Conduct disorder	4–6
Substance misuse disorder	2–3

Sources: Michaud P-A, Fombonne E (2005) Common mental health problems. In: Viner R (ed.) *ABC of Adolescence*, BMJ Books, Blackwell; Costello et al (2003) *Archives of General Psychiatry* 60:837–844; Ford et al (2003) *Journal of the American Academy of Child and Adolescent Psychiatry* 42:1203–1211); Fombonne E (2003) *Journal of Autism and Developmental Disorders* 33:365–382.

distress or escape from an interpersonal crisis, to suicide. About 7–14% of adolescents will self-harm, depending on its definition.

Eating disorders are common during adolescence. About 40% of females and 25% of males begin dieting in adolescence because of dissatisfaction with their body. With anorexia nervosa and bulimia there is a morbid preoccupation with weight and body shape.

These conditions are considered in Chapter 23.

Health risk behaviour

During adolescence, young people begin to explore 'adult' behaviours including smoking, drinking, drug use, violence and sex. These behaviours, often referred to as 'risk-taking' behaviours, may reflect the adolescent's search for pleasure and excitement by participating in new and enjoyable experiences, as well as exerting independence from parents or rebelling against parents' wishes and lifestyle. There is also considerable pressure to fit in with peers.

Adolescents do not always understand the risks involved and may behave as if they are immune from harm. Participating in these activities may also deflect attention away from themselves to mask shyness or anxiety. Unfortunately, health risk behaviours started in adolescence tend to continue into adult life.

Sexual health

The average age for first sexual intercourse is 16 years, with a fifth of 14-year-olds having had intercourse. Having sexual intercourse at an early age is often associated with unsafe sex. This may be because of a lack of knowledge, lack of access to contraception, inability to negotiate obtaining contraception, being drunk or high on drugs or unable to resist being pressurised by their partner.

Risk-taking behaviour in adolescents can result in sexually transmitted diseases (STDs) or unplanned pregnancy. STDs may present with urethral or vaginal discharge, urinary symptoms, pain on micturition, abdominal or loin pain, or postcoital vaginal bleeding. Chlamydia is asymptomatic in 50% of cases and can lead to later infertility. In young teenagers it is more likely to present with a vaginal discharge. Studies have shown that up to a third of sexually active teenage girls have a sexually transmitted infection. They are also at risk of HIV infection.

Management of sexually transmitted diseases

A sexual history should involve questions related to risk of STDs: number of partners, any partners during travel abroad, contraception used and whether vaginal, oral or anal sex, any discharge, lower abdominal pain, last menstrual period, urinary symptoms. However, many sexually transmitted infections are asymptomatic, especially in younger teenagers.

If indicated, swabs should be taken for virology and microbiology (to look for HPV (human papillomavirus), HSV (herpes simplex virus), chlamydia and gonorrhoea. HIV testing may be indicated.

Treatment regimens vary depending on prevalent antibiotic resistance. Chlamydia can be treated with azithromycin or doxycycline, gonorrhoea with a cephalosporin. Metronidazole can be added for pelvic inflammatory disease. It is advisable to inform and treat partners.

Contraception

Most adolescents who are sexually active *are* using contraception, albeit sometimes haphazardly. In the UK, contraception is used by only half at first intercourse. Condoms, followed by oral contraceptive pill, are the commonest form of contraception used. As teenagers have a relatively high failure rate in their ability to use condoms correctly and with the oral contraceptive pill from irregular use, the 'double Dutch' method of condom and oral contraception is often advocated to protect against both sexually transmitted infections and pregnancy.

Adolescents with chronic disease, e.g. diabetes, even without microvascular complications, are generally started on lower doses of the contraceptive pill. Some medications prescribed in adolescents are potentially teratogenic (e.g., retinoids for acne) and may therefore need to be combined with an oral contraceptive pill or depot hormonal implant.

Emergency contraception

Emergency contraception (the 'morning after pill') can provide significant protection from pregnancy for up to 72 hours after unprotected intercourse. Emergency contraception is available from a pharmacist without prescription for those 16 years and over, and on prescription for those under 16 years. If taken within 72 hours it has a 2% failure rate. Side-effects include nausea and lethargy. However, knowledge of emergency contraception is poor amongst most young people.

Teenage pregnancy

The UK has the highest rate of teenage pregnancy in western Europe. Teenage girls may present with complaints such as abdominal pain, fatigue, breast tenderness or appetite changes rather than late or missed menstrual period.

Becoming a teenage mother can be a positive life choice and is influenced by culture. There may be considerable support from the extended family, and this may work well. However, in those where the pregnancy was unintended or who are emotionally deprived and want to be a mother to be loved, or who are unsupported and live in poverty, there may be many adverse consequences for the mother and child. Children of teenage mothers have a higher infant mortality, a higher rate of childhood accidents, illness and admission to hospital, being taken into care, low educational achievement, sexual abuse, and mental health problems. Deprivation, from the mother's lack of financial and emotional support and the paucity of her own education and life experiences, is the strongest risk factor. Protective factors are having a supportive family, religious belief and a stable, long-term relationship with the partner.

Health promotion

The reasons to undertake health promotion in adolescents are:

- it is the period for starting health risk behaviours (smoking, alcohol, drug misuse, sexual health and risk-taking)
- health risk behaviours started in adolescence often continue into adult life
- health behaviours may have a direct effect on their lives, e.g. teenage pregnancy, road traffic accidents
- increasing morbidity, e.g. obesity and diabetes.

The main areas for health promotion are:

- health risk behaviours
- mental health
- violent behaviour
- physical activity, nutrition and obesity
- parent–adolescent communication.

There are a number of approaches to health promotion for adolescents:

1. Provide suitable information in a user-friendly way for teenagers. An example is the website Teenage Health Freak (www.teenagehealthfreak.org) (Fig. 28.4).
2. By society as a whole, e.g. banning cigarette advertising, making emergency contraception available in pharmacies. These can be very effective. However, there is increasing evidence

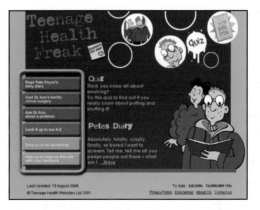

Figure 28.4 The website Teenage Health Freak promotes health in a user-friendly way to teenagers.

Summary

The main health problems of adolescents

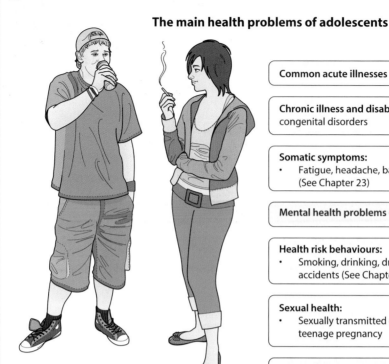

> **Common acute illnesses**

> **Chronic illness and disability** including previously fatal congenital disorders

> **Somatic symptoms:**
> * Fatigue, headache, backache and abdominal pain (See Chapter 23)

> **Mental health problems** (See Chapter 23)

> **Health risk behaviours:**
> * Smoking, drinking, drug abuse, road traffic accidents (See Chapters 1 and 23)

> **Sexual health:**
> * Sexually transmitted disease, contraception, teenage pregnancy

> **Eating disorders** (see Chapter 23) **and obesity** (see Chapter 12)

that improving the socioeconomic circumstances of young people would be the most effective intervention for health promotion. Also, as adolescents often embark on more than one risk behaviour, tackling the underlying problem may reduce other risk-taking behaviours; e.g. a programme to reduce bullying in a whole school may also reduce other behaviour such as drug misuse.

3. Training programmes to improve adolescents' ability to accept or reject certain courses of behaviour. Can be effective for the individual, but is time-consuming and expensive.

4. Health promotion by professionals. Exhorting adolescents not to smoke, to eat a balanced diet, use contraception, etc., has not been found to be effective, and may be counter-productive. However, health professionals do have a role in health promotion at an individual level. It is likely to be most effective if targeted at those who are receptive or contemplating change in their health risk behaviour.

Further reading

Viner R 2002 ABC of Adolescence. BMJ Books

Appendix

Growth charts

These are examples of growth charts used in the UK (Fig. A.1a, b, c and d).

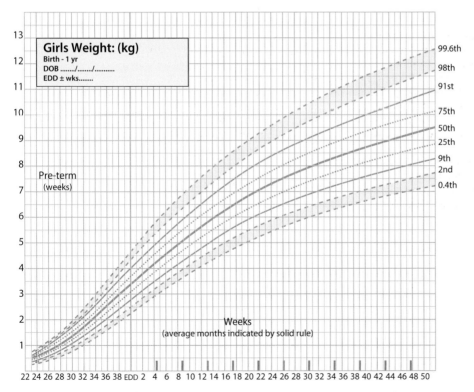

Figure A.1 Growth charts. **(a)** Weight chart for female infants in the first year of life. (Chart © Child Growth Foundation.)

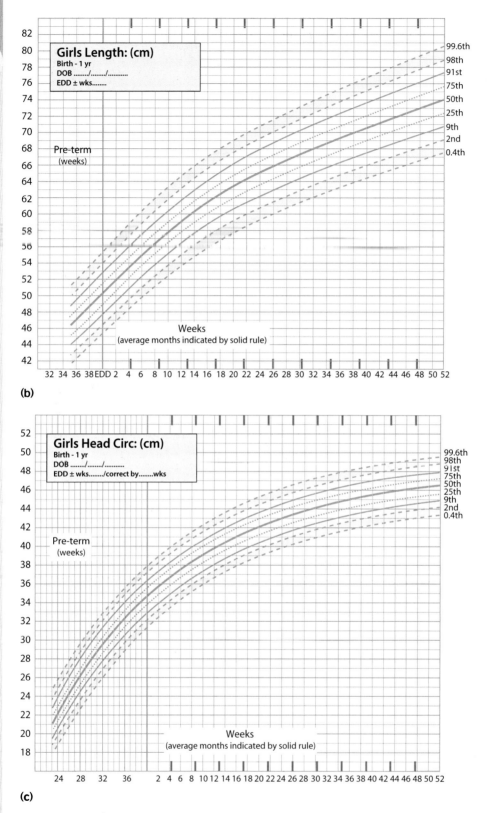

Figure A.1 (cont'd) Growth chart for female infants in the first year of life. **(b)** Length. **(c)** Head circumference. This nine centile UK growth chart shows the 0.4 and 99.6 centile lines. The interval between each pair of centile lines is the same (−2/3 standard deviation). (Chart © Child Growth Foundation.)

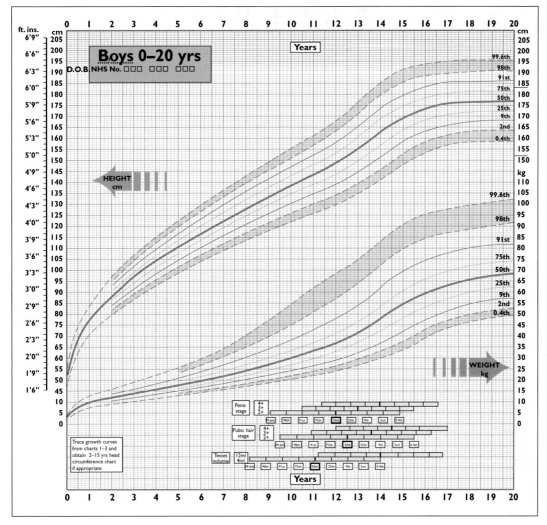

Figure A.1d Growth chart of males from birth to 20 years using the nine centile UK chart. This shows the 0.4 and 99.6 centile lines. The interval between each pair of centile lines is the same (2/3 standard deviation). (Chart © Child Growth Foundation.)

Gestational age assessment of newborn infants

(a) External appearance

External sign	0	1	2	3	4
Oedema	Obvious oedema of hands and feet; pitting over tibia	No obvious oedema of hands and feet; pitting over tibia	No oedema		
Skin texture	Very thin gelatinous	Thin and smooth	Smooth; medium thickness. Rash or superficial peeling	Slight thickening. Superficial cracking and peeling especially of hands and feet	Thick and parchment-like; superficial or deep cracking
Skin colour	Dark red	Uniformly pink	Pale pink; variable over body	Pale; only pink over ears, lips, palms, or soles	
Skin opacity (trunk)	Numerous veins and venules clearly seen, especially over abdomen	Veins and tributaries seen	A few large vessels clearly seen over abdomen	A few large vessels seen indistinctly over abdomen	No blood vessels seen
Lanugo (over back)	No lanugo	Abundant; long and thick over whole back	Hair thinning especially over lower back	Small amount of lanugo and bald area	At least half of back devoid of lanugo
Plantar creases	No skin creases	Faint red marks over anterior half of sole	Definite red marks over > anterior half of sole; indentations over < anterior 1/3	Indentations over >anterior 1/3 of sole of foot	Definite deep indentations over >anterior 1/3 of sole
Nipple formation	Nipple barely visible; no areola	Nipple well defined; areola smooth and flat, diameter <0.75 cm	Areola stippled, edge not raised, diameter <0.75 cm	Areola stippled, edge raised, diameter >0.75 cm	
Breast size	No breast tissue palpable	Breast tissue on one or both sides, <0.5 cm diameter	Breast tissue both sides; one or both 0.5–1.0 cm	Breast tissue both sides; one or both >1 cm	

(b) Neurological examination

(c) Graph for reading gestational age from total score

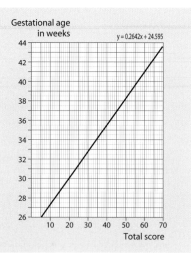

Figure A.2 Scoring system for assessment of gestational age in newborn infants (Dubowitz examination). This is a method of assessing gestational age according to external appearance **(a)** and neurological examination **(b)**. The infant's gestational age (± 2 weeks) is determined from the total score using a conversion graph **(c)**. (Adapted from Dubowitz L M S, Dubowitz V, Goldber C, Clinical assessment of gestational age in the newborn infant. *Journal of Pediatrics* 1970; 77: 1–10.)

Blood pressure chart

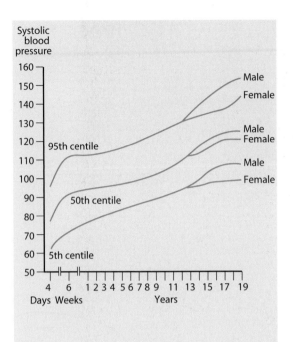

Figure A.3 Systolic blood pressure according to age. Blood pressure charts are also available according to height. (Data from de Swiet M, Fayers P, Shinebourne E A, Blood pressure in a population of infants in the first year of life: the Brompton Study. *Pediatrics* 1980; 65: 1028–1035 and de Man S A et al, Blood pressure in childhood: pooled findings of six European studies. *Journal of Hypertension* 1991; 1(9): 109–114.)

Peak flow chart

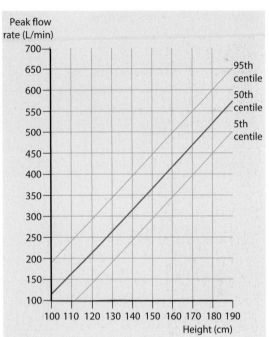

Figure A.4 The normal range of peak flow measurements according to height. (Reproduced with permission from Godfrey S, Kamburoff P L, Nairn J R, Spirometry, lung volumes and airway resistance in normal children aged 5 to 18 years. *British Journal of Diseases of the Chest* 1970; 64: 15–24.)

Normal ranges: haematology

Age	Hb (g/dl)	MCV (fl)	WBC ($\times 10^9$/L)	Platelets ($\times 10^9$/L)
Birth	14.5–21.5	100–135	10–26	150–450 at all ages
2 weeks	13.4–19.8	88–120	6–21	
2 months	9.4–13.0	84–105	6–18	
1 year	11.3–14.1	71–85	6–17.5	
2–6 years	11.5–13.5	75–87	5–17	
6–12 years	11.5–15.5	77–95	4.5–14.5	
12–18 years:				
Male	13.0–16.0	78–95	4.5–13	
Female	12.0–16.0	78–95	4.5–13	

Normal ranges: clinical chemistry

As the normal range for tests varies between laboratories, this must be checked with the local laboratory. (Values adapted with permission from Addy D P, *Investigations in Paediatrics*, WB Saunders, London, 1994 and other sources.)

Test		Normal range (plasma or serum)	
Alanine aminotransferase (ALT)		<40 U/L	
Albumin	Neonate*	25–35 g/L	
	Child	35–55 g/L	
Alkaline phosphatase (ALP)	Neonate*	150–700 U/L	
	1 month–1 year	250–1000 U/L	
	2–9 years	250–850 U/L	
	Years	Females	Males
	10–11	250–950 U/L	250–730 U/L
	14–15	170–460 U/L	170–970 U/L
	>18	60–250 U/L	50–200 U/L
Ammonia	Neonate	<100 µmol/L	
	Infant/child	<40 µmol/L	
Amylase	Neonate	<50 IU/L	
	1–3 months	<100 IU/L	
	>1 year	<130 IU/L	
Aspartate aminotransferase (AST)		<50 U/L	
Blood gas (arterial, not preterm)	pH	7.35–7.45 L (hydrogen ion 35–44 nmol/L)	
	PO_2	11–14 kPa (82–105 mmHg)	
	PCO_2	4.5–6 kPa (32–45 mmHg)	
	Bicarbonate	18–25 mmol/L	
	Base excess	–3 to +3 mmol/L	
Calcium (total)	24–48 h	1.8–3.0 mmol/L	
	>1 week	2.15–2.60 mmol/L	
Calcium (ionised)	24–48 h	1.00–1.17 mmol/L	
	>1 week	1.18–1.32 mmol/L	
Chloride		96–110 mmol/L	
Creatine kinase	Infant/child	60–300 U/L	
Creatinine	Infant*	20–65 µmol/L	
	1–10 years	20–80 µmol/L	
Creatinine clearance	1–3 months	27–69 ml/min/1.73 m^2	
	3–6 months	61–84 ml/min/1.73 m^2	
	6–12 months	77–126 ml/min/1.73 m^2	
	>2 years	110–200 ml/min/1.73 m^2	
C-reactive protein		<10 mg/L	
Ferritin	Child	15–150 µg/L	
Gammaglutamyl transferase (GGT)	1–12 months	<80 U/l	
Glucose	1 day	>2.6 mmol/L	
	>1 day	2.6–5.5 mmol/L	
	Child	3.0–6.0 mmol/L	
Glycosylated haemoglobin (HbA$_{1C}$)	5–16 years	3–6%	
17-Hydroxyprogesterone (17-OHP)	>2 days	0.7–12 nmol/L	
	Child	0.4–4 nmol/L	
Iron	Infant	5–25 µmol/L	
	Child	10–30 µmol/L	
Lactate (fasting)		0.5–2.0 mmol/L	
Magnesium		0.6–1.0 mmol/L	
Osmolality		275–295 mosm/kg	
Phosphate	Neonate*	1.4–2.6 mmol/L	
	Infant	1.3–2.1 mmol/L	
	Child	1.0–1.8 mmol/L	
Potassium	Infant	3.5–6.0 mmol/L	
	Child	3.3–5.0 mmol/L	
Protein (total)	Neonate*	54–70 g/L	
	Infant	59–70 g/L	
	Child	60–80 g/L	
Pyruvate		40–70 µmol/L	
Sodium		133–145 mmol/L	
Thyroid-stimulating hormone (TSH)	>1 week	0.3–4.5 mU/L	
Thyroxine (T$_4$, total)	Child	85–180 nmol/L	
Urea	Neonate*	1.0–5.0 mmol/L	
	Infant	2.5–8.0 mmol/L	
	Child	2.5–6.5 mmol/L	
Urate		120–350 µmol/L	

*Depends on gestational age.

Index

Index

497

Index